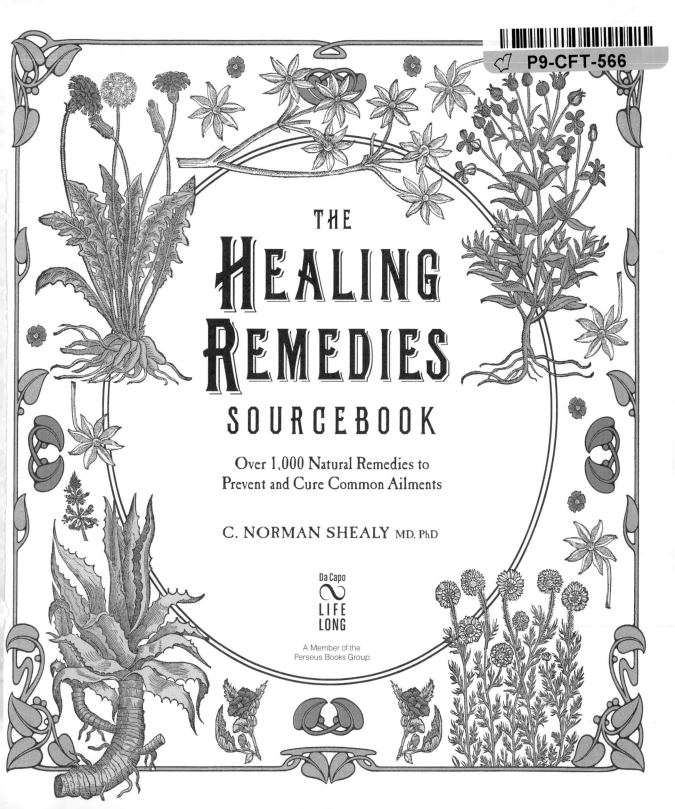

THE
HEALING
REMEDIES
SOURCEBOOK

Over 1,000 Natural Remedies to
Prevent and Cure Common Ailments

C. NORMAN SHEALY MD, PhD

Da Capo
∞
LIFE
LONG

A Member of the
Perseus Books Group

CONTRIBUTORS

C. NORMAN SHEALY MD. PhD is the founder of the American Holistic Medicine Association and a world-renowned neurosurgeon. He is the director of the Shealy Institute in Springfield, Missouri—a center for comprehensive health care and pain and stress management. He has written many books, including *Miracles Do Happen* and *The Self-Healing Workbook*, and has also acted as consultant editor on *The Complete Family Guide to Alternative Medicine*.

KAREN SULLIVAN is the author of many books on alternative health and nutrition, including *In a Nutshell: Vitamins and Minerals*. She has also acted as general editor on *The Complete Illustrated Guide to Natural Home Remedies* and lectures widely on women's health and general health issues.

SHEILA LAVERY writes widely on healthcare for several magazines and newspapers. Her work, which often focuses on children's health issues, has also been included in various encyclopedias of alternative health. She specializes in herbalism and aromatherapy, and she is the author of *In a Nutshell: Aromatherapy*.

EVE ROGANS began studying Traditional Chinese Medicine in 1981 and has undergone clinical training in China. She is the author of *In a Nutshell: Chinese Medicine*, and she works in a private practice where she specializes in pediatric acupuncture.

NON SHAW is a professional herbalist. She teaches herbalism, massage, and Bach Flower Remedies and has written the herbalism and Bach Flower Remedy sections in a range of health reference books. She writes for several health and women's magazines and is co-founder of a publication for independent herb users.

MARY CLARK has been a practitioner of healing and esoteric arts for over 20 years. She has studied Ayurveda, nutrition, herbalism, aromatherapy, and stress management and is trained in astrology and consulting the *I Ching*, with a focus on medical diagnosis. She uniquely combines approaches in her work for various corporations including Forbes, Sony, and Barnes & Noble.

PIPPA DUNCAN is former editor of one of the U.K.'s leading health magazines and now works for a variety of monthly publications, specializing in children's health. She has contributed to several reference books on family healthcare, including *The Complete Family Guide to Alternative Medicine*.

SPECIAL THANKS TO

Maria Anderson, Philip Auchinvole, Tony Bannister, Jan Boyle, Glyn Bridgewater, Stephanie Brotherstone, Deena Bunn, Kimberley Bunn, Adam Carne, Rob Chappell, Judith Cox, Naomi Denny, Juliette Denny, Nina Downey, Rebecca Drury, Cathy Glendinning, Paul Golding, Rachel Could, Paul Harley, Deborah Heath, Julia Holden, Simon Holden, Natalie Jerome, Carolyn Jikeimi-Roberts, Mette Lauritzen, Jan Lewington, Kay Macmullan, Jack Martin, Jim McClean, Norma McClean, Henry Milne, Helen Omand, Elin Osmond, Wendy Oxberry, Sunny Pitcher, Caron Riley, Vincent Riley, Warren Saunders, Michelle Sawyer, Stephen Sparshatt, Sarah Stanley, Andrew Stemp, Neil Strowger, Jenny Sullivan, Bethany Sword, Lauren Sword, Sheila Sword, Gav Tuffnell, Mary Watson, Derek Watts, Louise Williams, Robert Williams

Editor in Chief: C. Norman Shealy
General Editor: Karen Sullivan

Printed and bound in China by
South China Printing Co. Ltd.

Cataloging-in-Publication data for this book is available from the Library of Congress.

First published in 1998 by HarperCollins*Publishers*

First Da Capo Press edition 2012

ISBN: 978-0-7382-1591-4

Published by Da Capo Press
A Member of the Perseus Books Group
www.dacapopress.com

Da Capo Press books are available at special discounts for bulk purchases in the U.S. by corporations, institutions, and other organizations. For more information, please contact the Special Markets Department at the Perseus Books Group, 2300 Chestnut Street, Suite 200, Philadelphia, PA, 19103, or call (800) 810-4145, ext. 5000, or e-mail special.markets@perseusbooks.com.

1 3 5 7 9 10 8 6 4 2

CONTENTS

INTRODUCTION

THE INCREASED USE OF NATURAL medicines and remedies over the past decade has prompted one of the most exciting developments in healthcare in our time. Many of the tenets of modern medicine have been challenged, and the crisis that conventional healthcare is now facing is the result of its own philosophy. The main premise of conventional medicine is that curing disease will lead to good health. This ignores the fundamental concept that pathology is individual to the sufferer, and that prevention is ultimately more important than treatment for the population at large.

This idea is borne out by the fact that modern medicine is simply not as efficient or effective as we have been led to believe; indeed, evidence suggests that it may cause and create more fatal diseases than it cures, and despite the huge sums of money invested, the populations of the U.K., Australia, the U.S., and most of Europe do not live as long or as healthily as people from other cultures, where healthcare investment is substantially lower.

Adverse drug reactions and side-effects are one of the 10 most common reasons for hospitalization in the U.S. The information provided to doctors and physicians throughout the course of their careers is largely funded by the pharmaceutical industry, which earns billions each year from sales of prescription and over-the-counter medicines. As a result, we, in the West, have been encouraged to adopt a "pill-popping" approach to health—taking an average of 26.5 million pills per hour. Sleeping tablets, analgesics (painkillers), antihistamines, sedatives, and antidepressants rank among the top 20 drugs prescribed by physicians, and more than 52 million aspirin or acetaminophen tablets are taken each day in the U.S.

Perhaps the most alarming result of this over-dependence upon drugs is the fact that we have stopped taking responsibility for our own health. When we have a headache, we take a painkiller; when we have a cold, we might take an antihistamine. We suppress the symptoms of health conditions because we want to feel better; we no longer accept the logic that pain or discomfort is a message from our body that something is wrong. We have become used to the idea that someone or something else can deal with our health problems. By taking a pill or conventional medicine in some form, we do experience a relief from symptoms, but what is important to remember is that the cause of the pain or illness remains. By treating the symptoms, or suppressing them, we are doing nothing to treat the root cause. Eczema sufferers apply ointments and creams to the surface of the skin; they may take anti-inflammatories or antihistamines to ease the itching, but the cause of the eczema is still there and the body's reaction has been masked by drugs. They have not been cured. Their illness has merely been controlled. Recently, this trend has begun to change. Scares about the side-effects and long-term effects of immunization, abuse of painkillers, antihistamines, and antibiotics have proved that conventional medicine, despite its many miracles, has been overused and we have become far too dependent on it. Many of us are no longer happy to accept the risks of prescription drugs, and are realizing that there are natural, healthy alternatives. With the increased interest in diet, emotional health and well-being, and exercise, we are becoming more in tune with our bodies and are choosing to listen to the messages they give. Even more importantly, we are taking steps to prevent illness rather than simply treat it when it does arise, and for this reason we are willing to try natural substances that not only treat health conditions, at cause level, but work with the body to keep it well. Natural remedies are more likely to make you feel better, more vital, and more alert; they have fewer side-effects and because they work actively to prevent illness, they are, perhaps, the answer to the healthcare crisis that has been spiraling out of control.

Our understanding of how different cultures approach healthcare is blossoming. Figures show that many common Western illnesses, such as eczema, asthma, and digestive problems simply do not exist to the same degree in other countries. We have a greater understanding of how disease can be prevented and cured using herbs, oils, homeopathic remedies, food, vitamins and nutritional supplements, and other substances that encourage our bodies to work at their optimum level.

The sale of natural products has increased hugely. Our approach to our health is changing dramatically, and this increased interest is being fed by a broad range of products from around the world that are now available in our local stores. Our growing understanding of holistic treatment has encouraged us to examine the healing practices of cultures from around the world, and from each we can gather invaluable information about diet, lifestyle, illness, health, and well-being. The modern clinical emphasis on separating different aspects of our physical, mental, and spiritual health has resulted in a dehumanizing of medicine. By treating the whole person, holistic therapies can restore the proper balance and promote a sense of complete well-being, inside and out.

This book concentrates on the remedies that form the basis of eight international therapeutic disciplines: homeopathy, aromatherapy, Chinese herbal medicine, herbalism, Ayurveda, flower essences, folk or traditional medicine (also called home remedies), and nutrition. These remedies can be used to encourage and enhance good health and to treat and prevent illnesses, both chronic and acute. Many of these remedies are derived from plants, which have a wide variety of therapeutic uses; indeed, up to 140 conventional drugs in use today are based on plants and herbs.

A large number of these remedies have been in use for thousands of years, and it was the practice of herbalism and other disciplines that made it possible for so many of our conventional drugs to be created. However, pharmaceutical companies isolate and often synthesize the active ingredient of a plant or herb, and many practitioners believe that this causes side-effects and other problems that do not occur when the substance is taken in its whole, natural form.

Isolating the active ingredients of plants produces powerful and often toxic drugs, while medical herbalism offers a gentler, safer, and less disruptive effect, allowing the body to undertake its own natural healing process.

There are over 1000 remedies outlined in this book, many of which you can grow or purchase from a reputable health store. Others will be items from your larder—everyday goods with healing and therapeutic properties that may surprise you. Each of the remedy sources has a data file of features, cautions, and other useful information, and there are often recipes for practical applications. Each of the main eight disciplines is also introduced, which helps you to understand how, for instance, the use of something like cinnamon or ginseng differs between Western and Chinese herbalism, and between folk medicine and Ayurveda. You'll learn how a rose aromatherapy oil is different from a rose flower essence, how vitamin C and healthy bacteria can encourage good health, and how belladonna, a poisonous substance, can be taken in tiny dilutions to relieve fevers and other problems. You'll discover natural alternatives to caffeine and sleeping pills, laxatives, and antacids, in remedies that strengthen your mind and body, lift your mood, calm your nerves, and enhance your resistance to infection and illness.

Around 200 common ailments are also discussed in detail, with practical examples of how you can use the remedies from around the world to cure or prevent them. We are on the brink of an exciting new era in healthcare, and with the benefit of these remedies, presented in easy-to-follow files, grouped by the discipline in which they are most often used, you and your family can experiment with safe substitutes to conventional medicines by following the comprehensive instructions. These remedies are the medicine of the future, and this is the essential guide for anyone who wants to take responsibility for their own health. By using only a few of these remedies, you can live longer and with a better quality of life. These are the secrets of good health from around the world; experiment with care and you'll be amazed at the results.

KAREN SULLIVAN, London

How to Use This Book

THIS EXHAUSTIVE AND GLORIOUSLY illustrated reference work is dedicated to the whole spectrum of alternative healing remedies. Aimed at the general reader, this comprehensive book covers the origins, methods, principles, and remedies of eight alternative therapies—Ayurveda, Aromatherapy, Flower Remedies, Chinese Herbal Medicine, Herbalism, Homeopathy, Vitamins and Minerals, and Traditional Home and Folk Remedies.

PART ONE: Therapies and Healing Remedy Sources. Eight chapters cover the different therapies. In each case, the background and history of the therapy are covered, together with how it works, information on visiting a practitioner, and extensive guidelines for self-help. Following the introduction to the therapy, the major remedies and remedy sources are covered with details on how they should be taken. "Therapy Connections" highlights the remedy sources which are common to more than one therapy, giving a full picture of the properties and various uses of one particular remedy source.

PART TWO: Treating Common Ailments. Over 160 pages of common ailments and the relevant remedies with which they can be treated. Caution boxes will make clear the situations in which the remedies are not suitable. Cross-referencing directs the reader back to Part One, where the source of the remedy, its properties, and uses are outlined in detail.

PART THREE: Reference Section. A useful and comprehensive index.

PART 1
THERAPIES & HEALING REMEDY SOURCES

AYURVEDA

AYURVEDA IS A HOLISTIC SYSTEM OF medicine, meaning that our mind, body, and spirit are all taken into consideration in the diagnosis and treatment of illness. In the West we have long believed that each of us has the same anatomy, physiology, and disease process, but it has become increasingly clear that this approach does not take into account our very prominent differences—including our mental attitudes, our lifestyles, and our fundamental energy or spirit. Ayurveda is based on the philosophy that we are all unique, so it addresses each of these things in its treatment of people as individuals, and teaches that all illnesses affect the body and the mind, in isolation from each other.

WHAT IS AYURVEDA?

Ayurvedic medicine is the traditional system of medicine practiced in India and Sri Lanka. Like traditional Chinese Medicine, Ayurveda is a complete system of healthcare, designed to contribute to a way of life, rather than an occasional treatment.

The word "Ayurveda" means "science" or "wisdom" of life, and it embraces elements as diverse as medicine, philosophy, science, spirituality, astrology, and astronomy. Although Ayurveda has been practiced for over 3,000 years, it is a sophisticated and advanced system of living that is as relevant today as it was so many years ago. In fact, as we begin to realize the limitations of

our conventional Western approach, it becomes clear that Ayurveda can offer much to treat and prevent many modern diseases that conventional medicine has been unable to treat. Some of these include ME (myalgic encephalomyelitis), stress-related disorders, arthritis, impotence, asthma, eczema, and chronic illness. It offers natural herbal remedies to counter imbalances in the body, and detoxification, diet, exercise, meditation, spiritual guidance, and wide-ranging techniques to improve mental and emotional health.

PRANA – THE ENERGY OF LIFE

The fundamental belief in Ayurveda is that everything within the universe is composed of energy, or "prana." Like everything else, we too are comprised of energy, which changes according to our circumstances, our environment, our diets and lifestyles, and the world around us. Some of these changes can be positive, and others negative, and in order to ensure that most of the changes are positive, we must live in a way that encourages energy balance. Energy controls the functions of every cell, thought, emotion, and action, so every aspect of our lives, including the food we eat and the thoughts we think, affects the quality of our energy, and consequently our health.

A HISTORY OF AYURVEDA

Over 3,000 years ago, 52 great *Rishis*, or seers, of ancient India discovered through meditation the "Veda," or the knowledge of how our world and everything within it works. Contained within the knowledge of the Veda were the secrets of sickness and health. These secrets were organized into a system called Ayurveda, the sophistication of which is apparent in the most famous of all ancient Ayurvedic texts, the *Charaka Samhita*. The knowledge of the Rishis had three main components: etiology (the science of the cause of illness and disease), symptomatology (the study of symptoms), and finally medication (the process of treating individuals to cure disease or relieve pain).

The beliefs were founded on Hindu philosophy, and were expanded and enhanced by the teachings of the Lord Buddha (d. 483 B.C.E.), who taught that the mind could be enriched through correct thinking. Today Buddhism is one of the fastest-growing belief systems in the West. The eightfold path of Buddhism encompasses:

- right understanding
- right action
- right concentration
- right thought
- right livelihood
- right effort
- right mindfulness
- right speaking

Another important Ayurvedic text, the *Sushruta Samhita*, offers guidance on surgery, surgical equipment, suturing, and the importance of hygiene during and after an operation. Detailed medical information is teamed with commonsense advice on how to live a healthy and meaningful life.

The Texts

Throughout much of their history, the Indians came into contact with the Persians, Greeks, and Chinese, with whom they exchanged information. About 900 B.C.E. the Ayurveda, written in India, combined descriptions of disease with information on herbs and "magic." The first great known Hindu physician, Charaka, practiced about 1000 B.C.E. Sushruta, in the 5th century C.E., noted the relationship of malaria to mosquitoes, and of plague to rats, knew of more than 700 medicinal plants, and described more than 100 surgical instruments. He treated fractures, removed tumors and kidney stones, and delivered babies by Cesarean section.

In Vedic philosophy our lives become meaningful when we strive to fulfill our potential, but that cannot be achieved without basic good health.

CAUSES OF DISEASE

Ayurvedic practitioners believe that disease may be triggered by many external causes, including planetary influences, acts of god, fire and accidents, harmful gases (which we would today call pollution), poisons and toxins, and evil spirits. As well as this, there are two other main causes of illness, an imbalance of the "tri-doshas" (vátha, pitta, and kapha, *see page 10*) and mental imbalance.

The purpose of Ayurveda is to enable people to avoid serious illness by understanding how we become ill. For the most part, it works on a preventive basis, but when we do become ill it offers a wide range of treatments to help the body heal itself. Every Ayurvedic remedy is free of side-effects, is made from natural substances, and is nontoxic. In order to benefit from Ayurveda, it is not necessary to understand or believe in the complex spirituality that goes hand-in-hand with the system. All that is necessary is an open mind and a desire to be healed.

HOW DOES IT WORK?

Our constitutions are very important in Ayurveda, and each of us is individual, according to our specific energies. We inherit many aspects of our constitution, and we can live a healthy and happy life if we strive to attain a good quality of spirit (with no envy, hatred, anger, or ego), and maintain a healthy diet and lifestyle.

Your constitution is determined by the state of your parents' doshas at the time of your conception, and each individual is born in the "prakruthi" state, which means that you are born with levels of the three doshas that are right for you. But, as we go through life, diet, environment, stress, trauma, and injury cause the doshas to become imbalanced, a state known as the "vikruthi" state. When levels of imbalance are excessively high or low it can lead to ill health. Ayurvedic practitioners work to restore individuals to their "prakruthi" state.

THE FIVE ELEMENTS

The universe consists of five elements, Ether (space), Air, Earth, Fire, and Water. Our bodies consist of a combination of these elements. All five elements exist in all things, including ourselves.

ETHER corresponds to the spaces in the body: the mouth, nostrils, thorax, abdomen, respiratory tract, and cells.

AIR is the element of movement so it represents muscular movement, pulsation, expansion and contraction of the lungs and intestines—even the movement in every cell.

FIRE controls enzyme functioning. It shows itself as intelligence, fuels the digestive system, and regulates metabolism.

WATER is in plasma, blood, saliva, digestive juices, mucous membranes, and cytoplasm—the liquid inside cells.

EARTH manifests in the solid structures of the body: the bones, nails, teeth, muscles, cartilage, tendons, skin, and hair.

The five elements also relate to our senses:
- Sound is transmitted through Ether;
- Air is related to touch;
- Fire is related to sight;
- Water is related to taste; and
- Earth is connected to smell.

Ayurveda teaches that all organic matter is formed from the Earth element, which "gave birth" to other matter. All five elements may be present in all matter: Water, when it is frozen, becomes solid like Earth; Fire melts it back to Water; Fire can turn Water to steam, which is dispersed within the Air and the Ether.

THE THREE DOSHAS

There are three further bio-energies, called doshas, which exist in everything in the universe, and which are composed of different combinations of the five elements. The three doshas affect all body functions, on both a mental and a physical level. Good health is achieved when all three doshas work in balance. Each one has its role to play in the body.

- **VÁTHA** is the driving force; it relates mainly to the nervous system and the body's energy.

- **PITTA** is Fire; it relates to the metabolism, digestion, enzymes, acid, and bile.

- **KAPHA** is related to Water in the mucous membranes, phlegm, moisture, fat, and lymphatics.

The balance of the three doshas depends on a variety of factors, principally correct diet and exercise, maintaining good digestion, healthy elimination of body wastes, and ensuring balanced emotional and spiritual health.

We will be made up of a combination of two or all three types of dosha, although we may tend to be predominantly one. Some sub-groups include vátha-pitta, vátha-kapha, or pitta-kapha.

THE FUNDAMENTAL QUALITIES

The principle of qualities in Ayurveda is similar to the Chinese concept of yin and yang, in that every quality has its opposite, and good health depends on finding a balance between the two extremes of qualities such as slow and fast, wet and dry, cloudy and clear. For example, hot and cold exist together as a pair of qualities, and everything in between is composed of levels of heat and cold. Heat relates to pitta, an imbalance of which can cause problems such as fevers, heartburn, or emotional disturbances, such as anger or jealousy. If you have an excess of pitta, you need to reduce your heat quality by eating fewer pitta foods, such as onions, garlic, and beef, and introduce more "cooling" foods, such as eggs, cheese, and lentils.

THE HEALING REMEDIES SOURCEBOOK

AGNI AND DIGESTION

In Ayurveda, good digestion is the key to good health. Poor digestion produces "ama," a toxic substance that is believed to be the cause of illness. Ama is seen in the body as a white coating on the tongue, but it can also line the colon and clog blood vessels. Ama occurs when the metabolism is impaired as a result of an imbalance of "agni." Agni is the Fire which, when it is working effectively, maintains normality in all the functions of the body. Uneven agni is caused by imbalances in the doshas, and such factors as eating and drinking too much of the wrong foods, smoking, and repressing emotions.

MALAS

Malas represent the effective elimination of waste products and there are three main types: *Sharkrit* or *pureesha* (feces); *Mootra* (urine); *Sweda* (sweat). Ama is a fourth type of waste, which cannot be eliminated, and an accumulation of which causes disease.

THE SEVEN TISSUES

Imbalance in the doshas also causes imbalance in the seven body tissues, or "dhatus." These are: plasma (rasa), blood (raktha), muscle (mamsa), fat (madas), bone (asthi), marrow and nerves (majja), and reproductive tissues (shukra). The dhatus support and derive energy from each other, so when one is affected the others also suffer.

AYUVEDIC TREATMENT

SHODANA

In Ayurvedic medicine, it is essential to detoxify the body before prescribing restorative treatment. Shodana is used to eliminate disease, blockages in the digestive system, or any causes of imbalance in the doshas. Where shodana is required the practitioner can use "panchakarma" therapy, and sometimes a preparatory therapy called "purwakarma." Purwakarma breaks down into two types of preparatory treatment, known as "snehana" and "swedana":

- **Snehana** involves massaging herbal oils into the skin to encourage elimination of toxins. Blended oils are used to treat specific disorders, such as stress, anxiety, insomnia, arthritis, or circulation problems. Oils can also be massaged into the scalp for depression, insomnia, and memory problems. Snehana can sometimes involve lying in an oil bath, which is thought to be even more effective at allowing you to absorb the properties from herbal oils.

- **Swedana** means sweating. It is sometimes used in conjunction with the oil treatment, but on a separate day. Steam baths are used to encourage the elimination of toxins through the pores, and, together with the oil treatments, they make the detoxification process much more effective.

PANCHAKARMA

This is a profound detoxification. It is traditionally a fivefold therapy, but all five aspects are used only in very rare cases. You may need only two or three of the following treatments:

- **Nirhua vasti** (*oil enema therapy*). The oil is passed through a tube to the rectum, using gravity, rather than pressure, so that it does not cause damage. Oil enemas are often used to eliminate vátha- or pitta-oriented problems, such as in the treatment of constipation, irritable bowel syndrome, diarrhea, indigestion, and fungal infections.

- **Ánuvasana vasti** (*herbal enema*). The practitioner makes a herbal decoction and passes it through the tube. The selection of a herbal enema rather than an oil one depends on the patients problem and the contraindications.

- **Vireka** (*herbal laxative therapy*). Vireka is used as a normal part of any detoxification therapy, and is also used to treat pitta-oriented disease, such as gastro-intestinal problems, and vátha problems, such as constipation and irritable bowel syndrome. It also helps with inflammatory skin complaints, fluid retention, liver problems, and energy problems.

- **Vamana** (*therapeutic vomiting*). This is a traditional treatment for respiratory and catarrhal problems such as bronchitis, sinusitis, and asthma, but it is rarely used today.

- **Nasya** (*herbal inhalation therapy*). This treatment involves inhaling the vapor from medicinal herbs infused in boiling water. It is used mostly to eliminate kapha-oriented problems, ear, eyes, nose and throat disorders, headaches, migraine, neuralgia, sinusitis, catarrh, and bronchitis.

SAMANA

After the detoxification process, the practitioner may prescribe herbal or mineral remedies to correct imbalances in the doshas. These are to stimulate agni and restore balance in the doshas. They are not prescribed to eradicate disease, because the disease is just a symptom of doshic imbalance. Herbal remedies are usually prescribed in liquid form or as dried herbs, although they can also come in powder or tablet form.

Prescriptions are usually made up of groups of herbs, to which you add eight cups of water and boil until the liquid is reduced to one cup. You may have to take the remedy two or three times a day.

Your practitioner will also advise on lifestyle, food, and exercise. There is no single healthy diet in Ayurveda—just a diet that is best for you. It is important to eat to suit your constitution, and the practitioner may prepare a diet sheet for you to use.

PLANT POWER

In many cases the whole plant is used in an Ayurvedic treatment; in others, only part. All plants are associated with the following properties and effects:

- **THE THREE DOSHAS.** Plants can be used to increase or decrease an influence as required.
- **SHAD RASA (the tastes).** Every plant contains one or more of the six basic tastes, which are sweet, acidic, salty, pungent, bitter, and astringent.
- **GUNAS (the properties).** The gunas are distinctive characteristics that can be related to matter, thoughts, and ideas. There is a belief that everything in the universe is made up of complementary opposites.

There are 20 gunas: hot and cold, hard and soft, oily and dry, light and heavy, dull and sharp, subtle and gross, slimy and rough, unmoving and mobile, turbid and transparent, solid and liquid. The properties of each guna are related to the doshas, and specific substances, which are characterized by specific gunas, can increase or decrease dosha influence throughout the body. The properties of each guna can affect the doshas.

Many herbs are used in Ayurvedic preparations, and are sold as essences, pills, powders, pastes, and potencized remedies. Often they are herbs that are known and used in the West, although they are used differently in Ayurvedic medicine.

It is usually safe to combine taking Ayurvedic herbal remedies and orthodox medicines. However, you should inform your Ayurvedic practitioner of any medication you are currently taking or have taken in the past.

OTHER USEFUL AYURVEDIC TREATMENTS INCLUDE:

- Meditation
- Breathing exercises
- Marma puncture (rather like acupuncture; adjusting energy levels in the body by stimulating energy points in the body, which can stimulate some of its functions and maintain health)
- Marma therapy, applying pressure or massage to marma points
- Yoga
- Unblocking chakras, which are centers of energy located along the midline of the body which distribute energy to the 107 marma points on the body
- Rejuvenation therapy, or rasayana, which helps to promote and preserve health and longevity in the healthy, and to cure disease in the sick
- Psychotherapy or counseling

VATHA is a combination of the elements Air and Ether, with Air being the most dominant. Its qualities are light, cold, dry, rough, subtle, mobile, clear, dispersing, erratic, and astringent. Vátha is the lightest of the three doshas, portrayed by the color blue. Predominantly vátha people are thin with dry, rough, or dark skin; large, crooked or protruding teeth; a small, thin mouth, and dull, dark eyes.

Characteristics:

- Constipation
- Frequent, sparse urination
- Little perspiration
- Poor long-term memory
- Rapid speech
- Anxiety and depression
- High sex drive (or none at all)
- Love of travel
- Dislike of cold weather

PITTA is mostly Fire with some Water. Its qualities are light, hot, oily, sharp, liquid, sour, and pungent. Pitta is "medium" and portrayed by the color red. Pitta types seem to conform to a happy medium, and are of medium height and build, with soft, fair, freckled, or bright skin; soft, fair, light brown, or reddish hair that goes prematurely gray; small, yellowish teeth, and an average-sized mouth.

Characteristics:

- Clear, sharp speech
- Light, uninterrupted sleep
- Intelligent
- Clear memory
- Jealous
- Ambitious
- Passionately sexual
- Interested in politics
- Dislikes heat
- Loves luxury
- Loose stools, diarrhea
- Strong appetite
- Great thirst

KAPHA is a combination of mostly Water and some Earth. Its qualities are heavy, cold, oily, slow, slimy, dense, soft, static, and sweet. Kapha is the heaviest of the doshas, and is portrayed by yellow. Kapha people tend to be large-framed and often overweight, with thick, pale, cool, and oily skin; thick, wavy and oily hair, either very dark or very light; strong white teeth, and a large mouth with full lips.

Characteristics:

- Slow speech
- Needs lots of sleep
- Sluggish, steady appetite
- Heavy sweating
- Large, soft stools
- Business-like
- Good memory
- Passive, almost lethargic
- Dislikes cold and damp
- Likes good food, familiar places

WHAT CAN AYURVEDA TREAT?

- Allergies
- Anxiety
- Arthritis
- Back pain
- Bronchitis
- Circulation problems
- Colds
- Digestive complaints
- Dyslexia
- Eczema
- Headaches
- High blood pressure
- Insomnia
- Irritability and emotional stress
- Obesity
- Skin problems
- Water retention
- Ayurveda will keep the immune system strong and capable of fighting off infection, and able to address chronic disorders

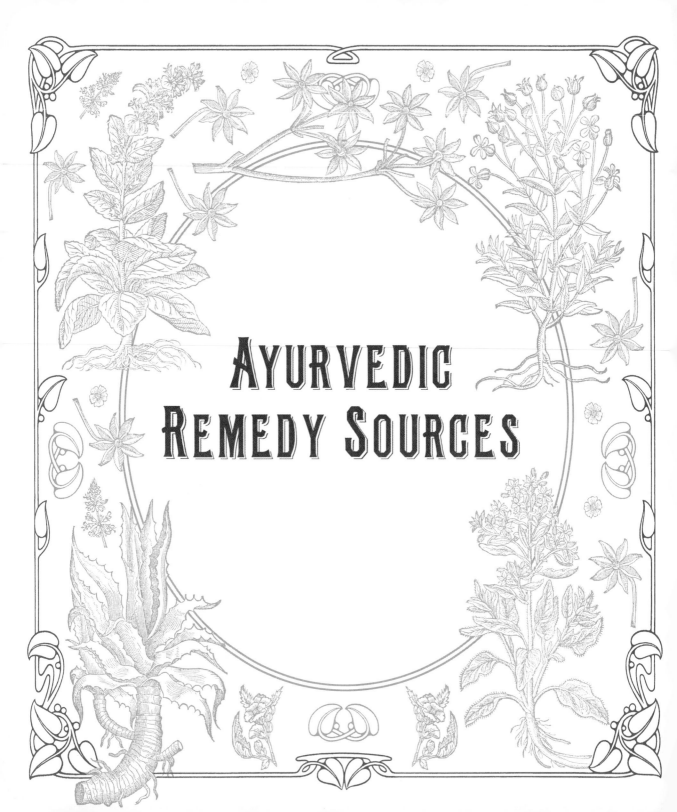

Ayurvedic Remedy Sources

ACHILLEA MILLEFOLIUM
YARROW *Gandana*

Yarrow is a sacred plant to many cultures. Yarrow balances emotional upsets, and is a frequent addition to treatments during menopause.

PROPERTIES

Yarrow is bitter, pungent, astringent, cooling, and drying. It acts as a diaphoretic, antispasmodic, anti-inflammatory, antiphlogistic, antiseptic, and tonic. Yarrow is carminative, alterative, sedative, vulnerary, and emmenagogic.

Part of Plant Used Leaves, stalks, flowers, and fruit.
Conditions Treated Used for hemorrhages, ulcers, measles, colds, fever, nosebleeds, abscesses, vaginitis, varicose veins, headache, menopause, hemorrhoids, gout, cellulite, acne, sunburn, smallpox, and chicken pox.
Form Taken Skin patches, lotion, bath, compress, massage oil.
Used with Other Herbs? Angelica, cedarwood, cinnamon, clove, lavender, lemon, licorice, myrrh, myrtle, sarsaparilla, St. John's wort, turmeric.

HOW TO USE

- For wound treatment, simply press fresh leaves and flower tops into cuts and scrapes on the way to washing and bandaging them.
- Place the seeds in a pot and add boiling water.
- As an infusion to relieve menstrual cramps or hot flashes, steep 2 teaspoons of the dried herb in a cup of boiling water for about 10 minutes. Add honey to taste, and drink warm.

CAUTION
- Do not administer yarrow to children under two years old.
- Those with sensitive skin may be irritated when exposed to the sun while using yarrow.
- It should not be used in cases of high vátha.

ACORUS CALAMUS
CALAMUS ROOT *Vacha*

Also known as sweet flag or myrtle flag, this rhizome is a reddish, hairy root, known throughout Asia for its medicinal properties.

PROPERTIES

This herb is pungent and bitter, with astringent qualities. It is a stimulant, a heating/drying agent which warms vátha and decreases kapha states. It can be used as a decongestant and expectorant. Calamus root is emetic and anticonvulsive; it is a bronchio-dilator, and increases circulation to the brain.

Part of Plant Used The root.
Conditions Treated Calamus strengthens the adrenals, improves muscle tissue, helps circulation, and is useful in periods of weakness. It has a beneficial effect on gingivitis (gum disease), and a massage with calamus oil will stimulate lymphatic drainage.
Form Taken Use in a compress or as massage oil.
Used with Other Herbs? Mixes well with ginger, yarrow, lemon, orange, cinnamon, and also with cedar.

HOW TO USE

- Calamus reduces kapha and vátha, and increases pitta.
- Calamus root is often used to improve the memory.
- A simple formula for boosting your brain power: mix ¼ of a teaspoon of the powdered root with a ½ teaspoon of honey. Take internally every morning and evening. Use any time you are experiencing mental stress and overstimulation. A great help at exam time!

CAUTION
- Calamus can cause bleeding disorders, such as nosebleeds and hemorrhoids, if used in excess.
- Use only the recommended dose.
- Calamus can have a very strong and long-lasting odor. It may be appropriate to use it in conjunction with rosemary, lavender, or a sweet-smelling herb.

ALLIUM CEPA
ONION *Dungri*

Onion and its relative garlic are members of the lily family. They are some of the oldest-known medicinal plants, rich in trace elements, minerals, and sulfur.

PROPERTIES

Onion is a pungent, sweet bulb with heating and drying qualities. It is an excellent stimulant, carminative, and expectorant.

Part of Plant Used The bulb.
Conditions Treated Onion has been used to treat a broad spectrum of ailments, including nerve rejuvenation, colds, skin disease, parasites, bronchial disorders, asthma, joint problems and arthritis, cysts and growths, fluid retention.
Form Taken Onion can be peeled and eaten raw, cooked, powdered, juiced, taken as a tea, decoction, infusion, in food, and as an oil.
Used with Other Herbs? Combines well with ginger, black pepper, cumin, coriander, eucalyptus.

HOW TO USE
- Onion reduces kapha and vátha, and increases pitta. Its stimulating effects aid in the secretion of digestive juices.
- Onion juice has been used to treat infected wounds, amebic dysentery, and, at one time, juice applied to the ear was said to cure deafness!
- Onion may be used directly on the skin for natural relief from burns.

CAUTION
- Nursing mothers beware: onion in your breast milk may cause colic in your infant.
- Some people have allergies to onion and may develop a skin rash. If one appears, discontinue use.
- Consult a physician before consuming large quantities of onion for medicinal purposes.
- Some people have trouble digesting raw onion. If this is the case, steam or blanch the onion before eating.

ALLIUM SATIVUM
GARLIC *Lashuna*

Garlic is one of the oldest-known medicinal plants. Ayurvedic practitioners prescribed garlic liberally for cancer and leprosy.

PROPERTIES

Garlic is an excellent stimulant, carminative, and expectorant. The juice is disinfectant, rejuvenative, and antispasmodic. Garlic has a rejuvenating effect on all tissues and systems.

Part of Plant Used The bulb.
Conditions Treated Garlic has been used to treat a broad spectrum of ailments, including colds, skin disease, parasites, joint problems and arthritis, cysts and growths, and fluid retention. Like onion, garlic helps eliminate lead and other heavy metals from the body. It is beneficial to diabetics and cancer patients.
Form Taken Garlic cloves can be chewed, cooked, powdered, taken as a tea, decoction, infusion, in food, and as an infused oil.
Used with Other Herbs? Ginger, black pepper, cumin, coriander, eucalyptus.

HOW TO USE
- Garlic reduces kapha and vátha, and increases pitta.
- Its stimulating effect aids digestion.
- Garlic juice has been used to treat infected wounds and amebic dysentery.
- Garlic may be used as a natural antibiotic.

CAUTION
- Nursing mothers beware: garlic in your breast milk may cause colic in your infant.
- Some people have allergies to garlic and may develop a skin rash. If one appears, discontinue garlic use.
- Consult a physician before consuming large quantities of garlic for medicinal purposes.

ALOE VERA
ALOE VERA *Kumari*

Aloe's fame as a treatment for burns and scalds goes back to Alexander the Great, who used an island off Somalia for the sole purpose of obtaining the "amazing wound-healing" plant.

PROPERTIES
Aloe vera has bitter, cooling, sweet qualities. It is astringent, and an excellent blood cleanser.

Part of Plant Used The leaf, the gel, the juice.
Conditions Treated Aloe vera relieves inflammation, soothes muscle spasm, purifies the blood, and cleanses the liver. Fresh aloe gel scooped or expressed from the spongy leaves of the plant can be spread on the skin to heal burns, scalds, scrapes, sunburn, and wounds.
Form Taken Drink aloe juice for internal conditions, and apply the gel externally. To soothe wounds, clean the wound with soap and water. Cut several inches off an older leaf, slice it lengthwise, and apply the gel to the wound.
Used With Other Herbs? Barberry, cinnamon, cloves, licorice, St. John's wort.

HOW TO USE
- Aloe vera is good for all doshas; it will bring balance equally to kapha, pitta, and vátha.
- Cover the leaves with vegetable oil. Any vegetable oil can be used as the base. Allow the mixture to soak for 60 days, then strain. Keep the oil in a dark glass container. The oil will keep indefinitely.

CAUTION
- Aloe vera gel can cause skin irritation in some people. If irritation occurs, discontinue use.
- Aloe vera contains a powerful laxative—anthraquinone—which can cause diarrhea and intestinal cramps. If you use aloe juice or supplements as a laxative, use under the guidance of a physician, and never exceed the recommended dosage.

ANGELICA
ANGELICA *Choraka*

In the West, angelica has been associated with magic and sorcery for centuries. Chinese angelica, or dong quai, has been used in Asia for thousands of years, and is enjoying renewed popularity as a gynecological aid.

PROPERTIES
Angelica is pungent, sweet, heating, and moisturizing. It is stimulant, expectorant, tonic, emmenagogue, carminative, and diaphoretic. It has antibacterial properties, and has been used to induce menstruation and abortion.

Part of Plant Used The roots, leaves, and seeds.
Conditions Treated Amenorrhea, menstrual cramps, PMS, anemia, headaches, colds, flu, hiccups, arthritis, rheumatism, poor circulation, adrenal excess, digestive disorders, heartburn, bronchitis, poor blood clotting, poor liver function.
Form Taken As an inhalant, nose drops, in a vaporizer, tea, tincture, massage oil.
Used with Other Herbs? Rose, St. John's wort, yarrow, vetiver, fennel, cumin, chamomile.

HOW TO USE
- In general, angelica balances all three doshas. If used in excess, or in high pitta states, it will increase pitta.
- It is a wonderful expectorant and digestive aid.
- You can prepare the leaves and seeds as an infusion for a mild treatment, or use the root in a decoction for a stronger effect.

CAUTION
- Fresh angelica roots are poisonous. Drying eliminates all danger.
- Do not use with hypertension or heart disease.
- Angelica can increase photosensitivity; use a sunscreen if spending time outdoors.
- Pregnant women should avoid angelica because of its history as an abortifacient.

APIUM GRAVEOLENS
CELERY SEED *Ajwan*

Celery seed, or ajwan, grows wild in India all year round. Traditional Ayurvedic practitioners prescribe celery seed to reduce high vátha states—indigestion, nervous stomach, and ungrounded emotions. In aromatherapy, celery seed oil can be used to counteract jet lag and exposure to smog and toxic environments.

PROPERTIES
Celery seed has pungent, salty qualities, and a heating/moisturizing effect. It is used as a stimulant, expectorant, antispasmodic, and lithotrophic.

Part of Plant Used The bulb.
Conditions Treated The common cold, coughs, sinus congestion, respiratory infections, bronchitis, laryngitis, arthritis, digestive problems, high blood pressure, insomnia, diseases of the liver and spleen, and irregular menstruation.
Form Taken As a food, a tea or infusion, steam, powder, massage oil, or gargle.
Used with Other Herbs? Basil, black pepper, camphor, eucalyptus, sandalwood.

HOW TO USE
- Celery seed reduces kapha and vátha, and increases pitta.
- It is most commonly used as a diuretic, since fluid retention aggravates high blood pressure, congestive heart conditions, premenstrual syndrome, arthritis, and gout.

CAUTION
- Celery seed may cause minor discomfort in some people. If you are experiencing a stomach upset or diarrhea while taking celery seed, discontinue use.
- Pregnant women should not take celery seed without a physician's approval because of its strong diuretic properties.
- Do not give celery seed to children under two years old.

BERBERIS VULGARIS
BARBERRY

Barberry has been in use as a healing herb for thousands of years. The Egyptians used it to prevent plagues—a testimony to its antibiotic properties.

PROPERTIES
Barberry is a stimulant, a respiratory aid, and is antibiotic, antibacterial, and antifungal. It decreases heart rate, shrinks tumors, stimulates intestinal movement, and enlarges blood vessels.

Part of Plant Used The berries, roots, and ground bark.
Conditions Treated Skin infections, urinary tract infections, diarrhea, dysentery, cholera, arthritis, conjunctivitis, high blood pressure, throat infections, mouth ulcers, abnormal uterine bleeding.
Form Taken Tea or infusion, gargle, eye wash, douche, compress, and powder.
Used with Other Herbs? Garlic, ginger, saffron, wild sunflower.

HOW TO USE
- Barberry can be used to treat a variety of symptoms in its decoction form. Drink up to one cup a day.
- For a compress to treat conjunctivitis, soak a clean cloth in the decoction (before you add any honey). Place over the eye.

CAUTION
- Barberry may stimuulate the uterus and should not be taken by pregnant women.
- Barberry is a very powerful herb, and should be used in small doses and under the supervision of a physician or alternative healthcare practitioner.
- If the dosage is too high, barberry can cause nausea, vomiting, hazardous drops in blood pressure, and dizziness.

BRASSICA NIGRA
MUSTARD *Rai*

Mustard is an annual plant cultivated as a spice all over the world. It has been used for centuries as a pungent condiment and healing herb by the Chinese, the Greeks, and the Ayurvedics.

PROPERTIES

Antiseptic, warming, carminative, antibacterial, and antiviral. Mustard aids digestion and eases gastric distention. It is an emetic, rubefacient, and a laxative.

Part of Plant Used The seed and pods.
Conditions Treated For centuries, mustard plasters have been used to treat chest colds and coughs. Mustard is also beneficial for backache, joint pain, digestive upsets, hiccups, and as a laxative. Mustard eases constipation, minor aches and pains, and muscle stiffness.
Form Taken As a spice or oil, in compresses and poultices.
Used with Other Herbs? Aloe vera, ginger, garlic, and onion.

HOW TO USE

- Mustard reduces pitta and kapha, and has a neutral effect on vátha.
- Mustard oil can be rectified with alcohol (1 part oil to 40 parts alcohol) and used as a lotion for joint pains, arthritis, and sluggish circulation.
- A mustard foot bath will clear blood congestion in the head, warm up cold feet, and lower a fever in the early stages of illness.

CAUTION

- Large amounts of mustard can cause irritation and inflammation. Do not let undiluted mustard oil come in contact with the skin.
- Do not use mustard plasters for more than 10–15 minutes at a time, or blistering and irritation can occur.

CARUM CARVI
CARAWAY *Sushavi*

This perennial plant is found in the wild in North America, Europe, and Asia. Caraway is best known in Europe in the making of rye bread, where the addition of caraway seeds aids in the digestion of starch. It is also a favorite addition to laxative herbs, tempering their violent effects.

PROPERTIES

Caraway is a pungent, heating/drying agent, known for its stimulant and carminative properties. As an antispasmodic, caraway will soothe the muscles in the digestive process. It can also relax uterine tissue and is therefore beneficial for menstrual cramps.

Part of Plant Used The seed.
Conditions Treated Caraway aids the digestive process, both internally and in external application. It soothes indigestion, gas, colic, flatulence, and accumulation of toxins and fluids. It is also beneficial as a scalp treatment. The oil can be used as an enema for intestinal parasites. A stomach massage with a very small amount of the oil will reduce flatulence. Caraway seeds can be added to any laxative to temper its strength and to soothe the colon.
Form Taken Teas, as an oil for stomach massage, in an inhaler, and as a spice to aid the digestion of starches.
Used with Other Herbs? Caraway blends well with dill, fennel, anise, basil, cardamom, and jasmine.

HOW TO USE

- Caraway reduces vátha and kapha, and increases pitta. It clears kapha mucus buildup and soothes vátha emotion. Caraway increases pitta digestive fire.
- Eat a teaspoonful of the seeds to aid digestion, or make an infusion.
- Finely crush 9 teaspoonsful of seeds using a pestle and mortar.
- Place the seeds in a pot and add boiling water.
- Allow the infusion to stand for 20 minutes, then strain and drink as needed, up to 3 cups a day.

CAPSICUM ANNUUM
CAYENNE PEPPER *Merchi*

This fiery red pepper, used the world over in cooking, is known to many Westerners by its Caribbean name, cayenne. Ironically, only a tiny amount of the world's red pepper supply comes from the Caribbean—India and Africa are the main producers.

PROPERTIES

Cayenne pepper assists digestion by stimulating the flow of saliva and stomach secretions. It is analgesic and warming, increasing circulation. It has strong digestive, carminative, and emetic properties.

Part of Plant Used The pod.
Conditions Treated Cayenne alleviates colds, gastrointestinal and bowel problems, and is used as a digestive aid. Externally, cayenne treats arthritis and muscle soreness. Creams containing cayenne are frequently used in the treatment of shingles.
Form Taken Raw, powdered, as a spice, oil, tea, or plaster.
Used with Other Herbs? Garlic, onion, coriander, lemon, ginger.

HOW TO USE

- Externally, cayenne can be used for arthritis and muscle soreness, and internally as a digestive aid and a treatment for colds, fever, toothache, diarrhea, and constipation. For a pain-relieving muscle rub, mix ½ of a teaspoon of cayenne powder or puréed fresh cayenne to 1 cup of warm vegetable oil.

CAUTION
- Do not give to children under two years old.
- Use rubber gloves when chopping cayenne peppers, as they may burn. If burning does occur, wash with vinegar several times, rinsing carefully.
- Pepper oil will cause severe pain on contact with sensitive tissues, such as eyes or genitals.

CASSIA ANGUSTIFOLIA
SENNA

The Chinese name for this herb is *Fan-Hsieh-Yeh*, or "foreign-country laxative herb." Senna has a very strong laxative effect on the body. Indian senna (*C. angustifolia*) is a close relative of North African and American senna, but its properties are much milder.

PROPERTIES

Bitter, pungent, cooling, and purging. It is cathartic, antiseptic, antispasmodic, cholagogue, and cleansing. Senna acts mostly on the lower half of the body.

Part of Plant Used The leaves and whole seed pods.
Conditions Treated Senna is the most powerful herbal treatment for constipation, especially when it is chronic. Do not use if you suffer from hemorrhoids. Senna has sometimes been used to reduce fevers, and is an ingredient in sore throat remedies.
Form Taken Used as a powder, tea, or supplement.
Used with Other Herbs? Anise, cardamom, cinnamon, coriander, fennel, ginger, nutmeg, orange.

HOW TO USE

- Senna reduces kapha and vátha, and increases pitta.
- A senna infusion will give you the benefits of senna's laxative power.
- For children or the elderly, senna pods have a more gentle laxative effect.

CEDRUS DEODARA
CEDAR *Devadaru*

The wood we know of for its insect-repellent qualities (the cedar chest which protects woolens from moths) is also, according to the Ayurvedics, an excellent treatment for dandruff. Considered a soothing tonic to the skin, cedar is often used in men's perfumes and toiletries, particularly aftershave lotions.

PROPERTIES

Cedar is bitter and pungent, with antiseptic, diuretic qualities. It is useful as a nervine and expectorant. Cedar has a heating, drying effect on the body. The astringent, tonic qualities in cedar make it an excellent antidote to oily skin, oily scalp, and dandruff.

Part of Plant Used The wood and bark.
Conditions Treated Bronchitis, urinary infections, fear and nervous tension, oily hair, hair loss, oily skin, dandruff, sensitive skin, as a rub for sore joints and muscles, and to provoke sluggish menstrual cycles.
Form Taken Oil for massage and inhalation; made into a tea or an infusion.
Used with Other Herbs? Blends well with camphor, sandalwood, vetiver.

HOW TO USE
- Cedar will reduce pitta and kapha, while increasing vátha.
- Cedar is an excellent air freshener, deodorizer, and insect repellent—add oil of cedar to water in an atomizer and spray the room, or add 10 drops to a tablespoon of vegetable oil and rub it onto skin.

CAUTION
- Cedar should not be taken by pregnant women, as it will stimulate the menstrual cycle, and acts as a possible abortifacient.

CENTELLA ASIATICA
GOTU KOLA *Brahmi*

According to tradition, the natives of Sri Lanka were the first people to use gotu kola. They noticed that elephants, animals renowned for their longevity, loved to eat the rounded gotu kola leaves. Hence the proverb "Two leaves a day keeps old age away." The Ayurvedics used gotu kola like ginseng, as a tonic for longevity.

PROPERTIES

Bitter, stimulating, cooling, and moistening. Gotu kola neutralizes blood acids and may lower body temperature. It acts as a nervine, a diuretic, and a rejuvenating tonic. It is excellent for hair growth and as a treatment for baldness.

Part of Plant Used The seeds, nuts, and roots.
Conditions Treated Gotu kola stimulates the central nervous system. It aids in the elimination of fluids, shrinks tissues, decreases fatigue and depression, and stimulates sexual appetite. Gotu kola is recommended for rheumatism, blood disease, mental disorder, high blood pressure, a sore throat, tonsillitis, cystitis, venereal disease, insomnia, and to relieve stress.
Form Taken Used as a massage oil, shampoo, poultice, tea, and skin cream.
Used with Other Herbs? Sandalwood, lemon.

HOW TO USE
- Gotu kola has a balancing effect on all three doshas.
- Gotu kola infusions, taken as a beverage, will improve circulation in the legs and treat varicose veins.
- They will also act as a soporific in cases of insomnia.
- Used as a compress, the infusion will relieve psoriasis.
- To make an infusion, pour 2 cups of boiling water over 1 teaspoon of the herb. Let steep for 10 minutes. Drink up to 2 cups a day, adding lemon or honey to taste if desired. If the results of a compress are disappointing, try strengthening the infusion used.

CINNAMOMUM CAMPHORA
CAMPHOR *Karpura*

When camphor is steam-distilled, it is fractionalized into blue, brown, and white camphors. Blue camphor is the heaviest and weakest, and it is used mostly in perfume distillation. Brown camphor contains strong carcinogens and should be avoided. White camphor has medicinal qualities and is the most readily available.

PROPERTIES

Camphor is a pungent, sour, heating substance. It has moisturizing properties which recommend it for use as an expectorant, decongestant, and bronchial dilator. Camphor is frequently employed for its twin analgesic and antiseptic qualities.

Part of Plant Used The twigs and leaves. Both have a strong camphor smell. Make sure that you purchase camphor which has been steam-distilled from natural sources.
Conditions Treated Camphor clears the mind and eases headaches. It alleviates joint and muscle pain. It acts on the nervous system and tissues, as well as the respiratory system. Camphor is indicated for bronchitis, asthma, coughs, arthritis, rheumatism, and gout. It also helps nasal and sinus congestion.
Form Taken Use as a massage oil, compress, salve, steam inhalation, and in lotions.
Used with Other Herbs? Use camphor in small doses only. Blends with rosemary, eucalyptus, and juniper.

HOW TO USE

- Camphor reduces kapha and vátha, and it increases pitta when used in excess.
- For bronchitis and colds, try a camphor inhalation. Half-fill an enamel pan or heat-proof dish with just-boiled water. Add 7 drops of oil of camphor. Use a towel to form a "tent" over the bowl. Inhale deeply for several minutes. Stop if you feel dizzy or if the steam is too hot for your skin.

CINNAMOMUM ZEYLANICUM
CINNAMON *Twak, Taj*

Cinnamon originally grew in southern Asia. Ancient Ayurvedic practitioners used it as a treatment for fevers, diarrhea, and to mask unpleasant flavors in other healing herbs. The Greeks used cinnamon to treat bronchitis, but the Europeans championed the use of cinnamon in baking.

PROPERTIES

Cinnamon is a pungent, sweet astringent, with stimulating, heating qualities. It acts as a diaphoretic, parasiticide, antispasmodic, aphrodisiac, analgesic, and diuretic.

Part of Plant Used The bark and leaf.
Conditions Treated Cinnamon is recommended for respiratory ailments, such as colds, sinus congestion, and bronchitis. As a digestive aid, it relieves dyspepsia, intestinal infections, and parasites. It aids circulation and helps to alleviate anemia.
Form Taken As a tea, spice, inhalant, massage oil, or powder.
Used with Other Herbs? Cardamom, orange, nutmeg, licorice.

HOW TO USE

- Cinnamon reduces vátha and kapha, and increases pitta.
- Because of its strong antibacterial effect, cinnamon can be used to treat minor scrapes and cuts.
- Cinnamon contains the natural anesthetic oil eugenol, which will help relieve the pain of minor wounds.

CAUTION
- Do not use cinnamon in cases of high pitta.
- Cinnamon will aggravate bleeding, and can be a skin irritant and a convulsive in high doses.
- Cinnamon bark oil in particular can be an irritant and is not recommended for use on the skin.
- Cinnamon infusions should not be given to children under two.

COMMIPHORA MYRRHA
MYRRH *Bola*

Myrrh is the gum from a shrub native to northeastern Africa and southwestern Asia. The shrub can grow to 30ft. (9m) tall. Myrrh exudes from natural cracks or man-made incisions in the bark. It leaves the tree as a pale yellow liquid, which hardens into a yellowish-red or reddish-brown substance which is collected for use. This resin or gum has been used for thousands of years for its healing properties.

PROPERTIES
Myrrh is an alterative. It is analgesic, emmenagogic, rejuvenative, astringent, expectorant, antispasmodic, and antiseptic. Its tonic effects benefit all tissues of the body.

Part of Plant Used The sap or gum.
Conditions Treated Myrrh is a treatment for amenorrhea, dysmenorrhea, menopause, coughs, asthma, bronchitis, arthritis, rheumatism, traumatic injuries, ulcerated surfaces, anemia, pyorrhea, excessive weight, halitosis, gum disease, sore throat, canker sores, and mouth ulcers. Myrrh is used to clean wounds, as a douche, to promote lung drainage, and to treat hemorrhoids.
Form Taken As a lotion or salve, massage oil, gargle, incense, plaster, or infusion.
Used with Other Herbs? Frankincense, juniper, cypress, geranium, aloe, pine.

HOW TO USE
- Myrrh reduces kapha and vátha, while increasing pitta.
- Its antiseptic and antifungal properties recommend it for sore throats, swollen gums, and cold sores. Myrrh oil can be used directly on sore gums, or to make a gargle.

CAUTION
Do not use myrrh in cases of high pitta.

CORIANDRUM SATIVUM
CORIANDER *Dhanyaka, Dhania*

Coriander is a bitter, pungent herb, with a sweet, pleasant taste. Its energy is cooling and moisturizing. It has strong stimulant and alterative properties. Coriander acts as a diuretic and diaphoretic. Coriander stimulates the plasma, blood, and muscles. It is thought to be an aphrodisiac because of its phyto-estrogen content.

PROPERTIES
Coriander is a bitter, pungent herb, with a sweet, pleasant taste. Its energy is cooling and moisturizing. It has strong stimulant and alterative properties.

Part of Plant Used The seeds and leaves.
Conditions Treated Coriander alleviates urinary infections, cystitis, rashes, hives, burns, digestive disorders, such as gas pains, vomiting, and indigestion. Coriander is beneficial for respiratory problems—it eases allergies and hay fever.
Form Taken Used as a spice, tea or infusion, a compress, douche, shampoo, and massage oil.
Used with Other Herbs? Used with lemon, cajeput, lavender, cardamom, clove, nutmeg, jasmine, sandalwood, cypress.

HOW TO USE
- Coriander reduces all three doshas.
- Its antifungal, antibacterial properties were noted by the Romans, who used coriander to preserve meats.
- Like cinnamon, coriander powder can be sprinkled on cuts and scrapes to prevent infection.
- The infusion makes an excellent digestive aid.

CAUTION
- In high doses, coriander may cause kidney irritation.
- During pregnancy, use only under recommendation from your physician.

CROCUS SATIVUS

SAFFRON *Kesar, Nagakeshara*

Saffron is a small, perennial crocus with purple flowers cultivated in Spain, France, Sicily, Iran, and India. The young plant does not flower for the first few years. When it matures, it produces flowers with golden stigmas which are quite expensive to harvest.

PROPERTIES
Saffron is warming, digestive, stimulant, and rejuvenating. It has anodyne, antispasmodic properties; it is frequently used as an emmenagogue and expectorant.

Part of Plant Used The stigmas or threads.
Conditions Treated Aids digestion and improves appetite. Benefits menstrual pain and irregularity, menopause, impotence, infertility, anemia, enlarged liver, umbago, rheumatism, cough, asthma, gastrointestinal complaints, colic, and chronic diarrhea.
Form Taken Whole threads as a spice, in oils, infusions, and food. The oil can be used as a massage oil, perfume, or bath.
Used with Other Herbs? Cedarwood, champa, lavender, rosewood, sandalwood.

HOW TO USE
- Saffron can be used to balance all three doshas.
- A saffron infusion can be helpful for irregular menstruation and menstrual pains.
- Steep 6–10 stigmas in ½ cup of boiling water. Take 1 cup a day, unsweetened.

CAUTION
- Do not use during pregnancy, as the herb can promote miscarriage.
- Saffron can be narcotic in large doses—do not exceed the medicinal amount indicated. A dose of ½oz. (10–12g) can be fatal for humans.

CUMINUM CYMINUM

CUMIN *Jeera*

Cumin seeds are pungent, savory brown seeds with a flavor common to Indian and Middle Eastern cooking. Heating the seeds, by cooking or infusing, aids the digestive power of the cumin. Cumin is very rich in vitamins and minerals, and is an antidote to weakness and fatigue.

PROPERTIES
Cumin has a pungent, bitter effect, with neutral to cooling properties. It acts as a blood cleanser, a carminative, aiding in the absorption of nutrients to the system. Cumin is a physical and sexual stimulant. It is antispasmodic, alterative, and acts as a lactagogue and immune builder.

Part of Plant Used The seed.
Conditions Treated Digestive disorders and gas pains, anemia, migraine, allergies, nervous conditions, low breast milk, and lack of sexual drive. Cumin builds up the immune system of people who suffer severe allergies.
Form Taken In a compress, as a spice and infusion, in massage oil, and as an inhalation.
Used with Other Herbs? Because of its overpowering smell, use cumin in small amounts when mixing with other herbs. Cumin is frequently used with lemon, black pepper, coriander, lavender, and rosemary.

HOW TO USE
- Cumin reduces kapha and pitta, and increases vátha.
- To relieve abdominal pain, add the seeds to food.
- Abdominal pain can also be treated with a cumin seed poultice.
- Strain, dry, then crush the seeds with a heavy object (a clean stone, rolling pin, or hammer).

CAUTION
- An excess of cumin may cause nausea.

CURCUMA LONGA
TURMERIC *Haridra, Haldi*

Turmeric holds a place of honor in Ayurvedic medicine. It is a symbol of prosperity, and was believed to be a cleanser for all the systems in the body. Turmeric was prescribed as a digestive aid, a treatment for fever, infections, dysentery, arthritis, jaundice, and it has been used as a basic ingredient in curries for thousands of years.

PROPERTIES

Antiseptic, warming, pungent, bitter, and astringent. Turmeric acts as a stimulant, an alterative, and carminative, with vulnerary, antibacterial properties. Turmeric rhizomes are ground to make the familiar yellow powder.

Part of Plant Used The roots.
Conditions Treated Indigestion, poor circulation, cough, amenorrhea, pharyngitis, skin disorders, diabetes, arthritis, anemia, wounds, bruises, and all immune system deficiencies. Because of its energizing effect on the immune system, turmeric is being studied for use in the treatment of HIV and AIDS.
Form Taken As a massage oil, in facial creams and lotions, in compresses, or as a food or spice.
Used with Other Herbs? Ginger, musk, wild sunflower.

HOW TO USE
- Reduces kapha and vátha, and increases pitta.
- Reduces fat, purifies blood, and aids circulation.
- It benefits digestion, and can help rid the body of intestinal parasites.

CAUTION
- Do not use in cases of hepatitis, extremely high pitta, or pregnancy.
- Turmeric is said to reduce fertility, and would not be recommended for someone trying to conceive.

ELETTARIA CARDAMOMUM
CARDAMOM *Elaichi*

Cardamom is a stimulating plant which eases the brain and the respiratory and digestive systems. Its sweet, warming energy brings joy and clarity to the mind, and is particularly good for opening the flow of prana, or vital energy, through the body. Added to milk, cardamom will neutralize mucus-forming properties; added to coffee, it detoxifies caffeine.

PROPERTIES

Cardamom is a stimulant, an expectorant, a diaphoretic, and has aphrodisiac properties. Its qualities are pungent and sweet, with heating/moisturizing effects on the doshas. Cardamom aids in the digestion of fats and starches, stimulates, and calms acid stomach and acid regurgitation.

Part of Plant Used The seeds and root.
Conditions Treated Cardamom aids respiratory problems, such as coughs, colds, bronchitis, asthma, and loss of voice. It also benefits the digestive system in cases of vomiting, belching, and indigestion. Cardamom's stimulating effects bring mental clarity and good humor.
Form Taken Tea, as an additive to milk and food, as a bath, inhalation, or massage oil.
Used with Other Herbs? Cardamom blends well with orange, anise, caraway, ginger, and coriander.

HOW TO USE
- Cardamom reduces kapha and vátha, and stimulates pitta.
- Because of its soothing nervine properties, it will calm a fluttery high vátha state by kindling agni (fire).
- Cardamom removes excess kapha mucus from the stomach and lungs.
- Basundi, a milk-based digestive aid, is also a dessert.

CAUTION
- Do not use with ulcers, or in high pitta states.

EUGENIA CARYOPHYLLATA
CLOVES *Lavanga*

Clove is the bud of a tropical evergreen tree. Now common as a kitchen spice, clove was a rare, prized substance for thousands of years.

PROPERTIES

Clove has pungent and heating properties. It functions as an analgesic, expectorant, stimulant, and carminative. Clove has antifungal properties useful for treating athlete's foot, and it deodorizes the mouth and breath.

Part of Plant Used Dried flower buds (either whole or powdered).

Conditions Treated Clove is recommended for colds, coughs, asthma, laryngitis, pharyngitis, toothache, indigestion, vomiting, hiccups, low blood pressure, and impotence. Clove tones muscles, and expectant mothers are recommended to eat cloves in the last month of pregnancy to strengthen the uterus.

Form Taken As an oil, compress, inhalation, massage oil, lotion, spice, and tea.

Used with Other Herbs? Cardamom, cinnamon, lavender, ginger, orange, bay leaf.

HOW TO USE

- Cloves reduce kapha and vátha, and increase pitta.
- Clove has long been used to fight bacteria, tooth decay, and anesthetize dental pain.
- For temporary relief of toothache prior to visiting your dentist, clean your teeth gently and thoroughly. Dip a Q-tip in pure clove oil. Apply it to the affected tooth and surrounding gum area.

CAUTION

- Clove should not be given to children under two, or nursing mothers, and should be used with care by pregnant women. External use of the oil may cause a rash.

GLYCYRRHIZA GLABRA
LICORICE *Mulathi*

Licorice is one of the most popular healing herbs in Ayurvedic medicine. It has been used for ulcers and malaria, to treat throat and respiratory problems, and to soothe rashes and infections. Due to its strong, sweet taste, the herb is sometimes used in recipes to mask the unpleasant taste of another herb.

PROPERTIES

Licorice is sweet and astringent. It is a demulcent, expectorant, and germicide, with laxative and alterative properties. It has been used with muscle problems because of its anti-inflammatory, antiarthritic properties. Licorice is antibacterial and antiviral.

Part of Plant Used The root and bark.

Conditions Treated Strengthens the nerves, promotes the memory, treats asthma, bronchitis, throat problems, digestive disorders, disorders of the spleen, liver disease, Addison's disease, inflamed gall bladder, colds, coughs, constipation, ulcers, and gastritis. Licorice powder has also been used externally to treat genital herpes and cold sores.

Form Taken As a powder, tea or infusion, food, or oil.

Used with Other Herbs? Black pepper, clove, fenugreek, ginger, long pepper, sage, turmeric.

HOW TO USE

- Licorice reduces both vátha and pitta.
- The herb, a common treatment for bronchitis and colds, may be chewed directly, taken as a tea, or made into a medicated ghee, or clarified butter, preparation.

CAUTION

- Licorice may increase blood pressure slightly and can cause mild adrenal stimulation. In pregnant and nursing women, or cases of high blood pressure or high adrenal function, it should be used only on the advice of a physician.

INULA HELENIUM
WILD SUNFLOWER
Elecampane, Suria-Mukhi

Traditional Ayurvedic and Chinese herbalists have long used the dried root of the wild sunflower, or elecampane, to treat bronchial infections, asthma, and whooping cough.

PROPERTIES

Wild sunflower is a sweet, bitter, pungent herb with warming, drying qualities. It acts as an expectorant, a tonic for the nervous system, a rejuvenative, and a galactagogue (induces milk secretion). Elecampane's antibacterial and antifungal qualities support its use in the effective expulsion of intestinal parasites.

Part of Plant Used The roots.
Conditions Treated Colds, bronchial infections, coughs, lung congestion, and infection. It aids digestive disorders, such as amebic dysentery, pinworms, hookworms, and giardiasis. It stimulates the brain, kidneys, stomach, and uterus, and eases sciatica. Wild sunflower has been used to treat menstrual cramps.
Form Taken Inhalations, massage oils, and lotions.
Used with Other Herbs? Cedarwood, cinnamon, lavender, frankincense, musk, tuberose.

HOW TO USE

- Elecampane increases pitta, and reduces kapha and vátha with its warming, drying qualities. A decoction treats both respiratory and digestive upsets.

CAUTION

- Traditionally used to stimulate the uterus so should be avoided by pregnant women. Some people develop a rash when in contact with the herb or its oil. If so, discontinue use. Do not give wild sunflower to children under two years of age.
- Use of the herb may cause photosensitivity in some people.

HYPERICUM PERFORATUM
ST. JOHN'S WORT

St. Johns wort is a bushy, flowering shrub found the world over. The leaves and flowers have long been used for their diuretic, emmenagogic, and antidepressant qualities. The ancient Greek scholar, Galen, describes the herb as the antidote to intestinal worms.

PROPERTIES

Bitter, astringent, sweet, and cooling. St. John's wort has moisturizing, vulnerary, antispasmodic, anti-inflammatory properties. It is an expectorant, a nutritive tonic, and a nervine.

Part of Plant Used The leaves and flowers.
Conditions Treated Spinal problems, skin problems, joint pain, problems associated with aging, trauma, and eczema. St. John's wort has been indicated for stomachache, colic, congestion in the lungs, insomnia, anemia, headache, jaundice, catarrh, burns, wounds, and sores. It can be used to treat carcinoma, bedwetting, melancholy, depression, uterine cramping, and menstrual problems.
Form Taken As a massage lotion, compress, or salve; as a tea, tincture, or infusion.
Used with Other Herbs? Angelica, chamomile, rosewood, yarrow.

HOW TO USE

- St. Johns wort reduces pitta and kapha, and increases vátha. An oil extract of St. John's wort can be used internally for stomachache, colic, or intestinal disorders. Externally, the oil will soothe wounds, burns, and treat skin cancer. Put the fresh leaves and flowers in a glass jar, and fill it with olive oil. Close the jar and leave it for six to seven weeks, shaking it often. The oil will turn red. Strain the oil through a cloth. If a watery layer appears when the oil has stood for a while, decant or siphon it off. Stored in a dark container, the oil will keep for up to two years.

MEDICAGO SATIVA
ALFALFA

Alfalfa is grown the world over, primarily as food for livestock. The ancient Chinese, noticing their cattle preferred grazing in alfalfa, started to sprout alfalfa shoots to use as a vegetable.

PROPERTIES
Alfalfa is bitter and astringent, with cooling properties. It is high in chlorophyll and nutrients. It alkalizes and detoxifies the body, aids the liver, and is good for anemia, ulcers, diabetes, hemorrhaging, and arthritis. Alfalfa promotes pituitary gland function and contains antifungal agents.

Part of Plant Used The leaves, petals, flowers, and sprouts.
Conditions Treated Alfalfa leaves help to reduce blood cholesterol levels and clean plaque deposits from arterial walls. It has been used to treat anemia, colitis, sciatica, and rheumatism. Sip the infusion for a natural breath freshener.
Form Taken Take as a tea, supplement, or in sprouts.
Used with Other Herbs? Fenugreek, garlic, ginger, saffron, turmeric.

HOW TO USE
- Alfalfa reduces both kapha and váthа, and has a neutral effect on pitta.
- It is a great detoxifier and can be used on a regular basis to cleanse the system and provide refreshing chlorophyll.
- The tea can be used to reduce cholesterol.

CAUTION
- Never eat alfalfa seeds because they contain high levels of the toxic amino acid canavanine. Over time, eating the seeds could result in impaired functioning of the platelets and white blood cells. The alfalfa plant also contains saponins, chemicals which may affect red blood cells. In recommended doses, alfalfa is considered completely safe. Pregnant and nursing women should consult a physician before use.

MYRISTICA FRAGRANS
NUTMEG *Jaiphala*

Nutmeg is a tropical evergreen tree native to Indonesia. The brown, wrinkled fruit contains a kernel which is covered by a bright red membrane.

PROPERTIES
Warming, stimulant, rejuvenating. Nutmeg improves appetite and digestion. It is highly aromatic, carminative, and has strong hallucinogenic properties when ingested in large quantities.

Part of Plant Used The kernel of the seed.
Conditions Treated Nutmeg is calming and sleep-inducing, making it an excellent remedy for insomnia and other sleep disorders. It has been used to treat diarrhea and vomiting. Nutmeg strengthens the heart and eases menstruation. In small quantities, it acts on the stomach, improving digestion and appetite, while dispeling flatulence or acid stomach. Nutmeg has been used to ease kidney trouble.
Form Taken Whole or as a powder, as a tea, spice, massage oil, or an inhalation.
Used with Other Herbs? Balsam, bay, cinnamon, cumin, lavender.

HOW TO USE
- Licorice reduces both váthа and pitta.
- The herb, a common treatment for bronchitis and colds, may be chewed directly, taken as a tea, or made into a medicated ghee, or clarified butter, preparation.

CAUTION
- Can be very toxic if eaten. Eating as few as two nutmeg kernals can cause death. Use only in the medicinal amount. Consult a physician before using nutmeg medicinally. Pregnant women and people in high pitta condition should avoid nutmeg. Nutmeg has hallucinogenic properties.

OCYMUM BASILICUM
BASIL *Tulsi*

There are many different varieties of basil. The Indian variety is also known as basil krishna, because it is said that Krishna wore garlands of this herb around his neck to increase his detachment and his faith.

PROPERTIES

Basil acts as a diaphoretic, a febrifuge (a fever reducer), and a nervine. Basil is antibacterial, antiseptic, antifungal, and antispasmodic. Basil stimulates the immune system by increasing the production of antibodies.

Part of Plant Used The leaves and oil.
Conditions Treated Basil can provide relief for colds, coughs, asthma, sinus congestion, headaches, arthritis, rheumatism, and fevers. Basil oil kills intestinal parasites, and as such is recommended for abdominal conditions, parasites, and stomachache. A basil poultice can be used to treat ringworm infections.
Form Taken Basil can be drunk as a tea or juice, cooked into medicated ghee, used as an inhalation, massaged as a therapeutic oil, or made into a compress or poultice.
Used with Other Herbs? Basil is wonderful when used in conjunction with camphor, rosemary, juniper, lemon, eucalyptus, myrtle, lavender, bergamot, lime, and clary sage. Great fragrances!

HOW TO USE

- Basil reduces kapha and vátha, and increases pitta.
- It has a strong effect on the emotions, and can ease fear or sadness.

CAUTION

- Avoid use when in a high pitta condition, because basil increases pitta. Use with care during pregnancy, as basil has been used as a menstruation promoter and labor inducer.

PIPER LONGUM
LONG PEPPER *Pippali*

Native to India and Java, these peppers are gathered and stored to ripen for use, in order to preserve the greatest heat potency. Long pepper, or *pippali*, is the primary ingredient in Ayurvedic medicine to treat kapha disorders.

PROPERTIES

Long pepper is a pungent, heating stimulant. It has strong digestive, carminative, and emetic properties. Long pepper acts as a decongestant and expectorant. It is analgesic and warming, and increases the circulation.

Part of Plant Used The fruit (pepper).
Conditions Treated Asthma, bronchitis, throat problems, digestive disorders, disorders of the spleen. Externally, long pepper can be used for arthritis and muscle soreness. Taken internally, it is useful as a digestive aid and a treatment for colds, fever, toothache, diarrhea, and constipation.
Form Taken As a powder, tea or infusion, food, or oil.
Used with Other Herbs? Black pepper, fenugreek, ginger, turmeric.

HOW TO USE

- Long pepper restores kapha and vátha to balance, invigorating sluggish kapha, and warming vátha's coolness.
- Its warming action increases pitta.
- Use a *pippali* and rock salt tea to clear sore throats, sinus congestion, coughs, and hiccups.

CAUTION

- Long pepper should not be given to children under two years old. Use rubber gloves when chopping peppers, as they may burn the fingertips. If burning should occur, wash with vinegar several times, rinsing carefully. Pepper oil can linger for several hours, and will cause severe pain if it comes in contact with sensitive tissues, such as eyes or genitals.

PIPER NIGRUM
BLACK PEPPER
Marich, Mari

In Ayurvedic traditions, black pepper or *marich* is named after the Sanskrit word for the sun. Black pepper contains very potent solar energy, and is a powerful digestive stimulant. Black pepper is rajasic, or energy-producing, in nature.

PROPERTIES

Black pepper has a heating and drying effect. The taste is pungent and bitter—both properties good for balancing an overabundance of kapha.

Part of Plant Used The pepper kernel and the oil made from it.

Conditions Treated Black pepper stimulates the plasma and the blood, nervous system, spleen, and reduces fat. It is beneficial for chronic indigestion, toxins in the colon, sinus congestion, and can stimulate the circulation to help warm cold hands and feet.

Form Taken Take as a spice, as an oil, tea, or compress.

Used with Other Herbs? Black pepper combines well with orange, ginger, cypress, anise, sandalwood, lemon, and basil.

HOW TO USE

- Reduces kapha, increases pitta and vátha.
- Use in cooking as a stimulant—black pepper's qualities are enhanced by heating.
- The oil can be used to clear sinus congestion and stimulate fat reduction.

CAUTION
- Do not use in high pitta state or in cases of inflammation of the digestive organs. Overuse of stimulant herbs can impair your body's natural balancing systems. If you find you are attracted to adding pepper to most of your food, then start cutting back.

SANTALUM ALBUM
SANDALWOOD *Chandana*

Sandalwood is a small tree which grows primarily in southern Asia. While the aromatic wood is used to make scented carvings, the medicinal properties are in the oil, which can be pressed from the wood, or extracted with alcohol or water.

PROPERTIES

Bitter, sweet, astringent, cooling, moisturizing. Sandalwood is alterative, hemostatic, antipyretic, antiseptic, antibacterial, carminative, sedative, antispasmodic, and aphrodisiac. It works as a nervine, an expectorant, a diuretic, a disinfectant, and a moisturizer. It also helps to regenerate tissues.

Part of Plant Used The wood.

Conditions Treated Sandalwood has been used to treat cystitis, urethritis, vaginitis, acute dermatitis, herpes, bronchitis, palpitations, gonorrhea, sunstroke, dry skin, acne, laryngitis, nausea, tuberculosis, depression, insomnia, prostatitis, nervousness, anxiety, and impotence. Sandalwood can cure skin problems that are bacterial in origin.

Form Taken In perfumes and massage oils; as a gargle, lotion, bath, inhalation, compress, or douche.

Used with Other Herbs? Clove, geranium, musk, myrrh, tuberose, vetiver.

HOW TO USE

- Reduces pitta and vátha, and has a neutral effect on kapha.
- A sandalwood decoction will reduce fever if taken internally; externally, it can be used to treat acne and other skin problems.
- To make a decoction, boil 1 heaped teaspoon of sandalwood in 1 cup of water. Cover and boil for several minutes. Strain and cool. Drink 1 or 2 cups a day, a tablespoon at a time. For external use, apply to freshly washed skin, and let dry. Repeat three times a day or as needed.

TRIGONELLA FOENUM-GRAECUM
FENUGREEK *Methica*

Fenugreek is another healing herb whose qualities were brought to the attention of humans by animals. Farmers noticed that sick cattle would eat fenugreek plants even when they would not eat anything else.

PROPERTIES

Antiseptic and warming. Fenugreek has expectorant qualities. It is anti-inflammatory, antiseptic, and soothing. The soothing expectorant qualities aid in promoting menstruation, as well as easing coughs, sore throats, and digestion (encouraging flow in the body).

Part of Plant Used The seeds.
Conditions Treated Constipation, digestive disorders, bronchitis, inflamed lungs, fevers, high cholesterol, eyestrain, sore throats, wounds, boils, rashes. It stimulates the uterus, promotes water retention and weight gain, reduces blood sugar levels, and lowers cholesterol.
Form Taken As a spice, tea, massage oil, inhalant, poultice, or plaster.
Used with Other Herbs? Peppermint, lemon, anise.

HOW TO USE
- Fenugreek reduces kapha and vátha, and increases pitta.
- Fenugreek helps asthma and sinus problems by reducing mucus.
- The seeds can be eaten by nursing mothers to increase milk production.
- A fenugreek poultice can be used to treat boils and rashes.
- Gargling a fenugreek decoction will soothe sore throats.

CAUTION
- Fenugreek seeds may cause water retention and weight gain. Because of its use as a uterine stimulant, fenugreek should not be taken by pregnant women. Do not give fenugreek to children under two.

VATTIVERIA ZIZANOIODES
VETIVER

Vetiver is a grassy plant known for its grounding, centering properties. In India, it is sown wherever there is soil erosion, to hold down the earth and prevent further damage to the land. Modern herbalists use it to enable an individual to connect to the earth and feel his or her purpose. It is helpful during emotionally stressful times and has been used as a tonic for women suffering from PMS.

PROPERTIES

Warming, sweet, and bitter. Vetiver is an antiseptic tonic, grounding, regenerating, and strengthening. It is an aphrodisiac, and can be used to repel moths.

Part of Plant Used The leaves and roots.
Conditions Treated Arthritis, root chakra blockage, nervousness, insomnia, rheumatism, stress, disconnectedness, anorexia, postnatal depression, aging skin, fatigue, menopause, loss of appetite.
Form Taken As a lotion, bath, massage oil, in patches and perfumes.
Used with Other Herbs? Angelica, citrus, cinnamon, lavender, sandalwood, sage, yarrow.

HOW TO USE
- Vetiver reduces vátha, and increases both kapha and pitta.
- Vetiver oil is particularly useful for jet lag, and for grounding and clarity while traveling.
- Use as a base 2fl. oz. (60ml) apricot kernel oil. Add 5 drops vetiver oil, 5 drops geranium oil, and 2 drops juniper or grapefruit oil. Apply this mixture liberally all over your skin before traveling.

CAUTION
- Vetiver has a very strong smell. Do not allow it to overpower any blend you are making with it.

ZINGIBER OFFICINALIS
GINGER *Ardraka*

Ginger is native to India, where the ancient Ayurvedics used it to preserve food, as a digestive aid, and as a spiritual and physical cleanser. Garlic was shunned on the days leading up to religious festivities, but plenty of ginger would be consumed in order to be sweet-smelling and purified for the gods.

PROPERTIES

Ginger is a pungent, sweet herb with warming/drying qualities. It acts as a stimulant, diaphoretic, antidepressant, and expectorant.

Part of Plant Used The root.

Conditions Treated Ginger is recommended for colds, coughs, flu, indigestion, vomiting, belching, abdominal pain, motion sickness, laryngitis, arthritis, hemorrhoids, headaches, impotence, diarrhea, heart disease, and memory loss.

Form Taken As a food, tea, gargle, and compress. Also used as a massage oil.

Used with Other Herbs? Black pepper, eucalyptus, juniper, cedar, coriander, all citrus fruits.

HOW TO USE
- Its muscle-relaxant, heating pitta qualities can warm uterine walls, soothing menstrual cramps.
- It is also frequently used as an antidote to travel sickness.
- For motion sickness (on land, sea, or in the air), use a few drops of ginger oil on a small bandage and place behind the ear.

CAUTION
- Do not use in cases of high fever, bleeding, with inflammatory skin conditions, or if ulcers are present. Ginger in large doses can bring on menstruation. Pregnant women with a history of miscarriage should exercise caution and consult their physician before use.

Chinese Herbal Medicine

CHINESE MEDICINE IS AN ANCIENT system of healing—acupuncture and Chinese herbal medicine grew up in tandem over 2,000 years. It is based on the philosophy of a very different civilization from our own, a civilization that perceived people as either "in harmony" or "out of harmony" with themselves and their surroundings. Traditional Chinese Medicine (TCM) sees disease in terms of patterns of disharmony, and so attempts to restore the balance in the person who is sick. Energy is believed to flow through channels called meridians, through which disease may be treated.

WHAT IS CHINESE HERBAL MEDICINE?

TCM uses terminology that sounds strange to most Westerners. Instead of talking about rheumatic diseases or neurological diseases, it classifies diseases as being caused by Wind, Heat, Dampness, or Cold. Instead of talking about rheumatism in the knee joint, it may classify it as Cold-Damp in the Stomach meridian. Western medicine focuses on a specific cause for a specific disease, and when it isolates that cause or agent it tries to control or destroy it. Chinese medicine is also concerned with the cause, but it focuses on the patient's response to that disease entity, both physiological and psychological. All the relevant information, including symptoms that may not seem related to the patients main complaint, is collected together to enable the

YIN AND YANG

Chinese medicine is based on the philosophy of yin and yang. These are the dual forces in the universe, seen both within nature and in human beings. They are used to explain the ongoing process of natural changes—yang is more prevalent during the day, while yin forces are more prevalent at night. There is no absolute yin or yang in living things—a cold

yin-type illness may have aspects of yang, such as sharp, forceful contractions. Yin and yang both depend on each other and keep each other under control. However, it is when they go seriously out of balance and do not correct themselves that there is disease.

Everything has a yin and a yang aspect—for instance:

ITEM		YIN		YANG	
Time	Breath	Night	Inside	Day	Back/Upper/
Season	Temperature	Fall/Winter	Inhalation	Spring/	Outside
Energy	Moisture	Passivity/	Cold	Summer	Exhalation
Body	Direction	Stillness	Wet/Damp	Activity/	Hot/Dry
		Front/Lower/	Downward	Movement	Upward

practitioner to discover the pattern of disharmony within that person, which can then be addressed by Chinese medicine. For instance, two patients coming with asthma may have completely different diagnoses according to Chinese medicine. The one with a pale face, prone to catching colds (Lung Qi Deficiency) will be given a completely different herbal formula to the patient who has a dry cough, thirst, and breathlessness on exertion (Lung Yin Deficiency). TCM does treat the same diseases—to a large extent people have the same problems the world over—it just perceives them in an entirely different way.

A SHORT HISTORY

The earliest herbal formulas in China were found to have been written down in the 3rd century B.C.E. In fact, the main book of the theory of Chinese medicine—the *Yellow Emperor's Inner Classic*—was compiled in the 1st century C.E., and is still taught in schools of TCM. Over the centuries, leading physicians have written down both herbal and acupuncture formulas, which explains the vast bulk of Chinese medicine reference books. The Imperial Grace Formulary of the Tai Pang Era (around 985 C.E.), for example, contains 16,834 entries, many of which are still commonly referred to today.

The early herbal formulas were very simple and elegant, while the later ones are much more complicated. Either type can be useful, depending on the patient and the physician's preferred manner of working. A practitioner of TCM, or someone practicing Chinese herbal medicine specifically, will diagnose the patient's pattern of disharmony, find the tried and tested prescription which is closest to that patient's pattern, and add or subtract herbs to make it more suitable for that individual. Herbs are seldom used singly; they are usually combined in prescriptions containing 4–16 substances.

THE CHINESE THEORY OF LIFE

The Chinese believe that every living being is sustained by a basic Life Force, called "qi" (pronounced "chee"). Human beings receive their qi from a mixture of the influences of both Heaven and Earth. Therefore, we do have an element of the divine in us, which separates us from the animals. Chinese medicine works with the qi that we have to make us better. It may unblock the flow of qi in the body if it is stuck, or it may nourish qi if it is deficient. We are born with a fixed amount of qi inherited from our parents (Yuan Qi—source, or genetic, qi). This is used both as our "reserve tank" and as a catalyst in most of the chemical processes of the body. We can nourish our Yuan Qi, though we cannot add to it. We may, however, deplete it through bad living practices—long-term lack of sleep or good food, drugs, drink, or years of excessive sex. The Chinese believe that this source qi is stored in the Kidneys (where its substance is called Jing or essence), and its functions include the control of sexual and reproductive activity in the body. We get our day-to-day qi from the air we breathe (Gong Qi) and the food we eat (Gu Qi).

Qi permeates the entire body; it directs the blood, nerve, and lymphatic systems (Ying Qi). It protects us from catching viruses (Wei Qi), and fights them if they get into the body. It transforms the food we eat into bodily substances—blood, tears, sweat, and urine—keeps organs in their proper place, and prevents excessive loss of sweat. Qi keeps the body warm and is naturally the source of movement and growth, as it has all these functions. We also use it in TCM to describe the functions of any Organ—for instance, Lung qi may be "weak" or Liver qi "blocked."

MERIDIANS AND ORGANS

Although qi is everywhere in the body, it does have main pathways along which it flows, nourishing and warming the organs and body parts, and harmonizing their activity. These channels are called the meridian system (Jing-Luo). Most acupuncture points are sited along these channels, and most herbs that a practitioner of Chinese medicine prescribes enter one or more of the meridian pathways. There are 12 main meridians, and these correspond to the 12 main organs in the body, such as the Liver, Heart, Stomach, Kidneys, Spleen, and so on. These meridians are bilateral—there is an identical pair on each side of the body. Some are more yin meridians, with functions more to do with storing the vital essences of the body. These are the Kidneys, Liver, Spleen, Heart, Lungs, and Pericardium. The other six are more yang meridians, with functions more to do with transportation of fluids and food. These are the Bladder, Gall bladder, Stomach, Small Intestine, Large Intestine, and the Triple Burner (a mechanism which regulates the overall body temperature and the Upper, Middle, and Lower parts (Jiaos) of the body). There are also six extra meridians, one of which runs up the front center line of the body—the Ren Mai, or Conception Vessel, and one of which runs up the spine—the Du Mai, or Governor Vessel.

When a practitioner of Chinese medicine talks about an organ being out of balance, he or she usually refers to the meridian related to that organ, not necessarily the physical organ itself. For instance, the Liver meridian runs from the big toe, up the inside of the leg, through the genitals, and then deep into the Liver organ itself. There can be problems along the course of the meridian, and there is also a sphere of influence which each organ has within the body. The Liver controls the free flow of qi generally in the body, including the evenness of emotions, digestion, and menstruation. It also stores the blood, rules circulation in the tendons, has the major influence on the eyes, and manifests in the nails. It is therefore possible to see how diseases in these areas of the body may be treated via the Liver meridian.

In illness, different meridians exhibit different tendencies of disharmony—for instance, the Spleen has a tendency to deficiency causing Damp. This creates symptoms such as diarrhea or lassitude (tiredness). The Liver, on the other hand, has a tendency toward Rising yang, creating red sore eyes, migraines, and high blood pressure. It is these disharmonies that Chinese herbal medicine can address.

CONSULTING A CHINESE HERBALIST

When you consult a practitioner of Chinese herbal medicine, he or she will first of all ask you in detail about your presenting condition—when it first appeared, your symptoms, what makes it worse or better. You will then be asked about your past medical history and your general health, for example:

- your appetite, diet, digestion, stools, and urination
- your sleep patterns, any pain—headaches, backache—ear, nose, and throat (ENT) problems
- intake of drugs, alcohol, nicotine
- body temperature (more hot or cold), circulation, and perspiration
- energy levels, mental, and emotional states
- gynecology—menstruation, pregnancies, menopause

Finally, your practitioner will take both radial (wrist) pulses and look at your tongue, in order to help him or her to make a diagnosis according to Chinese medicine. The practitioner may search through some books to check on the herbal prescription most suited to your condition, and will then write down a prescription. This will include anything from 4 to 20 herbs, and their dosages in grams or in *qian* (Chinese measurements). The names of the herbs will be in English, Latin, Pinyin (anglicized Chinese), or in Chinese characters. Your practitioner will then make up the prescription for you or refer you to a herbal supplier to have it made up elsewhere.

Chinese herbs are mostly made of plant parts—leaves, flowers, fruit, or fruit peel, twigs, roots, bark, or fungus. There are some minerals, such as gypsum, but these are less commonly used. There are also animal parts in Traditional Chinese Medicine, such as snake, mammal bones, or deer horn. However, their importation has now been forbidden, and herbal practitioners find alternatives to prescribe.

PREPARATIONS AND TREATMENT

There are many different ways of taking herbs. Individual herbs can be added to foods or taken as a tea, but Chinese herbs are rarely taken singly—they are much more effective when made into a composite prescription.

Decoctions Packets of dried herbs are boiled for around 30 minutes, down to 2 cups, and then often boiled again to last two days. They smell worse than they taste!

Powders One teaspoonful of cooked, freeze-dried herbs is taken two or three times a day, mixed with a little cold water to a paste; then a little boiling water is added. This is somewhat unpalatable but easy and effective.

Tinctures One teaspoon of liquid taken two or three times a day. These are more palatable but not as strong as decoctions or powders.

Pills and capsules These are used-for patent remedies (prescriptions which have not been changed to suit the individual). They are easy to swallow, but you have to take a lot more than with Western drugs—sometimes eight tablets at a time.

Syrups These are patent remedies, mainly good for coughs or children's tonics.

Plasters These are used for rheumatic ailments (Wind-Damp); they are very effective for relieving local pain and stiffness. Treatment generally means taking herbs two or three times a day until the problem is gone.

At first you will need to see your practitioner every one or two weeks so that he or she can alter the prescription as your symptoms improve. You may experience slight nausea, diarrhea, or digestive upset as your system becomes used to the herbs. In this case, you will need to halve your dosage and build it up again slowly; your practitioner may add more digestive herbs in order that you may tolerate it better. After that, you may be able to see or even telephone your practitioner once a month in order to report on progress, and so that the prescription can be changed accordingly. Herbal medicines should not be taken without review for more than 30 days.

THE HERBS USED

PATENT HERBAL PREPARATIONS

These are sold as over-the-counter remedies for colds and flu, coughs and phlegm, even strep throat infections, as well as for rheumatic ailments, pain, and bruising from trauma. Patent remedies used for anything else must be diagnosed by a herbal practitioner, even tonics; for instance, do you need to tonify the qi, blood, yin, or yang? It is important to consult a herbal practitioner if you intend to use a patent remedy over a long period of time, such as a long-term tonic for an elderly person. Tonics should not be taken during an episode of cold or flu (Wind Invasion), as they tend to drive Wind deeper into the body.

Chinese herbs are hardly ever used singly—they are used mainly in combination with other herbs to make a balanced prescription. Some of the most commonly used herbs involved in those prescriptions follow in the next section. Each herb also has a particular range of dosages assigned to it—when comparing it to other herbs in a prescription, one can see whether it is used in an average dose, or whether one would use a smaller or larger dose in that prescription. Both these features mean that it is important to consult a qualified herbalist before using the herbs, either in a herbal pharmacy or privately through your state's Chinese Medicine Association.

CHILDREN AND BABIES

Chinese herbal medicine can be very effective for children and babies. Children's dosages are usually half or a quarter of those given for adults. There are ways of encouraging children to take the herbs, either by involving them in the preparation of the prescription, or by sweetening it with honey, or by offering a cookie afterward! There are certain herbal powders especially formulated for babies.

PREGNANCY

Many herbs are expressly forbidden in pregnancy, whilst some are especially good for pregnant women. There are several which may help to prevent miscarriage. Take only herbs prescribed by a qualified practitioner when pregnant.

CAUTION

Some patent remedies containing animal products may still be sold. They are now illegal in this country, so please check with the pharmacy first. Always go to a reputable practitioner (consult your state's Chinese Medicine Association). Some herbal patents for insomnia and mental disturbance contain mineral substances, such as oyster shell or magnetite. In excess, these can cause indigestion, so use them for a limited amount of time and find alternative prescriptions.

SAFETY NOTE

If prescribing herbs over a long period of time, it is important that the practitioner pays particular attention to any liver or kidney symptoms which may arise during the course of the treatment. A very few individuals may experience idiosyncratic reactions to herbs—these are usually due to genetic abnormalities and the herbs would not cause a reaction in most other individuals. Regular liver function tests are sometimes advised by practitioners, but their value in these cases is still a matter of debate.

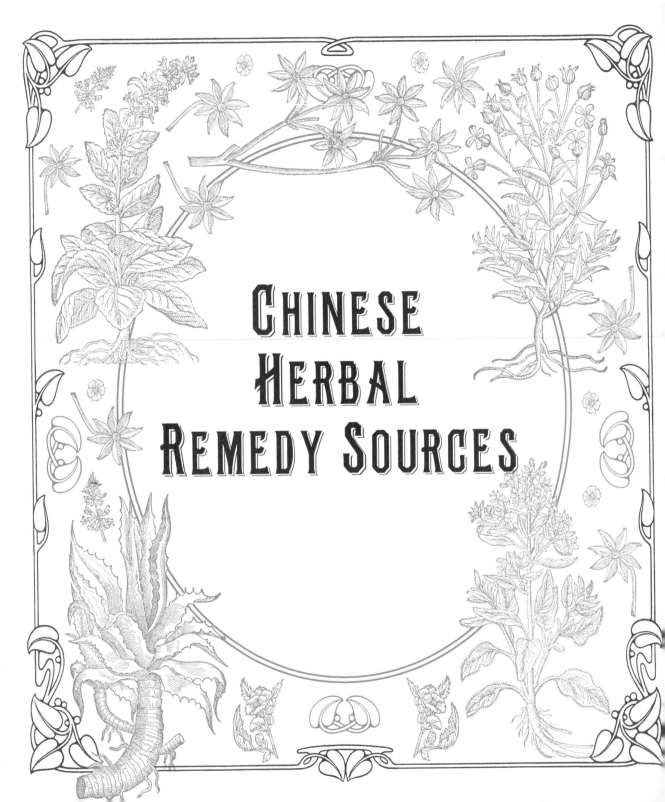

CHINESE
HERBAL
REMEDY SOURCES

HERB TASTES AND FUNCTIONS

A BRIEF NOTE ABOUT TASTES

In the next section, we will mention the taste of each herb. In TCM, taste partly determines therapeutic function, so it is important to know what it signifies:

ACRID—Pungent or acrid substances disperse and move qi (energy).
• Acrid herbs mainly affect the Lung functions.

BITTER—These herbs reduce excess qi, drain and dry excess moisture.
• Bitter herbs mainly affect the Heart organ.

SALTY—These herbs purge (drain through the bowels) and soften.
• Salty herbs mainly affect the Kidney organ.

SWEET—Sweet substances tonify, harmonize, and strengthen qi, and may sometimes moisten.
• Sweet herbs mainly affect the Spleen organ.

SOUR—Sour substances are astringent and prevent or reverse the abnormal leakage of fluids and energy.
• Sour herbs mainly affect the Kidney organ.

BLAND—Bland substances have none of these tastes. They primarily leech out Dampness and promote urination.
• This helps both the Spleen and the Kidneys.

ACANTHOPANAX GRACILISTYLUS

Wu Jia Pi

This herb dispels Wind Dampness from the muscles, joints, and bones. Wind Dampness causes rheumatic and arthritic ailments. Wu Jia Pi also treats Damp Cold conditions where the circulation is obstructed, as in the swelling of the legs or stiff knee joints. The dried herb, or a decoction, can be taken in wine.

HOW TO USE

Wu Jia Pi is a warm drying (acrid) herb which tonifies the Liver and Kidneys. These meridians decline as we get older, so it is especially helpful in treating rheumatism, arthritis, or stiffness in the elderly or those suffering from long-term illness. It is particularly helpful when the smooth flow of qi and blood is obstructed. It is also good for developmental delays in the motor functions of children. It is also used for difficulties with urination, and edema.

PROPERTIES Acrid, Warm

CHANNELS Liver, Kidney

FUNCTIONS AND USES
• Dispels Wind Dampness, and strengthens the sinews and bones: use for chronic Wind Cold Damp Painful Obstruction (Bi syndrome) when deficiency of the Liver and Kidneys causes weak sinews and bones.
• Transforms Dampness and reduces swelling: use for water retention.

CAUTION
• Use with caution in yin deficiency with heat signs, as it dries and heats further.

AGASTACHE RUGOSA

Huo Xiang WRINKLED GIANT HYSSOP, PATCHOULI

This herb transforms Dampness, a "pathogenic influence" which creates stagnation in the Middle Burner (Spleen and Stomach), with various digestive or fluid-retaining effects. Huo Xiang helps the Spleen to recover its function of transporting and transforming food in the body.

HOW TO USE

Huo Xiang is used specifically for stuck digestion, leading to bloating either above or below the navel, nausea, fatigue, lack of appetite, and a moist white coating on the tongue. It is the main herb in the patent formula Huo Xiang Zheng Qi Wan, which is used for gastric flu.

PROPERTIES Acrid, slightly Warm

CHANNELS Lung, Spleen, Stomach

FUNCTIONS AND USES

- Fragrantly transforms Dampness: this means that it tonifies the Spleen so that it transforms the Dampness obstructing the middle area, which is interfering with the Spleen's normal digestive functions.
- Harmonizes the Middle Burner and stops vomiting; also used for morning sickness.
- Releases the exterior and expels Dampness, as in gastric flu.

CAUTION

- No herbs used for getting rid of damp (shown by a thick tongue coating or by the presence of phlegm) may be used deficient yin with heat signs (shown by a peeled tongue)—they will further dry the patient up and make the condition worse.

ALPINIA OXYPHYLLA

Yi Zhi Ren BLACK CARDAMOM

This herb warms Internal Cold. Yi Zhi Ren is a cardamom, and all cardamoms warm the Middle area. Yi Zhi Ren also warms the Kidneys and controls fluids coming from that area—which makes it good for urinary incontinence, or frequency and enuresis (bed-wetting) from Cold-Deficient Spleen and Kidneys.

HOW TO USE

- Yi Zhi Ren is helpful in spermatorrhea, when men cannot hold the sperm or when it leaks out.
- When the Spleen yang is weak and Cold it does not transform the feces properly, leading to diarrhea.
- There may also be vomiting, Cold abdominal pain (better with warmth), excessive saliva, and a thick, unpleasant taste in the mouth.
- It is very good to relieve drooling.
- Yi Zhi Ren is a valuable herb for warming the system, from infancy to old age.

PROPERTIES Acrid, Warm

CHANNELS Kidney, Spleen

FUNCTIONS AND USES

- Warms the Kidneys, firms the Jing-essence and holds in urine: this herb is used when the yang aspect of the Kidneys is Deficient and cannot hold sperm or urine in place.
- Warms the Spleen and stops diarrhea: Cold, Deficient Spleen or Stomach patterns causing diarrhea and other digestive symptoms.

CAUTION

- Contraindicated for spermatorrhea, frequent urination, or vaginal discharge due to heat.

ANGELICA DABURICA

Bai Zhi

Bai Zhi belongs to a group of Warm, Acrid herbs that release exterior conditions; that is, superficial illnesses caused by viruses, with symptoms in the skin or muscle layers. The herbs mainly affect the sweating mechanism, either causing the body to sweat, or if necessary stopping it from sweating.

HOW TO USE

- Bai Zhi is used mainly for sudden headaches (Wind-caused headaches), especially those along the Stomach channel, i.e. the front of the head, the forehead.
- It is particularly good for headaches caused by sinusitis, and to help the sinusitis itself.
- It is very good for ulcerated boils in cases where the pus is not yet discharged—use it with Jie Geng.
- It is often added to prescriptions for vaginal discharge, especially for a white (Cold) discharge rather than a yellow, smelly one (Hot type).

PROPERTIES Acrid, Warm
CHANNELS Lung, Stomach
FUNCTIONS AND USES

- Expels Wind and alleviates pain: use for externally contracted Wind Cold patterns, especially those with head symptoms.
- Reduces swelling and expels pus: use in the early stages of a sore in order to reduce swelling.
- Expels Dampness and alleviates discharge. It is used for treating leukorrhea (vaginal discharge) from Damp Cold in the lower abdominal area.
- Helps to open up the nasal passages.

CAUTION
- Contraindicated in deficient blood or deficient yin patterns because it is very drying. Use cautiously if sores have already burst.

ANGELICA SINENSIS

Dang Gui CHINESE ANGELICA

Dang Gui is such a widely used herb that it has entered the Western herbal pharmacy. In TCM it is used to treat patterns of Blood Deficiency, and therefore affects mostly the Heart and Liver, which direct and store the Blood, respectively.

HOW TO USE

Dan Gui is unusual among Blood-tonifying herbs in that it both nourishes and invigorates blood circulation, and is therefore not cloying, as Shu di Huang can be. It is good for Blood-Deficient symptoms such as pale complexion, tinnitus, blurred vision, and palpitations, and is commonly used for all menstrual disorders, such as irregular menstruation, amenorrhea, or dysmenorrhea (painful menstruation). It is essential for pain in general as it moves the Blood—abdominal pain, traumatic injury, and even arthritic pain associated with Blood Deficiency (pain according to TCM may be caused by Stagnant Blood).

PROPERTIES Sweet, Acrid, Bitter, Warm
CHANNELS Heart, Liver, Spleen
FUNCTIONS AND USES

- Tonifies the Blood and regulates the menses.
- Invigorates the Blood and disperses Cold: an important herb for stopping pain due to Blood stasis.
- Moistens the intestines and unblocks the bowels: like all tonifying herbs, Dang Gui is moistening—in this case it is also directed to the intestines.

CAUTION
- Use with caution for diarrhea or abdominal swelling due to dampness contraindicated for yin deficiency.

ATRACTYLODES MACROCEPHALA

Bai Zhu

This herb is one of a group that treat Qi Deficiency, as as we replenish our day-to-day energy from air and food, the two main organs involved are Lungs and Spleen.

HOW TO USE

Bai Zhu is a major tonifying qi herb in cases of diarrhea, vomiting, fatigue, lack of appetite, lack of strength in the limbs, and is one of the herbs in the seminal tonifying prescription of the "Four Gentlemen" (Si Jun Zi Wan). It also helps Damp disorders such as edema and reduced urination, and is used in the Jade Screen prescription for spontaneous sweating due to Qi Deficiency. It is used for any type of threatened miscarriage when combined with other appropriate herbs.

PROPERTIES Sweet, Bitter, Warm

CHANNELS Spleen, Stomach

FUNCTIONS AND USES

- Tonifies the Spleen and benefits the qi: use Bai Zhu to treat Spleen and Stomach Deficiency.
- Strengthens the Spleen and dries Dampness: use for digestive disorders, water retention and even for treating Damp Painful Obstruction (rheumatic ailments).
- Firms the exterior and stops sweating.
- Strengthens the Spleen and calms the fetus: for restless fetus when due to Spleen Deficiency not holding the fetus in.

CAUTION

- Contraindicated in cases of yin deficiency with heat signs of injured fluids.

ASTRAGALUS MEMBRANACEUS

Huang Qi MILK-VETCH ROOT

This herb treats Qi Deficiency, and as we replenish our day-to-day energy from air and food, the two main organs involved are Lungs and Spleen (the main digestive organ in TCM).

HOW TO USE

Huang Qi is for Spleen-Deficient symptoms such as lack of appetite, fatigue, and diarrhea. Its action is also upward and outward, so it helps prolapsed uterus or uterine bleeding, but is also used in prescriptions to help the immune system fight viruses. It is used for frequent colds and helps excessive sweating. It is good for edema and pus-filled sores that have not yet discharged, and is also used in postnatal fever from severe loss of blood.

PROPERTIES Sweet, slightly Warm

CHANNELS Lung, Spleen

FUNCTIONS AND USES

- Tonifies the Spleen and benefits the qi: use for all Deficient Spleen patterns.
- Raises the yang qi of the Spleen and Stomach: use for prolapse—it makes things go up.
- Tonifies the Protective Qi (Wei Qi) and firms the exterior: goes to the outside of the body, and regulates the opening and closing of the pores.
- Benefits Water and reduces swelling.
- Tonifies the qi and Blood: particularly for severe loss of blood.

CAUTION

- Contraindicated for full heat conditions or yin deficiency with fire—it heats too much.

AUKLANDIA LAPPA
Mu Xiang COSTUS ROOT

Mu Xiang regulates and invigorates the qi when it becomes stuck or "stagnant," optimizing the function of the gastrointestinal tract and helping stop pain.

HOW TO USE
Mu Xiang primarily helps digestive symptoms and pain. It is for Spleen or Stomach Stagnation symptoms such as lack of appetite, epigastric (above the navel), or abdominal pain or swelling, nausea, and vomiting. It is also used for Liver and Gall Bladder Stagnation, symptoms such as pain, swelling, or soreness in the flanks (sides). It is very good for diarrhea, dysentery, and tenesmus (a spasm of the rectum where one feels the need to defecate without being able to) due to Stagnation of qi in the Intestines rather than Deficiency. However, it also helps a Deficient Spleen regain its normal functions of transportation and transformation.

PROPERTIES Acrid, slightly Bitter, Warm
CHANNELS Gall Bladder, Large Intestine, Spleen, Stomach

FUNCTIONS AND USES
- Promotes the movement of qi and alleviates pain: use for Spleen, Stomach, Liver, or Gall Bladder Stagnant Qi (pain is always a result of Stagnant Qi or Blood).
- Regulates Stagnant Qi in the Intestines.
- Strengthens the Spleen and prevents Stagnation: use Huang Qi with tonifying herbs to prevent their cloying side-effects.

CAUTION
- Contraindicated in cases of yin deficiency or depleted fluids.

CANNABIS SATIVA
Hou Ma Ren HEMP

Huo Ma Ren comes into the category of Descending Downward: it facilitates the expulsion of the stool in cases of constipation. Huo Ma Ren is ungerminated cannabis seeds, but does not have the effects that smoking cannabis leaves or resin has.

HOW TO USE
Huo Ma Ren is a moist laxative and therefore works gently by lubricating the Intestines. As it is mild in nature it is suitable for debilitated patients, the elderly, and those who are weakened by a febrile (feverish) disease or after childbirth. Also, as it is moistening, it is good for Blood Deficiency and general lack of fluids. One would often add Blood-nourishing herbs, such as Shu di Huang and Dang Gui for constipation due to Blood Deficiency, as in the elderly.

PROPERTIES Sweet, Neutral
CHANNELS Large Intestine, Spleen, Stomach
FUNCTIONS AND USES
- Nourishes and moistens the Intestines: as it does not have a harsh effect, it is most suitable for constipation in the weak and elderly.
- Nourishes the yin: it mildly tonifies the yin and can be used in cases of Yin Deficiency with constipation. The yin is often depleted during a long illness like ME (or post-viral syndrome); also commonly in the elderly.
- Clears Heat and promotes healing of sores: use as an auxiliary herb for sores and ulcerations, taken orally or applied topically (locally).

CAUTION
- Long-term use may possibly result in vaginal discharge. Overdose may lead to nausea, vomiting, and diarrhea.

CARTHAMUS TINCTORIUS

Hong Hua SAFFLOWER FLOWER

This herb invigorates (or "regulates") the Blood, treating problems associated with Blood stasis. In TCM, these problems include pain and internal masses or growths.

HOW TO USE

Hong Hua is used for any Blood stasis patterns. These may include such gynecological problems as amenorrhea, post-partum dizziness, or fibroids. It may also include other tumors if they are caused by congealed blood, and many skin diseases, such as Kaposi's sarcoma, and scarlet fever. As it helps stuck Blood pain it is good for wounds or painful sores. It helps to bring out a measles' rash fully and is useful for pain in the limbs. It also helps joint pain in arthritis.

PROPERTIES Acrid, Warm

CHANNELS Heart, Liver

FUNCTIONS AND USES

- Invigorates the Blood and unblocks menstruation: it expels congealed Blood in the meridians and is not just for menstrual problems.
- Dispels Blood stasis and alleviates pain: it enters the Blood level of the channels (as opposed to qi or organ level).

CAUTION

- As with many blood-moving herbs, do not take this during pregnancy.

CINNAMOMUM CASIA

Gui Zhi CINNAMON TWIGS

Gui Zhi belongs to a group of Warm, Acrid herbs that release exterior conditions; that is, superficial illnesses caused by viruses, with symptoms in the skin or muscle layers. These mainly cause sweating, or stop sweating where necessary.

HOW TO USE

Gui Zhi is used mainly for colds and flu, and commonly in combination with Bai Shao, when there is too much sweating in a cold condition and the patient is becoming weak. It is often added to prescriptions for rheumatic complaints in the joints and limbs, especially the shoulders, caused by Cold Obstruction causing pain, where it sends warmth through the channels. Use for edema, where it sends warm yang energy through the meridians to move and transform the settled fluid. It is often used with licorice (Gan Cao) for palpitations and shortness of breath due to Deficient Heart yang. It can be used for menstrual cramps or irregular menstruation caused by Cold.

PROPERTIES Sweet, Warm

CHANNELS Lung, Bladder

FUNCTIONS AND USES

- Adjusts the body's sweating in externally caused Cold conditions.
- Warms the meridians and disperses Cold: use for rheumatic ailments; also for gynecological problems caused by Cold obstructing the Blood.
- Moves the yang and transforms qi: use for water retention (edema) from Cold, where poor circulation of yang qi has failed to move the fluids in the body.

CAUTION

- Contraindicated in warm diseases, either from fever, deficient yin with heat signs, or heat in the blood with vomiting.

CITRUS RETICULATA

Chen Pi TANGERINE PEEL

This herb regulates and invigorates the qi when it becomes stuck or "stagnant," optimizing the function of the gastrointestinal tract and helping stop pain.

HOW TO USE

Chen Pi is a very important herb as it "awakens the Spleen." It is for stagnant qi patterns with symptoms like epigastric (above the navel) or abdominal bloating, fullness, belching, nausea, and vomiting. It is very good for a lot of sticky sputum and other Phlegm Damp symptoms, such as loss of appetite, fatigue, loose stools, and a thick, greasy tongue coating. It is therefore used for disorders affecting both the Spleen and the Lungs. It is particularly important for putting into tonifying prescriptions to make them more digestible.

PROPERTIES Acrid, Bitter, Warm, Fragrant
CHANNELS Spleen, Stomach, Lung
FUNCTIONS AND USES
- Regulates the qi and strengthens the transportation function of the Spleen: it promotes the movement of qi in general, while directing it down.
- Dries Dampness and transforms Phlegm: use for. a stuffy feeling in the chest and diaphragm.
- Helps prevent stagnation.

CAUTION
- Contraindicated in dry cough due to Yin or Qi Deficiency, as it is drying (fragrant) and warm. Use with caution with a red tongue or yellow phlegm (symptoms of heat).

CONDONOPSIS PILOSULA

Dang Shen CODONOPSIS ROOT

This herb is similar to Ren Shen: it treats Qi Deficiency, affecting primarily the Lungs and Spleen (the main digestive organ in TCM). It is less expensive than Ren Shen.

HOW TO USE

- Dang Shen does basically the same work as Ren Shen, but is not as strong. In prescriptions it is used in place of ginseng to tonify the qi of the Spleen and Lungs, while ginseng is preferred for more serious situations, such as a patient who is barely conscious.
- It is used for lack of appetite, fatigue, tired limbs, diarrhea, vomiting, and prolapse—all symptoms of Spleen Qi Deficiency. It is also used for Lung Deficiency with chronic cough, shortness of breath, or copious sputum due to Spleen Deficiency. As it tonifies fluids, it is used in diabetes and the aftermath of febrile illnesses. It is the main herb in the seminal qi tonic prescription Si Jun Zi Wan ("Four Gentlemen"). Like all the qi tonics, it is sweet and cloying, and must therefore be combined with qi-moving herbs.
- Tonifies the Lungs.

PROPERTIES Sweet, Neutral
CHANNELS Lung, Spleen
FUNCTIONS AND USES
- Tonifies the Middle area, benefits the qi, and strengthens the Stomach and Spleen: use for all Deficient Qi patterns.
- Strengthens the qi and nourishes fluids.

CAUTION
- Long-term use may possibly result in vaginal discharge. Overdose may lead to nausea, vomiting, and diarrhea.

COIX LACHRYMA JOBI

Yi Yi Ren
SEEDS OF JOB'S TEARS

This is one of the Chinese herbs that transform Dampness, but it is more active on the Lower Burner than the Middle Burner.

HOW TO USE

Like Fu Ling, Yi Yi Ren clears Dampness by promoting urination, but its Spleen-strengthening function is not as strong, and it works more on the Lower Burner (Kidneys) than on the Middle Burner (Spleen and Stomach). Use with Spleen-tonifying herbs to get rid of water retention; it may be used for Lung or Intestinal abscesses to help get rid of pus.

PROPERTIES Sweet, Bland, slightly Cold

CHANNELS Spleen, Lung, Kidney

FUNCTIONS AND USES

- Promotes urination and leeches out Dampness: for edema or water retention in the legs.
- Clears Wind Dampness: this means Painful Obstruction syndrome, such as arthritic conditions.
- Clears Heat and expels pus: use when sores have become full of pus; pushes pus out.
- Strengthens Spleen and stops diarrhea: use when the Spleen is deficient, causing Damp diarrhea.
- Clears Damp Heat: for any digestive problems with a greasy yellow tongue coating.

CAUTION
- Use with caution during pregnancy.

CORNUS OFFICINALIS

Shan Zhu Yu CORNELIAN
CHERRY FRUIT, DOGWOOD FRUIT

Shan Zhu Yu stabilizes and binds. It is sour and astringent, and helps keep in bodily substances which may leak, such as urine.

HOW TO USE

Shan Zhu Yu is used for leakage of fluids due to weak Jing-essence, with symptoms such as excessive urination, incontinence, spermatorrhea, and premature ejaculation. In shock, it helps Liver and Kidney Deficiency, with such symptoms as lightheadedness, dizziness, sore and weak low back and knees, or impotence. It is useful for excessive uterine bleeding when the cause is Deficiency. It is one of the six herbs in the basic yin-tonifying prescription Liu Wei di Huang Wan (Six Flavor prescription), so if carefully combined it may tonify yin or yang.

PROPERTIES Sour, slightly Warm

CHANNELS Kidney, Liver

FUNCTIONS AND USES

- Firms the Kidneys and retains the Jing-essence.
- Absorbs sweating and supports collapse: use for devastated yang and qi, as in shock.
- Tonifies and builds the Liver and Kidneys.
- Stabilizes the menses and stops bleeding.

COPTIS CHINENSIS

Huang Lian COPTIS RHISZOME, GOLDEN THREAD

This herb clears Heat: this includes febrile conditions and illnesses with Heat signs. It is one of the "Three Yellows," which are often used together for severe infections.

HOW TO USE

Huang Lian deals with Damp Heat in the Middle Burner (digestive organs), and also the Heart and Pericardium. This latter leads to symptoms such as very high fever with delirium and disorientation. It can also be used to treat painful, red eyes and sore throat. It is very good with the infectious diseases still prevalent in the developing world. It is used for violent diarrhea and acid regurgitation from Stomach Heat. A decoction may be placed on sore, red eyes, boils, anal fissures, conjunctivitis, and used locally it is good for treating trichomoniasis, a protozoan infection of the vagina.

PROPERTIES Bitter, Cold
CHANNELS Heart, Liver, Stomach, Large Intestine
FUNCTIONS AND USES
- Clears Heat and detoxifies Fire Poison.
- Clears Heat and drains Dampness, especially in the Stomach and Intestines—dysentery, vomiting.
- Clears Heart Fire: symptoms such as irritability and insomnia.
- Stops Hot bleeding.
- Drains Stomach Fire: digestive dysfunction.

CAUTION
- Do not use for deficient yin patterns, where the fluid may be deficient anyway—Huang Lian would dry out more. Like all the clearing heat herbs it is Cold in energy, so it is contraindicated in any diseases cause by Cold.

CRATAEGUS PINNATIFIDA

Shan Zha HAWTHORN FRUIT, CRATAEGUS

This herb relieves digestive problems resulting from over-indulgence in greasy foods, and helps to promote efficient digestion by increasing gastrointestinal secretions and enzymatic functions.

HOW TO USE

Shan Zha is used for abdominal distention, belching, pain, and reduced appetite. It is also used for children who fail to thrive. It is especially useful if the symptoms are accompanied by diarrhea or chronic dysentery. It is particularly indicated for postnatal abdominal pain and menstrual pain when the cause is congealed Blood, and hernias with testicular pain and swelling. Recently it has also been used for hypertension (high blood pressure), coronary artery disease, and high cholesterol.

PROPERTIES Sour, Sweet, slightly Warm
CHANNELS Liver, Spleen, Stomach
FUNCTIONS AND USES
- Reduces and guides out food stagnation: for obstruction due to meat or greasy foods.
- Transforms Blood stasis and dissipates knottedness: enters the Blood level and is used for treating Blood stagnation disorders.
- Stops diarrhea: when the herb is slightly charred, it has an astringent effect.

CAUTION
- Use with caution in cases of Spleen and Stomach Deficiency without food stagnation, and in diseases with acid regurgitation.

CUSCUTA CHINENSIS

Tu Su Zi CHINESE DODDER SEEDS

This herb tonifies the yang, and as they are the basis of all the body's yang, it mainly affects the Kidneys. In TCM, the Kidneys house the body's reserves, and the Kidney yang is also responsible for sexual and endocrine disorders.

HOW TO USE

Tu Su Zi helps the Jing-essence so is good for impotence, nocturnal emissions, and premature ejaculation, as well as such Kidney Yang Deficient symptoms, such as sore lower back and knees, frequent urination, incontinence, and vaginal discharge. It is used for such Liver and Kidney Deficient symptoms as tinnitus (ringing in the ears), dizziness, blurred vision, or spots in front of the eyes. It stops leaking, so it is good for diarrhea or loose stools from Deficiency, and it also helps prevent threatened or habitual miscarriage.

PROPERTIES Acrid, Sweet, Neutral

CHANNELS Kidney, Liver

FUNCTIONS AND USES

- Tonifies the Kidneys and benefits the Jing-essence: unlike most Kidney yang herbs, which are heating and therefore drying, Tu Su Zi is also moistening, so helps preserve the yin fluid.
- Tonifies the Liver and Kidneys and improves vision: use for patterns of Deficient Liver and Kidney yin and yang.
- Benefits the Spleen and Kidneys and stops persistent diarrhea.
- Calms the fetus.

CAUTION

- Although this is a neutral herb, it leans more toward tonifying the yang and should therefore not be use for Fire from Yin Deficiency.

CYPERUS ROTUNDUS

Xiang Fu NUT-GRASS RHIZOME

This herb regulates and invigorates the qi when it becomes stuck or "stagnant," optimizing the function of the gastrointestinal tract and helping stop pain in various parts of the body, particularly menstrual and digestive pain.

HOW TO USE

Xiang Fu is a very widely used herb, as it has the ability to disperse stuck qi and to harmonize the energy, both in digestive and in gynecological disorders. It is particularly suitable for pain in the sides, fullness in the epigastrium (above the navel), pain and stuffiness in the chest, lack of appetite, wind and indigestion, as well as vomiting and diarrhea due to Liver Qi invading the Spleen. It is also for swollen, tender breasts (due to PMS), and is an important herb for breast lumps. It is essential in prescriptions for dysmenorrhea (menstrual cramps) or irregular menstruation, and can be used in pregnancy for treating Liver Qi stagnation patterns.

PROPERTIES Acrid, slightly Bitter, slightly Sweet, Neutral

CHANNELS Liver, Triple Burner

FUNCTIONS AND USES

- Moves qi and regulates Liver Qi: in pathology, the Liver energy has a tendency to become "constrained," resulting in pain above the navel and around the ribs.
- Regulates menstruation and alleviates pain: according to TCM, the Liver is one of the main organs involved in gynecology, and the cause of menstrual pain is frequently due to "constrained Liver Qi."

THE HEALING REMEDIES SOURCEBOOK

GASTRODIA ELATA

Tian Ma GASTRODIA RHIZOME

This herb has a sinking action—that is to say it takes qi down strongly.

HOW TO USE

Tian Ma is a very important herb for treating internal Liver Wind, with symptoms such as childhood convulsions or tantrums, epilepsy, spasms, or seizures. It is used for headaches, dizziness, and migraines caused by Wind Phlegm patterns, as well as Wind Stroke (stroke) with hemiplegia and numbness in the extremities. It is also good for rheumatic ailments in the lower back and limbs.

PROPERTIES Sweet, Neutral

CHANNELS Liver

FUNCTIONS AND USES

- Calms the Liver, extinguishes Wind, and controls tremors. There are two kinds of Wind in TCM, external—which brings in cold or flu, or arthritic symptoms, and internal—which is generated by dysfunction of the Liver. This herb treats the second.
- Extinguishes Wind and alleviates pain: especially Wind Mucus head pain.
- Disperses painful obstruction caused by Wind Damp.

CAUTION
- May be toxic in large doses.

EUCOMMIA ULMOIDES

Du Zhong EUCOMMIA BARK

This herb belongs to a group that tonify the yang, and as the Kidneys are the basis of all the body's yang, it mainly affects the Kidneys. In TCM, the Kidneys house the body's reserves, and the Kidney yang is also responsible for sexual and endocrine disorders.

HOW TO USE

Du Zhong is an expensive herb—it is necessary to kill the tree in order to get the bark. The Liver rules the sinews, the Kidneys rule the bones, so it is used for weak, sore, or painful lower back and knees, chronic fatigue, spermatorrhea (leaking of sperm), and frequent urination. Yang Deficient symptoms are always accompanied by Cold. It is the main herb for lower back pain caused by Qi and Blood Stagnation. It helps prevent miscarriage with bleeding during pregnancy, or when the fetus is restless, and it has recently been used for dizziness and lightheadedness due to hypertension from rising Liver yang.

PROPERTIES Sweet, slightly Acrid, Warm

CHANNELS Kidney, Liver

FUNCTIONS AND USES

- Tonifies the Liver and Kidneys, strengthens the tendons and bones.
- Aids the smooth flow of qi and Blood: use to promote circulation.
- Calms the fetus: use for Cold (lack of yang) Deficient Kidney patterns during pregnancy.

CAUTION
- Contraindicated for Heat from Yin Deficiency.

FRITILLARIAA THUNBERGII

Zhe Bei Mu FRITILLARIA BULB

Like Ban Xia, this herb transforms Phlegm, which in TCM is the accumulation of thick fluid mainly in the respiratory and digestive tracts, but which may occur in the muscles and other body tissues.

HOW TO USE

Zhe Bei Mu is a Cold herb which treats Phlegm Heat (as opposed to Ban Xia, which is warming), characterized by yellow sputum or sputum which is difficult to bring up. It is also indicated for Phlegm Fire coagulating and causing lumps in the breast or neck, and for Lung abscesses. Chuan Bei Mu is another form of this herb which is milder and not so cooling, and may be used for many types of cough, including dry Yin-Deficient ones.

PROPERTIES Bitter, Cold

CHANNELS Lung, Heart

FUNCTIONS AND USES

- Clears and transforms Phlegm Heat: use for acute Lung Heat patterns with productive yellow sputum.
- Clears Heat and dissipates nodules: use for Phlegm Fire which congeals and causes neck swellings.

CAUTION
- Ineffective in coughs due to Phlegm Cold.

GLYCYRRHIZA URALENSIS

Gan Cao LICORICE ROOT

This herb is one of a group that treats Qi Deficiency and tonifies the Spleen. As we replenish our day-to-day energy levels by breathing in air and eating food, the two main organs involved are Lungs and Spleen (the main digestive organ in TCM).

HOW TO USE

Gan Cao is a very useful herb, primarily because it is sweet and mild, so that it moderates the violent properties of other herbs in a prescription and makes them more digestible. Furthermore, it enters all 12 channels, so it can lead other herbs into those channels. It is used for Spleen Deficiency with shortness of breath, tiredness, and loose stools, and for Blood Deficiency with an irregular pulse and palpitations. It is used for any coughing and wheezing, and is good for spasms or cramps in the abdomen or legs. It is also useful for strep throat infections.

PROPERTIES Sweet, Neutral (raw), Warm (toasted)

CHANNELS All 12 channels

FUNCTIONS AND USES

- Tonifies the Spleen and benefits the qi.
- Moistens the Lungs and stops coughing: because it is neutral, it can be used to treat either Heat or Cold in the Lungs.
- Clears Heat and detoxifies Fire Poison: use Gan Cao for sores or sore throats with pus.

CAUTION
- Contraindicated for cases of excess Dampness, nausea, or vomiting. May cause high blood pressure or edema if taken for an extended period of time.

LEDEBOURIELLA SESLOIDES

Fang Feng

Fang Feng belongs to a group of Warm, Acrid herbs that release exterior conditions; that is, superficial illnesses caused by viruses, with symptoms in the skin or muscle layers.

HOW TO USE

Fang Feng means in English "guard against wind," so it is used particularly in ailments where Wind is predominant, according to TCM. This means it causes sweating (Acrid quality) in colds and flu. It is also useful in arthritis, where the pain moves about from joint to joint (Wind type of arthritis). It treats numbness and trembling caused by Wind and Phlegm blocking the channels.

PROPERTIES Acrid, Sweet, slightly Warm
CHANNELS Bladder, Liver, Spleen
FUNCTIONS AND USES
- Releases the Exterior and expels Wind: use for headaches, chills, and body aches from externally contracted Wind Cold.
- Expels Wind Dampness and alleviates pain: use for Exterior Wind Damp Painful Obstruction (rheumatic ailments).
- Expels Wind: Fang Feng alleviates trembling of the hands and feet.

CAUTION
- Contraindicated in cases of Deficient Blood with spasms—it does not tonify the blood and produces sweating, so one would have to add tonifying blood herbs to stop it depleting the Blood further. Contraindicated for cases of Deficient Yin with heat signs. Yin is the fluid in the body and it keeps the body cool, so Deficient Yin can produce a "false heat" such as in menopausal sweats. As Fang Feng produces more sweat it would deplete the yin fluid even further—it needs to be carefully contraindicated.

LINGUSTICUM CHUANXIONG

Chuan Xiong SZECHUAN LOVAGE ROOT, CNIDIUM

This herb invigorates (or "regulates") the Blood, treating disorders associated with Blood stasis. In TCM, these problems include pain and internal masses or growths.

HOW TO USE

Chuan Xiong is an important herb for gynecology, as many gynecological problems are caused by Stagnant Blood circulation—problems such as dysmenorrhea (menstrual cramps), amenorrhea (lack of menstruation), difficult labor, or retained placenta. It is also used for chest, flank, and epigastric (above the navel) pain caused by Stagnant Qi and Blood. It is a leading herb for externally caught Wind disorders (viruses), with symptoms such as headaches, migraines, and dizziness. It is useful for arthritis and a variety of skin problems caused by Wind, including itching. It is an essential herb used in combinations for treating all types of headaches.

PROPERTIES Acrid, Warm
CHANNELS Liver, Gall Bladder, Pericardium
FUNCTIONS AND USES
- Invigorates the Blood and promotes the circulation of qi: use for any Blood stasis patterns, especially in gynecology.
- Expels Wind and alleviates pain: it goes to the top and exterior parts of the body.

CAUTION
- Contraindicated in yin deficiency with Heat signs (it is warming), headaches due to rising Liver yang, Qi Deficiency (it does not tonify), or excessive menstrual bleeding (it moves blood further).

LONICERA JAPONICA

Jin Yin Hua HONEYSUCKLE, "GOLD SILVER FLOWER"

Jin Yin Hua is one of a group of herbs that clears Heat: this includes febrile conditions and any illnesses with Heat signs, such as fever, inflammation, red eyes, aversion to heat, and hot skin eruptions.

HOW TO USE

Jin Yin Hua has a strong effect against many pathogenic bacteria. It is especially useful against salmonella (food poisoning), and is effective against many streptococcus or staphylococcus infections. It is good for painful, hot swellings, particularly of the breast (mastitis), throat (viral or bacterial tonsillitis), or eyes (conjunctivitis). It is also used in "summer-heat diseases," where the hot weather produces fevers, sweating, and thirst. It is used for bad dysentery and bacterial urinary tract infections.

PROPERTIES Sweet, Cold

CHANNELS Large Intestine, Lung, Stomach

FUNCTIONS AND USES

- Clears Heat and relieves toxicity: use Jin Yin Hua for hot, painful sores.
- Expels External Wind Heat: use for the early stages of febrile illnesses.
- Clears Damp Heat from Lower Burner: use for dysentery or cystitis.

CAUTION

- Contraindicated in cases of diarrhea due to Spleen and Stomach Deficiency—it is for strong infections and does not tonify weakness. Contraindicated in sores which do not have infected pus, but clear liquid inside.

LYCIUM BARBARUM

Gou Qi Zi CHINESE WOLFBERRY, MATRIMONY VINE FRUIT

This herb treats patterns of Blood Deficiency, and in TCM the two organs most affected by this disorder are the Heart and Liver, which direct and store the Blood, respectively.

HOW TO USE

Gou Qi Zi is used for such Liver and Kidney Deficient symptoms as sore back and weak knees, impotence, leaking of sperm, and diabetes, particularly in the elderly, when the yin is in decline. It is used for Liver and Kidney Deficiency which leads to Blood and essence failing to nourish the eyes, so is good for failing or blurred vision, dizziness, dry, or sore eyes. As it enriches the yin of the Lungs, it is good for consumptive coughs.

PROPERTIES Sweet, Neutral

CHANNELS Liver, Lung, Kidney

FUNCTIONS AND USES

- Nourishes and tonifies the Liver and Kidneys: because this herb is neither Hot nor Cold, it is commonly used in treating Liver and Kidney Deficiency with patterns of Yin and Blood Deficiency.
- Benefits the Jing-essence and brightens the eyes: Jing (ancestral qi) is held in the Kidneys, while the Liver meridian goes to the eyes.
- Moistens the Lungs.

CAUTION

- Contraindicated in full Heat disorders, especially exeternal (viruses), and in cases of Spleen Deficiency with loose stools.

OPHIOPOGON JAPONICUS

Mai Men Dong
OPIOPOGON TUBER

This herb tonifies the yin, and it therefore moistens and nourishes fluid. Any of the major organs may suffer from a Yin Deficiency, so Mai Men Dong is an important herb for their revitalization.

HOW TO USE

Mai Men Dong particularly strengthens the yin in the Upper part of the body, so it is good after febrile illness when the mouth is parched, and there is severe thirst or recurring fever. It is used for an irregular pulse and palpitations from the same causes of injury to the fluids or Blood. It is particularly for a dry cough, with or without mucus, and for Stomach Yin Deficiency, which includes stomach aches, "dry" vomiting, and a shiny tongue with little coating. It is also for diabetes, as well as being used to brighten vision and strengthen the lower back. Like Tu Su Zi, it is added to prescriptions to moisten, but only in Yin-Deficient patterns.

PROPERTIES Sweet, Bitter, slightly Cold
CHANNELS Lung, Stomach, Heart
FUNCTIONS AND USES
- Moistens the Lungs and stops coughing.
- Tonifies the Stomach yin and generates fluid.

CAUTION
- Contraindicated in case of deficiency without Heat signs. Like all tonifying yin herbs, it aids Dampness and should therefore not be used for cold, phlegmy coughing or Deficient Spleen with loose stools or a thick, greasy tongue coating.

PAEONIA LACTIFLORA

Bai Shao WHITE PEONY ROOT

Bai Shao is a cooling herb with a sinking action—which means it takes qi down strongly. It is useful when the Liver is not fulfilling its function of making the Blood and qi flow smoothly.

HOW TO USE

Bai Shao has many uses and is an important herb. It treats headaches and dizziness due to rising Liver yang, and flank, chest, and abdominal pain from constrained (stuck) Liver Qi, or disharmony between the Liver and Spleen, which normally have a close relationship in the upper abdomen. Generally, this herb "softens" the Liver, treating spasms in the abdomen, or cramps in the hands or feet. It is good for menstrual irregularity or pain, or uterine bleeding, and, as it preserves the yin fluids and treats vaginal discharge and leaking of sperm. It treats excessive sweating in an external illness, or night sweating in Yin Deficiency.

PROPERTIES Bitter, Sour, Cool
CHANNELS Liver, Spleen
FUNCTIONS AND USES
- Pacifies the Liver yang and alleviates pain: use for patterns of Liver yang rising, constrained Liver Qi or disharmonies between the Liver and the Spleen.
- Nourishes the Blood and regulates the menses.
- Adjusts the Ying and Wei: this refers to the balance between the inner and outer qi levels, which control the opening and closing of the pores.
- Preserves the yin.

CAUTION
- Exercise caution with diarrhea due to Cold from deficiency, as it is a cold herb.

PANAX GINSENG

Ren Shen GINSENG ROOT, "MAN ROOT"

Ren Shen is an expensive herb as it takes six or seven years to cultivate. It is calming and has a proven effect on stress.

HOW TO USE

Ren Shen is invaluable because it tonifies both the qi (lack of energy) and the yin (lack of fluid). It is used after shock, with shallow respiration, shortness of breath, cold limbs, profuse sweating, and a weak pulse. It is good for Lung problems, such as labored breathing and wheezing, and Spleen Qi Deficient problems such as lethargy, lack of appetite, bloating, and diarrhea, or, more severely, prolapse of the stomach, uterus, or rectum. It calms the Heart when there are palpitations, and in cases of anxiety, insomnia, or forgetfulness. As it is so expensive, it is usually substituted by Dang Shen in prescriptions.

PROPERTIES Sweet, slightly Bitter, slightly Warm

CHANNELS Lung, Spleen

FUNCTIONS AND USES

- Strong tonifier of Root Qi: helps to revive an unconscious person.
- Tonifies the Lungs and benefits the qi.
- Strengthens the Spleen and tonifies the Stomach.
- Ren Shen generates fluid and stops thirst: use for diabetes when the qi and Blood have been injured by high fever and sweating.
- Benefits the Heart Qi and calms the spirit.

CAUTION

- Contraindicated for Yin Deficiency with Heat signs (it is slightly warming), heat excess or no significant Qi Deficiency. Overdose can lead to headache, insomnia, and a rise in blood pressure.

PANAX NOTOGINSENG

San Qi NOTOGINSENG ROOT, PSEUDOGINSENG ROOT

This herb is used for bleeding or hemorrhage. Generally this herb is not used alone, but with other herbs that treat the cause of the bleeding, such as Hot Blood, Yin Deficiency, Spleen Deficiency, or stasis of the Blood.

HOW TO USE

San Qi has long been used in battle—soldiers carried this black powder with them to stem wounds. It may be taken on its own or in a prescription. It is used for all kinds of internal and external bleeding, such as vomiting blood, nosebleed, blood in the urine or stool, uterine bleeding, or trauma-induced bleeding. It is good for chest and abdominal pain, as well as joint pain caused by congealed Blood. It can also be used after heart attacks to get rid of debris in the coronary artery, and is very useful after injuries, for swelling and pain due to falls, fractures, bruises, and sprains.

PROPERTIES Sweet, slightly Bitter, Warm

CHANNELS Liver, Stomach, Large Intestine

FUNCTIONS AND USES

- Stops bleeding and transforms Blood stasis: because this herb can stop bleeding without causing Blood stasis, it is very widely used.
- Reduces swelling and alleviates pain: San Qi is a first choice for traumatic injuries.

CAUTION

- Contraindicated during pregnancy. Use with caution in patients with Blood or Yin Deficiency.

PHELLODENDRON AMURENSE

Huang Bai, Huang Bo

AMUR CORK TREE BARK, CYPRUS ROTONDIS, "YELLOW FIR"

This herb is one that clears Heat: this includes febrile conditions and any illnesses with Heat signs. It is one of the "Three Yellows," which are often used together for severe infections.

HOW TO USE

Huang Bai is particularly good for Damp Heat symptoms in the bottom third of the body, such as yellow, smelly vaginal discharge, foul-smelling diarrhea, or dysentery. It is also used for red, swollen, and painful legs, and Damp Heat jaundice. It can be used for menopausal symptoms of hot sweats, or for afternoon fevers at the end of a long illness or when withdrawing from illicit drugs. It is good for leg ulcers which require antibiotics. It is a weaker (and cheaper) version of Huang Lian in its antimicrobial effects.

PROPERTIES Bitter, Cold
CHANNELS Kidney, Bladder
FUNCTIONS AND USES

- Drains Damp Heat, particularly in the Lower Burner: use Huang Bai for Damp Heat leukorrhea (vaginal discharge).
- Detoxifies Fire Poison, i.e. toxic sores with pus in them.

CAUTION

- Contraindicated in cases of Spleen Deficiency, with or without diarrhea (Spleen Deficiency must be diagnosed by a qualified TCM practitioner).

PINELLIA TERNATA

Ban Xia PINELLIA RHIZOME

This herb is one that transforms Phlegm, which in TCM is the accumulation of thick fluid mainly in the respiratory and digestive tracts, but which may occur in the muscles and other body tissues.

HOW TO USE

Ban Xia is one of the main herbs for drying Damp, and is used for abdominal and epigastric (upper abdominal) bloating and nausea, or for a stifling feeling in the chest due to Phlegm Damp—it is often used with Chen Pi. It can be added to prescriptions to avoid nausea from other herbs. It reduces any lumps or obstructions caused by Phlegm in the body.

PROPERTIES Acrid, Warm
CHANNELS Lung, Spleen, Stomach
FUNCTIONS AND USES

- Dries Dampness, transforms Phlegm, and helps rebellious qi to descend; it is one of the main herbs for coughs with sputum. It helps the Spleen to dry out and so produce less mucus.
- Harmonizes the Stomach and stops vomiting: it takes qi down so helps Phlegm Dampness in the Stomach that rebels upward and causes vomiting.
- Dissipates nodules and reduces lumps: use for nodules caused by Phlegm lingering, such as goiter or lumps in the breast.

CAUTION

- Contraindicated in bleeding, coughs due to Yin Deficiency (dry coughs) or depleted fluids—it is very drying. Use with caution. In very large amounts, it is somewhat toxic (causing nausea), but can be cured by ginger.

PLATYCODON GRANDIFLORUM

Jie Geng BALLOON FLOWER ROOT

This herb relieves coughing and wheezing. Like other cough remedies, it treats the manifestation (presenting symptoms) of the problem, and therefore needs to be combined with other herbs that treat the root cause.

HOW TO USE

Like Xing Ren, Jie Geng can be used for a wide variety of coughs, especially for coughs caused by external pathogens, either Wind Cold or Wind Heat. It is useful for loss of voice, especially when this is caused by external Heat drying up the fluids in the throat. However, when combined carefully, it can be used for loss of voice due to Phlegm Heat or Yin Deficiency. It is often put into other prescriptions to direct herbs to the chest and head areas.

PROPERTIES Bitter, Acrid, Neutral
CHANNELS Lung
FUNCTIONS AND USES

- Circulates the Lung Qi, expels Phlegm and stops coughing: Jie Geng can be used to treat a wide variety of coughs, depending on the other herbs with which it is combined.
- Benefits the throat and opens the voice: used in many cases of sore throat and loss of voice, especially those caused by external Heat.
- Makes herbs go to the upper body.
- Promotes the discharge of pus: use for expelling pus associated with Lung abscess or throat abscess.

CAUTION

- Contraindicated in coughing blood (Hemoptysis), as it makes things go up and would make the condition worse.

POLYGALA TENUIFOLIA

Yuan Zhi CHINESE SENEGA ROOT, POLYGALA

Yuan Zhi nourishes the Heart and calms the Spirit, or Shen, which is said to reside in the Heart. When the Shen is calm, personality is at its most potent.

HOW TO USE

Yuan Zhi is used for insomnia, anxiety, palpitations, and forgetfulness. However, it differs from Suan Zao Ren in that it is most effective in cases when the patient thinks too much (excessive brooding), or for restlessness and disorientation. "Phlegm misting the Heart" implies quite serious psychological or psychiatric disturbances, when the Spirit is not clear and the patient loses touch with reality. It is also used for seizures and epilepsy. It is useful for coughs with copious sputum, especially when difficult to expectorate, and is applied topically for abscesses, sores, and swollen and painful breasts.

PROPERTIES Bitter, Acrid, slightly Warm
CHANNELS Heart, Lung, Kidney
FUNCTIONS AND USES

- Calms the Spirit and quietens the Heart: use for pent-up emotions.
- Expels Phlegm and clears the orifices: when "mucus envelops the orifices of the Heart," with consequent emotional problems.
- Helps expel Phlegm from the Lungs.
- Reduces abscesses and dissipates swellings: use in powdered form, applied topically or mixed into a glass of wine.

CAUTION

- Contraindicated during pregnancy. Use with caution in patients with Blood or Yin Deficiency.

POLYGONUM MULTIFLORUM
He Shou Wu
FLEECEFLOWER ROOT

This herb treats patterns of Blood Deficiency, and in TCM the two organs most affected by this disorder are the Heart and Liver, which direct and store the Blood, respectively.

HOW TO USE

He Shou Wu is very commonly used, as it both tonifies and preserves the Kidney Jing-essence without being cloying. It is particularly used for premature graying or when the hair falls out (the name means "black hair"), as well as for dizziness, blurred vision, spots in front of the eyes, and a weak lower back and knees. It stops premature ejaculation, leaking of sperm, and vaginal discharge. Used raw, it is good for goiter and neck lumps—and as it moistens, is useful for constipation. It treats chronic malaria and prevents hardening of the arteries.

PROPERTIES Bitter, Sweet, Astringent, slightly Warm
CHANNELS Liver, Kidney
FUNCTIONS AND USES
- Tonifies the Liver and Kidneys, nourishes the Blood and Jing-essence: used for treating Yin and Blood Deficiency.
- Firms the Jing and stops leakage: this refers to male sexual problems.
- Relieves Fire toxicity: use He Shou Wu raw for carbuncles and sores.
- Moistens the Intestines and unblocks the bowels.
- Expels Wind from the skin by nourishing the Blood: use for rashes that appear suddenly.

CAUTION
- Contraindicated for Spleen Deficiency, Phlegm, or diarrhea.

POLYGONUS MULTIFLORUM
Ye Jiao Teng
FLEECEFLOWER VINE

Ye Jiao Teng nourishes the Heart and calms the Spirit, which is said to reside in the Heart. It is therefore useful in tackling disturbed emotions.

HOW TO USE

Ye Jiao Teng is good for Yin or Blood Deficiency patterns with insomnia, irritability, or emotional and nervous patients who cannot eat. It is especially useful for dream-disturbed sleep, and helps one feel comfortable in oneself. It also nourishes the Blood in the four limbs when the circulation is blocked or weak due to Blood Deficiency, and is used for such symptoms as generalized as weakness, soreness, and aching or numb limbs. As it nourishes the Blood in the channels (meridians), it is also used externally as a wash for itching and skin rashes.

PROPERTIES Sweet, slightly Bitter, Neutral
CHANNELS Heart, Liver
FUNCTIONS AND USES
- Nourishes the Heart and Blood, and calms the Spirit.
- Activates Blood circulation and unblocks the channels.
- Alleviates itching: use as an external wash.

CAUTION
- Contraindicated with diarrhea.

PORIA COCOS
Fung Ling TUCKAHOE, HOELEN, BREAD ROOT

Fu Ling is a widely used herb that transforms Dampness, a "pathogenic influence" which creates stagnation in the Middle Burner, with various digestive or fluid-retaining effects.

HOW TO USE
Fu Ling both strengthens the Spleen and gets rid of Dampness. It is good for difficulty with urination, diarrhea, or edema (water retention), all symptoms of Dampness in the system. It helps with loss of appetite or bloating. Other symptoms of Phlegm include headaches or dizziness, and as it calms the Spirit it is good for palpitations, insomnia, or forgetfulness. It is a main ingredient in the qi-strengthening prescription Si Jun Zi Wan ("Four Gentlemen") and is also essential in the main yin-tonifying prescription, where it stops a person becoming too moist from the yin (fluid) tonifying herbs.

PROPERTIES Sweet, Bland, Neutral

CHANNELS Heart, Spleen, Lung

FUNCTIONS AND USES
- Promotes urination and leeches out Dampness by causing urination.
- Strengthens the Spleen and harmonizes the Middle area: helps prevent Dampness building up.
- Strengthens the Spleen and transforms Phlegm (congested fluids which can cause Heart palpitations and other symptoms).
- Quietens the Heart and calms the Spirit.

PRUNUS ARMENICA
Xing Ren APRICOT KERNEL

This herb is primarily used to treat coughing and wheezing. As it treats the manifestation (presenting symptoms) of the problem, it needs to be combined with other herbs that treat the root cause.

HOW TO USE
Xing Ren may be used for many kinds of coughing, whether from Heat or Cold, Exterior or Interior, depending on the combination with other herbs. Because the herb is moist in nature, it is useful for externally caught dry cough. It can be combined with Huo Ma Ren or Dang Gui for constipation due to Deficient Qi and dry Intestines.

PROPERTIES Bitter, slightly Warm, slightly Toxic

CHANNELS Lung, Large Intestine

FUNCTIONS AND USES
- Stops coughing and calms wheezing: Xing Ren is used widely for many kinds of cough.
- Moistens Intestines and unblocks the bowels: a secondary benefit due to the high oil content of Xing Ren.

CAUTION
- Use with caution for children and in cases of diarrhea.

PRUNUS PERSICA
Tao Ren PEACH KERNEL

This herb invigorates (or "regulates") the Blood, treating problems associated with Blood stasis. In TCM, these disorders include pain and internal masses or growths.

HOW TO USE

Tao Ren is a very strong herb. It breaks through Blood and is an important herb for hard abdominal masses and tumors, and for epigastric lumps such as enlarged Liver or Spleen, if there is Stagnant Blood present. It also treats congealed Blood amenorrhea and abdominal pain, or pain from injuries. It is good for psychosis caused by congealed Blood (according to TCM) or post-partum psychosis, and treats Lung and Intestinal abscesses. Like many seeds, it is useful for constipation caused by dry Intestines.

PROPERTIES Bitter, Sweet, Neutral
CHANNELS Heart, Liver, Lung, Large Intestine
FUNCTIONS AND USES
- Breaks up Blood stasis: it is a stronger herb than Hong Hua.
- Moistens the Intestines and moves stools.

CAUTION
- Contraindicated during pregnancy.

RADIX REHMANNIA GLUTINOSA
Sheng di Huang
CHINESE FOXGLOVE ROOT

Sheng di Huang is one of a group of herbs that clear Heat: this includes febrile conditions and any illnesses with Heat signs. It can be used to treat diabetes by addressing the Heat cause.

HOW TO USE

Sheng di Huang is a very moistening as well as cooling herb. Therefore it is used in febrile illnesses where the Heat over a period has dried up the fluids in the body, causing thirst, irritability, and a scarlet tongue. It is also used, often with Bai Shao, when Heat in the Blood level causes hemorrhage from the vessels, leading to bloody urine, nosebleeds, and vomiting of blood. Untreated diabetes causes excessive thirst and urine—Sheng di Huang treats the Heat cause and helps the body replace the fluids.

PROPERTIES Sweet, Bitter, Cold
CHANNELS Heart, Liver, Kidney
FUNCTIONS AND USES
- Clears Heat and cools the Blood: use in all febrile conditions where there is a very high fever, thirst, and a scarlet tongue. Also in hemorrhage when Heat enters the Blood level.
- Nourishes the yin and generates fluids: treats low-grade, long-term fever with dry mouth, constipation, and night sweats.
- Cools Heart Fire blazing: mouth and tongue ulcers, irritability, insomnia.

CAUTION
- Contraindicated in cases of Spleen Deficiency with Dampness—Sheng di Huang is too moistening. Also contraindicated in the presence of Phlegm.

RHEUM PALMATUM

Da Huang RHUBARB ROOT AND RHIZOME

Da Huang comes into the category of Descending Downward: it facilitates the expulsion of stools in cases of constipation. This downward action clears Heat.

HOW TO USE

Da Huang (rhubarb) is a purgative. It has a strong downward action and clears Heat by acting as a powerful laxative. It treats Damp Heat jaundice, dysentery, and cystitis in the same way. It is good for Stagnant Blood complaints such as endometriosis, amenorrhea (lack of menstruation), and appendicitis.

PROPERTIES Bitter, Cold
CHANNELS Heart, Large Intestine, Liver, Stomach
FUNCTIONS AND USES
- Drains Heat and purges accumulations: use for Full Heat conditions where there is fever, thirst, constipation, abdominal pain, a full pulse, and yellow fur on the patient's tongue.
- Drains Damp Heat via the stools.
- Clears Full Heat from the Blood: use for "reckless" bright red Blood that is flowing strongly, e.g. bleeding hemorrhoids (piles), nosebleeds.

CAUTION
- Contraindicated in the first stage of infectious diseases. Also contraindicated for Qi or Blood Deficiency—it doesn't tonify weakness but may be added to a tonifying prescription to clear heat. Contraindicated for Cold—it is a Cold herb. Extreme caution should be exercised during pregnancy, during menstruation, and postpartum (after birth); it has a strong downward action.

REHMANNIA GLUTINOSA

Shu di Huang CHINESE FOXGLOVE ROOT COOKED IN WINE

This herb treats patterns of Blood Deficiency, and in TCM the two organs most affected by this disorder are the Heart and Liver, which direct and store the Blood, respectively.

HOW TO USE

Shu di Huang is a very important herb—it is both a Blood and a yin tonic. Blood Deficient symptoms include a pale complexion, dizziness, palpitations, and insomnia; also menstrual problems such as irregular bleeding, uterine bleeding, and amenorrhea (no menstruation). Kidney Yin Deficient patterns include night sweats, heat in the bones, nocturnal emissions (wet dreams), diabetes, and tinnitus (ringing in the ears). Jing Deficiency includes such Kidney symptoms as low back pain, weakness of the knees and legs, lightheadedness, deafness, and also premature graying of the hair.

PROPERTIES Sweet, slightly Warm
CHANNELS Heart, Kidney, Liver
FUNCTIONS AND USES
- Tonifies the Blood: Blood Deficient symptoms are similar to those of anemia.
- Nourishes the yin: use for treating Kidney Yin Deficient patterns.

CAUTION
- Use with caution in cases of Spleen and Stomach Deficiency, or Stagnant Qi or Phlegm. As with many tonifying herbs, it nourishes the moist substances in the body, so overuse can lead to bloating and loose stools: It must be carefully combined.

SCHISANDRA CHINENSIS
Wu Wei Zi SCHISANDRA FRUIT

Wu Wei Zi stabilizes and binds. It is a Sour and Astringent herb, and helps to keep leaking fluids and other substances within the body.

HOW TO USE

Wu Wei Zi is used for chronic coughs, wheezing, and asthma, especially with mucus, although it can also be used for dry coughs, as it nourishes the yin fluid. At the other end of the body, it is used for leaking of sperm, and urinary frequency or incontinence, vaginal discharges, especially watery and white (Cold), and daybreak diarrhea due to Spleen and Kidney Deficiency. It is indicated for excessive day or night sweating, with thirst and dry throat, but in common with other herbs in this category, it is not for sweat caused by outside infections. It also treats diabetes, the "wasting-thirsting" syndrome. Furthermore, it "holds the Heart yin in place," treating symptoms such as palpitations, irritability, dream-disturbed sleep, insomnia, forgetfulness, and fear of ghosts and of going outside. Basically, it helps keep a person feeling sane and calm.

PROPERTIES Sour, Warm
CHANNELS Heart, Kidney, Lung
FUNCTIONS AND USES
- Absorbs the leakage of Lung Qi and stops attacks of coughing.
- Firms the Kidneys, binds up Jing-essence and stops bouts of diarrhea.
- Absorbs sweating and generates fluids.
- Quietens the Spirit and calms the Heart.

CAUTION
- Contraindicated for external conditions, and the early stages of coughs and rashes—it will keep the "exterior pathogenic factor" inside.

SCUTELLARIA BAICALENSIS
Huang Qin SKULLCAP ROOT

This herb is one that clears Heat: this includes febrile conditions and any illnesses with Heat signs. It is one of the "Three Yellows," which are often used together for severe infections.

HOW TO USE

Huang Qin mainly clears Heat in the chest and abdominal areas, so it is used for virulent diseases with high fever, irritability, thirst, cough, and expectoration (coughing up) of thick, yellow sputum. It can also be used topically on a dressing to clear red, hot swellings. It is used for dysentery and smelly diarrhea; also for febrile diseases which have a Damp element—symptoms such as a feeling of heaviness on the chest, and thirst with no desire to drink. It may be used for Damp Heat jaundice. It is one of the main herbs used in pregnancy to prevent miscarriage, and if toasted can stop Hot Bleeding from the nose, uterus, chest area, or in stools.

PROPERTIES Bitter, Cold
CHANNELS Heart, Lung, Gall Bladder, Large Intestine
FUNCTIONS AND USES
- Clears Heat, particularly in the Upper Burner (the upper third of the body, chest area).
- Clears Damp Heat: especially in the Stomach or Intestines. It is also used for Damp Heat in the Lower Burner, with symptoms such as cystitis.
- Clears Heat and calms the fetus.

CAUTION
- Contraindicated for tuberculosis, which is a Heat Deficiency of the lungs, not a full heat, Cold diarrhea or any Cold in the abdomen, threatened miscarriage from a Cold condition.

STEPHANIA TETRANDRA

Han Fang Ji STEPHANIA ROOT

Like Wu Jia Pi, this herb dispels Wind Dampness from the muscles, joints, and bones. Whereas Wu Jia Pi is a Warm herb, however, Han Fang Ji is Cold. Wind Damp causes rheumatic and arthritic ailments.

HOW TO USE

As a Cold herb, Han Fang Ji treats hot, painful swollen joints, such as in an acute attack of rheumatoid arthritis. It has an analgesic (pain-relieving) and anti-inflammatory effect. It is very good in treating edema, especially of the lower body and legs, gurgling or ascites in the abdomen. It may also treat acute edema of the upper body (water on the lung).

PROPERTIES Bitter, Acrid, Cold

CHANNELS Bladder, Spleen, Kidney

FUNCTIONS AND USES

- Expels Wind Dampness and alleviates pain: use for Wind-Damp-Heat in the channels, causing painful hot joints.
- Promotes urination; very effective at reducing edema—use Han Fang Ji whenever Damp collects.

CAUTION
- Use with caution in cases of Yin Deficiency, as it is very drying.

ZIZIPHUS SPINOSA
Suan Zao Ren
SOUR JUJUBE SEED

This herb nourishes the Heart and calms the Spirit, which is said to reside in the Heart. Laboratory tests have proved that Suan Zao Ren has a sedative effect. It is used to treat emotional problems.

HOW TO USE

Suan Zao Ren is one of the main herbs used for calming the Heart by nourishing the Blood, treating symptoms such as irritability, insomnia, palpitations, and anxiety. It is also very good for both spontaneous and night sweating, and is used both in menopausal syndromes and withdrawal from addictive drugs, as well as many kinds of emotional problems.

PROPERTIES Sweet, Sour, Neutral

CHANNELS Liver, Gall Bladder, Heart, Spleen

FUNCTIONS AND USES

- Nourishes the Heart yin and the Liver Blood, and calms the Spirit.
- Prevents occurrence of abnormal sweating.

CAUTION
- Caution should be exercised in cases of severe diarrhea or Heat excess.

TRADITIONAL HOME AND FOLK REMEDIES

EVERY CULTURE, ACROSS THE CENTURIES, has had its own understanding and ways of healing. Local plants, customs, and beliefs determined the form it took, which varied not only across countries but also between villages. Even today, away from the convenience of conventional physicians, local communities around the world practice their own form of medicinal healing using plants, age-old wisdom, and an instinctive and learned knowledge of their bodies as the tools.

A RETURN TO OLD WAYS

With the advent of technology and the growing dependence upon the miracles of modern medicine, most of us have lost the art of looking after ourselves. We have become dependent upon physicians, prescription drugs, store-bought preparations, and, through that, have lost an understanding of our bodies and how they work. Somewhere along the line we have put not only our faith but our independence in the hands of others. When we have a cold, a rash, even painful joints, we go straight to the medicine cabinet, or call to arrange an appointment at the doctor's office. The use of natural preparations, and the number of people addressing minor complaints

in their own homes, hit an all-time low over the past decades, and only now are we experiencing a renaissance of natural healing and home remedies, as it becomes clear that conventional medicine, for all its wonders, is not the answer to everything.

Busy Western physicians have little time to spend diagnosing their patients, and our Western approach to pathology and anatomy is based on the theory that we are all the same. Individual personalities, lifestyles, emotions, spirituality, and indeed physical bodies are not taken into consideration for most conventional treatment, but we have now learned that it is the complex combination of these very things that can make us sick or well. Treatment, therefore, needs to examine a wider picture.

In the past, many of us had the knowledge and the wherewithal to treat ourselves, using foodstuffs in our larders and plants growing in our yards and fields. There would have been a village healer or physician who could be called upon in times of emergency, but for day-to-day and common ailments, treatment was undertaken at home. While our understanding of biochemistry could not match that of a modern physician, our knowledge of how plants and various substances work in our bodies, and, indeed, how our bodies respond in various situations, and to different treatments, was much more profound. Women instinctively treated their children and their families—recognizing a bad temper as the onset of illness, perhaps, and being capable of addressing the cause of an illness according to a more general knowledge of our holistic being.

Today, most drugs on the market tend to deal with symptoms, rather than the root cause of an illness. Conditions and symptoms such as asthma, eczema, ME (CFS), headaches, and menstrual problems are controlled rather than cured. We take a tablet to ease the pain of a headache, but we do not stop and consider why we have a headache. In the past, we had a much greater general understanding of the causes and effects of illness, and a much more instinctive approach to treatment. Folk medicine and home remedies kept the majority of people healthy and it is that tradition to which many people are increasingly returning today.

CONVENTIONAL MEDICINE AND THE FOLK TRADITION

Physicians' offices are overwhelmed by the constant needs and demands of people suffering from minor illnesses. Conventional medicine has its place, and no one can deny that it has extended our lifespans and improved our chances of surviving serious illnesses. But it has its own drawbacks, one of the first and foremost being our dependence upon it. The majority of us are not able to listen to our bodies, and to take responsibility for our own health, in our own environment. Even conventional physicians welcome simple remedies to deal with the recurrent hazards of everyday life—coughs and colds, sore throats, cuts, bruises, skin infections, and many others— because it takes the pressure off medical systems and allows them to spend more time with more serious cases.

In the past, when conventional medicine did not have as much to offer and people could not afford to visit a physician, there was a commonsense approach to minor ailments. Indeed, many of the same remedies used have been adopted and adapted by conventional Western medicine. The popularity of these remedies is, quite simply, due to the fact that they are effective. They do, on many occasions, work better or at least as well as some of the pharmaceuticals of the modern age, and treatment is less likely to be complicated by side-effects. Their wider use means that we are less dependent upon conventional medical expertise and more self-confident. The power shifts from the physician back to the patient, which is both time- and cost-effective for everyone, and gives us a stake in our own health. Once learned, folk and home remedies can be used again and again.

PREVENTING ILLNESS

Natural medicine in the home is more than just first aid for common and minor ailments. It can be preventive, using some of the most common items in the larder—onions, garlic, thyme, mint, sage, chamomile—to protect against many illnesses. Modern research—particularly over the last three decades—is now justifying the use of plants and household items, things that have been used for centuries in both folk medicine and traditional cookery. For example, mint calms the digestive system; lemon is a great detoxifier, helping the liver and kidneys to function effectively; rosemary has profound antiseptic powers and is a natural stimulant; and caraway seeds will prevent flatulence. By incorporating some of these elements in your day-to-day meals, you not only add flavor and variety, but also provide the systems of your body with nourishment and support. These remedies have a beneficial effect on our general health and deal with specific problems, something that conventional drugs do not. Most available drugs work to address specific systems and do nothing for our overall health; many of them have side-effects that are more dangerous than the symptoms they are addressing. Traditional folk and home remedies tend to work with our bodies, allowing them to heal themselves by keeping them strong and healthy.

A HISTORICAL PERSPECTIVE

Whenever possible, a system of folk medicine is best understood as a dynamic in a historical context. The Aztecs in Mexico provide a good example of how conventional medical systems can go hand in hand with folk medicine, feeding from one another and allowing both to grow according to the needs of the population.

Aztec establishment (as opposed to folk) medicine was highly organized, with a herbarium, a zoo, an intellectual elite, and a training and certification academy. It was based on a complex theoretical structure and experimental research. Some segments of the population, however, had only limited access to this medicine. They relied instead on traditional treatments and medicines.

Aztec establishment medicine was eliminated when the Spanish conquerors killed the medical personnel and introduced their own medicine. This intrusive system became the new medicine of the Aztec establishment. The system still offered limited access. Some elements of the European approach, however, were compatible with the folk medical practice of the Native Americans and were therefore incorporated into a new folk system. Mexican folk medicine thrived and continued to incorporate elements of the new establishment medicine.

Similarly, Native North American systems were the establishment medicine in their own societies before conquest. Europeans brought diseases that decimated populations and challenged indigenous medical systems. The social and moral bases of the systems came under attack by missionaries and governments, even as immigrants began to adopt the ideas and materials from native systems. Again, this intrusive medicine became the establishment medicine, and Native American medicine, incorporating some Euro-American elements, became folk medicine.

DISCOVERING PLANT BENEFITS

The history of using plants for medicine and healing goes back to the beginning of humankind. In their search for nourishment, primitive humans sampled many kinds of plants. Those that were palatable were used for food, while plants with toxic or unpleasant effects were avoided or used against enemies. Other plants that produced physiological effects such as perspiration, defecation, healing, or hallucinations were saved for medicinal purposes and divination. Over the course of thousands of years, people have learned to use a wide variety of plants as medicines for different ailments.

More than 4,000 years ago, the Chinese emperor Qien Nong (Chi'en Nung) put together a book of medicinal plants called *Ben Zao* (*Pen Tsao*). It contained descriptions of more than 300 plants, several of which are still used in medicine. The Sumerians, at the same time and later, were recording prescriptions on clay tablets, and the Egyptians were writing their medical systems on rolls of papyrus. The oldest such document, known as the *Papyrus Kabun*, dates from the time of King Amenemhet III (1840–1792 B.C.E.) and contains information about women's diseases and medical conditions.

The most famous of these medical papyri, the so-called *Ebers Papyrus*, reports voluminously on the pharmaceutical prescriptions of the era. It includes specific information on how plants are to be used, for example, in the treatment of parasite worms or of stomach ailments. Some of these plants are still used today—in folk and conventional medicine.

The Greeks and the Romans derived some of their herbal knowledge from these early civilizations. Their contributions are recorded in Dioscorides' *De Materia Medica* and the 37-volume natural history written by Pliny the Elder. Some of these works are known to us through translations into Arabic by Rhazes and Avicenna. The knowledge of medicinal plants was further nurtured by monks in Europe, who grew medicinal plants and translated the Arabic works. The first recognized apothecaries opened in Baghdad in the 9th century. By the 13th century, London became a major trading center in herbs and spices.

In the Dark Ages, the belief of the Christian Church that disease was a punishment for sin caused a great setback in medical progress. Women in childbirth welcomed the pain as an opportunity to atone for their sins. Only in monasteries did herbals and other documented sources of natural medicine continue to be painstakingly translated.

The Renaissance provided a new forum for the development of the folk tradition. William Caxton printed dozens of medical manuals, and Nicholas Culpeper translated the entire physicians' pharmacopoeia *The English Physician and Complete Herbals* in 1653. It is still in print. The advent of alchemy, and the split between the "new philosophy" of reason and experiment, and the previous tradition of "science" (ancient medical doctrines, herbalism, astrology, and the occult) ended the golden age of herbals. Witch hunts disposed of village "healing women," women were forbidden to study and all nonprofessional healers were declared heretics. The use of herbs became associated with magic and the occult, an uneasy alliance that has been difficult to shake. Herbalism was effectively dropped from mainstream medical training, though folk advice and treatment from the apothecary herbalist continued to be available, especially in less well-off areas.

Folk medicine and home remedies do not provide a miracle cure, but almost anyone can benefit from the prudent use of herbs, plants, and household items as a form of restorative and preventive medicine. Most plants offer a rich source of vitamins and minerals, aside from having healing properties, and can be an important part of the daily diet, eaten fresh, or perhaps drunk as a tisane. A herbal tonic is useful, for example, in the winter months, when fresh fruit

TRADITIONAL FOLK MEDICINE TODAY

The term "folk medicine" refers to the traditional beliefs, practices, and materials that people use to maintain health and cope with disease, outside of an organized relationship with academic, professionally recognized, and established medical systems and treatments.

The beliefs and practices that make up a system of folk medicine are very closely related to the history and traditions of a recognizable social group. Many people practice folk medicine today, generally working in an environment where they share the belief system of their patients, and their approach to maintaining health and treating disease.

The growing concern about the side-effects of medicinal drugs, including the tragedies caused by compounds like thalidomide, has meant that herbalism has been called upon once more to provide natural medicines. In particular, pregnant women, children, people with chronic conditions that have refused to be shifted by orthodox medicine, and those with immunosuppressed conditions have had successful—and, most importantly, safe—treatment without the use of toxic drugs. Environmental pollution, food additives, contaminated water, and many other factors put massive stress on our bodies and immune systems, and it is now more important than ever to take a step back from chemical preparations and find ways to support our bodies against the demands of contemporary living.

As research into the active constituents of herbs continues, increasing numbers of ancient treatments and tonics are being rediscovered and recognized, and brought back into widespread use. The global transportation network means that we now have access to treatments used in countries around the world—bringing us a variety of amazing plants such as ginseng, guarana, tea tree oil, aloe vera, and ginkgo biloba.

Much of the pharmacopeia of academic medicine—including aspirin (from the white willow)—has been derived from folk remedies, even as academic medicine has disparaged the folk reasons for their use. In the past, this process has mostly been haphazard, but since the Second World War there has been an intensified, systematic investigation of tribal and folk medicines in the search for new preparations. More than 120 current prescription drugs are obtained from plants, and about 25 percent of all prescriptions contain one or more active ingredients from plants. There are plenty of herbal remedies already in use within orthodox medicine; for example, components of the yew tree have been used successfully to halt cancer, and the rosy periwinkle is used to control leukemia, especially leukemia in children.

Comparison and evaluation of folk and academic medical systems and practices is difficult. On the one hand, indiscriminate interpretation of folk medicine may result in inappropriate rejection of proven establishment methods—for example, some immunization, and drugs required to treat chronic and serious illness that may not have existed in the past. On the other hand, the dangerous aspects of folk medicine have often been emphasized, usually without recognizing the contributions of folk to conventional medicine and the similarities between them.

Today, there is a greater understanding of the power of natural remedies, and their use is being slowly accepted and indeed encouraged—particularly for ailments that people can safely and appropriately treat at home, such as headaches and upset stomachs, or sore throats. Disorders of the liver, heart, kidneys, etc., as well as severe illness—particularly in small children—are too serious for home treatment, and should be referred to a professional practitioner.

and green vegetables are not a regular part of our diets. Or plants like echinacea or garlic can be taken daily to improve the general efficiency of the immune system.

Some of the most common conditions that respond to home treatment include: hay fever, colds and respiratory disorders, digestive disorders (like constipation and ulcers), cardiovascular disease, headaches, anxiety, depression, chronic infections, rheumatism, arthritis, skin problems, anemia, and many hormonal, menstrual, menopausal, and pregnancy problems. On top of that are minor ailments such as scrapes, bruises, burns, swellings, sprains, and bites and stings.

Herbs do influence the way in which the body works, and although they are natural, they will have a profound effect on its functions. It is essential that you read the labels of any herbal products you have purchased, and follow carefully the advice of your herbalist. More is not better, although herbs don't have the side-effects of orthodox drugs, they have equally strong medicinal properties and can be toxic when taken in excess, causing liver failure, miscarriage, and heart attack, among other things.

TREATING YOURSELF AT HOME

There are a variety of forms in which treatment can be offered, depending on the condition and your individual needs. Look at the "Preparing Remedies" box alongside. Many remedies are easily and quickly made. Some can be prepared in advance and stored for future use.

CAUTION

Symptoms which could indicate a serious medical problem, and for which professional advice should be sought immediately, include: unusual or persistent headaches; chronic pain; blood in the urine; feces; or mucus; persistent fatigue or weight loss; and bleeding between menstrual periods. That is not to say that home remedies cannot be used to treat the pain and discomfort of serious problems—folk and home treatment can go hand in hand with conventional medicine, and many remedies are safe to take alongside medication.

PREPARING REMEDIES

TISANES Tisanes are mild infusions, usually prepackaged and sold in the form of a tea bag, which are boiled for a much shorter period than an infusion.

POWDERS Plants in this form can be added to food of drinks, or put into capsules for easier consumption. Make your own powder by crushing dried plant parts.

PILLS Plant remedies only rarely take this form, since it is difficult to mix more than one herb and control the quantities. Some of the more common remedies will be available from professional herbalists or health food stores, or you can press your own with a domestic press.

COMPRESSES AND POULTICES
Compresses and poultices are for external use, and can be extremely effective; the active parts of the herb reach the affected area without being altered by the digestive process. A poultice is made up of a plant which has been crushed and then applied whole to the affected areas. You can also boil crushed plant parts for a few minutes to make a pulp, which will act as a poultice, or use a powdered herb and mix with boiling water. Because they are most often applied with heat and use fresh parts of the plant, they are more potent than compresses. Poultices are particularly useful for conditions like bruises, wounds, and abscesses, helping to soothe and to draw out impurities. A compress is usually made from an infusion or decoction, which is used to soak a linen or muslin cloth. The cloth is then placed on the affected area, where it can be held in place by a bandage or plastic wrap. Compresses can be hot or cold and are generally milder than poultices.

ESSENTIAL OILS Often used in other therapies, like aromatherapy (*see page 127*), the essential oils of a plant are those which contain its "essence," or some of its most active principles. Useful for making tinctures and ointments.

BATHS Plants and other items can be added to bath water for therapeutic effect—inhalation (through the steam) and by entering the bloodstream through the skin. An oatmeal bath, for instance, would work topically on eczema, and a chamomile bath would both soothe skin, and calm and relax.

INHALATIONS Warm, moist air can relieve many respiratory problems and allow the healing properties of plants and other products to enter the bloodstream through the lungs. To prepare an inhalation, half-fill a big bowl with steaming water, and add a herbal infusion or decoction, or 2–3 drops of an essential oil.

TINCTURE

Powdered, fresh, or dried herbs are placed in an airtight container with alcohol and left for a period of time. Alcohol extracts the valuable or essential parts of the plant and preserves them for the longest possible time.

1   You can make your own tincture at home by crushing the parts of the plants you wish to use (about 1oz. [25g] will do).
2   Suspend the plants in alcohol (about 1–1²/₃ cups. [600ml] of vodka or any 40 percent spirit) for about two weeks, shaking occasionally. Dried or powdered herbs (about 4oz. [100g]) may also be used, with the same amount of alcohol.
3   After straining, the tincture should be stored in a dark glass airtight jar. Doses are usually 5–20 drops, which can be taken directly or added to water.

DECOCTION

The roots, twigs, berries, seeds, and bark of a plant are used, and much like an infusion, they are boiled in water to extract the plants' ingredients. The liquid is strained and taken with honey or brown sugar as prescribed.

1   Put 1 teaspoonful of dried herb or 3 teaspoonfuls of fresh herb (for each cup) into a pan. Fresh herbs should be cut into small pieces.
2   Add some water to the herbs. If making large quantities, use 1oz. (30g) dried herb for each 2 cups. (500ml) of water. The container should be glass, ceramic, or earthenware. Metal pans should be enameled. Do not use aluminum.

3   Bring to the boil and simmer for 10–15 minutes. If the herb contains volatile oils, cover the pan. Strain, cool, and refrigerate. The decoction will keep for about three days.

INFUSION

Effectively another word for tea, an infusion uses dried herbs, or in some instances fresh, which are steeped in boiled water for about 10 minutes. Infusions may be drunk hot, which is normally best for medicinal teas, or cold, with ice.

1   Put 1 teaspoonful of the herb or herb mixture into a china or glass teapot, for each cup of tea that is required. Add boiling water.
2   Add 1 cup of boiling water to the pot for each teaspoonful of herb that has been used. Keep the pot covered and always use the purest water available, which will ensure that the medicinal properties of the plant are effectively obtained. Strain the infusion and drink hot or cold—either sweetened or unsweetened. Use licorice root, honey, or brown sugar to sweeten. Infusions should be made fresh each day, if possible. Infusions are most suitable for plants from which the leaves and flowers have been used, since their properties are more easily extracted by gentle boiling.

OINTMENT

For external use, ointments and creams are often prescribed. You can make your own by boiling the plant parts to extract the active properties, and adding a few ounces (grams) of pure oils (such as olive or sunflower).

1   Make 2 cups (500ml) of infusion or decoction (depending on what is appropriate for the herb), and strain. Reserve the liquid.
2   Pour 6 tablespoons oil (90ml) into a pan. Mix 3oz. (75g) of fat into the oil. If a perishable base fat is used (such as lard), a drop of tincture of benzoin should be added for each 2 tablespoons (30g) of base. Add the liquid.
3   Simmer until the water has evaporated. Stiffen the mixture with a little beeswax or cocoa butter to make a cream. Melt in slowly.

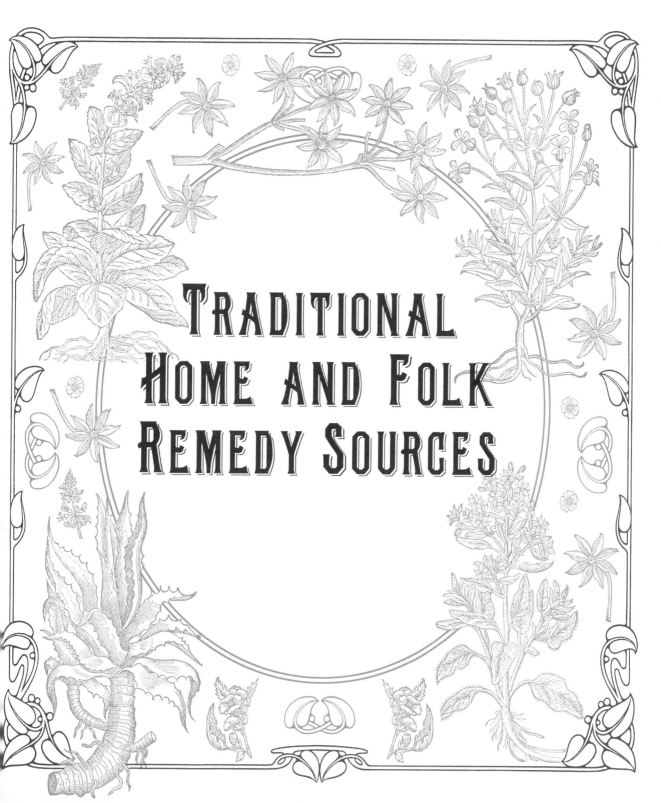

Traditional Home and Folk Remedy Sources

ALLIUM CEPA
ONIONS

The onion is by far the most important bulb vegetable in terms of its healing properties. It is used both in its green stage as a scallion, or green onion, and in its mature stage as a bulb—the tightly packed globe of food-storage leaves containing the volatile oil that is the source of the onion's pungent flavor. Thought to have originated in Asia, the onion has been cultivated since ancient times. The bulb of the onion is used in cooking and medicinally; like garlic, it warms the body and stimulates the circulation. Onions have long been considered the mainstay of every household remedy chest.

USES
- Apply fresh onion to an abscessed tooth or a boil to draw out infection and help to encourage circulation to the area, which will facilitate quick healing.
- Mix onion juice with honey to relieve the symptoms of a cold.
- Taken daily, onions can help to prevent cancers of the digestive tract.
- The regular consumption of onions can reduce nervous debility.
- Onion poultices are used to treat bronchitis and can also help in the treatment of acne and boils.
- Onions are often recommended for gastric infections; onions will be effective cooked and raw.

PROPERTIES
- Onions cause the body to "weep," which helps to release toxins
- Onion increases blood circulation and can relax the muscles
- Expectorant and diuretic
- Helps to reduce serum cholesterol after a fatty meal
- May provide some protection against cancer
- Antibiotic, draws out infection
- Warming
- Strengthens the lungs

ALLIUM SATIVUM
GARLIC

Garlic belongs to the onion family, and is one of the best-known and most-used medicinal plants. It has a strong odor, which many people find off-putting, but its health-giving and preventive properties make it well worth suffering the effects.

USES
- Fresh garlic, eaten daily, can reduce chronic acidity of the stomach.
- Eat crushed garlic for sexual debility.
- May help to reduce attacks of allergic asthma and hay fever.
- Garlic-infused oil can be used as a chest rub for respiratory or digestive ailments, or in the ear to reduce inflammation.
- Fresh garlic, eaten regularly, will reduce the need for antibiotics.
- Garlic syrup can be used to treat bronchitis, lung infections, and digestive disorders.

PROPERTIES
- Cleanses the blood and helps create and maintain healthy bacterial balance (flora) in the gut
- Helps to bring down fever
- Antiseptic
- Antibiotic
- Antifungal
- Tones the heart and circulatory system
- Boosts the immune system
- May help to reduce high blood pressure
- May prevent some cancers, in particular stomach cancer

TIP
The smell of garlic on the breath can be reduced by eating an apple, drinking a little fresh lemon juice, or eating fresh parsley.

APIUM GRAVEOLENS
CELERY

Hippocrates, the father of medicine, wrote that celery could be used to calm the nerves, and, indeed, its very high calcium level is likely to be the reason for this phenomenon. The seeds, leaves, and edible root of the plant are used. Celery is best eaten raw, and its juice is particularly useful. The seeds are rich in iron and many vitamins, including A, B, and C, and can be used in the treatment of liver problems and high blood pressure.

USES

- Eat the seeds to treat arthritis (for which they act as an anti-inflammatory) and to relieve muscle spasms (antispasmodic action).
- Grated, raw celery can be used as a poultice to apply to swollen glands.
- Raw whole celery can be eaten regularly to reduce high blood pressure, and to act as a tonic for the liver.
- Celery juice or an infusion of celery seeds may be drunk to alleviate sciatica.
- Drink celery juice before meals to suppress the appetite. Chew celery seeds after a meal as a digestive.

PROPERTIES

- Celery helps to reduce high blood pressure
- Digestive, reducing spasm in the intestinal tract and acting as an anti-inflammatory agent
- Purifies the blood
- May help in the treatment of arthritis and rheumatic disorders; in Japan, rheumatic patients are sometimes put on a celery-only diet
- Celery seeds also have anti-inflammatory properties
- Stimulates the thyroid and pituitary glands

CAUTION

Because celery may cause the uterus to contract, it should not be eaten during pregnancy.

ARMORACIA RUSTICANA
HORSERADISH

Horseradish is a member of the mustard family, and is native to southeastern Europe. It is widely cultivated for its pungent, fleshy root. Japanese horseradish, or wasabi (Wasabidjaponica), is used both for cooking and for therapeutic purposes, and the grated rhizomes are often sold as a dry, green-colored powder.

USES

- Apply tincture of horseradish root to skin eruptions, including those associated with acne, to draw out the infection and encourage healing.
- Add some horseradish root to your toothpaste to clean teeth effectively, kill bacteria, and control mouth ulcers.
- Eat fresh horseradish, mixed with a little lemon juice, for the relief of sinus infections and nasal blockages.
- Eat freshly grated horseradish root for edema and swelling associated with PMS.
- A horseradish poultice can be applied to chilblains and hemorrhoids to encourage healing and improve the circulation of the blood.

PROPERTIES

- Diuretic
- Stimulant
- Clears nasal passages
- Antiseptic
- Stimulates blood flow

TIP

Too much horseradish taken internally can cause night sweats and occasionally diarrhea and abdominal cramping.

AVENA SATIVUM
OATS

Oats are a cereal plant, and are both extremely nutritious and useful therapeutically. Oats are one of the best sources of inositol, which is important for maintaining optimum blood cholesterol levels. Eaten daily, they provide a wealth of excellent effects.

USES

- Eat raw oats as a source of fiber to ease constipation.
- Oatmeal (unrefined) can be eaten on a regular basis to reduce the effects of stress and nervous disorders.
- Cooked oats will relieve fatigue.
- A compress of oatmeal or an oatmeal bath soothes eczema and other problem skin conditions.
- Boil a tablespoon of oats in ½ pt. (250ml) of water for several minutes and drain; use as a nerve tonic and for its nourishing properties.
- Use the tincture for stress, addictions, eating disorders, and depression.
- Eat oats dairy to lower blood cholesterol and to experience tonic effects.

PROPERTIES

- A tonic for general debility, and used in the treatment of anorexia, also helpful for convalescence and fatigue
- Oats lower blood cholesterol levels
- Oats help to control hormonal activity
- Cleansing—internally and externally; may protect against bowel cancer when taken internally
- Used in the treatment of eczema
- Extremely rich in B vitamins and minerals
- Antidepressant, and can be used to treat depression, stress, and nervous disorders

CAUTION
Oats contain gluten, which causes an allergic reaction in some individuals.

ASPARAGUS OFFICINALIS
ASPARAGUS

A herbaceous perennial of the *Liliaceae* family, asparagus is cultivated for its tender shoots, which appear in early spring. In 1806, the French chemist Louis Nicolas Vauquelin, who discovered the elements chromium and beryllium, isolated asparagine, the first amino acid to be discovered, from the asparagus plant. Asparagus is a liver tonic, and promotes elimination (through the urine).

USES

- Drink asparagus water (the water remaining after steaming asparagus spears) for urinary complaints, arthritis, and rheumatism.
- Freshly cooked asparagus will tonify the liver, and may be used in cases of liver congestion and conditions such as hepatitis to encourage healing.
- Asparagus tincture can be added to food and drinks to encourage the elimination of urine.

PROPERTIES

- Encourages the flow of urine, making asparagus a useful diuretic
- Acts as a tonic to the liver
- Aids digestion
- May help control the symptoms of PMS, including breast tenderness and abdominal bloating

CAUTION
Asparagus is high in purines, and anyone suffering from gout should avoid it.

BRASSICA OLCRANEA
CABBAGE

Cabbage has traditionally been used for medicinal purposes as well as for cooking. It has anti-inflammatory properties, and contains chemicals which can prevent cancer. The ancient Greeks used fresh white cabbage juice to relieve sore or infected eyes, and juice from the cabbage stem is a good remedy for ulcers.

USES

- Make cabbage a regular part of your diet to reduce the risk of cancer.
- A cabbage poultice can be applied to boils and infected cuts to draw out the infection and disperse pus.
- Applied to bruises and swelling, macerated cabbage leaves will encourage healing.
- Dab white cabbage juice on mouth ulcers, and gargle for sore throats.
- A warm cabbage compress, on the affected area, reduces the pain of headaches and some kinds of neuralgia.

PROPERTIES

- An excellent anti-inflammatory
- Cabbage contains lactic acid, which acts to disinfect the colon
- Used to reduce the pain of headaches and rheumatic disorders
- Soothes eczema and other itching or weeping skin conditions
- Anticancerous
- Red cabbage leaves are the basic ingredient of a good cough syrup

CAUTION

Do not eat red cabbage raw, because the high levels of iron can interfere with gut absorption and irritate the gut, causing constipation. Avoid cabbage if you suffer from goiter, or take maoi antidepressants. Red cabbage (cooked) can cause constipation and irritation of the colon, due to the large quantities of iron.

CAMELLIA SINENSIS
TEA

Tea is the beverage made when the processed leaves of the tea plant are infused with boiling water. Native to Southeast Asia, the tea plant is a small, shrub-like, evergreen tree that belongs to the family *Theaceae*, its seeds contain a volatile oil, and its leaves contain the chemicals caffeine and tannin.

USES

- The fluoride in tea may be beneficial in preventing dental caries.
- Tea may help in the treatment of diarrhea, dysentery, hepatitis, and gastroenteritis.
- The flavonoids contained in tea may destroy harmful bacteria and viruses.
- Cold, steeped tea bags placed over the eyes will soothe soreness and irritation. Tea's astringent properties also make tea bags useful for treating minor injuries and insect bites.
- The leaves of green and black tea may be beneficial in the prevention of heart disease and stroke.

PROPERTIES

- Provides folic acid (vitamin B9), some potassium, and also magnesium
- Contains fluoride (a trace)
- Acts on the nervous system to control the respiratory and digestive systems
- Diuretic and astringent
- Antioxidants called polyphenols have beneficial effects on the circulatory system, while flavonoids act on the immune system

CAUTION

Tea can interfere with the effectiveness of drugs such as allopurinol (for the treatment of gout), antibiotics, antiulcer drugs, and the drug theophylkline, prescribed for asthma. It can prevent the absorption of iron and interfere with the effectiveness of sedative drugs. Drinking tea to excess can cause constipation, indigestion, dizziness, palpitations, irritability, and insomnia.

CAPSICUM ANNUUM
VAR. ANNUUM
RED PEPPER

The red pepper is also known variously as bell pepper, sweet pepper, and capsicum. It is one of five different types (grossum type) of Capsicum *annuum* var. *annuum*; the peppers from which the spices cayenne and chili are produced are longum peppers.

USES

- Peppers increase perspiration and therefore have a cooling effect on the body.
- They may be effective in the treatment of varicose veins, asthma, and digestive complaints.
- Peppers reduce sensitivity to pain by irritating the tissues and increasing blood supply to the affected area, which then effectively numbs the pain.
- Cayenne acts as a tonic for those suffering from tiredness and cold. It can also induce a feeling of well-being. It is an expectorant and has been effective in treating catarrh and sinus problems.

PROPERTIES

- Peppers are an excellent source of vitamin C (a fresh green pepper contains 10 percent vitamin C)
- All peppers also contribute small amounts of iron and vitamin A: the largest amounts of vitamin A are found in fresh red peppers, while paprika and chili powder are also very rich in this vitamin
- Peppers are a good source of potassium, and have low levels of sodium and fiber

CAUTION

Pungent peppers, such as chili peppers, may cause skin irritation and painful inflammation when used in excess or when in contact with the eyes and broken skin. The seeds are particularly powerful. Strong peppers may also temporarily irritate the urinary system as the oils are excreted in urine.

CITRUS LIMON
LEMON

Lemons are the most widely grown acid species belonging to the citrus group of fruit. They rank third among all citrus fruit in tonnage produced, and have been used for generations for their therapeutic properties. Lemons are rich in vitamin C, and have a cleansing effect on the digestive system. They have a wide range of therapeutic properties, making them the mainstay of any good home remedy chest. The leaves and the whole fruit may be used, according to requirements.

USES

- Blood purifier, improves the body's ability to expel toxins; useful for skin problems like acne and boils
- Rich in vitamins B and C
- Antifungal
- Antacid
- Antiseptic
- Aids digestion
- One of the most powerful natural styptics; use on cuts and grazes to stop bleeding
- Antibacterial and antiviral properties. Lemons are excellent for halting the progression of infections

PROPERTIES

- The high potassium content of lemons will encourage the heart action, so lemons are a useful tonic for anyone with heart problems.
- Lemons are a natural insecticide and will discourage mosquitoes and flies.
- Drink fresh lemon juice (lemon in hot water will do) to cleanse the system. For a lemon drink, boil 3 sliced lemons in 1 pt. (600ml) water, until the liquid is reduced by half. Add honey to taste.
- Drink lemon juice in hot or warm water first thing in the morning as a liver tonic.
- Lemon juice taken in hot water will ease stomach acidity; when drunk before going to bed, it may help to relieve cramp and "restless legs" syndrome.

CITRUS PARADISI
GRAPEFRUIT

The grapefruit is an evergreen tree, *Citrus paradisi*, of the *Rutaceae* family, and its fruit is the largest of the commercially grown citrus fruit. Like all citrus fruit, grapefruit is rich in vitamin C and potassium. Pink grapefruit is rich in vitamin A, and acts as a natural antioxidant. Grapefruit is an excellent cleanser for the digestive and urinary systems, and the peel has many therapeutic properties.

USES

- Eat grapefruit seeds to rid the body of worms.
- Grapefruit pith and membranes lower cholesterol in the blood.
- Drinking grapefruit juice can encourage healthy skin; used in the treatment of acne for its mild exfoliating properties.
- Grapefruit juice cleanses the kidneys and helps to eliminate toxins from the body.
- Aromatherapy massage with grapefruit oil is invigorating and uplifting, and may help to treat depression.
- Local massage, with a few drops of essential oil blended in a carrier oil, will relieve the severity of a headache.
- Drinking grapefruit juice with iron supplements or foods rich in iron increases the absorption of iron in the body.
- Detoxifies the liver, and can ease chronic liver conditions. May help to reduce the severity of a hangover.

PROPERTIES

- Grapefruit cleanses the digestive and urinary systems, and is therefore often recommended by naturopaths
- Reduces appetite
- Aids in the breakdown of fats in the body
- Strengthens the respiratory system and aids respiration
- Invigorating tonic
- Relieves symptoms of colds and flu
- May help in the treatment of osteoarthritis

CUCUMIS SATIVIS
CUCUMBER

The cucumber, *Cucumis sativis*, is a vine fruit that can be eaten fresh or pickled. A member of the *Cucurbitaceae* family, it is related to melons and squash. Cucumbers were native to northwestern India but have long been distributed throughout Asia, Europe, and Africa. Cucumber is a popular vegetable, which has been widely used in folk medicine to reduce heat and inflammation. It is a rich source of vitamin C, and can be used externally to cool and cleanse.

USES

- Drink cucumber juice or eat fresh cucumber to soothe heartburn or to improve an acid stomach.
- Drink 3–5fl. oz. (100–150ml) of cucumber juice every two hours for a gastric or duodenal ulcer.
- For strained or inflamed eyes, place a slice of cucumber on each eyelid to reduce swelling and soothe.
- Apply fresh cucumber or cucumber juice to sunburned skin to cool it down.
- Ground dried cucumber seeds are used to treat tapeworm.
- Cucumber juice, drunk daily, may help to control eczema, arthritis, and gout.
- Skin conditions respond to cucumber. Include fresh cucumber in your diet as much as possible.
- Cucumber juice acts as a kidney tonic.
- Use cucumber ointment on inflamed skin.
- Fresh cucumber juice, or the whole raw vegetable, is a mild diuretic and is cleansing. Use to treat lung and chest infections, and to bring down fever.

PROPERTIES

- Diuretic
- Cooling
- Cleansing, particularly for skin disorders
- Used in the treatment of gout and arthritis
- Anti-inflammatory—soothes inflammatory skin conditions
- May help to treat lung and chest disorders
- Drink cucumber juice for inflammatory conditions such as arthritis

DAUCUS CAROTA
CARROT

The carrot is a member of the *Umbelliferae* family, which also includes celery and parsnip. Carrots were first used as medicinal herbs rather than as vegetables, and they have the dual purpose of acting as therapeutic agents, and providing the best source of beta carotene (a form of vitamin A) in the human diet.

USES

- Drink fresh, raw carrot juice daily to energize and cleanse the body. It will help to relieve the effects of stress and fatigue, and boost the body after illness.
- Carrot soup is a traditional home remedy for infant diarrhea—it soothes the bowel and slows down bacterial growth.
- Raw, grated carrots or cooked, mashed carrots can be applied to wounds, cuts, inflammations, and abscesses to discourage infection and encourage healing.
- Dried carrot powder will restore energy, and can help to treat infections, glandular problems, headaches, or joint problems.
- The antioxidant qualities of carrots will help to prevent some of the damage caused by smoking.

PROPERTIES

- Energizing
- Carrot cleanses the system of impurities
- Contains calcium, which will encourage health of skin, hair, and bones
- May help in the treatment of eye problems
- Useful in the treatment of respiratory conditions
- Carrot may help to relieve skin disorders
- May help to overcome many glandular disorders

CAUTION

Eating an excessive quantity of carrots may cause the skin to yellow temporarily. Carrot seeds are a nerve tonic and will also induce abortion; avoid during pregnancy.

EUGENICA CARYPHYLLATA
CLOVES

Cloves are the dried buds of a tree of the myrtle family, *Syzygium aromaticum*. The tree, which may reach a height of 40ft. (12m), produces abundant clusters of small red flower buds that are gathered before opening and dried to produce the dark brown, nail-shaped spice, clove. Whole and ground cloves used as food seasonings account for half the world production of cloves.

USES

- Oil of cloves can be placed directly on a sore tooth or mouth abscess to draw out the infection and ease the pain. Chew cloves for the same effect.
- Dab a tiny amount of neat oil on insect bites.
- Clove tea is warming, and can encourage the body to sweat, which is helpful for high fever or vomiting.
- Oil of cloves may be used during a long labor to hasten birth.
- Clove tea can be used to soothe wind and ease nausea—particularly the nausea of travel sickness.
- Inhale an infusion of cloves to clear the lungs and refresh the airways.
- A clove and orange pomander can be hung in cupboards as an effective insect repellent.

PROPERTIES

- Antiseptic and powerfully analgesic—particularly to the gums and teeth
- Cloves are warming, and useful for people who are prone to colds
- Anti-inflammatory, when used locally on swellings
- Cloves are calming to the digestive system
- Eliminate parasites from the body

CAUTION

Cloves can cause uterine contractions, and should not be used in pregnancy.

FICUS CARICA
FIG

Figs comprise a large family of deciduous and evergreen tropical and subtropical trees, shrubs, and vines belonging to the mulberry family, *Moraceae*. The most important fig is *Ficus carica*, the tree that produces the edible fig fruit. Figs are a nutritious and sustaining food, with a long history of medicinal use. For example, there are several references in the Bible to figs being used to treat infections.

USES

- Eat dried figs to ease constipation.
- To bring a boil to a head, split a fig, heat it, and place it directly on the boil. This is a particularly good method for treating boils and ulcers in the mouth.
- Fig juice can be drunk daily as a cancer preventive.
- Digestive troubles can be eased by eating fresh figs after light meals or just prior to heavy meals.
- Roasted figs can be used as a poultice on boils and hemorrhoids in order to encourage healing and to draw out infection.
- Fresh figs can soothe respiratory ailments by acting as an anti-inflammatory agent.
- Boil four or five fresh figs in about 1 pt. (500ml) of water; bring to the boil, strain, cool, and drink the liquid for sore throats.

PROPERTIES

- Highly alkaline
- Contains a powerful healing agent
- Soothes mucous membranes, particularly in the respiratory system
- The stem of the fresh fruit is antifungal, and can be used to treat warts
- Anticancerous
- Contains ficin, which aids the digestion
- Contains a bactericide
- Reduces body heat, and helps to ease inflammation

GLYCYRRHIZA GLABRA
LICORICE

Licorice is a pretty blue-flowered perennial, grown mainly in Europe. The roots are crushed, ground, and boiled to extract the juice, which is then thickened to produce hard black sticks of paste known as black sugar. The bittersweet flavoring is used in candy and tobacco, as a soothing ingredient in cough drops and syrups, as a laxative, and in the manufacture of shoe polish. Licorice is also an excellent source of iron.

USES

- Licorice syrup can be used to treat persistent coughs, and to reduce the incidence of asthma attacks.
- A strong infusion can protect against and heal ulcers. Drink it three times each day.
- Steep licorice root with a blend of other soothing herb teas to treat gastric disorders, and to stimulate kidneys and bowel.
- Used with other strengthening herbs such as ginseng for exhaustion.
- Licorice is used in creams or pastes for the relief of inflamed psoriasis and hot and weepy skin conditions.

PROPERTIES

- Expectorant and anti-inflammatory, making it excellent for stubborn coughs and lung infections
- Mild laxative
- Adrenal tonic
- Detoxifies the body. In the Far East, licorice is used to rid the body of poisons such as salmonella or as an antidote to overuse of drugs
- Raises blood pressure. Can be used in the treatment of low blood pressure

CAUTION

Large doses of licorice can cause water retention and exacerbate high blood pressure. Avoid in pregnancy.

HAMAMELIS VIRGINIANA
WITCH HAZEL

Witch hazel is a common tree grown in the U.S. Its leaves or roots are used for medicinal purposes. The common name arose as a result of the remarkable medicinal properties of the alcoholic extract from the leaves and bark of the plant, which is used on bruises and inflammations, and as a rubbing lotion.

USES

- Drink an infusion two or three times daily when there is inflammation (such as that of arthritis or rheumatism, sprains, or bruising) and for internal bleeding.
- Apply externally (as a decoction, tincture, or cream) for the treatment of bruising, hemorrhoids, or varicose veins.
- Use as a compress for sprains and strains.
- Dilute one part witch hazel to 20 parts boiled, cooled water, and use as an eye wash for sore and inflamed eyes.
- Add to the bath to reduce the aches and pains of rheumatic conditions.
- Witch hazel ointment can be used for painful joints, bruising (applied very gently), and local pain.

PROPERTIES

- Analgesic
- Antiseptic—witch hazel can be used as a facial wash, and diluted to wash cuts and grazes
- Helps to control diarrhea when taken internally, and can encourage the health of the digestive tract
- Witch hazel soothes swellings, and reduces inflammation and bleeding, internally and externally
- Will encourage healing of bruises, sprains, and bleeding hemorrhoids

HORDEUM SATIVUM VULGARE
BARLEY

Barley is rich in minerals (calcium and potassium) and B-complex vitamins, which makes it useful for convalescents or people suffering from stress. Barley has been used for its restorative qualities, in medicine and in cooking, for thousands of years. Malt is produced from barley.

BARLEY WATER

- Add 2 tablespoons of pearl barley to 1 pt. (500ml) of water and boil for 10 minutes.
- Strain, and add barley to a fresh pint of water.
- Boil for another 10 minutes.

USES

- Barley water can be used in the treatment of respiratory disorders, and eases dry, tickling coughs.
- Barley water can be used for urinary tract infections and cystitis, and can ease flatulence and colic.
- Cooked barley is easily digested and nutritious, and is a traditional remedy for constipation and diarrhea.
- Barley water reduces acid in the spleen if drunk twice a day for a month.
- Make a poultice of barley flour to reduce inflammation of the skin.
- Barley may help to prevent heart disease, as it promotes the normal functioning of the heart and is able to stabilize blood pressure.
- Eat in soups and stews when convalescing.
- Barley poultices can be applied to soothe inflamed skin

PROPERTIES

- Nutritious
- Anti-inflammatory, particularly to the urinary and digestive systems
- Used in the treatment of respiratory disorders
- Taken daily, it may lower cholesterol levels

THE HEALING REMEDIES SOURCEBOOK

JUGLANS REGIA
WALNUT

Walnut is the common name for about 20 species of deciduous trees in the walnut family, *Juglandaceae*. The fruit has an outer leathery husk and an inner hard and furrowed stone, or nut. Walnuts are rich in protein, and high in potassium and other minerals such as zinc and iron. The bark of the walnut tree is used to treat gum disease, among other things.

USES

- Eat daily while convalescing to relieve fatigue and generally strengthen the body.
- Fresh walnuts and walnut oil can encourage circulation, and because they are rich in potassium, will keep the heart healthy.
- to Add walnut bark to the bath for rheumatism, and sore and aching muscles and joints.
- Apply walnut bark tincture, in a little carrier oil, to swellings and skin problems, in order to encourage healing.
- Eat walnuts for heartburn and diarrhea.
- Fresh walnuts can help to soothe the colic and dispel gas in the abdomen.
- Walnut oil, added to salads and vegetables, will help to ease the discomfort of irritable bowel syndrome and act as a mild laxative.

PROPERTIES

- The bark of the walnut tree is astringent and cleansing
- Walnut bark strengthens the gums and acts as an anti-inflammatory
- The bark discourages milk flow in nursing mothers
- The nuts are aphrodisiac and mildly laxative
- The nuts prevent worms
- The nuts are soothing and a natural digestive

LACTOBACILLUS
YOGURT

Yogurt is a fermented, slightly acidic food product made from milk. Its origins are unknown (although the name is Turkish), and it resembles the many other fermented milk foods made throughout the world, such as kefir and kumiss. Unlike many of these foods, however, yogurt is usually made from a concentrated milk and is soured by a specific bacillus, *Lactobacillus bulgaricus*. As a food, yogurt is a rich source of protein, and contains all of the vitamins and minerals found in milk.

USES

- Live yogurt should be eaten to increase beneficial bacteria following a course of antibiotics. Eat daily for two to three weeks.
- Make your own yogurt. Add 3 teaspoons of live yogurt to 1 pt. (600ml) of milk. Leave to set.
- Apply live yogurt to areas affected by thrush; it can also be used internally as a douche.
- Daily intake of yogurt may prevent heart disease.
- Cleanse the skin with yogurt, which is a natural moisturizer.

PROPERTIES

- Live yogurt is antifungal, and can be used in the treatment of thrush
- Live yogurt may help to reduce cholesterol levels
- Encourages the growth of healthy bacteria in the bowels, which aids absorption of nutrients and helps to prevent infection
- Helps to produce vitamin B
- Yogurt stimulates bowel movements
- Helps to prevent and control the growth of cancerous cells

CAUTION

Live yogurt is not effective when mixed with sweeteners; for best effect make your own yogurt and flavor with a little unpasteurized honey and banana.

LINUM USITATISSIMUM
FLAXSEED

Flax is a group of annual and perennial plants from the *Linaceae* family. Several varieties of one species, *L. usitatissimum*, are grown primarily for their fiber, used in making linen, or for their seeds, the source of linseed oil. The seeds contain a remarkable healing oil which can be used both internally and externally. Flaxseed is also known as linseed, but should not be confused with the "boiled" linseed oil available from building merchants. As far back as Hippocrates, flaxseed tea has been used to treat sore throats, hoarseness, and bronchial spasms.

USES

- Apply the oil to sprains to reduce inflammation and ease the pain.
- Mix flaxseed with lime water to reduce the pain of burns.
- Flaxseed (linseed) tea can be used for mild constipation, and to encourage kidney function. The tea also works to ease kidney pains and cramping.
- The tea can be drunk during bouts of bronchitis to reduce inflammation of the lungs and prevent spasm.
- Add lemon and honey to flaxseed tea to encourage its action and improve taste.

PROPERTIES

- Mildly laxative
- Tonic for the kidneys and encourages their action
- Encourages healing
- Analgesic
- Antispasmodic

CAUTION
Commercially produced linseed oil is used in protective coatings such as paints and varnishes because it has a drying action. It is not suitable for human consumption.

MALUS SPECIES
APPLE

The apple has many uses in traditional medicine, and the old adage "To eat an apple going to bed will make the physician beg his bread" has been justified by its many health-giving properties. Research shows that apples are excellent detoxifiers, and apple juice—even store bought—can destroy viruses in the body.

USES

- Eat raw apples regularly, as a detoxificant, for gout and rheumatism.
- To prevent viruses from settling in, and to reduce their duration, eat an apple (or drink a glass of apple juice) three times a day.
- Raw, peeled, and grated apples can be used as a poultice for sprains.
- For indigestion, heartburn, and other digestive disorders, eat an apple with meals.
- Use an apple poultice for treating rheumatic and weak eyes.
- Two apples a day can reduce cholesterol levels by up to 10 percent.
- As a treatment for intestinal infections, hoarseness, rheumatism, and fatigue, increase your daily intake to as much as 2lb. (1kg).
- For curative purposes, as an alternative to eating the whole fruit, drink 2 cups (500ml) of naturally sweet apple juice a day.

PROPERTIES

- Cleans teeth and strengthens gums
- Lowers cholesterol levels
- Antiviral action
- Detoxifies
- Protects from pollution, binding to toxins in the body and carrying them out
- Neutralizes indigestion
- Prevents constipation
- Soothing and antiseptic

NASTURTIUM OFFICINALIS
WATERCRESS

Watercress is a floating or creeping water plant of the mustard family, *Cruciferae*. A perennial, it grows best in fresh water, particularly in cool streams and ponds, and in wet soil. Its round, edible leaves are pungent to the taste, and commonly used as salad greens or as a garnish. It is a rich source of vitamin C.

USES

- Sometimes recommended for gall bladder complaints and anemia.
- The bruised leaves are said to remove pimples and to fade freckling. Eat to help skin eruptions.
- Eat fresh daily: may help to prevent migraine. Eat with a meal if you have a tendency toward heartburn or dyspepsia.
- High levels of potassium may help to prevent insomnia—eat some fresh leaves an hour before bedtime, and often throughout the day.
- Watercress may help in the treatment of edema.
- It is used to treat respiratory ailments such as coughs, catarrh, and bronchitis—eat fresh until symptoms improve. It can be useful as a preventive measure for chronic respiratory conditions.
- Watercress may strengthen the whole body system in cases of debility caused by chronic illness.

PROPERTIES

- Contains benzyl mustard oil, which is powerfully antibiotic, but does not harm our healthy bacteria (flora)
- Beneficial to the health of the intestines
- Encourages immune activity in the body
- Provides good supplies of the vitamins C, A, and B (thiamine and riboflavin), iron, potassium, and calcium
- Stimulates digestion

OLEA EUPOPEA
OLIVE

The olive is a handsome, long-lived, evergreen, subtropical tree, and has been cultivated for at least 4,000 years for its edible fruit and valuable oil. It is native to the eastern Mediterranean region, where its culture may have been begun by Semitic people as long ago as 3500 B.C.E. Its leaves and the oil of its fruit are used in cooking and medicinally, and studies show that it has powerful anticholesterol action in the body, making it a useful addition to any home medicine cabinet.

USES

- Rub olive oil into patches of eczema, dandruff, and psoriasis to reduce itching and encourage healing.
- Olive oil, taken daily, can reduce the risk of heart disease and help to slow down the degenerative effects of aging.
- Drink a little extra virgin olive oil to cure a hangover.
- Olives and olive oil, as part of a daily diet, will help to prevent and treat circulatory problems, and lower cholesterol levels.
- Eat olives for constipation.
- Olives are said to counteract poisoning from mushrooms or fish—drink a little extra virgin, cold-pressed oil when symptoms present themselves.

PROPERTIES

- Antioxidant
- Anticancerous
- Emollient—particularly useful for skin conditions
- Olive oil can be used to treat constipation
- Soothes the itching of eczema, and moisturizes dry skin, hair, and scalp
- Olive oil is rich in vitamin E, and is now known to help lower cholesterol levels in the body
- It may reduce the risk of circulatory disease and nervous disorders
- Useful in the treatment of gastric disorders because it reduces the secretion of gastric juices

OYRZA SATIVA
RICE

Rice is the cereal that is a staple food to more than half of the world's peoples. It also has important medicinal uses, for which the rhizomes, seeds (the grains), and germinated seeds are used. White rice is the grain that is left after the bran and germ have been removed; brown rice retains the bran and germ. Rice is available as a breakfast cereal (the grains are "puffed" during manufacture), and is fermented to produce rice wine, called saki by the Japanese.

USES

- Eat rice daily if you suffer from chronic dyspepsia—excellent for heartburn, particularly that associated with pregnancy.
- Use rice bran for the treatment of hyperalcuria.
- Use rice flour to make a poultice for relieving inflammation of the skin, including acne, measles, burns, and hemorrhoids.
- A natural diuretic—increase your intake prior to menstruation if you suffer from bloating and symptoms of PMS. Eaten regularly, rice can prevent edema.
- The seeds are used to treat urinary ailments.
- Rice water helps to overcome stomach upsets.

PROPERTIES

- Rice contains high levels of carbohydrates (87 percent of white, uncooked rice)
- Rich in B vitamins (folic acid and pyridoxine), iron, and potassium. Brown rice also contains the B vitamin thiamine, which is present in the bran
- White rice has 1 percent of fat; in brown rice the amount of fat is higher
- Rice contains low amounts of sodium and is also free from cholesterol
- A natural tonic
- Diuretic
- Digestive
- Controls sweating
- Lowers blood pressure
- Anti-inflammatory

PERSICA AMERICANA GRATISSIMA
AVOCADO

Avocados are the fruit of a small, subtropical tree. They are rich in vitamins A, some B-complex, C, and E vitamins, and potassium, and because they contain some protein and starch, as well as being a good source of monounsaturated fats, they are considered to be a perfect—or complete—food. Traditionally, avocados have been used for skin problems. The pulp has both antibacterial and antifungal properties.

USES

- An avocado paste can be applied to rashes and rough skin to soothe and smooth.
- To make a face mask, mash a ripe avocado with a little olive oil and apply to the skin.
- Avocado oil can be used as a base oil for massage.
- Eat an avocado each day when convalescing.
- The pulp, applied to grazes and shallow cuts, and covered with sterile gauze, can prevent infection entering the body and encourage healing.
- Eat regularly for digestive and circulatory problems.
- The flesh of a ripe avocado soothes sunburned skin.

PROPERTIES

- Excellent restorative food, particularly during convalescence
- Traditionally used for sexual problems
- Helps with skin disorders
- Antioxidant
- Used to treat circulatory problems
- Digestive
- Antibacterial
- Antifungal

CAUTION

Do not eat avocados or take any product containing avocado if you have been prescribed maoi antidepressants.

THE HEALING REMEDIES SOURCEBOOK

PIPER NEGRUM
BLACK PEPPER

Black pepper, a traditional seasoning for food, is a warm, aromatic, and comforting spice with therapeutic uses. The fruit, or corns, of the vine and the essential oil extracted from them are used. Black pepper is the whole, sun-dried, unripened fruit of the vine; white pepper is the ripe fruit, from which the skins have been removed.

USES

- Black pepper is useful for treating indigestion and flatulence—add to food daily for preventive action.
- Its essential oil eases muscular aches and pains, and is used to treat colds and flu.
- When used as a homeopathic remedy for fever, pepper can help to lower the body temperature.
- Pepper is an effective emetic and expectorant, and can be taken internally, or rubbed onto the chest (a tiny amount of oil in a suitable carrier oil), to prevent catarrh and to encourage healing.
- In Ayurvedic medicine, black pepper mixed with ghee is used to treat nasal congestion, sinusitis, and inflammation of the skin.

PROPERTIES

- Stimulating
- Expectorant
- Anesthetic
- Tranquilizing
- Analgesic

CAUTION
The essential oil may irritate those with sensitive skin. Large amounts of black pepper used regularly may result in overstimulation of the kidneys. When using black pepper for medicinal purposes, follow the recommended dosage.

PRUNUS AMYGDALMUS DULCIS AND PRUNUS AMYGDALMUS AMARA
ALMOND

The almond tree produces the oldest and most widely grown of all of the world's nut crops, and is indigenous to western Asia and North Africa. Of the two major types of almonds grown, the sweet almond (*P. dulcis*) is cultivated for its edible nut. The bitter almond (*P. amara*) is inedible but contains an oil—also present in the sweet almond, and in the ripe kernels of the apricot and peach—which, when combined with water, yields hydrocyanic (prussic) acid and benzaldehyde, the essential oil of bitter almonds. The oil is used in making flavoring extracts and in some sedative medicines.

SPECIAL NOTE
Eat almonds with foods rich in vitamin C to encourage maximum absorption.

USES

- Combine almond milk with barley water for urinary problems.
- Almond milk is an excellent tonic during convalescence.
- Drink almond milk daily to reduce frequency of digestive disorders, and to relieve respiratory problems.

PROPERTIES

- Sweet almonds are high in protein
- Almonds reduce inflammation: used in the treatment of bronchitis
- Rich in protein, fat, zinc, potassium, iron, B vitamins, and magnesium
- Aids respiration
- Acts as a digestive

SINAPIS ALBA
MUSTARD *Brassica Nigra*

Black and white mustards are used for culinary and medicinal purposes. The leaves, flowers, seeds, and oils of the black mustard are used, while only the seeds of the white mustard are useful. Black mustard powder is an important herbal remedy because it draws blood to the surface of the skin quickly, which means that it is "rubefacient," and warming. Mustard oil is used as an ingredient in liniments, stomach stimulants, and emetics.

USES

- Taken internally, mustard encourages the circulation, eases stomach and liver problems, and is able to stimulate the heart.
- Eat fresh mustard leaves when convalescing—they are nutritious and will help to encourage healing.
- A mustard foot bath (1 teaspoon of mustard powder added to a bowl of hot water) is a traditional remedy for colds, circulatory problems, and headaches.
- A mustard poultice on the chest relieves infection and congestion.
- Mustard essential oil can be used externally for neuralgia.

PROPERTIES

- Rich in calcium and iron
- Mustard helps to restore bacterial balance in the intestines
- Mustard greens are rich in vitamin A, iron, and zinc
- White mustard relieves pain, and is a diuretic and an antibiotic
- Mustard flour is an antiseptic and a deodorizer
- Mustard oil can be used for pain relief of arthritic conditions and chilblains

CAUTION

Mustard seeds can burn the skin; use carefully. Avoid contact with the mucous membranes, and with sensitive skin.

SOLAN URN LUBEROSUM
POTATO

The potato plant is native to the Americas. It was supposedly endowed with powers such as the ability to cure impotence, and so long as the plant remained rare in Europe, its price often reached astronomical heights. Potatoes have been used for medicinal purposes for hundreds of years, and are extremely nutritious, supplying fiber, B vitamins, minerals, and vitamin C. The peels are high in potassium, and potato-peel tea has been traditionally used around the world for high blood pressure. The juice of raw potatoes is most useful, and can be added to soups, juices, or stews to disguise the taste.

USES

- The juice of the raw potato can be used for stomach ulcers and to relieve the inflammation of arthritis.
- Make a potato poultice for healing a bruise or sprain of any kind.
- Raw, grated potatoes can relieve the pain of a burn.
- Apply hot baked potato pulp for tennis elbow and other joint pain.
- Boiled potato peel is said to be useful for inflammation of the prostate. Apply as a poultice to the affected area.
- Eaten daily, potatoes can help to prevent premature aging and heart disease.

PROPERTIES

- Alkaline, which helps to detoxify the body
- Anti-ulcer
- Helps relieve inflammation and pain
- The skin contains chlorogenic acid, which can help to prevent cell mutation, causing cancer

CAUTION

Poisonous alkaloids are present in most nightshade plants, including the common potato, but it is perfectly safe to eat if cooked, and in small amounts when raw. Sprouting potatoes are poisonous and should not be eaten.

VACCINIUM OXYCOCCUS VAR. PALUSTRIS
CRANBERRY

Cranberries are small acidic berries which are rich in vitamins C and A, and contain an excellent infection-fighting ingredient. The commercial cranberry, *Vaccinium macrocarpon*, is a creeping evergreen plant of the heath family, whose red, acidic fruit is used in sauces and jellies served with savory and sweet foods and in a variety of fruit juice beverages.

USES

- Cranberries contain a substance which affects the acidity of the urine and acts as a bactericide. A daily glass of cranberry juice will prevent and treat cystitis, and discourage kidney stones. Fresh cranberries and cranberry juice are used in the treatment of prostate problems and urinary tract infections.
- Crushed cranberries, boiled in distilled water and skinned, can be added to a cup of warm water to overcome an asthma attack. The berries contain an active ingredient similar to that in the drugs used to control asthma.

PROPERTIES

- An antiseptic action on the urinary system
- Used to control asthma
- Improves the health of the circulatory system
- Aids in the treatment of kidney stones

CAUTION

Cranberries contain large amounts of oxalic acid, and should not be eaten raw.

ZEA MAYS
CORN

Archeological evidence indicates that a type of primitive corn was used as a food in Mexico at least 7,000 years ago. The kernels of corn have a translucent, horny appearance when immature and are wrinkled when dry. The ears are eaten fresh or frozen, or are canned. Corn, or maize, is known primarily as a staple food, but it also has therapeutic properties. The corn silk (stigmas and styles of female flowers), fruit, seeds, and oil are used.

USES

- Corn silk refers to the hairs covering the corn. A tea made by infusing corn silk in hot water may help in the treatment of kidney stones. Drink three times a day.
- Corn silk is also a good cleanser of the urinary tract. A little of it eaten raw, with or without the corn kernels, will benefit the whole urinary system and may help to prevent cystitis.
- Corn and its products may be beneficial in the treatment of bedwetting in children, disorders of the prostate and cystitis, and inflammation of the urethra.

PROPERTIES

- Corn provides carbohydrates, B vitamins (thiamine and riboflavin), vitamin C, vitamin A, potassium, and zinc
- Stimulating and cooling
- Used in Chinese medicine for treating urinary and kidney problems
- Corn silk cleanses the kidneys and the urinary tract

CAUTION

People suffering from pellagra (a niacin-deficiency disease) may be advised to eliminate corn and corn products from their diet. Some people are allergic to corn—if you suffer a rash, headaches, or any other symptoms, avoid corn and corn products.

BICARBONATE OF SODA
BAKING SODA

Baking soda is a white powder that is traditionally used as a raising agent for baking. It is used in many natural remedies, and on its own for its soothing and neutralizing properties.

USES

- Salt and baking soda in the bath may reduce the effect of minor exposure to X-rays.
- A paste of baking soda and water can be applied to diaper rash to reduce skin inflammation and irritation.
- Drink a solution of baking soda and hot water (1 teaspoon to 1 cup [250ml]) to reduce flatulence and ease indigestion.
- For bee stings, extract the sting and apply a paste of baking soda and water to neutralize it.
- The juice of half a lemon mixed with 1 teaspoon of baking soda and warm water will help ease a headache. Drink every 15 minutes until the pain begins to recede.
- Brush your teeth with baking soda, a natural whitener which reduces agents causing bad breath.

PROPERTIES

- Anti-inflammatory, particularly useful for skin conditions
- Natural bleach for teeth
- Alkaline (neutralizes acids)

CAUTION
Baking soda should be used only externally on children and babies. Consult a physician before taking baking soda if you have high blood pressure or heart trouble.

BREAD

Bread—particularly wholegrain bread—is an excellent source of carbohydrates and B-complex vitamins, which maintain the health of the nervous system and ensure the healthy functioning of body systems. Traditionally, bread was used as a poultice, and applied as a styptic to stop the bleeding of wounds.

USES

- Apply cold bread to closed eyes to reduce the inflammation of conjunctivitis and soothe itching.
- Apply a warm bread poultice to infected cuts to reduce itching and pain.
- Apply fresh bread to shallow wounds to help stop the bleeding.
- Ease the pain, and help to bring out a boil by applying a hot bread poultice.
- Eat wholegrain bread while convalescing and when under stress—it is rich in B vitamins that feed the nervous system and contains three times as much fiber as white bread.

PROPERTIES

- Nutritious
- Anti-inflammatory
- Styptic (stops bleeding)

HONEY

Honey is the sweet liquid produced by bees from the nectar of flowers. The source of the nectar the honey is made from determines its color and flavor. For centuries, honey has been used as an antiseptic, for external and internal conditions, and as a tonic for overall good health. Each country has a distinctive type of honey, dependent on the local flowers upon which the bees feed.

USES
- Honey water can be used as an eye lotion (particularly good for conjunctivitis and other infectious conditions).
- Gargle with honey water to soothe a sore throat and ease respiratory problems.
- Honey and lemon mixed together are a traditional remedy for coughs.
- Mix with apple cider vinegar as a tonic or "rebalancer." This may also help to relieve the symptoms of arthritis and reduce arthritic deposits.
- Honey ointment can soothe and encourage healing of sores in the mouth or vagina.
- Honey is an excellent moisturizer, and can be rubbed into the skin as a revitalizing mask.
- Honey warmed with a little milk can be used as a gentle sedative.

PROPERTIES
- Soothes raw tissues
- Helps to retain calcium in the body
- Honey helps to balance acid accumulations in the body (because of the significant amount of potassium it contains)
- Sedative
- Antifungal

CAUTION
Unpasteurized honey should not be eaten by pregnant women, and only sparingly by children. However, ensure that you buy cold-pressed honey, because heated honey contains additives and loses its healing properties.

ACETIC ACID
VINEGAR

Vinegar (from the French *vinaigre*, "sour wine") is an acidic liquid obtained from the fermentation of alcohol, and used either as a condiment or a preservative.

USES
- Sip first thing in the morning, and just prior to meals to reduce appetite and encourage efficient digestion.
- Drink a glass of warm apple cider vinegar with honey a half-hour before bed to encourage restful sleep.
- Vinegar can be drunk (warm with a little honey) to treat digestive disorders and urinary infections.
- Apply vinegar to wasp stings to ease discomfort.
- Coughs, colds, and infections will respond to a cup of warm water with 2 tablespoons of vinegar and some honey. Arthritis and asthma may also be treated with the same drink, adding slightly more vinegar.

PROPERTIES
- Helps to make more efficient use of calcium in the body, and can help to encourage strong bones, hair, and nails
- Vinegar is antiseptic, astringent, and excellent for urinary tract infections

INHALATION
Vinegar is antispasmodic, and is useful for treating the bronchospasms common to bronchitis sufferers. Bronchitis is the inflammation of the bronchi, which link the windpipe to the lungs. It causes production of thick phlegm, and gives rise to bouts of coughing. Inhaling the steam given off by hot cider vinegar will soothe spasms. Pour some apple cider vinegar into a pan and put it on the cooker to heat. Bring to the boil and simmer for a few minutes. Remove from the heat and pour into a medium-sized bowl. Take the bowl to your kitchen table and sit down with it in front of you. Drape a large towel over your head and the bowl, making a tent. Inhale deeply while the steam continues to be produced. This will also help catarrh.

HYDROGEN DIOXIDE
WATER

Pure water is a clear, colorless liquid made up of oxygen and hydrogen. Water is the most common substance on the Earth's surface, covering more than 70 percent of the planet. It is also present in the atmosphere as a gas (water vapor or steam). Water is essential to life on Earth and constitutes a large part of most living things. Human beings are comprised of about 75 percent water. Water is necessary for maintaining the correct osmotic pressure in cells, and is needed for many other body processes, such as transporting nutrients and waste products around the body in the blood (blood is about 80 percent water). Water that has been cooled or heated to form ice, hot water, or steam can be used to treat minor complaints.

USES

- Drink plenty of fresh water if you suffer from edema.
- Drink water to counter the effects of a hangover, and during illness to encourage the expulsion of toxins. People who drink excessive amounts of alcohol or coffee, or who smoke, should drink at least eight glasses of water daily.
- It can help to prevent tooth decay when sufficient fluoride is present.
- Water acts as a diuretic and a mild laxative—it adds water to stools and may stimulate muscle contraction in the digestive tract.
- Hard water may play a role in preventing hypertension and heart disease.
- Ice reduces swellings and is particularly beneficial for sprains. Ice packs help to relieve backache.
- Cold compresses placed around the throat may ease an attack of croup.
- Children suffering from croup will get relief when placed in a steamy bathroom. This is best achieved by running the hot water faucet or the shower.
- Swallowing cracked ice may be beneficial in relieving morning sickness and motion sickness.
- A hot compress can help to reduce skin inflammations caused by infection. Dip a face cloth or other thick cloth in hot water and wring out before applying.
- Bathing in warm water can encourage relaxation. Hot baths may help to soothe muscular aches and pains. A cool bath can be soothing for sufferers of prickly heat.

PROPERTIES

- Essential for life
- Dilutes toxins in the body, and expels them
- A natural diuretic
- Salt water is antiseptic
- Aids kidney action
- Prevents constipation
- May contain some naturally occurring fluoride
- Prevents dehydration

CAUTION

Water should be filtered before it is drunk if it contains impurities. Bottled mineral waters may be high in sodium.

THE HEALING REMEDIES SOURCEBOOK

HERBALISM

SINCE BEFORE RECORDED HISTORY humans have used plants for food, medicines, shelter, clothing, dyes, weapons, musical instruments, and transportation. The cultural development of different countries and the rise and fall of empires have often been linked to the understanding and exploitation of plants. Herbalism, the use of plants for medicinal purposes, has been common to all peoples of the world. Our understanding of herbalism has been passed down by word of mouth from generation to generation.

It is the most natural thing in the world to use local flora for food and medicine, and list this knowledge for posterity. All native cultures have a well-developed understanding of local plants, and most of the world, even today, relies on herbal expertise for its primary healthcare. Shamans, wise women, bush doctors, traditional healers, and native medicine workers carry on a tradition thousands of years old.

Herbalism is the oldest, most tested, and proven form of medicine in the world. The *Ebers Papyrus* of the ancient Egyptians lists 85 herbs, some of which, like mint, are used in a similar way today. The Chinese herbal, *Pen Tsao*, contains over a thousand herbal remedies. The Assyrian and Babylonian scribes wrote herbal recipes on clay tablets. The Greek Hippocrates (477–360 B.C.E.) mentions herbs, remedies, and treatment stratagems which are still valid. Indeed, there is much practical and theoretical knowledge to be rediscovered. Globally, herbal lore is a treasure chest beyond price.

In the West, the Saxons wrote the *Leech Book of Bald*, a mixture of remedies and ritual. Their nine sacred herbs included yarrow, marigold, and hawthorn. A modern practitioner of herbal medicine would rate them equally highly. The golden age of herbals was precipitated by the development of the printing press. Culpeper printed the *London Dispensary* (1653) in English (it had previously been printed in Latin), and later published his *Complete Herbal*—a book, he boasted, from which any man (or woman) could find out how to cure themselves for less than three pennies! Culpeper's herbal was immensely popular and is still available, having gone through over 40 reprints.

Botanical medicine was regarded as fringe medicine for many years. It was valued as a starting place for modern research, but thought to have nothing to offer Western society as a therapy in itself. Pharmaceutical companies identified the active therapeutic principles of many plants, synthesized commercial analogues, and patented new drugs. But in doing so they often missed the major principles of using natural sources for therapeutic purposes. Herbalism, when practiced properly, is marked by a completely different attitude from orthodox medicine. It is a holistic system that uses plants, or plant parts, in a nonintrusive way. Herbalists believe that the constituents of a plant work synergistically to stimulate the natural healing process.

THE TENETS OF HERBALISM

- The whole plant is better than an isolated extract.
- Treat the whole person not just the symptoms.
- Practice minimum effective treatment and minimum intervention.
- Strengthen the body; encourage it to heal itself.

Today, there is a worldwide renaissance in therapeutic systems which use herbs as their major source of medicines. Modern science is validating traditional practices, precipitating a general reappraisal. Tibetan, Chinese, Native American, Indian, and Western systems are all examining their philosophical roots in a cross-cultural examination which is enriching to all. Many people now use herbs because they are felt to be safer, cheaper, more natural, and to have fewer side-effects. This is not always the case. Any substance can trigger an idiosyncratic response. Herbs must be given with knowledge and responsibility. But by following a few rules and using common sense, we add to our health, our sense of belonging, and our pleasure at being on the planet.

MODERN HERBALISM

Modern herbalism is practiced on two levels. These differ in the range of herbs which can be used, the results that can be achieved, and the amount of responsibility taken for treatment:

AS A PROFESSION

Western consultant medical herbalists act in just the same way as orthodox practitioners. They are trained in orthodox medical diagnosis and can provide a complete alternative. They also work with physicians to offer a complementary service. A medical herbalist will sometimes use some powerful herbs which are restricted by law, or only available after a personal consultation, in the same way as an orthodox practitioner will use prescription-only medicines. A good medical herbalist will have undergone extensive training and he or she will certainly belong to an established body of practitioners.

AS A SELF-HELP SYSTEM

Herbs are ideal as a simple system of home care for first aid, everyday ailments, the management of chronic conditions, strengthening of the body, and preventive treatment. Herbs can be safely taken as long as a few simple rules are followed (*see The Rules of Safe Home Treatment, page 92*).

HERBALISM AND CONSERVATION

One hundred years ago, a person could have walked into the garden or local woods and returned with a remedy for a baby's gripe, a stomachache, sprained ankle, stiffening gout, or any number of ailments. Today, we can walk into the local store and find the shelves full of natural ingredients from all corners of the world—from carrots and cabbage to precious spices like cinnamon. This array would have been the envy of a medieval apothecary; but while the stock is available, the knowledge is scarce. The culture of responsibility, self-care, and interaction with nature has largely been lost. It must be rediscovered if herbs and their proper uses are to be properly understood.

A herb has a taste, color, smell, texture, and history. The antiseptic calendula lotion applied to a spot was once an orange marigold growing clear and open-faced in a sunny meadow. The lavender used to reduce the tension of a pounding headache and bring sleep once shimmered in a soporific violet-purple haze on a French mountainside. Such pictures are part of the heritage of healing, and help us to remember and understand the actions of herbs and the way they work within the body.

Part of the beauty of herbalism lies in the many different possible methods of taking herbs. The skill in choosing the best method for a specific individual and condition is part of the art of caring. Hand baths, foot baths, skin washes, rubs, massage oils, eye washes, compresses, and fomentations are undervalued. Local treatments allow the herb to act exactly where it is needed, avoid affecting the whole system, and are comforting and effective. Remember that in all herbal preparations it is best to use organic herbs.

USING HERBS AT HOME

To be able to care for yourself and your family by making natural remedies is a pleasure, and the benefits are legion. The organic chemistry of remedy-making is an extension of cooking, and the same principles and skills apply. For success, use the best-quality ingredients, practice absolute cleanliness, and follow the instructions carefully.

THE HEALING REMEDIES SOURCEBOOK

PREPARATION

THE FRESH PLANT

The easiest way to take a herb is to pick it directly from the plant. Leaves can be used in salads, sandwiches, or soups. Chickweed, chicory, dandelion, and marigold make excellent salad additions. Nettle is traditional for green soup. Elderflower fritters are fun. Chewing a few fresh leaves of marjoram will help clear the head. Horseradish leaves will clear sinuses. Sage eases mouth sores and sore throats. Fresh leaves can also be used to make water infusions (teas), decoctions, tinctures, infused oils, and creams.

Follow standard recipes and dosages. Most recipes give the amounts for dried herbs. When using fresh material, add one-third more, as fresh plants contain a considerable amount of water.

IMMEDIATE RESPONSE

For cuts, grazes, and stings, pick four or five leaves (dock is traditional when stung on countryside walks as it is so readily available) and rub the leaves together between the hands to bruise them and release the juices. When damp, apply to the affected area and hold in place. Poultices can be made in the same way.

It is important to remember that several herbs may be recommended for a particular ailment; all are slightly different. For example, would rose, lavender, rosemary, or chamomile be best for your headache? Would a cool compress be best, or a long soak in a rosemary bath? Knowledge of the herb, the individual, and the different methods must be combined to prescribe remedies that will be really effective.

WHERE TO GET HERBS

Many herbs and herbal products are freely available. Plants or seeds can be bought from garden centers (always check the Latin name) and grown in the garden or in a window-box.

Dried herbs are available from herb stores and some wholefood outlets. Always specify the herb (the Latin name if possible) and the part of the plant to be used—root, bark, leaf, or flower.

Herbal products, remedies, tinctures, tablets, etc. are available from wholefood stores, and some pharmacies and general food stores. Read the label and instructions carefully.

Regarding plants picked from the wild, countries have different rules and some plants are protected by law. Check the legal situation and get permission from the landowner. Check identification carefully and pick the minimum required, with proper regard for conservation. Never gather roots from the side of the road, by recently sprayed crops or foliage, or from sickly-looking plants.

PREPARATIONS

Most herbs are sold in dried form. In this form they can simply be powdered and sprinkled on to food (half a flat teaspoon twice daily), but most are prepared further. Herbs are prepared for:

AVAILABILITY AND PRESERVATION—so that seasonal plants are available all year round.

CONVENIENCE, EASE OF USE—compressed tablets are often more convenient to take than a cup of tea.

SPECIFIC USE, TO AID THE ACTION OF THE HERB—for example, infused oils for rubs, honey for adding a soothing and demulcent quality to thyme.

- Consider the whole body first. Is medication needed? Consider a change of rest, diet, or exercise before prescribing the patient any remedy.

- Use simple remedies internally and externally. This will encourage the body to heal itself.

- Make a list. Know what you are taking and what to expect. Keep a note of all remedies taken. This will be useful if you need help later.

- Take as recommended. Remember the herbal tenet of minimum effective dosage and intervention. Stick to the standard dosages. Doubling does not double effectiveness; it may put an extra burden on a body that is already sick.

- TLC. Use lots of Tender Loving Care. A positive and loving attitude helps to make the illness more bearable, and may even speed up the healing process.

- Monitor progress after a few days.

- Stop treatment if there is any adverse reaction. Remember, people are all individuals; children, especially, respond quickly, so be alert for changes or new symptoms.

- Seek professional help if in any doubt. Assessing your own symptoms is different from making a diagnosis, which needs an objective eye.

THE REMEDIES

HERBAL REMEDY CARRIERS

Herbal remedies come in a variety of forms:

Tinctures are the most common type of internal remedy prescribed by herbalists. They are made by soaking the flowers, leaves, or roots of the herbs in alcohol to extract and preserve their properties. Tinctures keep well, and are easy to store. Because they are highly concentrated, you need only take a small amount at a time.

Infusions are less concentrated and are an easy way to take herbs at home. The herbalist prescribes fresh or dried flowers, leaves, or green stems of the herbs, which you make with water into a "tea"—a rather misleading word, as it suggests a pleasant drink, which is rarely the case with prescription herbs. Sweeten with honey if you find the taste unpalatable. The properties of some herbs—for example, comfrey, marshmallow, and valerian root—are destroyed by heat, so they should be infused or "macerated" in cold water for up to 12 hours. These are quicky assimilated and gentle to use for children, convalescents, and those with delicate digestion.

Decoctions are similar to infusions, but are made from tougher materials such as roots, bark, nuts, and seeds. Using the same proportions, place the herb and water in a saucepan and bring to the boil, simmer for 10–15 minutes, strain, and drink hot.

Tablets and capsules are taken in the same way as a conventional drug, and are useful for people who would rather not taste the remedy.

Creams and ointments are applied externally to soothe irritated or inflamed skin conditions, or ease the pain of sprains or bruises. Cream moistens dry or cracked skin, and massaging the ointment into bruises and sprains helps to ease the pain. In both cases the active ingredients of the herb pass through the pores of the skin into the blood stream to encourage healing.

Compresses, either hot or cold, help with aches, pains, and swollen joints. Fold a clean piece of cotton into an infusion of the prescribed herb and apply to the point of pain. Repeat as the compress cools or, in the case of cold compresses, until the pain eases.

Poultices, made from bruised fresh herbs or dried herbs moistened into a paste with hot water, are also good for painful joints or drawing out infection from boils, spots, or wounds. Place the herb on a clean piece of cotton and bandage on to the affected area. Leave in place for around two hours or until the symptoms ease.

Suppositories and douches are sometimes prescribed for rectal problems such as piles, or vaginal infections, respectively. The suppositories will come ready-made for you to insert. Douches are made from an infusion or decoction that has been allowed to cool.

Herbal baths are perhaps the most pleasant of the herbal remedies, and are a useful supplement to other forms of treatment. The heat of the water activates the properties of the volatile oils so that they are absorbed through the pores of the skin and inhaled through the nose. In both cases they pass into the bloodstream, and when inhaled they also pass through the nervous system to the brain, exerting a healing effect on both mind and body.

SEEING A PROFESSIONAL

Professional consultant medical herbalists are usually trained in orthodox diagnosis and can treat all of the ailments treated by a family physician or general practitioner. Accredited members of organizations such as the National Institute of Medical Herbalists have undergone four years of university or university-standard study and two years of supervision. They will understand all the indications and contraindications of herbs, and any problems which may arise from taking orthodox drugs. They will refer to other specialists if necessary.

It is becoming more common for a patient to register with a herbalist in the same way as one would register with a physician—for a check-up and then to be on the records should the need arise. Such patients have yearly checks to maintain optimum health. Whole families register, as herbalism is especially suited to children and the elderly.

A consultation will take about an hour and consider all aspects of health, diet, exercise, and lifestyle. Your herbalist will take a "holistic" view, which means taking into consideration everything that affects your health on a physical, mental, and spiritual level.

You will be asked questions about:
- age
- career
- personality, priorities
- concerns
- appetite
- sleeping patterns
- previous medicines and illnesses
- bowel movements
- family
- symptoms
- any other aspect that is relevant

As well as what you say, your therapist will want to know how you feel and will note your appearance. The condition of your hair, skin, and facial expression, your posture, and how you move all provide important clues that will help with the diagnosis. There may also be a physical examination. Treatment will then be prescribed by the therapist.

Before a first visit it is worth spending some time considering your health and expectations. It is useful to make a list of relevant points in your medical history and questions you want to ask, as these can easily be missed or forgotten in the stress of a first meeting. If for any reason you do not get along with the practitioner, try another one. It is important that there is a relationship of mutual trust and respect.

Many of the herbs prescribed will be familiar, but some will be unknown to you. After a consultation, a herbalist is able to prescribe herbs which are limited by law and not freely available over the counter to the general public.

METHODS AND DOSAGES

WATER – INFUSIONS (TEAS)

Standard strength

1oz. (25g) herb to 2 cups (500ml) water; or 1 teaspoon herb to 1 cup water

Dose

Some herbs have specific indications and dosages; other herbs are not recommended at certain times, for example, early pregnancy or when breast-feeding. Read the indications and contraindications of each herb carefully.

Standard adult dose

- 1 cup three times a day for normal conditions
- 1 cup up to six times a day, or every two hours, for acute conditions
- Drink 1 cup twice a day as a long-term strengthening tonic

Children's dose

Reduce proportionally. Give a child of seven half the standard adult dose. At six months, use 1 teaspoon of the standard strength tea. For breastfeeding infants, give the remedy to the mother.

Brewing times

To some extent this depends on personal taste, but the following is a good guide:

- up to 3 minutes for flowers and soft leaves
- up to 5 minutes for seeds and leaves
- up to 10 minutes for hard seeds, roots, and various barks

Water infusions at the standard strength are used as teas, gargles, lotions for the skin, compresses, and fomentations. Dilute with an equal amount of water for hand or foot baths, douches, and enemas.

WATER – DECOCTIONS

Standard strength

1½oz. (40g) herb to 3 cups (750ml) water

Method

- Put herb in saucepan
- Add 3 cups (750ml) water
- Put on a tight lid
- Bring to the boil, then turn down as low as possible and simmer for 10–15 minutes
- Strain thoroughly
- Discard herb
- Pour decoction into a clean bottle
- Will keep in a refrigerator for two or three days

Dose

- ⅓ cup twice a day for normal conditions, and as a tonic
- ⅓ cup three to six times a day for acute conditions

Decoctions can be diluted with an equal amount of water and used in the same ways as water infusions for hand baths, gargles, etc.

WATER – SIMPLE SYRUPS AND HONEYS

Method

- Make standard decoction with 1½oz. (40g) herb and 3 cups (750ml) water
- Return to heat, remove lid, and simmer gently till liquid is reduced to 1 cup (250ml), which may take a few hours
- Add 2¼ cups (600g) honey or 2 cups (500g) sugar, stirring until completely dissolved
- Pour into clean bottle, label, and date

Standard adult dose

- 2 teaspoons 3 to 6 times a day

Children under five

- 1 teaspoon three times a day

Syrups and honeys can be used to sweeten other herbal preparations, or added to food or drink. They are ideal for children because they are sweet.

ALCOHOL – TINCTURES

A tincture is an alcohol-based herbal preparation. Tinctures can be made with fresh or dried herbs. The absolute strength of the alcohol needed varies slightly depending on the herb, but the method given below is sufficient for standard home use.

Method

To make 1¼ cups (300ml) of tincture:
- Chop 2 tablespoons (12g) dried or 1oz. (25g) fresh herb
- Put in large glass jar
- Cover with ¾ cup (200ml) alcohol, such as vodka or brandy, and 6 tablespoons (100ml) water
- Put on a lid and leave for two weeks
- Shake occasionally
- After two weeks, strain well through a muslin bag
- Squeeze out the liquid
- Pour into clean, amber glass bottle. Label and date
- Keep in a cool place away from children
- Will keep indefinitely

Standard adult dose
- 1 teaspoon 3 times a day, standard
- 5 drops to 1 teaspoon a day as a tonic
- 1 teaspoon 6 times a day for acute conditions

A tincture can be diluted with water: 2 teaspoons to 1 cup water can be used as a skin lotion, wash, foot bath, gargle, compress, or douche.

OIL – LINIMENT

A liniment is a soothing rub to relieve fatigued and stiff muscles and joints. Put the fresh herb in a jar and cover with olive oil. Leave for up to six weeks. Strain the mixture through a cloth. Stand until the oil separates off: use this.

OIL

Oil is soothing and nourishing for the skin, and acts as a lubricant to carry the active principles of the herbs in rubs, massage oils, and salves. There are two methods of infusion, hot and cold. Hot is used for thyme, rosemary, comfrey root, and spices such as cayenne, mustard, and ginger. Cold is used for flowers.

INFUSED OIL

Method

To make 1 cup (250ml):
- Chop 3 tablespoons/¼ cup dried herbs or spices, or 6 tablespoons/½ cup fresh herbs
- Put half into a clean pan with a lid
- Cover with 1 cup (250ml) pure vegetable oil (a pure and light vegetable oil is best).
- Put in a water bath and simmer gently for two hours (it is important that direct heat is not used, as this might burn the oil)
- Strain
- Throw away used herbs
- Put remaining half of unused herbs in pan
- Cover these with the oil (it will have changed color, having picked up some of the quality of the herbs)
- Replace lid and return pan to water bath for another couple of hours. Strain
- Pour oil into clean bottles, label, and date

This double method makes a strong infused oil which can be used as it is, mixed with tincture for a liniment, or thickened with beeswax (for a thin cream, use 1 part beeswax to 10 parts infused oil; for a thick salve, use 1 part beeswax to 5 parts infused oil).

ALCOHOL – SPICED OR TONIC WINE

A good way to make a strengthening remedy for everyday use is to make a tonic wine. Spiced wines make good aperitifs, to stimulate and improve digestion.

Method
- 1oz. (25g) herb(s)
- 1–2oz. (25–50g) spices, depending on taste
- 8½ cups (2l) of wine
- Stand for two weeks
- Strain and bottle

Dose
- ¼ cup twice a day before meals (warm water can be added)

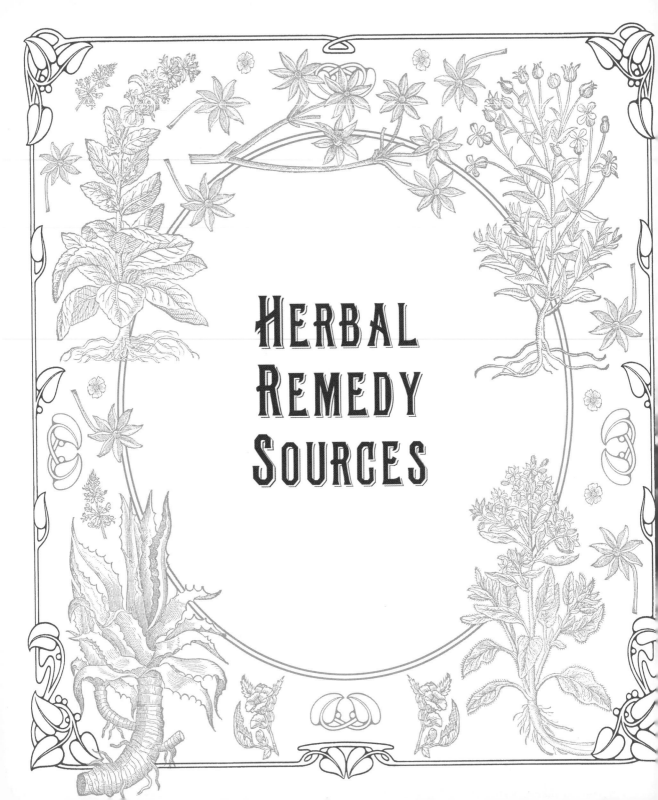

Herbal Remedy Sources

ACHILLEA MILLEFOLIUM
YARROW

A common wild plant with feathery leaves and white or pink flowers. Often found on lawns. In Greek myth, achillea is said to have been used by Achilles to treat his army's wounds.

USES

- Early stages of fevers, especially with hot, dry skin.
- Catarrh, sinusitis, hay fever, and dust allergies.
- For high blood pressure, with hawthorn and linden.
- With a little ginger for cold feet.
- Internal and external use for varicose veins and spontaneous bruising.
- Useful for thrombosis, to prevent blood clots.
- Supportive for people undergoing radiotherapy and intestinal infections.
- Diarrhea, liverishness, colic, and weak digestion.
- Irregular menstrual bleeding, cramps, and vaginal discharges.
- Helps pelvic circulation.

PROPERTIES

- Diaphoretic
- Anti-inflammatory
- Antiseptic
- Antispasmodic
- Styptic
- Gentle bitter tonic

NOTES AND DOSAGES

- Standard doses (*see pages 94–95*). Take freely for fevers and acute complaints.
- For a bath, simmer a handful of fresh leaves in 2 cups (500ml) water for 15 minutes.
- Strain and add to your bath water.

CAUTION

Avoid large does in pregnancy, small amounts are safe, but if in doubt consult a professional herbalist. Some people develop an allergic rash if they handle the fresh herb in sunlight.

AGRIMONIA EUPATORIA
AGRIMONY

A common wild plant with slender spikes of bright yellow flowers. The whole herb is used. Culpeper recommended it for gout "used outwardly in an oil or ointment, or inwardly, in a syrup or juice."

USES

- As a tea or tincture for indigestion, heartburn, diarrhea, and liverish feelings. Especially helpful for people suffering from food allergies—on a long-term basis.
- With St. John's wort and horsetail for bed-wetting and chronic cystitis.
- As a lotion for the cleansing of wounds.

AGRIMONY DIGESTIVE TONIC

Combine equal parts of agrimony, raspberry leaf, and lemon balm (*Melissa officinalis*). Store away from the light. Make a tea from 1 teaspoon of the mixture to 1 cup of boiling water, and drink freely for colicky pains with looseness and nervous diarrhea.

PROPERTIES

- Astringent and tonic
- Tones and strengthens the digestive system and liver
- A wound herb

NOTES AND DOSAGES

- Standard doses (*see pages 94–95*).
- Agrimony makes a tasty substitute for normal tea.

CAUTION

May aggravate constipation, but otherwise a safe and gentle herb to use.

ALCHEMILLA VULGARIS
LADY'S MANTLE

A wild plant of wayside and meadows. Grows well in shady gardens, and bears sprays of greenish-yellow flowers.

USES

- Heavy menstrual bleeding, either alone or with an equal part of shepherd's purse or yarrow. Also for bleeding in the middle of the menstrual cycle and for irregular menstruation.
- To prevent menstrual cramps and for PMS, taken during the second half of the menstrual cycle.
- Thrush and other vaginal discharges, taken as a tea or douche.
- Traditional treatment for infertility in women with no obvious cause.
- Children's diarrhea.

LADY'S MANTLE AND CHAMOMILE WASH

Make a strong tea with 1 cup of boiling water to 1 teaspoon of lady's mantle and 2 teaspoons of chamomile flowers. Infuse in a covered vessel for 15 minutes. Use this as a soothing wash for itchy genitals, in men and women.

PROPERTIES

- Astringent
- Tones and strengthens the womb

NOTES AND DOSAGES

- Standard doses. It is a pleasant drinking tea.

CAUTION

Do not use in pregnancy except under professional guidance, but otherwise a safe herb. Always seek medical advice for bleeding in mid-menstrual cycle.

ALLIUM SATIVUM
GARLIC

The familiar cooking herb. Garlic can be harvested about six to eight months after planting, in the summer. Bulbs not needed immediately can be dried in the sun and stored.

USES

- Beneficial in cases of thrombosis, hardening of the arteries, high blood pressure, and high cholesterol.
- For chest infections, asthma, flu, colds, and ear infections. Combines well with echinacea.

GARLIC OR ONION MILK

Put 1 onion or 3 cloves of garlic, thinly sliced, into a pan with 2 cups of milk (cow's, goat's, sheep's, soy milk, or nut milk). Simmer over a very low heat for 20 minutes. Strain. Can be stored in a refrigerator for 2 or 3 days. Dose: Infants 2 to 4 teaspoons every four hours. Young children can drink freely if feverish and croupy.

PROPERTIES

- Antiseptic
- Antibiotic
- Expectorant
- Fungicide and antihistamine
- Lowers blood pressure

NOTES AND DOSAGES

- Tablets are easy to take. Follow the instructions on the box. Mix chopped garlic with an equal amount of honey and take 1 teaspoon 3 to 6 times daily. Half dose for children. The infused oil can be applied to the skin, ear, and chest, to fight infections. Regular dietary use benefits the circulation.

CAUTION

Safe to use but may be too hot for some constitutions, in which case use with milk. Enteric-coated tablets are available. These are easier on the digestion.

ALOE VERA
ALOE VERA

A succulent, tropical plant that has been used for centuries to heal both externally and internally. Aloes are resistant to drought, taking in water very easily and losing moisture very slowly.

USES
- Applied to burns and sunburn, ringworm, infected cuts, acne, shingles, eczema, wrinkles, and areas of dry, itchy skin.

ALOE GEL
Wash the leaves. Cut into 2in. (5cm) lengths. Slice each piece in half, to expose the largest amount of gel. Wrap each piece in plastic wrap and date. To use: remove plastic and apply the gel side of the leaf to the skin; smear over the affected area, or hold in place with a bandage.

PROPERTIES
- Soothing
- Cooling
- Antiseptic
- Antifungal

NOTES AND DOSAGES
- Aloes are easily grown as a house plant. Cut the leaf and apply the gel directly to the skin, or take 1 tablespoon, twice daily, as an internal medicine. The cut leaves will keep and can be used again. There are many excellent preparations of aloe in the stores—follow the instructions on the packet. The fresh aloe is unsurpassed for burns, irritable rashes, and sunburn. Keep some in the freezer for immediate use.

CAUTION
The gel is safe, but preparations of the whole leaf are strongly laxative and should not be used for long periods or in pregnancy.

ALTHEA OFFINCIALIS
MARSHMALLOW

A wild plant easily grown in gardens. Use the root and leaves. It grows up to 4ft. (1.5m) tall, with pale pink flowers. Its name comes from the Greek word *altho*, meaning "to cure."

USES
- For acid stomach, heartburn, ulcers, hiatus hernia, and irritable bowel.
- Helps nonproductive and dry coughs.
- Irritable bladder.
- Dry skin, taken as a tea.
- Powdered root mixed into a cream or added to water to make a paste for insect bites and weeping eczema.

MARSHMALLOW PASTE
This is an especially effective preparation for insect bites and stings. Take enough marshmallow root powder to cover the affected area, and add cold water to make a stiff paste. Apply thickly and allow to dry. Wash off and replace the paste every 2 or 3 hours.

PROPERTIES
- Soothing
- Mucilaginous

NOTES AND DOSAGES
- Can be taken freely. For best results soak 1oz. (25g) cut root or leaf in 2 cups (500ml) cold water overnight. Strain and drink 3 cups daily.

ANGELICA ARCHANGELICA AND ANGELICA SINENSIS
ANGELICA ROOT

A tall, stately plant, popular in large gardens. The root should be dug up in the fall of the plant's first year, dried quickly, and stored in an airtight container. It will retain its medicinal properties for several years.

USES

- Tincture or decoction for convalescence, persistent fevers, indigestion, and weak digestion in general, colic and cramping pains, coughs, poor circulation, and general weakness with feelings of cold.
- Chinese angelica (Dang Gui or *Angelica sinensis*) is an especially good tonic for women. In China it is called "women's ginseng." It is used for menstrual cramps and pains, anemia, and general debility in women.

CANDIED ANGELICA

Cut the stems into 1in. (2.5cm) lengths and simmer in sugar water until they are soft. Strain. Simmer in a sugar syrup (2 cups [500g] sugar in 1 cup [250ml] water) for an hour. Strain and allow to dry. Sprinkle with powdered sugar and store in an airtight tin. Dose: 2in. (5cm) strip every few hours.

PROPERTIES

- Warming and restorative
- Antiseptic
- Diuretic
- Diaphoretic
- Expectorant

CAUTION

Angelica root is contraindicated in diabetes, as it increases the sugar level in the blood. Avoid large doses in pregnancy, except as advised by a qualified herbalist. The amounts taken in food are harmless. Some people's skin is sensitive to handling the fresh plant.

ARCTIUM LAPPA OR ARCTIUM MINUS
BURDOCK

A common wayside plant with large leaves and purple flowers. The root is commonly used.

USES

- For "eruptive" and stubborn skin conditions, especially when hot and inflamed-looking—for example, acne, spots, boils, rashes, psoriasis, rheumatism, and gout.

PICKLED BURDOCK ROOT

Wash the root and cut into small rounds. Simmer in water until soft. Strain and put into a clean jar. Pour hot cider vinegar over the root. Label and date. Dose: As a tonic, chew a piece first thing every morning. As a digestive, chew a piece 20 minutes before your meals.

PROPERTIES

- Blood cleanser
- Alterative
- Diuretic
- Lymphatic cleanser

NOTES AND DOSAGES

- Take 2 teaspoons of dried root, decocted, daily, or 1 teaspoon of the tincture twice daily for some months. For lack of appetite, take the tincture 3 times daily, before meals, in a little water or fruit juice, 5–10 drops for children and 20 drops for adults. Pickled burdock root makes a good daily tonic, digestive, and blood strengthener. It is a useful way to use the roots after weeding.

CAUTION

Large doses may cause a cleansing rash. It is best to start with small doses and then slowly increase them. Avoid in early pregnancy except with expert advice.

ARCTOSTAPHYLOS UVA-URSI
AVA URSI LEAVES

A small evergreen shrub of moors and mountains, also known as bearberry. The leaves are astringent and have a high tannin content.

USES

- For cystitis, together with soothing herbal remedies such as marshmallow.
- With horsetail or nettle for irritable bladder with persistent frequency.
- With lady's mantle or shepherd's purse for thick, white vaginal discharges.
- Take along with agrimony for diarrhea.

PROPERTIES

- Diuretic
- Urinary antiseptic
- Astringent

NOTES AND DOSAGES

- For tea, use 1 teaspoon dried leaves to 1 cup water and infuse for 10 minutes.
- For acute cystitis, take 1 cup of tea, or 1 teaspoon of tincture, 2 or 3 times daily for up to a week.
- Take in combination with the suggested herbs for long-term use.

CAUTION

Do not use during pregnancy or breast-feeding, or during kidney disease. Do not use for more than two weeks without consulting a professional herbalist.

ASTRAGALUS MEMBRANACEUS
ASTRAGALUS

A herbaceous perennial plant of the pea family. The root is used for therapeutic purposes.

USES

- Decoction or tincture for chronic fatigue, persistent infections, night sweats, multiple allergies, and glandular fever.
- Modern research shows that the herb helps to counteract tiredness and lack of appetite in patients undergoing chemotherapy and radiotherapy for cancer.
- Soothing and healing for stomach ulcers.

PROPERTIES

- Helps to strengthen the immune system
- A famous Chinese tonic

NOTES AND DOSAGES

- Standard doses (*see pages 94–95*). Called Huang Qi.
- The root can be bought in Chinese herb stores.
- It is often used as a soup stock with other nourishing herbs for people with severe immune deficiencies.
- Immune-enhancing soups can be made using astragalus root, which has a mild, sweet taste.

CAUTION

A safe herb for home use, but severely debilitated patients should always be seen by a professional herbalist, who will prescribe according to the individual's condition and circumstances. Always tell the hospital if you are taking herbal medicine in conjunction with their treatment.

CALENDULA OFFICINALIS
MARIGOLD FLOWERS

A popular garden plant with orange or yellow flowers. Do not confuse it with French and African marigolds (*Tagetes* species), which must not be taken internally.

USES

- Digestive colic, stomach, and duodenal ulcers.
- Speeds post-operative healing, reduces adhesions.
- Children's infections and fevers; as a gargle for sore throats and tonsillitis.
- Wash, cream, or compress for boils, spots, inflamed wounds, painful varicose veins, leg ulcers, sore nipples in nursing mothers, and sore eyes.
- Douche or bath for thrush and vaginal infections.
- Lotion or cream for itchy skin rashes, grazes, cuts, broken chilblains, eczema, and fungal infections.

MARIGOLD TINCTURE

Also sold as calendula lotion. Compresses and fomentations: 2 teaspoons tincture to 1 cup water. Dip cloth into water, wring out. Use cold water to soothe and draw heat, for sprains, congestive pain, and hot joints. Use hot water (compress is called a fomentation) to relax and encourage circulation. For spasm, stiffness, and cold joints. Wrap around affected part. Cover.

PROPERTIES

- Lifts the spirits
- Antispasmodic
- Antiseptic
- Antifungal
- Healing and anti-inflammatory

NOTES AND DOSAGES

- Add 2 or 3 flowers to 1 cup of boiling water. Infuse for 10 minutes. Drink 3 cups a day, or 1 cup every 3 hours for acute complaints. Half dose for children over five years old. Give infants 3 or 4 teaspoons of a weak tea in fruit juice.

AVENA FUTUA
WILD OATS

A wild grass, and the origin of cultivated oats (*Avena sativa*). The whole plant (called oat straw) is used, picked while still green. Cultivated oats may be substituted.

USES

- Weakness and nervous exhaustion. A good remedy for helping to "keep on the go."
- Restless sleep from overexcitement.
- With valerian to ease the symptoms of withdrawal from tranquilizers.

OAT WATER

Take 2 teaspoons of porridge oats and rub well between your fingers. Add to 1 cup of cold water. Stir well and leave for 20 minutes. Stir again and pass through a tea strainer. Makes a soothing drink for diarrhea, cystitis, and stomach upsets caused by antibiotics.

PROPERTIES

- Nourishing and restorative to nerves and reproductive organs
- Antidepressant
- Strengthening

NOTES AND DOSAGES

- For oat straw, make a tea with 2 teaspoons to 1 cup of water. Infuse for 15 minutes.
- For oats in general, buy the tincture. Use 20 drops every 2 hours when you need to keep going or 1 teaspoon 3 times daily for weakened states.
- Eating porridge is beneficial to the nervous system and helps lower cholesterol levels.
- For a bath, fill a muslin bag with porridge oats and hang it under the hot faucet, so that the water flows through it.
- Preparations of oats for making baths can also be bought at general and herbal pharmacies.

CAPSICUM MINIMUM
CAYENNE

The kitchen spice, also called chili pepper. There are many different types of pepper spices made from red peppers, varying in strength from the mild paprika to the hottest cayenne.

USES

- Poor circulation, chills, and inefficient digestion in the elderly.
- Externally for cramps and muscle spasm, aches and pains, cold and stiff joints, post-shingles neuralgia, and for unbroken chilblains.

OAT WATER

Make an infused oil using: 1 dessertspoon cayenne pepper, 2 dessertspoons powdered mustard seed, 2 teaspoons powdered ginger root, 1 cup unblended vegetable oil, sunflower or grapeseed oil. Use as a rub for cold joints and muscle spasm.

PROPERTIES

- Circulatory stimulant
- Antispasmodic
- Carminative

NOTES AND DOSAGES

- People with poor circulation can add capsicum to any herbal medicines, with benefit.
- Capsicum-based creams, liniments, and infused oils should only be used on small areas and rubbed in well.

CAUTION

Use only in very small quantities. A small pinch of the powder or 5–10 drops of the tincture is sufficient for a single dose. Avoid applying to inflamed areas. Avoid getting it into your eyes. Can aggravate acidity and heartburn.

CODONOPSIS PILOSULA
CODONOPSIS

A sprawling herb with yellow, bell-shaped flowers, grown in China. The roots of this plant are used for medicinal purposes. Codonopsis can be purchased in Chinese herbal pharmacies as Dang Shen.

USES

- For general debility, exhaustion, weakness, lack of appetite, chronic diarrhea, excessive perspiration, acidity, chronic coughs, asthma, and shortness of breath.
- Used as a decoction, a tincture, or as a powder sprinkled on food.

SOUP OF THE "FOUR GENTLEMEN"

This is a famous traditional Chinese digestive and energy tonic. It is made from codonopsis, white atractylodes (Bai Zhu), Chinese angelica (Dang Gui), poria (Fu Ling), and licorice. Add 1oz. (25g) of the herb mixture to 1 pt. (500ml) of water. Simmer for 15 minutes, strain, and drink daily.

PROPERTIES

- Soothing and strengthening
- An immune system tonic

NOTES AND DOSAGES

- Take 1oz (25g) of the powder daily, sprinkled onto soups or made into a decoction.
- Codonopsis is also known as the poor man's ginseng.

CAUTION

Safe but best used for long-term debility. Use other herbs in acute conditions.

CHAMOMILLA RECUTITA
CHAMOMILE

A wild plant with small, daisy-like flowers. It is the flowers that are most often used for therapeutic purposes. Chamomile is an aromatic plant, and it was used as a strewing herb in the Middle Ages.

USES
- Anxiety, tension, headaches, and insomnia.
- For any kind of digestive upset—acidity, heartburn, wind, and colic.
- Lotion, cream, or bath for itchy skin conditions.
- For restless and overexcitable children, and for most children's complaints, including fevers and teething troubles. Especially helpful for infants.

CHAMOMILE COMPRESS FOR SORE AND INFLAMED EYES OR SKIN

Put a handful of dried chamomile flowers into a bowl. Slowly pour on boiled water, stirring all the time until they make a mash. Allow to cool. Wrap in a length of cotton and apply. Leave on for at least 15 minutes.

PROPERTIES
- Calming and soothing
- Anti-inflammatory
- Antiseptic
- Antispasmodic
- Digestive

NOTES AND DOSAGES
- May be taken freely.
- As a sedative make a double-strength tea, using 2 teaspoons of flowers or 2 tea bags.
- Use a covered vessel, so the steam does not escape.

CAUTION
Can cause an allergic rash, but this disappears on stopping use of the herb.

CRATAEGUS OXYCANTHA OR CRATAEGUS MONOGYNA
HAWTHORN BERRIES AND FLOWERING TOPS

The berries and flowering tops of the common may tree. Hawthorn's Latin name comes from Greek words meaning hard (wood), sharp, and thorn.

USES
- Heart failure. If you are taking drugs for heart problems, seek professional advice before taking any herbal medicine.
- Irregular heartbeat.
- Helpful for angina and high blood pressure.
- With nervine herbs such as valerian and linden, for anxiety with palpitations.

HAWTHORN BRANDY

This is the nicest way of taking hawthorn as a heart-strengthening tonic. Pick the flowering shoots (with flowers and leaves), wash, dry, and pack into a large jar. Cover with brandy and leave in a cool place for two weeks. Strain off the liquid, bottle, and label. Dose: 4 teaspoons daily.

PROPERTIES
- Strengthens the heart
- Lowers blood pressure
- Relaxes arteries

NOTES AND DOSAGES
- Standard dose (*see pages 94–95*). Make a tea of the flowering tops or a decoction of the berries. Tincture: take 1 teaspoon in a little water twice daily. For heart disease, take this dosage for at least 6 months.

DIOSCOREA VILLOSA
WILD YAMS

The rhizome of a Mexican wild yam. The dried root retains its medicinal value for up to a year.

USES

- Stomach cramps, nausea, vomiting, hiccups, recurrent colicky pains, pain of diverticulitis, and gall bladder pains. With a little ginger for a quicker action.
- Menstrual cramps, and pain on ovulation.
- Menopausal symptoms, vaginal dryness.
- Useful for the treatment of rheumatoid arthritis.

DECOCTION FOR ARTHRITIC PAINS

Take 1oz. (25g) each of wild yam root and willow bark. Add to 6 cups (1.5l) water. Simmer together for 20 minutes. Strain. The decoction will keep in the refrigerator for two or three days. Dose: ½ cup 3 times daily, adding honey to taste.

PROPERTIES

- Anti-inflammatory
- Antispasmodic

NOTES AND DOSAGES

- Standard doses (*see pages 94–95*).
- Works especially well on persistent and recurrent problems.
- Wild yam is the starting point for synthesization of hormones for the contraceptive pill and for "natural progesterone," used in a prescription cream for menopause.

ECHINACEA AUGUSTIFOLIA AND ECHINACEA PURPUREA
ECHINACEA ROOT

Purple cone flower, a native plant of the U.S. Echinacea is the best way of ridding the body of microbial infections. It is effective against both bacteria and viruses.

USES

- For a weak immune system where patient suffers chronic tiredness and is susceptible to minor infections.
- For boils, acne, duodenal ulcers, flu, herpes, and persistent infections.
- As a gargle and mouthwash for sore throats, tonsillitis, mouth ulcers, and gum infections.

PROPERTIES

- Antiseptic
- Stimulates the immune system

NOTES AND DOSAGES

- For acute conditions, take large doses, 1 cup of the decoction or 1 teaspoon of the tincture every two hours for ten days.
- For chronic conditions use in combinations and take ½ cup of the combined decoction or 1 teaspoon of the combined tincture, 3 times daily.

EQUISETIUM ARVENSE
HORSETAIL

A weed which is common on damp ground. Horsetail reproduces by spores, like ferns. Galen, a physician of ancient Greece, used horsetail to heal sinews.

USES

- For irritable bladder with urgency and frequency.
- For blood in the urine.
- For bed-wetting problems, with cramp bark or St. John's wort.
- For arthritis.
- Strengthens nails and hair.
- Speeds healing after surgery.
- Compress for infected, weepy skin conditions.

PROPERTIES

- Styptic
- Diuretic
- Strengthens the bladder
- Antifungal

NOTES AND DOSAGES

- The healing properties of horsetail are due to its high content of silica and zinc.
- For a decoction, simmer 1 teaspoon in 2 cups of water for half an hour.
- Drink twice daily for one month.
- Make up a pitcher and keep it in the refrigerator.

CAUTION
Avoid large doses in early pregnancy.

FILIPENDULA ULMARIA
MEADOWSWEET

The leaves, stalks, and flowers of a wild plant common in damp meadows. The flowers are very fragrant, and the plant was a medieval strewing herb. Culpeper described it as a help to acquiring a "merry heart."

USES

- Acid stomach, heartburn, ulcers, and hiatus hernia. Combines well with comfrey, marshmallow, and chamomile.
- With peppermint or chamomile for indigestion, diverticulitis, and wind.
- Helpful for rheumatism and arthritis. Clears sandy deposits in urine.

TEA FOR ACID STOMACHS

Take equal parts of meadowsweet, chamomile flowers, and comfrey leaves, dried. Mix together and store in a clean jar. Use 1 teaspoon of the mixture to 1 cup boiling water. Allow the tea to steep for 10 minutes. Drink 3–6 cups daily.

PROPERTIES

- Antacid
- Astringent
- Anti-inflammatory
- Diuretic
- Calming for overactive digestive systems

NOTES AND DOSAGES

- Standard doses. Half dosages for children and elderly people. Will give quick relief for stomach pains, but best results come from long-term use.

CAUTION
Large doses and strong teas may cause nausea in some people.

FOENICULUM VULGARE
FENNEL

A familiar cooking herb—the leaves and seeds are used. Fennel has feathery leaves and grows to about 6ft. (2m.). It was traditionally reputed to instil strength and courage.

USES

- For colic, wind, and irritable bowel.
- For breast-feeding; helps milk flow and reduces colic.
- For anxiety, depression, and disturbed spirits.
- For arthritis and water retention or edema.
- For griping in infants, give the tea in teaspoon doses, as much as they will take, or add 2 teaspoons to milk formulas.

FENNEL EYE BATH

Fennel tea, diluted 1:1 with water and with the addition of a pinch of salt helps ease tired, dry eyes and maintain clear vision. As with any liquid used for the eyes, absolute cleanliness must be observed. Strain the tea through a very fine strainer before use, and make fresh every day.

PROPERTIES

- Warming
- Carminative
- Antispasmodic
- Antidepressant
- Promotes milk flow in nursing mothers

NOTES AND DOSAGES

- Standard doses.
- Fennel seed tea bags are easily available— remember to cover the cup to avoid losing any goodness.
- Traditionally taken during fasts to reduce hunger.

CAUTION
Remember that any blood in the urine should always be investigated by your physician.

FUCUS VESICULOSIS
BLADDERWRACK

A common dark brown seaweed found in the U.S. and Europe. Also called kelp.

USES

- A nourishing tonic.
- Obesity with tiredness and dry skin.
- Cellulite, chronic dry skin, and stubborn constipation. Regular use will delay the progress of arthritis and hardening of the arteries. A good tonic for old age.
- For children with slow mental and physical development.

BLADDERWRACK LINIMENT

To make an excellent liniment for rheumatism and arthritis add 1oz. (25g.) of dried bladderwrack to 2 cups (500ml.) of water. Simmer for a half-hour. Strain and add to an equal amount of comfrey infused oil (*see page 95*). Shake before use and rub in well twice daily.

PROPERTIES

- Nourishing and soothing.
- Stimulates the thyroid gland.

NOTES AND DOSAGES

- Take 1 tablet 3 times a day, or follow the instructions on the packet.
- When using powder, 1 or 2 teaspoons may be sprinkled on to cooked meals or soups.
- Half doses for children.

CAUTION
Avoid in overactive thyroid conditions, except with professional guidance. Not recommended for children under five. It is best to seek advice before using herbs for weight loss.

GINKGO BILOBA
GINKGO LEAVES

Leaves of the maidenhair tree, originally from China and often grown in parks. The tea, tincture, and tablets treat poor circulation, thrombosis, and varicose veins.

USES

- For poor circulation, thrombosis, varicose veins, cramp which comes on walking, white finger, and spontaneous bruising.
- Especially helpful for failing circulation to the brain in elderly people.
- Strengthens memory.
- Often improves deafness, tinnitus, vertigo, and early senile dementia.
- Helpful in asthma.

PROPERTIES

- Improves blood flow
- Strengthens blood vessels
- Anti-inflammatory
- Relaxes the lungs

NOTES AND DOSAGES

- The tea is best taken in large doses—at least 3 cups a day for some months. It is a pleasant drinking tea. Tablets are available—follow the dose on the packet.

GLYCYRRHIZA GLABRA
LICORICE ROOT

A sweet root used in confectionery and medicine (often mixed with other herbs for long-term use).

USES

- Irritable, dry coughs and bronchitis.
- Stomach, acidity, heartburn, ulcers, colitis, and intestinal infections.
- With other strengthening herbs for exhaustion.
- In creams for inflamed psoriasis and hot and weepy skin conditions.

PROPERTIES

- Soothing and anti-inflammatory
- Strengthening and up-building
- Expectorant

NOTES AND DOSAGES

- For bronchitis take ¼oz. (5g) of the powdered root 3 times daily with honey or in capsules, for up to 2 weeks. For a decoction use ½ teaspoon to 1 cup of water—take 3 cups daily. Half this for long-term use. Boiling the decoction for an hour and then drying it out in a low oven produces an extract that is easy to take.

CAUTION

Can cause water retention and raised blood pressure. Large doses can be laxative. Prolonged use should be avoided if you suffer from high blood pressure.

HARPAGOPHYTUM PROCUMBENS
DEVIL'S CLAW

The tuber from a South African plant, which survives in very arid conditions. Devil's claw contains a glycoside called harpagoside that helps to reduce inflammation in the joints.

USES

- Decoction or tincture for all types of arthritis, especially for inflamed joints and arthritis affecting a number of joints.
- For gout, lumbago, sciatica, and rheumatism.
- For itchy skin with no obvious cause.

DEVIL'S CLAW CAPSULES

Capsules are a good way of producing a customized remedy, and useful if you do not want to take a lot of liquid decoctions. Dose: two capsules three times daily. Buy 120 empty gelatin capsules from a herb store. Get out a flat dish and a coffee grinder. Powder 1oz. (25g.) chopped devil's claw in the coffee grinder (some stores sell it pre-ground). Put the powder in the dish. Fill each capsule by pushing the halves through the powder.

PROPERTIES

- Bitter tonic and anti-inflammatory

NOTES AND DOSAGES

- Decoction: ½ teaspoon to 1 cup of water, 2 cups a day. Tincture: 1 teaspoon twice daily. Tablets are available in most health food stores—follow the dosage on the box. For acute flare-ups, double the dosage for a week or two.

CAUTION
Avoid in pregnancy. May aggravate stomach acidity. Do not use in gastritis and with ulcers.

HAMAMELIS VIRGINIANA
WITCH HAZEL BARK AND LEAVES

A small U.S. tree often grown in gardens for its fragrant yellow spring flowers. The bark and leaves are used.

USES

- External use only for bruises, cuts, oily skin, spots, broken capillaries, piles, and painful varicose veins.
- As a compress for sprains, phlebitis, sunburn, and hot, swollen joints.
- As a compress and wash for hot and tired eyes.

WITCH HAZEL COMPRESS
Take 1oz. (25g.) cut bark and 2 cups (500ml.) water. Simmer together for 10 minutes. Strain and allow to cool. Dip a cloth into the decoction, wring, and apply for a half-hour, wetting it again as needed. Suitable for sunburn, swollen and inflamed joints, and aching varicose veins.

PROPERTIES

- Astringent
- Anti-inflammatory
- Antiseptic
- Styptic

NOTES AND DOSAGES

- Distilled witch hazel and other preparations are easily available. The decoction and tincture are stronger but tend to stain clothes. Dilute the tincture with 3 parts of water to use as a compress or lotion.

HYPERICUM PERFORATUM
ST. JOHN'S WORT

A common European wild plant, now a weed in many parts of the world. The tops of the plant are picked in full flower. It is easy to grow, but make sure you get the right species—perforatum has oil glands in the leaves which show up as transparent dots against the light.

USES
- Neuralgia, sciatica, and back pain.
- Pain from deep wounds.
- Mild depression. (Not for severe depression.)
- Tincture for shingles, cold sores, and herpes.
- Cream for sore skin, inflamed rashes, and cuts.

ST. JOHN'S WORT OIL

Pick the flowering tops. Put into a pestle, add a small amount of a pure, light vegetable oil such as sunflower oil. Pour just enough to cover, then pound together to crush, bruise, and start releasing the oil. Put into a large clear glass jar. Cover with more oil so that all of the herb is well covered. Shake well. Then add another inch of oil. Leave outside in direct sunlight for 20 days. The oil will turn red when it is ready. Use for skin, healing nerve damage, as a base for massage oils, or as a salve.

PROPERTIES
- Strengthens the nervous system and speeds healing
- Analgesic
- Antiviral
- Anti-inflammatory

NOTES AND DOSAGES
- Standard doses. It may be a week before depression begins to lift. The best preparations for external use are the infused oil and creams based on the infused oil (*see above*). For nerve damage, you may need to continue use for some months.

LEONURUS CARDIACA
MOTHERWORT

A European wild plant with a tall spike of small pink flowers. Self-seeds readily in the garden. Culpeper wrote, "...there is no better herb to drive melancholy vapors from the heart ... and make the mind cheerful, blithe and merry."

USES
- Anxiety with palpitations and irregular heartbeat.
- Tachycardia from an overactive thyroid.
- With skullcap or valerian, for tranquilizer withdrawal.
- With vervain for anxiety from stress and overwork.
- With sage for menopausal hot flashes.
- For menstrual cramps, taken on a regular basis.
- Take daily during the last two weeks of pregnancy to help with the birth.

MOTHERWORT AND LEMON BALM TEA

Make an infusion, or tea, by pouring a cup of boiling water on to 1–2 teaspoonful of the dried herb. Leave to infuse for 10–15 minutes. The tea should be drunk 3 times a day. Motherwort and lemon balm tea combines motherwort's sedative effect and lemon balm's antidepressant qualities. Mix together equal amounts of dried motherwort and lemon balm (*Melissa officinalis*) herbs. Store in a clean jar and label. Take as a regular tea for depression.

PROPERTIES
- Calms the heart and relaxes the womb
- Antispasmodic
- Emmenagogue

NOTES AND DOSAGES
- Standard doses of decoction or tincture. May take a few weeks to work.

LYCIUM BARBARUM OR LYCIUM CHINENSE
LYCIUM FRUIT

The bright red fruit of a Chinese shrub, grown in Europe as a hedging plant. It is a deciduous shrub, growing to 8ft. (2.5m.) tall and spreading to about 15ft. (5m.). Lycium bears pinkish flowers and grows well even in poor soil.

USES

- General weakness with vertigo, tinnitus, and recurrent headaches.
- For impotence and premature ejaculation.
- Convalescence, with equal parts of schisandra; improves skin color and restores strength.
- Failing eyesight.
- Aches and pains, especially backache, particularly in old age.

EYE – STRENGTHENING SOUP

Take 1oz. (25g.) lycium fruit, 3 chopped carrots, and a sliced onion. Add to 1pt. (500ml.) soup stock made with chicken or vegetable stock cubes. Simmer until the vegetables are cooked. Strain and blend. Take regularly to "nourish the vital essence and benefit vision."

PROPERTIES

- Tonic for old age and associated weakness

NOTES AND DOSAGES

- Also called wolfberry and the Duke of Argyle's tea plant. Chinese herbalists call the berries Gou-qi-zi. Tincture: ½fl. oz. (15ml.) with a little water daily. Dried fruit, ½oz. (10g.) daily chewed or in decoction. Traditionally, the berries are added to soup to help strengthen eyesight.

MENTHA PIPERITA
PEPPERMINT LEAVES

One of the most popular herb teas in the world. Easily grown in gardens, but is a rather invasive plant. Try growing it in a bucket buried in the ground, with the bottom knocked out.

USES

- Indigestion, colic, wind, nausea, vomiting, depressed appetite, menstrual cramps, and gall bladder pain. Adding a couple of drops of the essential oil to hot water, and drinking it, or sucking a strong peppermint sweet, is also effective.
- With elderflower and yarrow for colds, sinus problems, and blocked nose. Inhale the steam as you drink.

COOLING PEPPERMINT DRINK FOR HOT WEATHER

Make a weak peppermint tea using ½oz. (12g.) peppermint and 2 cups (500ml.) water. Add the juice of one lemon. Cool in the refrigerator, add ice and a sprig of fresh mint. Drink freely to avoid the debilitating effects of heat.

PROPERTIES

- Digestive
- Carminative
- Antispasmodic
- Mild stimulant
- Emmenagogue
- Cooling on the skin

NOTES AND DOSAGES

- Take freely. A small amount of peppermint may be added to most herb teas for flavor.

CAUTION

Avoid large does in pregnancy. The amounts taken in food are harmless. Not suited to infants; use catmint, which has the same properties and is more suitable.

PANAX GINSENG AND ELEUTHERO COCCUS SENTICOSUS
GINGSENG-SIBERIAN GINSENG ROOT

A famous tonic of the Far East, where it is very widely used. The word "ginseng" is said to mean "the wonder of the world."

USES

- Convalescence, exhaustion, lack of concentration, weakness in old age.
- With other strengthening herbs for getting rid of persistent infections.

GINSENG TONIC WINE

1oz (25g) powdered ginseng, 4 dried apricots, 8 blanched almonds, 4 cardamom pods (optional), 4 cups (1l.) red or white wine to taste. Put ingredients together, stand for 2 weeks, and strain. Drink a small glass (¼ cup) daily.

PROPERTIES

- Replenishes vital energy
- Strengthens the immune system
- Adaptogenic
- Increases concentration

NOTES AND DOSAGES

- Dose: 100mg. of powdered root, 300mg of cut root in decoction, or 20–30 drops of the tincture twice daily. Best suited to old and weakened people.

CAUTION

Not to be taken in pregnancy. May aggravate anxiety and irritability. Avoid with high blood pressure. Do not take large doses in conjunction with stimulants. Not for children, except under professional guidance.

PLANTAGO MAJOR OR PLANTAGO LANCEOLATA
PLANTAIN LEAF

The broad-leaved plantain or the ribwort plantain are common weeds of pathways and lawns. It was said to spring up wherever the English established a colony, giving rise to its common name of "white man's foot."

USES

- Running nose from allergies, irritation, and colds.
- Irritable bowel and irritable bladder.
- Compress or lotion for insect bites, allergic rashes, and infected eczema, cleaning wounds, drawing stings, and splinters.
- Soothes neuralgic pains and shingles rash.
- Cream or ointment for bleeding piles.
- The tea is a cooling drink for persistent fevers and is a useful addition to any medicine given to "hot" people.
- Mouthwash for sore and bleeding gums.

PLANTAIN LOTION

Finely chop sufficient fresh plantain leaves to fill a small jar. Add sufficient glycerin to cover the leaves. Stand for 2 weeks, stirring from time to time. Strain and store in a dark bottle. Makes a soothing and healing lotion for weeping and itchy rashes and insect bites.

PROPERTIES

- Soothing
- Healing
- Astringent

NOTES AND DOSAGES

- Double-strength tea (2 teaspoons per cup) for most purposes. Take it freely.

THE HEALING REMEDIES SOURCEBOOK

RHEUM PALMATUM AND RHEUM OFFICINALE
RHUBARB ROOT

Chinese rhubarb, also called turkey rhubarb. Edible garden rhubarb is a hybrid of this. *Rheum palmatum* is a perennial growing to a height of 6ft. (2m.), with 2ft. (60cm.) leaves.

USES

- Constipation, acute liver and gall bladder diseases.
- Feelings of congestion and fullness in the stomach.
- Stomach acidity.
- Gastroenteritis and diarrhea from food poisoning.
- Gout.
- Traditionally used in cancer.
- As a poultice for abscesses.

LAXATIVE WINE

Warm a glass of white wine (don't boil). Pour on to 1 teaspoon of chopped rhubarb root. Add a good pinch of cinnamon powder and stand overnight. Strain and drink.

PROPERTIES

- Laxative
- Astringent
- Bitter tonic
- Cooling

NOTES AND DOSAGES

- Half the standard dose: ½ teaspoon to 1 cup of water for decoction, or 30–40 drops of the tincture, 3 times daily.

CAUTION

Avoid in pregnancy, except as advised by a qualified herbalist. Not used in bowel spasm or when colicky pains are present. Avoid taking laxatives for long periods. Do not eat rhubarb leaves.

ROSMARINUS OFFICINALIS
ROSEMARY LEAVES

Late-flowering woody shrub. The whole plant smells, and it is almost impossible to pass by a rosemary bush without pinching a few leaves and rubbing them between the fingers to release the smell.

USES

- Depression.
- Headaches associated with gastric upsets. Take rosemary with chamomile for stress-related headaches.
- Poor circulation, taken regularly.
- A useful addition to any herbal medicine for conditions associated with cold and poor circulation.

ROSEMARY VINEGAR

Take 1oz. (25g) rosemary and 4 cups (1l) cider vinegar. Leave the rosemary to steep in the vinegar for two weeks. Shake occasionally. After two weeks, strain, bottle, label, and date. Use 2–4 teapoons in the final rinsing water when washing hair. For dandruff, massage rosemary vinegar thoroughly into the scalp 20 minutes before washing.

PROPERTIES

- Lifts the spirits
- Improves circulation
- Carminative
- Gentle bitter tonic

NOTES AND DOSAGES

- Standard doses used freely. Add 15 drops of essential oil to a bath to ease muscular tension, improve circulation, and boost spirits.

CAUTION

Avoid large doses in pregnancy, except as advised by a qualified herbalist. Do not use for treating headaches and migraines that feel "hot." The amounts taken in food are harmless.

RUBUS IDAEUS
RASPBERRY LEAVES

The leaves from the raspberry bush. Raspberries grow best in rich, moist, well-drained soil, and prefer a sunny position.

USES
- To promote an easy birth by tonifying the uterus.
- A mouthwash for sore mouths, sore throats, weak gums, and mouth ulcers.
- With marshmallow and peppermint for diverticulitis.
- Children's diarrhea and oral thrush. For infants, put raspberry leaf tea in a sterilized spray bottle and spray into the mouth 3 or 4 times daily.

RASPBERRY VINEGAR
This is made with the raspberry fruit. Fill a large jar with fresh raspberries. Cover with cider vinegar and stand in a cool place for two weeks. Strain and store in clean bottles. As a gargle for throats, dilute the vinegar with two parts of water to use.

PROPERTIES
- Astringent
- Antispasmodic
- Especially applicable to the womb

NOTES AND DOSAGES
- Standard doses. For tablets, follow the dose on the packet. To prepare for birth, the herb needs to be taken for at least 2 months. Continue for 3 or 4 weeks afterward to retone the womb quickly.

CAUTION
Avoid in early pregnancy except with professional advice—best taken during the last three months. Otherwise a safe herb.

RUMEX CRISPUS
YELLOW DOCK ROOT

A common wild plant, often used for blood and skin diseases. It contains anthraquinones, which act on the bowel and relieve constipation.

USES
- Chronic constipation.
- Liver congestion with poor fat digestion, and for feelings of heaviness which come on after eating.
- Stomach acidity, and for irritable bowel syndrome with constipation.
- Food poisoning and intestinal infections, to clear the source of irritation out of the digestive system.

LAXATIVE SYRUP
Take ½oz. (12g.) dried root, 1 cup (250ml.) of water and one stick of cinnamon. Simmer together for 20 minutes, then strain. Reduce over low heat to ¼ cup (50ml.). Add 4oz. (100g.) sugar. Stir over low heat until dissolved. Dose: 6 dessertspoons for adults; 3 for children and pregnant women.

PROPERTIES
- Astringent
- Laxative
- Bitter tonic
- Alterative

NOTES AND DOSAGES
- Make the decoction using ½oz. (12g.) yellow dock root to 2 cups (500ml.) water. For constipation, 1 cup of decoction or 2 teaspoons of tincture daily. More might be needed for short periods. Use half this dose for chronic conditions, for children, and for constipation in pregnancy.

CAUTION
Always consider dietary chances for stubborn constipation.

SALIX ALBA
WHITE WILLOW BARK

Bark from the willow tree. *Salix alba* is a 50ft. (15m.) silver-gray deciduous tree. A decoction or tincture of white willow treats arthritis, back pain, and lessens sexual desire.

USES

- All types of arthritis, especially with inflamed joints, and for gout. With celery seed for multiple painful joints.
- With cramp bark for inflammatory back pain, and lumbago.
- Chronic diarrhea.
- Take together with rosemary for headaches.
- Sexual overstimulation, wet dreams, and for premature ejaculation.
- Convalescence and low-grade recurrent fevers; feeling of being overheated in the evenings.

WILLOW BARK AND GINGER DECOCTION

Take 2 heaped teaspoons dried willow bark and 1 heaped teaspoon ginger powder. Add to 2 cups of water. Simmer together for 10 minutes. Strain. Add honey to taste and drink. Take freely, as needed, for chills, chronic diarrhea, and as a strengthening drink in convalescence.

PROPERTIES

- Anti-inflammatory
- Mild painkiller
- Anaphrodisiac
- Tonic

NOTES AND DOSAGES

- Take standard doses (*see pages 94–95*) and persist. Willow bark contains aspirin-like compounds, but it does not upset the stomach. It can be used to reduce dependency on aspirin and other anti-inflammatories.

SALVIA OFFICINALIS
SAGE LEAVES

The common garden and cooking herb. The purple or red variety is stronger, but any variety will suffice. Sow seeds in late spring, in well-drained soil. Choose a sunny position. The plant grows to about 2ft. (60cm.).

USES

- Depression and nervous exhaustion, post-viral fatigue, general debility.
- Anxiety and confusion in elderly people, or accompanying exhaustion and weakened states.
- For indigestion, wind, loss of appetite, and mucus on the stomach.

SAGE AND VINEGAR POULTICE

Bruise a handful of fresh sage leaves by flattening them with a rolling pin. Place in a pan and cover with cider vinegar. Simmer very gently until the leaves are soft. Wrap the leaves in a cloth and apply warm for bruises, swellings, and stings.

PROPERTIES

- Astringent
- Stimulant
- Antiseptic
- Carminative
- Antispasmodic
- Nervine
- Generally strengthening
- A woman's tonic

NOTES AND DOSAGES

- Traditionally, 1 cup a day maintains health in old age. For an extra strength, gargle, add 5 drops of tincture of myrrh (from pharmacies or herb stores) to 1 cup of sage tea. Sage tincture can be taken instead of the cold tea, for stopping night sweats—4 teaspoons daily, in a little water.

CAUTION

Avoid if allergic to salicylates (aspirin) Not suitable for children.

SAMBUCUS NIGRA
ELDERFLOWERS

The creamy white flowers from a small tree common in hedgerows and on wasteland. The tree is in flower for only three weeks in the summer. Elderflower ointment has long been a remedy for chilblains and chapped hands.

USES

- Take the tea or tincture for sinusitis, colds, running nose, hay fever, and flu.
- To break a fever with hot, dry skin—it will induce sweating, bring down the temperature, and protect the kidneys.

ELDERFLOWER NOSE WASH

Elderflower nose wash is useful for sinusitis and hay fever. Make a cupful of a strong infusion, allow it to cool to blood heat, and add a pinch of salt. Sniff the mixture up each nostril in turn, then allow it to run out or use a special nasal bath. Use daily during the hay fever season.

PROPERTIES

- Restorative for mucous membrane and sinuses
- Diaphoretic
- Diuretic
- Anti-inflammatory

NOTES AND DOSAGES

- The hot tea is taken freely, up to 1 cup every 2 hours, for colds and fevers; 3 cups a day for chronic colds and sinusitis. For children over five, use half doses. Eating fresh elderflowers will relieve the symptoms of hay fever, as will drinking a tea made with equal parts of elderflowers and eyebright (*Euphrasia officinalis*). To prevent hay fever, take 3 cups a day, starting two months before your regular season. For colds and runny noses in infants, add 3 or 4 cups of elderflower tea to their daily bath.

SCHISANDRA CHINENSIS
SCHISANDRA BERRIES

The red berries of an ornamental vine grown in China. The Chinese use schisandra berries to relieve spontaneous sweating.

USES

- Weakness with nervous exhaustion and sleeplessness; exhaustion from prolonged hard work.
- Loss of sex drive in women and men; restores softness to the skin.
- Dry and chronic coughs, and asthma.
- Night sweats.

SCHISANDRA WINE

Add 4oz. (100g.) dried schisandra berries to a bottle of rice wine. Store in a cool place for four weeks. Drink a small wine glass twice daily. For weak lungs with recurrent coughs, and to keep skin soft in old age.

PROPERTIES

- Astringent
- Nourishing
- Soothing expectorant

NOTES AND DOSAGES

- Called Wu Wei Zi in Chinese herbalism. Also available from specialist herb stores. Dose: tincture—take 1 teaspoon three times daily; dried berries—take ½oz. (10g.) daily by decoction.

SERENOA SERRULATA
SAW PALMETTO BERRIES

The fruit of a small palm-like plant grown in the West Indies and the U.S. The berries are gathered from early fall to the middle of winter, and dried for storage.

USES
- Prostate enlargement and cystitis.
- With damiana for weakness and impotence in men.
- Helps restore weight after severe illness.
- Failure to thrive in children, with marshmallow; take 10–15 drops of the combined tincture three times daily in fruit juice.

SAW PALMETTO AND NETTLE ROOT TINCTURE
Dig up, wash, and finely chop two or three handfuls of fresh nettle roots. Place in a jar and cover with saw palmetto tincture (available from specialist herb stores). Leave for two weeks, shaking from time to time. Strain and bottle. Dose: 30 drops, 3 times daily, for prostate problems.

PROPERTIES
- Strengthening tonic
- Urinary antiseptic
- Alterative
- Stimulates sex hormones

NOTES AND DOSAGES
- Decoction: ½ teaspoon of the crushed berries to 1 cup water. Adult dose: 1 or 2 cups daily. Tincture: 20–40 drops, in water, 3 times daily.

CAUTION
Avoid in early pregnancy except with professional advice. Always have suspected prostate problems medically checked.

SILYBUM MARIANUM
MILK THISTLE SEED

A tall, beautiful thistle that can easily be grown. The seeds resemble sunflower seeds. The seedheads are stored in a warm place to release the seeds.

USES
- For "liverishness" and liver disease, poor fat tolerance, pale stools, and to protect the liver when taking strong drugs and medicines.
- Depression which comes on following hepatitis.
- For treating gallstones and for inflammation.
- Useful for Candida and food allergies.
- High blood pressure with liverish symptoms.

PROPERTIES
- Strengthens and clears the liver and gall bladder.

NOTES AND DOSAGES
- Standard decoction: ½ cup 3 times daily for at least six months. Tablets are also available—follow the instructions on the box. Recent research indicates it may be useful in hepatitis C.

CAUTION
Liver disease should be treated by a professional.

SCUTELLARIA LATERIFOLIA OR SCUTELLARIA GALERICULATA
SKULLCAP

U.S. skullcap, which is easily grown in gardens, or European skullcap, which grows wild on river banks.

USES

- Anxiety, tension headaches, PMS; for exam nerves, and to help fight off post-exam depression.
- With valerian or chamomile and linden flowers for insomnia and disturbed sleep, and for tranquilizer withdrawal.

EXAMINATION TEA

Mix together equal parts of dried skullcap, linden flowers, and sage leaf. Store in a jar in a dark place. Make a tea in the normal way, using 1 teaspoon of the mixture to 1 cup of boiling water. Drink 1 cup before examinations or 3 cups a day whilst studying.

PROPERTIES

- Strengthens and calms the nervous system
- Antispasmodic

NOTES AND DOSAGES

- Standard doses (see pages 94–95). There are many relaxing tablets available at various stores containing skullcap and other herbs. Follow the dosage on the box.

CAUTION

Some years ago commercial preparations were found to contain germander, which is poisonous. Always buy your herbs and herbal preparations from a reputable firm.

SYMPHYTUM OFFICINALE
COMFREY

A common wild plant with large, bristly leaves and clusters of purple flowers. Comfrey root is used for treatment. One common name for comfrey is "knitbone," testifying to its healing powers.

USES

- Comfrey promotes rapid healing of cuts, wounds, sprains, and broken bones when taken as a tea or tincture, or used in poultices, creams, and liniments.
- Clean wounds well before applying comfrey.
- As a cream for cracked, dry skin.
- With chamomile and meadowsweet for hiatus hernia and stomach ulcers.

PROPERTIES

- Healing
- Mucilaginous

NOTES AND DOSAGES

- Standard doses (see pages 94–95). Add a few drops of a warming essential oil, such as black pepper, to the infused oil to make a good liniment for arthritis, bunions, and aches and pains arising from old injuries. Comfrey ointment is a traditional soothing and healing preparation for sprains, and aches and pains.

CAUTION

There has been suspicion of liver damage from using comfrey root and from eating large amounts of the herb. The herb tea and tincture are safe to use, but it is sensible to avoid them in pregnancy, during breast-feeding, and for infants. Preparations of the root are not taken internally.

TABEBUIA AVELLANEDAE
PAU D'ARCO

A tree from the South American rainforest. Also called lapacho and the Taheebo tree. It is particularly useful in the treatment of immunodeficiency diseases.

USES
- Immune deficiency with susceptibility to infections.
- Good for diarrhea and intestinal infections.
- Traditionally used for cancer. Recent research has shown that the herb may be helpful for breast, liver, and prostate cancers. May be taken in conjunction with orthodox cancer treatment.

TONIC SOUP
Make a decoction with ½oz. (12g.) Pau D'arco and 4 cups (1l.) water. Strain. Chop a small onion, two cloves of garlic, and a dozen oyster fungi. Simmer in the decoction until soft. Chop a small bunch of watercress and add to the soup just before serving. Eat daily for a weak immune system.

PROPERTIES
- Immune tonic
- Antibiotic
- Antifungal

NOTES AND DOSAGES
- Make half-strength decoctions, ½oz. (12g.) Pau D'arco to 2 cups (500ml.) water. Drink 3 cups daily. Tablets and capsules are available—follow the doses on the packet.

CAUTION
Large doses may cause nausea. People with blood clotting disorders should seek professional advice before taking the herb.

TANACETUM PARTHENIUM
FEVERFEW

A small-flowered daisy, easily grown in gardens. Use the leaves, which should be picked just before the plant flowers. Feverfew is good for period pains, vertigo, and arthritis. The name is a corruption of the word "febrifuge."

USES
- For migraine and arthritis.
- Combined with valerian for migraine linked with anxiety and tension.

FEVERFEW PREPARATIONS
There are many preparations of feverfew on the market, although many people still find that the fresh plant is the most effective.

PROPERTIES
- Anti-inflammatory
- Antispasmodic
- Emmenagogue

NOTES AND DOSAGES
- The best preparation is the tincture made from the fresh plant. Dose: 1 teaspoon in a little water at the first signs of a migraine; repeat after 2 hours if necessary. For repeated attacks and as a treatment for arthritis, take 1 teaspoon every morning. If you have a plant, 2 or 3 medium-sized leaves equal 1 teaspoon of tincture.

CAUTION
Not to be taken in pregnancy or during breast-feeding. Avoid giving to small children. Do not take if using blood-thinning drugs such as warfarin. Chewing the leaf can cause mouth ulcers in some people; if this is the case, use the tincture or capsules.

TARAXACUM OFFICINALIS
DANDELION LEAF

The leaves from the familiar weed, which can be picked at any time. The leaves can be cooked and eaten like spinach, and are good for a springtime cleansing tonic. Dandelion leaf tea relieves edema and water retention.

USES

- Tea for all types of water retention and edema, especially for swollen ankles which are associated with circulatory problems.
- Take with uva ursi or thyme for cystitis.

BLANCHED DANDELION LEAF

This stimulates digestion and is excellent to include in daily salad for cases of poor appetite, weak digestion, and liver, and for general convalescence. Put a large pot upside down over a growing plant to keep out the light. Leave for two weeks or until the leaves are white. Dose: two leaves daily.

PROPERTIES

- A powerful diuretic
- Nourishing

NOTES AND DOSAGES

- Use 2 or 3 teaspoons of the dried herb to 1 cup of boiling water. Drink freely. Take sufficient to produce a good flow of urine. Contains vitamins A and C and many trace minerals, and is especially high in potassium. The fresh leaves are a tasty salad ingredient.

TARAXACUM OFFICINALIS
DANDELION ROOT

The bitter dandelion root is a favorite in folk medicine, and particularly useful for stimulating a sluggish liver. The root of the dandelion is more effective than the leaves and stem in the treatment of liver problems. Coffee made from dandelion root is available, and it is thought to have a tonic effect on the pancreas, spleen, and female organs.

USES

- For all types of liver and gall bladder problems.
- For indigestion, loss of appetite, and constipation in pregnancy.
- For arthritis and stubborn skin disease in combination with burdock.
- Research shows that regular use helps reduce cholesterol.
- The liver plays a crucial role in detoxification and nutrition, hence dandelion root is helpful in most chronic and wasting diseases, and helps the body to cope with strong chemical drugs.

DANDELION COFFEE

Although dandelion is a wonderful plant, it does not always grow where it is wanted. When weeding, keep the long taproots. Scrub all the dirt off the roots, chop into pieces, and roast in a medium oven until dry and slightly burned. Make a decoction and take 1 or 2 cups a day as a liver strengthener and tonic.

PROPERTIES

- Liver tonic
- Promotes good digestion
- Alterative

NOTES AND DOSAGES

- At least 3 cups of decoction a day for 6 months. Tincture: 4–6 teaspoons daily. The decoction is best for liver problems.

TILTA EUROPEA
LINDEN

A tree often grown in parks and along streets. Its wood is good for carving, as it will take fine detail. Use the flowers, which are also called limeflowers. *Tilea europea* grows to 35m. (120 ft.). Its flowers are toxic to bees.

USES

- For anxiety, irritability, and insomnia. Long-term use strengthens the nervous system and improves tolerance of stress.
- Improves digestion, nervous indigestion.
- Induces sweating and reduces temperature in fevers. Suitable for children. Use at standard tea strength and take freely.

LINDEN FLOWER BATH FOR INFANTS

Especially good for dry skin and eczema with irritability. Take ½oz. (12g.) dried linden flowers and 2 cups (500ml.) water. Put into pan and bring to the boil, cover, and allow to stand for 15 minutes. Add to the baby's bath.

PROPERTIES

- Calming and soothing
- Strengthens nerves
- Antispasmodic
- Diaphoretic

NOTES AND DOSAGES

- Standard doses (*see pages 94–95*). May be taken freely. A popular everyday tea in France. Linden mixes well with other herb teas.

CAUTION
Old or improperly dried flowers are said to be somewhat narcotic. Reject stale-smelling and discolored flowers. Store carefully.

TURNERA DIFFUSA
DAMIANA

A small, strongly aromatic shrub grown in South America. The leaves are used for therapeutic purposes. They treat depression, anxiety, poor digestion, cystitis, and are a tonic for the reproductive system.

USES

- For impotence and sterility associated with anxiety, especially in men.
- For physical weakness, depression, mental stupor, and nervous exhaustion in both sexes.
- For prostatitis and relief of chronic cystitis.

DAMIANA COMBINATION FOR HERPES

Combine equal parts of tinctures of damiana and echinacea. Dose: 1 teaspoon every four hours. This will often avert an attack, if taken at the first signs. Alternatively, make a decoction with equal parts of the herbs and take ½ cup every four hours.

PROPERTIES

- Stimulant tonic for the nerves and reproductive system in both sexes
- Aphrodisiac

NOTES AND DOSAGES

- Take ½ cup of the tea or 1 teaspoon of the tincture twice daily. Alternatively, combine damiana with other herbs, such as wild oats or saw palmetto, and use 1 cup of the combination tea, or 1 teaspoon of tincture, twice daily.

CAUTION
Safe but quite stimulating. Do not exceed the recommended dose.

THYMUS VULGARIS
THYME

The popular thyme used in cooking recipes. Thyme is an attractive small perennial herb. It is easy to grow and thrives in the rock garden or a sunny well-drained border. There are many different garden varieties.

USES

- For any cough with infected or tough phlegm.
- Helpful, if taken regularly, in asthma.
- Specific for the treatment of whooping cough.

THYME SYRUP

Thyme makes an ideal antiseptic expectorant cough syrup. This recipe is for a tight chest and restless unproductive cough. Take ½oz. (12g.) thyme, 1oz. (25g.) chamomile, 1 teaspoon cinnamon, a pinch of cayenne or ginger (optional). Make a decoction, reduce, and add sugar or honey. Take as directed.

PROPERTIES

- Antiseptic
- Antibacterial
- Antifungal
- Expectorant
- Digestive tonic

NOTES AND DOSAGES

- Take freely. Large doses might be needed for coughs. For infants' coughs, 2 or 3 teaspoons of syrup up to 4 times daily. Make a chest rub from the infused oil. For children's worms, ¼–½ cup strong tea before breakfast, for 2 weeks.

CAUTION

Avoid large doses in pregnancy, except as advised by a qualified herbalist. The amounts taken in food are harmless. Asthma can be serious and should be treated by a professional.

ULMUS FULVA
SLIPPERY ELM BARK

The inner bark of a small U.S. tree, usually sold powdered. It smells rather like fenugreek, but tastes bland. It is very nutritious, as well as having healing properties.

USES

- Any sort of inflammation or irritation in the digestive tract: nausea, indigestion, wind, food allergies, stomach ulcers, acidity, heartburn, hiatus hernia, colitis, diverticulitis, and diarrhea. One of the most useful herbs for treating digestive problems.
- Mix with sufficient water to make a paste for drawing splinters.

SLIPPERY ELM AND CHAMOMILE POULTICE

Mix together 4 teaspoons each of slippery elm powder and dried chamomile flowers. Add hot water, slowly, stirring all the time to make a paste. Wrap the warm paste in light cotton and apply. Leave in place for a half-hour. Soothing and healing for any kind of painful swelling.

PROPERTIES

- Soothing
- Mucilaginous

NOTES AND DOSAGES

- Tablets flavored with carminative herbs are especially useful. Take 1 or 2 with a glass of water or milk before meals. For travel sickness and nausea in pregnancy, suck one tablet slowly. Stir 1 level teaspoon of powder into a drink, and take 3 times daily before meals.

VALERIANA OFFICINALIS
VALERIAN ROOT

The root of a wild plant with pretty pink flowers. In the Middle Ages, it was used as a spice and a perfume, as well as a medicine.

USES

- Anxiety, confusion, migraines, insomnia, and depression with anxiety.
- Useful when flying.
- Palpitations.

VALERIAN SLEEPING MIXTURE

Mix together equal amounts of tinctures of valerian root, dandelion root, and chamomile flowers (some specialist stores will make up the mixture for you). Store in a dark bottle and label. Adult dose: 1–3 teaspoons in a little water before bed for sleeplessness with tension or from indigestion.

PROPERTIES

- Sedative
- Nerve restorative
- Calms the heart
- Antispasmodic
- Carminative

NOTES AND DOSAGES

- The cold decoction is best: soak 1 teaspoon in 1 cup of cold water overnight. Dose: ½–1 cup. Tincture: 20–60 drops 3 times daily. More may be needed to help with tranquilizer withdrawal. Relaxing tablets containing valerian are widely available.

CAUTION

A safe herb in general use. Causes hyperactivity in some people. Very large doses can cause temporary giddiness. Do not take for long periods without examining why you are so tense. Tranquilizer withdrawl should only be undertaken with psychological support.

URTICA DIOICA
NETTLE

The common stinging nettle, which grows all over the world. Plants have either male or female flowers, which is suggested by the name *dioica*, meaning "two houses." Nettles produce a good textile fiber.

USES

- Iron deficiency anemia. Nourishing and building, good to take in pregnancy.
- For lethargy, weakness, and feelings of heaviness in the body.

NETTLE SOUP

Young nettle tops gathered in spring provide an unusual vegetable, which can be made into a nourishing soup. Pick 2 cups (500ml.) of the tops of young nettles, avoiding too much stem. Chop two medium potatoes, a carrot, and a small onion. Add the ingredients to twice as much water and boil until the potatoes are soft. Blend in a food processor. Serve seasoned to taste.

PROPERTIES

- Iron tonic
- Mild diuretic
- Antihistamine
- Strengthening
- Styptic

NOTES AND DOSAGES

- Standard doses (*see pages 94–95*). Leave to infuse for 15 minutes for best effect.
- The tops can be cooked as spinach or made into soup.
- Rubbing stiff joints with fresh nettles gives instant relief.

CAUTION

May be too drying for some people, in which case take with marshmallow.

VERBASCUM THASPUS
MULLEIN

A beautiful wild flower with a tall, thick spike of yellow flowers. Use the leaves and flowers. Mullein is demulcent, emollient, and astringent, good for lung complaints and diarrhea.

USES

- For deep and ticklish coughs and bronchitis. Helpful in asthma, by clearing sticky mucus.
- Mullein flower infused oil as ear drops for itchy ears and chronic earache, and as a salve for itchy eyelids.
- Mullein and garlic infused oil to soothe the pain of acute earache.
- Two drops of mullein flower infused oil, in a little juice, three times daily, is helpful for bed-wetting.

MULLEIN AND GARLIC INFUSED OIL

Pick the spike from a mullein in full flower. Make an infused oil (*see the instructions on page 95*). This is used for itchy ears. Fill a small jar with chopped garlic and cover it with the mullein oil. Leave overnight. Strain and use as drops for ear infections.

PROPERTIES

- A soothing expectorant
- Clears mucus
- Heals wounds

NOTES AND DOSAGES

- The tea gives the best results for coughs. Allow the mullein to infuse for a long time and drink freely.

CAUTION
Do not use eardrops if the eardrum has burst.

VERBENA OFFICINALISA
VERVAIN

An unprepossessing wild plant with a spike of small, pale pink flowers. Often missed. Vervain is a nourishing tonic.

USES

- Exhaustion and post-viral fatigue. Exhaustion from overwork. Vervain is a useful general tonic.
- Nervous depression.
- Fevers and flu, especially accompanied by headaches and nervous symptoms.
- Insomnia and excessive dreaming; also for feelings of paranoia.

SLIPPERY ELM AND CHAMOMILE POULTICE

Prepare a vervain flower remedy (*see page 206*) or buy a bottle of the prepared flower remedy stock. Add 4 drops of this remedy to 1 cup of vervain tea, standard strength. Drink 2 or 3 cups daily to relieve tiredness and tension resulting from overwork.

PROPERTIES

- Tonic
- Fever herb
- Nerve restorative
- Antispasmodic
- Carminative
- Diuretic
- Promotes milk flow
- Emmenagogue

NOTES AND DOSAGES

- Standard-strength teas taken every two hours in fevers, or 3 cups a day for chronic complaints. For worms and parasites, make double-strength tea and drink before breakfast for some weeks or until better. Vervain tea is an ideal restorative for people strained by overwork, especially mental work.

CAUTION
Avoid in pregnancy. Safe for children and when breast-feeding. Large doses of the tea can cause nausea.

VIBURNUM OPULUS
CRAMP BARK

The bark from the wild form of the guelder rose. Treats nervous complaints, cramp, spasms, heart disease, and rheumatism.

USES

- For any sort of cramping pains, colic, menstrual cramps, muscle spasm, and shoulder and neck tension.
- Back pain usually involves some muscle spasm—often a dramatic improvement with cramp bark.
- For children when bed-wetting is associated with tension and anxiety.

CRAMP BARK CAPSULES FOR MENSTRUAL CRAMPS

Grind 1oz. (30g.) cramp bark and 1 teaspoon ginger powder together in a coffee grinder until you have a fine powder. Fill standard-sized gelatin capsules, available from herb suppliers. Take 2 or 3 capsules as required for quick relief from pain.

PROPERTIES

- Relaxant
- Antispasmodic
- Mildly sedative

NOTES AND DOSAGES

- Best taken freely, 1 cup of the decoction or 1–2 teaspoons of the tincture 4 or 5 times daily. May be improved by the addition of a little ginger. For children, give 30 drops of tincture, in fruit juice, three times daily.

CAUTION

Safe in general use. Some people find that large doses will lower their blood pressure, making them feel a little faint.

VITEX AGNUS-CASTUS
AGNUS CASTUS BERRIES

The fruit of a pretty, half-hardy Mediterranean shrub. *Vitex agnus-castus* is also known as chaste tree, and is reputed both to increase sex drive, and also to damp it down, as indicated by its name!

USES

- PMS with irritability, breast pain, and water retention.
- Menopausal symptoms, especially with mood swings and depression. With sage for hot flashes.
- Helps restore a regular menstrual cycle when coming off the contraceptive pill or when the cycle has been disrupted.

AGNUS CASTUS PEPPER

The dried berries have a pleasant, peppery taste, and may be powdered in a coffee grinder and sprinkled on to meals. Dose: two good pinches or ¼ flat teaspoon. Agnus castus is still used in monasteries to help the monks keep to their vows of chastity, by balancing excess male hormones.

PROPERTIES

- Balances hormones

NOTES AND DOSAGES

- The best time to take the berries is first thing in the morning, before breakfast. One cup of the decoction or 20–30 drops of the tincture in a little water, taken daily, will usually suffice.

CAUTION

May cause chances in the menstrual cycle. This is a natural part of the way the herb works. Agnus castus may be taken in conjunction with hormone drugs, but it is best to seek the advice of a professional herbalist before doing so. Not to be taken with progesterone.

ZINGIBER OFFICINALE
GINGER

Ginger is the spice made from the rhizome, or enlarged underground stem, of the herbaceous perennial plant Zingiber officinale, a member of the ginger family. Native to southern Asia, ginger is widely cultivated in Africa, Asia, Australia, and the West Indies, particularly Jamaica.

USES

- For wind, colic, and irritable bowel.
- Good for chills, colds, and poor circulation.
- For fevers, added to elderflower or yarrow tea.

CRYSTALLIZED GINGER FOR TRAVEL SICKNESS AND NAUSEA

Peel a large piece of fresh ginger and chop it into small cubes. Make a syrup by dissolving 1 cup of sugar in 4 cups of water. Add the ginger and simmer gently until the root is soft. Leave in the syrup overnight, drain, and pack in sterilized jars.

PROPERTIES

- Warming
- Carminative
- Antispasmodic
- Diaphoretic
- Anti-emetic

NOTES AND DOSAGES

- More easily tolerated than cayenne. May be added to most remedies to improve absorption and activity. A mixture of ½ teaspoon of powder to 1 cup boiling water may be taken freely. Tincture: 5–20 drops in any herb tea. Crystallized ginger helps with the control of travel sickness.

CAUTION

Avoid taking ginger in acute inflammatory conditions or using locally on hot and inflamed areas. It will be too heating.

AROMATHERAPY

THE WORD AROMATHERAPY MEANS "treatment using scents." It refers to a particular branch of herbal medicine that uses concentrated plant oils called essential oils to improve physical and emotional health, and to restore balance to the whole person. Unlike the herbs used in herbal medicine, essential oils are not taken internally, but are inhaled or applied to the skin. Each oil has its own natural fragrance, and a gentle healing action that makes aromatherapy one of the most pleasant and popular of all the available complementary therapies.

HOW AROMATHERAPY WORKS

Aromatherapy is subtle but effective when used correctly and given time to work. While one treatment may prove immediately relaxing or reviving, the effects tend to be short-lived. Regular treatments are needed to rebalance body systems and if you have been stressed or ill, it could take several weeks of treatment before you notice an improvement. The practice of aromatherapy involves using more than just the aroma of certain plant oils to treat mind and body. It is concerned with getting essential oils into the body in order to alter body chemistry, support body systems, and improve moods and emotions. This is done most effectively by massaging oils into the skin. Manipulating the soft tissues of the body has been shown to release emotional and physical tension, relieve pain, promote healthy circulation, and restore the whole person to a balanced state of health.

Massage is the method of choice for professional aromatherapists. However, for home use oils can also be added to bathwater, or applied on hot or cold compresses to swollen, painful, or bruised areas.

When applied to the skin, essential oils start to work immediately on body tissues. The molecules in the oils are so small that they can be absorbed through the pores of the skin and into the bloodstream, by which means they are carried to every part of the body. However, aroma is important, and each essential oil has its own individual scent and healing property. Inhalation can reinforce the effects of oils applied to the skin, and it is a safe way to benefit from the healing properties of oils that could cause irritation. No one knows exactly how aromas affect the mind, but it has been theorized that receptors in the nose convert smells into electrical impulses which are transmitted to the limbic system of the brain. Smells reaching the limbic system can directly affect our moods and emotions, and improve mental alertness and concentration.

THE BENEFITS OF AROMATHERAPY

Aromatherapy benefits people rather than illnesses. It is gentle enough to be used by people of all ages and states of health. Aromatherapy is not recommended as a cure for any disease. Its most potent effect is that it relaxes mind and body, relieves pain, and restores body systems to a state of balance in which healing can best take place. It is also most effective when used as a preventive or to alleviate subclinical symptoms before they escalate into disease. The therapy has been shown to be particularly effective in preventing and treating stress and anxiety-related disorders, muscular and rheumatic pains, digestive problems, menstrual irregularities, menopausal complaints, insomnia, and depression.

ANCIENT ORIGINS OF A MODERN THERAPY

Aromatic plant oils have been used therapeutically for thousands of years. The ancient Vedic literature of India, and historic Chinese and Arabic medical texts, document the importance of aromatic oils for health and spirituality. In ancient Greece, Hippocrates, the "father of medicine," used fragrant fumigations to rid Athens of plague, and Roman soldiers kept up their strength by bathing in scented oil and having regular massages. However, the Egyptians were the most noted of the ancient aromatherapists. Physicians from all over the world are reputed to have traveled to Egypt to learn aromatic techniques.

Aromatherapy is believed to have come west at the time of the Crusades. Historical records show that essential oils were used during the plague in the 14th century. In the 16th and 17th centuries aromatherapy was popular among the great European herbalists. But it was not until the 18th and 19th centuries that scientists were able to identify many of the individual components of plant chemistry.

Research enabled scientists to extract the active components of medicinal plants. Ironically, this led to the development of pharmaceutical drugs and a rejection of plant medicine. However, in the 1920s the devotion of a French chemist, René Maurice Gattefossé, initiated a modest revival in plant oils. Gattefossé discovered that lavender oil quickly healed a burn on his hand, and went on to show that many essential oils were better antiseptics than their synthetic counterparts. He coined the term "*aromatherapie*" to encapsulate the healing effect of scented oils. Later, a French army surgeon, Dr. Jean Valnet, successfully used essential oils to treat soldiers wounded in battle and patients in a psychiatric hospital. In 1964 Valnet published Aromathérapie, still considered by many to be the bible of aromatherapy.

In the 1950s Marguérite Maury, an Austrian beauty therapist and biochemist, introduced the concept of using essential oils in massage, and established the first aromatherapy clinics in Britain, France, and Switzerland. From this varied history, aromatherapy has evolved to become one of the most valued of modern complementary therapies.

ESSENTIAL OILS AND HOW THEY WORK

Essential oils are extracted from the aromatic essences of certain plants, trees, fruit, flowers, herbs, and spices. They are natural volatile oils with identifiable chemical and medicinal properties. Over 150 essential oils have been extracted, each one with its own scent and unique healing properties. Oils are sourced from plants as commonplace as parsley and as exquisite as jasmine. For optimum benefits, essential oils must be extracted from natural raw ingredients and remain as pure as possible.

ESSENTIAL OILS IN ACTION

Despite considerable research, the chemistry of essential oils is not fully understood. Each oil is composed of at least 100 different chemical constituents, which are classified as aldehydes, phenols, oxides, esters, ketones, alcohols, and terpenes. There may also be many chemical compounds that have yet to be identified. The oils and their actions are extremely complex. All the oils are antiseptic, but each one also has individual properties—for example, they may be analgesic, fungicidal, diuretic, or expectorant. The collective components of each oil also work together to give the oil a dominant characteristic. It can be relaxing, as in the case of chamomile, refreshing, like the citrus grapefruit, or stimulating, like the aromatic rosemary.

METHODS OF EXTRACTION

Essential oils are extracted from plants by a simple form of pressure known as expression, or by distillation. Most oils are extracted by steam distillation. This involves water and plant material steaming the parts of the plant to be used in order to break down the walls of the cells that store the essence. The released essence, combined with the steam, passes to cooling tanks, where the steam condenses to a watery liquid, and the essential oil floats on top. The oil is skimmed off and bottled, and the remaining liquid is sometimes used as flower or herbal water.

Within the body, essential oils are able to operate in three ways: pharmacologically, physiologically, and psychologically. From a pharmacological perspective, the chemical components of the oils react with body chemistry in a way that is similar to drugs, but slower, more sympathetic, and with fewer side-effects. Essential oils also have notable physiological effects. Certain oils have an affinity with particular areas of the body. For example, rose has an affinity with the female reproductive system, while spice oils tend to benefit the digestive system. The oil may also sedate an overactive system, or stimulate a different part of the body that is sluggish. Some oils, such as lavender, are known as adaptogens, meaning they do whatever the body requires of them at the time. The psychological response is triggered by the effect that the aromatic molecules have on the brain.

Essential oils are not all absorbed into the body at the same rate. They can take 20 minutes or several hours, depending on the oil and the individual body chemistry of the person being treated. On average, absorption takes about 90 minutes. After several hours, the oils leave the body. Most oils are exhaled; others are eliminated in urine, feces, and perspiration.

BLENDING AND USING ESSENTIAL OILS

Essential oils can be used alone or blended together. Oils are blended for two reasons: to create a more sophisticated fragrance, or to enhance or change the medicinal actions of the oils. Blending changes the molecular structure of essential oils, and when they are blended well therapists can create a "synergistic" blend, where the oils work in harmony and to great effect. To create a blend, the therapist considers not only the symptoms and underlying causes of a patient's particular problem, but also the individual's biological and psychological make-up, and personal fragrance preferences. For therapeutic purposes, it is usual to mix only three or four oils together. If you want to blend oils at home, choose two or three oils which you believe complement each other. In general, oils from the same groups (citrus, floral, spicy, etc.), and those which share similar constituents, blend well. Using the proportions detailed overleaf, mix a blend using small amounts of the strongest scented oils and more of the lighter fragrances. You can use the recipes for suggested blends in the remedies section, or create some of your own. Be guided by your own likes and dislikes—the best blend for you is often the one you find most appealing.

CREATING BLENDS

To use oils on the skin, choose a light cold-pressed vegetable oil such as grapeseed, sweet almond, or sunflower oil. For hair treatments, choose a more penetrative oil, such as olive oil or jojoba. Where you need a slightly astringent oil, try hazelnut. Add your essential oils to the base oil a little at a time. Shake the bottle well and rub a little on the back of your hand to test the scent. Adjust the quantities until you achieve the blend you want. Add about 5 percent wheat germ oil to preserve the blend. Store blended oils in labeled dark bottles, out of children's reach, and use within three months.

USING ESSENTIAL OILS SAFELY

Aromatherapy is compatible with conventional medicine and most other forms of holistic treatment. However, if you are taking medication consult your physician. Some oils are not compatible with homeopathic treatment. Aromatherapy is safe to use at home for minor or short-term problems, providing you follow certain guidelines.

- Do not take essential oils internally.
- Do not put essential oils in the eyes.
- Keep all oils away from children.
- Do not apply oils undiluted to the skin, unless it is stated that it is safe to do so.

Consult a qualified practitioner for advice and treatment if you:

- are pregnant
- have an allergy
- have a chronic medical condition such as high blood pressure or epilepsy
- are receiving medical or psychiatric treatment
- are taking homeopathic remedies
- have a chronic or serious health problem, or if a problem becomes severe or persistent
- intend treating babies or very young children

AROMATHERAPY TECHNIQUES

There are many ways to use essential oils to good effect. The most common form of treatment among professional aromatherapists is to apply diluted essential oils to the body in a full body massage. But therapists also encourage the use of essential oils at home. When massage is not possible or appropriate, there are many other ways for people to benefit from aromatherapy.

MASSAGE

Massage in itself is nurturing and therapeutic, and the rubbing action releases the fragrance of the oils and ensures that they are well absorbed into the skin. When combined with the medicinal properties of the oils, massage forms a potent healing treatment that can be relaxing or energizing; it can soothe the nervous system, or stimulate the blood and lymphatic systems to improve physical and psychological functioning. It eases pain and tension from tired, taut, or overworked muscles, and lifts the spirits. Whenever possible, try to include massage in your home aromatherapy treatments.

Basic measurements

Dilute the essential oil in a cold-pressed vegetable carrier oil such as grapeseed, sweet almond, or sunflower oil. Use up to 5 drops of essential oil to 1 teaspoon of carrier oil for adults, half that strength for children under seven, and a quarter of the strength for children under three. The only essential oils suitable for babies are chamomile, rose, or lavender. Use only 1 drop to 1 teaspoon of carrier oil.

BATHS

Aromatic baths are a simple, useful, and versatile way to use essential oils at home. They can be used to enhance moods, relax or stimulate body systems, treat skin disorders, and ease musculoskeletal pain. Essential oils do not dissolve in water, but form a thin film on the surface. The heat of the water releases their vapor and aids absorption into the skin.

Basic measurements

Fill the bath with warm water before you add the oils. For adults, add 5–10 drops of essential oil to a full bath. Use less than 4 drops for children over two, and 1 drop for babies. Stir through the water with your hand.

STEAM INHALATIONS

Inhalations are most beneficial for throat and respiratory infection, sinus and catarrhal congestion, and headaches. They are also effective for those oils that could cause irritation if applied to the skin.

The steam releases the vapors of the oils. Steam inhalations are not always suitable for asthmatics or people with breathing difficulties, and they are not appropriate for treating children and infants.

Basic measurements

Add 3–4 drops of oil to a bowl of boiling water. Bend over the bowl, cover your head with a towel, and breathe deeply for a few minutes. You can also use this method as a facial sauna.

VAPORIZERS

These can be electric, or a ceramic ring that is heated by a light bulb, but most are ceramic pots warmed by a small candle. They are a natural way to scent, deodorize, or disinfect a room, and are one of the best ways to use oils for enhancing mood and balancing the mind. Vaporizers are also useful for when young children have breathing difficulties.

Basic measurements

Add water and 6–8 drops of oil to the vaporizer. Alternatively, add the oil to a bowl of water and place by a radiator.

CREAMS, LOTIONS, SHAMPOOS, AND GELS

One of the best ways to use oils for skin care and chronic skin complaints is to add them to a cream or lotion. This is more convenient and less greasy than massage, and it also means the oils can be applied when needed to wounds, bruises, or itchy skin. Adding oils to shampoos helps with everyday hair-care problems, and using essential oils with shower gels is excellent for fatigue and hangovers.

Basic measurements

Add 1 or 2 drops of essential oil to creams, lotions, and shampoos, and massage into the skin or scalp. Choose unscented products that are lanolin-free and made from good-quality natural ingredients.

GARGLES AND MOUTHWASHES

Although essential oils should not be swallowed, mouth-washes and gargles are excellent ways to use antiseptic oils to treat mouth ulcers, gum disease, throat infections, and bad breath. These methods are not suitable for children.

Basic measurements

Dilute 4–5 drops of essential oil in a teaspoon of brandy. Mix into a glass of warm water and swish around the mouth or use as a gargle. Do not swallow.

HOT AND COLD COMPRESSES

Compresses are an effective way of using essential oils to relieve pain and inflammation. They can be either hot or cold. Hot compresses are good for muscle pain, arthritis, rheumatism, toothache, earache, boils, and abscesses. Cold compresses benefit headaches, sprains, and swelling.

Basic measurements

Add 4–5 drops of essential oil to a bowl of hot or cold water. Soak a folded clean cotton cloth in the water, wring it out, and apply over the affected area. If using a hot compress, cover with a warm towel and repeat when it cools.

NEAT: A few essential oils—such as lavender, tea tree oil, and sandalwood—can be applied undiluted to the skin. Most oils should not be used neat as they can cause irritation.

NOTE: These are average safe dilutions for essential oils. In some of the following blends these measurements may vary slightly, but are still within safe guidelines.

AROMATHERAPY MASSAGE

The techniques of massage as we know it today in the West were developed in the 19th century by a Swedish professor, Pier Heidrich Ling, and his work is the basis for massage treatment today. Different strokes are appropriate for different areas of the body. Gentle strokes are used to commence a session to relax the superficial muscles, and more vigorous strokes then stimulate the deeper muscles.

Effleurage

Effleurage is designed to sensitize your partner and prepare for the later strokes. It is particularly effective for your face. Place your hands on your partner's cheeks, fingers downward. Then stroke gently toward the ears, using the minimum pressure required to maintain contact. You can use this sliding stroke to massage the whole body if you vary the pressure and speed.

Circling

Place both hands on your partner, a few inches apart, and stroke in a wide circular movement. Press into the upward stroke and glide back down. Your arms will cross as you make the circle, so just lift one hand over the other to continue. Circle lightly in a clockwise direction over the stomach to aid digestion.

Kneading

Place both hands on the area to be massaged with your fingers pointing away from you. Press into the body with the palm of one hand, pick up the flesh between your thumb and fingers, and press it toward the resting hand. Release and repeat with the other hand, as if you were kneading dough.

SEEING A PROFESSIONAL

A first appointment with an aromatherapist lasts between 60–90 minutes. It should take place in a warm, comfortable, subtly lit treatment room, containing a massage table, clean towels, and the therapist's stock of oils. The therapist may play soft music to create a relaxing atmosphere.

Every consultation begins with the therapist taking your case history. In order to provide safe, effective, holistic treatment, he or she needs to know about your medical history and if you have come with a particular problem. As well as finding out which oils would be best to use, aromatherapists need to know which to avoid. If you are pregnant, have sensitive skin, high blood pressure, epilepsy, or have recently had an operation, some oils would be unsuitable to use. Pregnant women, for example, should avoid certain oils including thyme, basil, rosemary, clary sage, and juniper, because they may harm the fetus or induce miscarriage. The therapist will ask about your stress levels, and if you are using medication or taking homeopathic remedies. It is also important for the aromatherapist to know what sort of mood you are in and what kind of day you have had. This interview takes about 20 minutes and you may be asked to sign a consent form at the end of it.

Treatment usually involves massage. For this you will be asked to undress down to your underwear and lie on the massage table covered with a towel to keep you warm and prevent you from feeling exposed. The aromatherapist will move the towel as he or she works around your body, but will not remove it completely.

The therapist uses the information you have provided when deciding on a suitable blend of oils. Generally, the oils you like best are the ones that work best for you. Using the chosen blend, the aromatherapist will begin your massage using gentle massage strokes and may also work on pressure points of the body. During the 30–45 minutes that it takes to give a full body massage the therapist will talk very little if at all, allowing you to relax completely.

At the end of your massage, you may be advised not to bathe or shower for several hours so that the oils can be fully absorbed. The therapist may conclude the visit by giving you oils to use at home.

THE HEALING REMEDIES SOURCEBOOK

Essential Oils

ANGELICA ARCHANGELICA
ANGELICA

The healing properties of angelica were so revered in antiquity that it was called the root of the Holy Spirit. There are over 30 varieties of angelica grown around the world; at least 10 are highly valued in Traditional Chinese Medicine. Angelica root and the seeds are used to produce the essential oil, which has a musky, sweet, woody scent.

PROPERTIES AND USES

Angelica is a tonic and stimulant that seems to strengthen the immune system. Detoxifying and diuretic properties stimulate the circulation and lymphatic systems to eliminate toxins from the body, making it useful for cellulite, arthritis, and fluid retention. It relieves indigestion and flatulence, and alleviates digestive problems caused by stress. Angelica's expectorant properties are beneficial in treating colds, bronchitis, and respiratory infections. It is good for dull, congested, or irritated skin. Angelica is also believed to have an affinity with the female reproductive system.

ANGELICA TRAVEL OIL

Add 5 drops angelica, 5 drops melissa, 5 drops peppermint, and 5 drops ginger to a small dropper bottle containing 2 tablespoons (30ml.) of sweet almond. Inhale or massage a few drops into the temples or around the back of the neck to relieve jet lag or headaches. A few drops massaged in a clockwise direction around the abdomen can ease stomachache.

CAUTION

Do not use during pregnancy or if you are a diabetic. Do not use on skin exposed to sunlight. Angelica oil attracts insects.

APIUM GRAVEOLENS
CELERY SEED

Best known as a salad vegetable in Europe, celery is grown in India, China, the Netherlands, and Hungary for its essential oil. Celery seeds are crushed to produce the warm, spicy, scented essential oil. Celery has been valued throughout history for its use as a diuretic and a digestive aid.

Blends well with lemon, peppermint, juniper, fennel, lavender, bergamot, pine, tea tree, cinnamon, and other spice oils.

DETOXIFYING MASSAGE BLEND

Add 4 drops celery, 3 drops juniper, 3 drops lemon to 4 teaspoons (20ml.) grapeseed oil, and use for a full body massage.

CAUTION

Do not use during pregnancy.

ANIBA ROSAEODORA
ROSEWOOD

Most rosewood oil comes from Brazil, where it is distilled from the heartwood of the rosewood tree. Although distillation from wild trees contributes to the destruction of the rainforest, cultivated trees are also used in the production of rosewood essential oil. But for the sake of preserving the rainforests, it may be best to keep this oil, with its subtle woody floral fragrance, for special occasions, or for when no other oil is suitable.

PROPERTIES AND USES

Rosewood is a tonic and an immune stimulant, useful for infections or viruses such as colds or glandular fever. It can be used as a mild painkiller, an antidepressant, and an aphrodisiac. As a tissue regenerator, it diminishes scars, wrinkles, and stretch marks. Because it is such a gentle oil rosewood benefits sensitive or irritated skin, and its antiseptic and bactericidal properties make it suitable for acne and wounds. The oil is also used to treat coughs and headaches, especially when they are accompanied by nausea. Rosewood is an emotionally uplifting and comforting oil that helps to rebalance the nervous system in times of stress. Rosewood is nonirritant, nontoxic, and nonsensitizing.

Blends well with rose, lavender, sandalwood, frankincense, basil, patchouli, cedarwood, and most woody, citrus, and floral oils.

REPLENISHING SKIN CARE OIL

Pour 4 teaspoons sweet almond oil into a small, dark glass bottle. Add 4 drops rosewood, 3 drops sandalwood, 3 drops frankincense. Seal and shake well. Smooth over face, neck, and dry skin patches, using gentle circular movements.

BOSWELLIA CARTERI
FRANKINCENSE

Frankincense, also known as olibanum, is distilled from the resin produced by the bark of a small North African tree. Wonderfully calming and richly fragrant, the oil has a history of use as a fumigant, in embalming, and as incense. It is considered a spiritual oil, used by many to encourage meditation.

PROPERTIES AND USES

Frankincense slows the breathing and calms the nervous and digestive systems, relieving anxiety, depression, nervous tension, emotional upsets, and stress-related digestive problems. As an immune stimulant and an expectorant, it can help respiratory and catarrhal conditions such as asthma, colds, chest infections, and chronic bronchitis. Frankincense has wound-healing, astringent, antiseptic, and anti-inflammatory properties,

making it ideal for treating cuts, scars, blemishes, and inflammation, and it is recommended for firming aging skin. Frankincense is helpful for cystitis, as it has an affinity with the genitourinary system. Irregular or heavy menstrual bleeding and nosebleeds can also benefit from its gentle healing properties.

Blends well with rose, lavender, geranium, neroli, orange, bergamot, mandarin, sandalwood, pine, black pepper, cinnamon, and other spice oils.

> **CAUTION**
> Safe to use during pregnancy. Do not take it internally and keep it out of children's reach.

CALENDULA OFFICINALIS
MARIGOLD

Calendula essential oil is not widely available, as the bright orange flowers of the common pot marigold yield only small amounts of oil. More common is infused oil of calendula, where the flowers are infused in warm oil, macerated, and strained. Marigold has had a variety of historical uses, treating anything from snake bites to toothache. The famous herbalists Nicholas Culpeper and John Gerard called the flower a "comforter of the heart and spirits."

PROPERTIES AND USES

As a soothing anti-inflammatory, antiseptic, and gentle astringent, calendula-infused oil is good for dry, cracked, or chapped skin, eczema, diaper rash, cracked nipples, and varicose veins. Because it helps to stop bleeding and has valuable wound-healing properties, it is a first-aid kit essential for cuts, grazes, wounds, and insect bites. Marigold has an affinity with the female reproductive system and has properties which help to regulate the menstrual cycle. The oil can also be used as a base for blending other essential oils.

Blends well with most floral and citrus oils.

CANANGA ODORATA
VAR. GENUINA
YLANG YLANG

This is extracted from a tropical tree that grows in the
Philippines, Indonesia, the Comoros, and Madagascar. The
name ylang ylang means "flower of flowers." The name suits
the heady floral fragrance of this oil, which is distilled from
the freshly picked flowers. Ylang ylang is a traditional tropical
remedy for infections and skin diseases, but is also well known
for its use in the Victorian hair preparation, Macassar oil.

PROPERTIES AND USE

Ylang ylang is a sedative, an antidepressant, and a tonic for
the nervous system. Depression, anxiety, tension, irritability,
and stress-related insomnia can all benefit from its soothing
properties. It helps to rebalance sebum production in oily
skin, acne, and both dry and greasy scalps. It can also be
used to calm irritated skin, as well as bites and stings. Ylang
ylang is reputed to be an aphrodisiac. It can be used to treat
sexual problems. It acts as a circulatory tonic and generally
rebalances body functions. It can help to reduce blood
pressure, and slow down breathing and heart rate in cases
of shock, panic, or rage.

Blends well with rosewood, rose, bergamot, vetiver,
frankincense, chamomile, lavender, and cedarwood.

CAUTION

Can cause nausea or headaches in high concentrations.
May irritate the skin of some hypersensitive people.

CEDRUS ATLANTICA
CEDARWOOD

The aromatic oil from the evergreen cedar tree was one
of the first oils to be used in ancient medicine and ritual.
Used by the ancient Egyptians for embalming, and by
the people of the Middle East since biblical times, the
wood still provides Tibetan monks with incense, burned
to aid meditation. Cedarwood oil is extracted by steam
distillation from the wood chips. It has a rich, woody,
masculine scent that is warming, physically cleansing,
and emotionally grounding.

PROPERTIES AND USES

The antiseptic, antiseborrheic, and mild astringent
properties of cedarwood make it a popular choice for
treating acne, oily skin eruptions, and dandruff. It has
diuretic properties which benefit the urinary system
and help to relieve cystitis, and it is also used for vaginal
infections and discharges. Cedarwood is an expectorant
and mucolytic, which explains its traditional use in the
treatment of catarrhal problems, especially bronchial
congestion and infections.

ANTIDANDRUFF TREATMENT

Add 6 drops cedarwood, 6 drops rosemary,
4 drops cypress oil to 3 tablespoons (50ml.) olive
oil. Massage into the scalp with your fingertips,
cover, and leave overnight, if possible. Shampoo
thoroughly. Use half the recipe for children.

CAUTION

Do not use during pregnancy. Several varieties of cedar
trees are used to produce oil that is sold as Cedarwood.
Some of this oil is very different from Cedrus atlantica.
Always make sure you buy atlas cedarwood oil.

CHAMAEMELUM NOBILE
ROMAN CHAMOMILE

Chamomile has a long history of use as a physical and emotional soother. It is one of the most gentle essential oils available, and particularly suitable for treating children. Massage can soothe fretful or colicky babies, and the diluted oil can be rubbed into the cheek to relieve teething pain. Of the many varieties of chamomile available, Roman chamomile is one of the most commonly used in aromatherapy.

PROPERTIES AND USES

Chamomile calms the nervous system and induces sleep. It has valuable anti-inflammatory, antiseptic, and bactericidal properties. Chamomile prevents and eases spasms, relieves pain, settles digestion, and acts as a liver tonic. It can be used to relieve headaches, toothache, menstrual cramps, arthritis, and neuralgia.

CHAMOMILE COMPRESS

Fill a bowl with ice-cold or hot water and add 4–5 drops of chamomile oil. Soak a clean face cloth or folded piece of clean cotton in the bowl, and wring it out. Apply the compress to the affected area until it has cooled or warmed to body temperature. Repeat. Note: Use a cold compress for rashes, cuts, headaches, sprains, or swellings; a hot compress for arthritic or rheumatic pain, boils, abscesses, earache, or toothache.

CAUTION

Do not use in the first three months of pregnancy. Do not allow chamomile essential oil to get into your eyes. Can cause dermatitis in some people. German chamomile may be used instead or Roman Chamomile, but not chamomile *Maroc Ormenis Multicaulis*, which is not true chamomile.

CINNAMOMUM ZEYLANICUM
CINNAMON LEAF

Cinnamon is grown in India, Sri Lanka, the Comoros, and the Seychelles, but the best cinnamon oil is believed to come from Madagascar. Cinnamon was used by the Greeks, Romans, and ancient Egyptians, and its medicinal properties have long been valued by the people of India and of China. The familiar warm, spicy fragrance is also reputed to enhance psychic ability.

PROPERTIES AND USES

Cinnamon stimulates a sluggish digestion, relieves flatulence and spasms, and combats intestinal infection. It acts as a respiratory and circulatory stimulant, helping with rheumatic problems and chest infections. It helps to fortify the immune system against chills and infections, and has a cooling effect on fevers. Cinnamon also has antiseptic, antimicrobial, and parasiticidal properties, making it good for head lice, scabies, and other skin infections. Cinnamon can relieve mental fatigue, improve poor concentration and nervous exhaustion, and help to lift depression.

Blends well with ylang ylang, frankincense, orange, benzoin, mandarin, lemon, basil, lavender, and ginger.

CINNAMON ROOM FRESHENER

Sprinkle a few drops on rolled cinnamon sticks and add to potpourri made from dried orange peel, orange oil, and basil for a room freshener that stimulates and refreshes the mind, relieves tension, and soothes the nerves.

CAUTION

Cinnamon leaf oil may cause skin irritation. Use only in a 1 percent dilution, and in moderation. Do not confuse with cinnamon bark oil, which is an irritant and should not be used in aromatherapy.

CITRUS AURANTIFOLIA
LIME

Limes were traditionally used as a digestive remedy and to prevent scurvy among sailors. Lime has a fairly wide application in modern aromatherapy. It has properties similar to those of lemon, and the two oils are often used interchangeably. The essential oil is expressed from the peel of the fruit, or steam-distilled from the whole fruit.

PROPERTIES AND USES

Lime acts as an appetite and digestive stimulant, and also helps to treat the symptoms of dyspepsia. Its antiseptic, antiviral, bactericidal, and fever-reducing properties make it valuable in fighting colds, flu, fever, and chest and throat infections. It also helps to strengthen the immune system. Oily skin and conditions such as acne, boils, and warts can also benefit from these properties. Lime has a restorative, tonic effect on the whole person. It also has notable antirheumatic properties, and is known to increase mental alertness and assertiveness.

Blends well with lavender, rosemary, clary sage, black pepper, bergamot, and other citrus oils.

STAY-ALERT DIFFUSER BLEND

Fill the dish of a pottery burner with water and add 4 drops lime, 2 drops black pepper, 2 drops peppermint. Light the night light and let the heat diffuse the oil into the air.

CAUTION

Lime increases the skin's sensitivity to sunlight. Do not apply to the skin within two days of exposure to the sunlight.

CITRUS AURANTIUM VAR. AMARA
CITRUS SINENSIS, ORANGE

Originally from China, oranges have a history of use in Traditional Chinese Medicine. Dried sweet orange is used to treat coughs and colds, while bitter orange is used to treat diarrhea. The outer peel of both bitter and sweet oranges is pressed to produce the sweet, fruity orange essential oil.

PROPERTIES AND USES

As a sedative orange is good for nervous tension and related insomnia, either blended with lavender, or alternated with lavender or sandalwood. It is also a cheering oil, which enlivens the mind and dispels depression. Orange has a normalizing effect on intestinal peristalsis, making it beneficial for painful spasms, constipation, and diarrhea. It also helps to normalize blood pressure and circulation, and stimulates the lymphatic system to relieve water retention. Orange helps to fight chills, bronchitis, colds, and flu, especially when mixed with complementary winter spice oils, such as cinnamon and clove.

Blends well with lavender, ylang ylang, neroli, cinnamon, black pepper, lemon, myrrh, and clove.

MASSAGE BLEND FOR CONSTIPATION

Mix 3 drops orange, 3 drops black pepper, 4 drops rosemary, 3 teaspoons (15ml.) sweet almond or grapeseed oil. Warm a little oil in the hands; massage into the abdomen clockwise.

CAUTION

Orange oil can increase skin sensitivity to the sun. May cause contact dermatitis in some people. Do not use more than four drops in the bath.

CITRUS AURANTIUM VAR. AMARA
NEROLI ORANGE BLOSSOM

The blossoms of the bitter orange tree yield this oil, which has an exquisite fresh floral fragrance. Neroli is named after an Italian princess, Anne-Marie of Nerola, who used it as a perfume. In folk traditions, orange flowers were included in bridal bouquets as a symbol of innocence and fertility, and to calm nervous couples on their wedding night.

PROPERTIES AND USES

Neroli tones the heart and circulatory system, and its carminative and antispasmodic properties can relieve digestive problems such as indigestion, diarrhea, flatulence, and stomach cramps. Neroli helps to tone the skin and improve elasticity. Added to cream or diluted in oil, it is used to prevent stretch marks, scarring, wrinkles, and to soothe sensitive skin. It is a gentle antidepressant and a nerve tonic, perhaps most helpful in treating anxiety, depression, nervous tension, and stress-related problems. As a sedative it can also help to combat associated insomnia.

Blends well with lavender, lemon, bergamot, rosemary, rose, ylang ylang, chamomile, geranium, benzoin, and most oils.

MASSAGE BLEND FOR HIGH BLOOD PRESSURE

Add 3 drops neroli, 3 drops celery, 4 drops rose to 1fl. oz. (25ml.) or 5 teaspoons grape seed or other vegetable oil and use for gentle massage.

CAUTION
Keep all essential oils out of the eyes and never take them internally.

CITRUS AURANTIUM VAR. AMARA
PETITGRAIN

Fresh and flowery petitgrain is often regarded as a cheaper alternative to neroli. It is distilled from the leaves and twigs of the bitter orange tree, whereas neroli comes from the blossom. Both oils have similar properties and fragrances, but petitgrain is also a valuable oil in its own right, with a revitalizing and restorative character.

PROPERTIES AND USES

Petitgrain can refresh or relax, depending on which oils it is blended with. It strengthens and tones the nervous system, and as such it can soothe many stress-related problems, such as nervous exhaustion and insomnia. Feelings of apathy, irritability, mild depression, anxiety, loneliness, and pessimism can all get a lift from petitgrain's antidepressant properties. This oil also has a tonic effect during convalescence, or when one is feeling "run down." It has a notable antispasmodic effect and helps to tone the digestive system, relieving flatulence and indigestion. Petitgrain is a deodorant, sometimes used to control excessive perspiration. It is also used to control the overproduction of sebum in the skin and has gentle antiseptic properties, making it ideal for many greasy skin and scalp conditions, especially acne and greasy hair.

INVIGORATING ROOM FRAGRANCER

Add 3 drops petitgrain, 3 drops lime, 2 drops cypress to a vaporizer dish filled with water. Light and burn for 10–15 minutes.

CAUTION
Keep out of reach of children.

CITRUS BERGAMIA
BERGAMOT

The bergamot tree was originally cultivated in Italy, where the fruit has a history of use in folk medicine. The refreshing essential oil is expressed from the peel of the fruit, which resembles a small yellow orange, when it is nearly ripe. Outside Italy, bergamot is perhaps best known as an ingredient in both Earl Grey tea and eau de Cologne.

PROPERTIES AND USES

Joyous and uplifting, bergamot is a powerful anti-depressant which has a wonderfully balancing effect on moods. As an antiseptic it is good for acne and boils. Other skin complaints, such as oily skin, eczema, and psoriasis, cuts, and insect bites, can also respond well to bergamot. The oil inhibits viral activity; when diluted in alcohol, it can be dabbed on cold sores, chicken pox, and shingles. The fragrance repels insects and the oil can be used to expel worms. Bergamot has an affinity with the genitourinary system. It is a diuretic and a powerful urinary disinfectant, particularly good for cystitis. It can also be used for thrush and other types of vaginal itching and discharge. As a digestive, bergamot is sometimes used to encourage appetite. It is also used to cool fevers.

Blends well with chamomile, geranium, lemon, sandalwood, myrrh, juniper, lavender, neroli, cypress, jasmine, and tea tree.

CAUTION
Bergamot increases the skin's sensitivity to sunlight. Never use undiluted on the skin. Avoid if you have sensitive skin. Mix with a carrier oil before adding to bath water to ensure it disperses well into the water.

CITRUS LIMON
LEMON

The ancient Greeks and Romans included lemon in their medicine chest and it has a history of use in European folk medicine. The essential oil which is expressed from the fresh peel has many varied applications, making it invaluable in the home aromatherapy kit.

PROPERTIES AND USES

Lemon can stimulate the body's defenses to fight all kinds of infection. It is beneficial in treating inflamed or diseased gums, mouth ulcers, sore throats, and acne. It helps to clear colds, flu, and bronchitis, and can be used to remove warts and verrucas, and to clear herpes blisters. The oil has a tonic effect on the circulation and is often used to treat varicose veins, poor circulation, high blood pressure, and fluid retention. Lemon is both diuretic and laxative, and has the ability to stop bleeding in minor cuts and nosebleeds. As an astringent it benefits greasy skin and can also be used to reduce a fever. Because it also counteracts acidity in the body, lemon helps to relieve acid indigestion, arthritis, and rheumatism. On an emotional level, refreshing lemon dispels depression and indecision.

Blends well with geranium, fennel, juniper, eucalyptus, sandalwood, and other citrus oils.

HANGOVER BATH OIL
Add 4 drops lemon, 2 drops fennel, 2 drops lavender to a warm bath and agitate the water with your hand. Relax for 10 minutes and inhale deeply.

CAUTION
Can irritate sensitive skin. Do not use before sunbathing. Dilute well for massage and bath blends, and do not use for more than a few days at a time.

CITRUS RETICULATA
MANDARIN

As the name suggests, mandarin oil originated in China, where the small, sweet fruit was traditionally given as a gift to the Mandarin. The essential oil is expressed from the peel. It has a delicate, fruity, floral aroma and a gentle healing action.

PROPERTIES AND USES

Mandarin is used mostly for treating digestive problems. It soothes indigestion and relieves intestinal spasms. It has a mild laxative effect and acts as a tonic for the stomach. It is gentle enough for children's digestive problems and hiccups. Mandarin also tones the liver, the body's main chemical processing and elimination organ. Because it is also a mild diuretic, mandarin can help to relieve fluid retention and stored toxins. The oil can be used as a skin toner for oily skin, acne, or congested pores. As a sedative it is also used to relieve nervous tension and insomnia during pregnancy, and can help to settle restless children.

Blends well with frankincense, chamomile, lavender, rosewood, neroli, and other citrus oils and spice oils, such as clove and cinnamon.

OIL TO PREVENT STRETCH MARKS
Add 4 drops mandarin, 3 drops neroli, 3 drops lavender to a bottle containing 1fl. oz. (25ml) or 5 teaspoonsful sweet almond oil and 1 teaspoonful wheat germ oil. Massage into the abdomen twice a day from the fifth month of pregnancy.

CAUTION
Mandarin may increase the skin's sensitivity to the sun.

CITRUS X PARADISI
GRAPEFRUIT

Refreshing grapefruit oil is expressed from the peel of the fruit, cultivated mainly in California, Florida, Brazil, and Israel. It has a fresh, tangy citrus scent that enlivens the mind and disperses feelings of gloom. Unlike many citrus oils, grapefruit does not increase the skins sensitivity to sunlight.

PROPERTIES AND USES

Grapefruit is diuretic, detoxifying, and cleansing to the kidneys. It also has a stimulating effect on the lymphatic system. Because of these properties, it helps to relieve fluid retention and eliminate the toxins that cause cellulite. It is also beneficial in a massage blend to ease stiff muscles after exercise. Grapefruit tones an oily skin and scalp, is helpful in treating acne and congested pores, and can be applied neat to cold sores. It also stimulates digestion and improves immunity to infection. As an antidepressant, grapefruit oil enlivens the mind, relieves anxiety, and combats nervous exhaustion.

Blends well with orange, lemon, sandalwood, bergamot, neroli, lavender, cypress, rosemary, geranium, juniper, cardamom, coriander, and other spice oils.

WAKE-UP SHOWER GEL
Mix 2 drops grapefruit, 2 drops petitgrain, 1 drop rosemary with a dollop of unscented shower gel and work to a lather with a sponge.

CAUTION
Do not take internally. Keep out of the eyes.

COMMIPHORA MYRRHA
MYRRH

Perhaps best known as one of the three gifts brought to the infant Jesus, myrrh was valued in ancient times as an ingredient in embalming preparations, incense, and as a medicine. According to legend, the soldiers of ancient Greece took myrrh ointment into battle to treat their wounds. Essential oil of myrrh has a musty, balsamic odor and is closely related to frankincense, with which it is often linked.

PROPERTIES AND USES

Myrrh has an excellent soothing, antiseptic, and healing effect on sore or inflamed gums, mouth ulcers, wounds, and cracked or chapped skin. It can speed the healing of weepy eczema, and because of its antifungal properties it can be used as a vaginal wash for thrush or in a foot bath for athlete's foot. Myrrh is also an expectorant and a lung tonic, good for coughs, colds, bronchitis, and flu. It stimulates, tones, and soothes the digestive system, and is often used for diarrhea, hemorrhoids, and indigestion. The oil is a uterine tonic, which can be helpful for menstrual irregularities. Myrrh relieves agitation, calms fears and uncertainties, and has a positive, balancing effect on the emotions.

Blends well with frankincense, sandalwood, mandarin, lavender, lemon, rose, eucalyptus, thyme, benzoin, geranium, peppermint, cypress, pine, and spice oils.

CHAPPED SKIN CREAM
Add 5 drops myrrh, 5 drops benzoin, 4 drops geranium to 1oz. (30g.) of good unperfumed, lanolin-free cream. Mix well and apply to the skin.

CAUTION
Do not use in high doses. Do not use at all during pregnancy.

CORIANDRUM SATIVUM
CORIANDER

Coriander is a highly aromatic annual herb. Coriander seeds were used by the ancient Greeks and have also been found in Egyptian tombs. The seeds and leaves are both used in cooking, and the Chinese use the whole herb for medicinal purposes. The essential oil, distilled from the crushed seeds, has a sweet and slightly musky, spicy, and woody aroma.

PROPERTIES AND USES

Coriander's pain-relieving properties make it suitable for headaches and neuralgia. It has a warming, antirheumatic effect, good for muscular pain and stiffness, arthritis, and rheumatism. Coriander is an effective digestive stimulant and tonic, used to relieve diarrhea, flatulence, nausea, painful spasms, and to stimulate appetite in cases of anorexia. It is also a nervous stimulant, beneficial for apathy, nervous exhaustion, and fatigue. The oil's stimulatory properties also work on the circulation. As such it is useful for hemorrhoids, poor circulation, and fluid retention. Coriander is an aphrodisiac which has a warming, stimulatory effect on the emotions.

Blends well with bergamot, sandalwood, petitgrain, pine, citronella, clary sage, ginger, and other spice oils.

CORIANDER MUSCLE RUB
Add 2 drops coriander, 4 drops juniper, 4 drops black pepper to 4 teaspoons (20ml.) grapeseed oil, and massage into tired and aching muscles.

CAUTION
Use in moderation. Keep all oils out of the reach of children.

CUPRESSES SEMPERVIRENS
CYPRESS

Ancient civilizations used the tall evergreen cypress tree as a source of incense for religious ceremonies and for medicinal purposes. The oil, which is distilled from the twigs and needles of the cypress, has a pleasant, smoky, wood aroma, and a number of therapeutic uses.

PROPERTIES AND USES

Cypress is an antispasmodic, useful in a vaporizer for respiratory problems such as bronchitis or asthma, or to prevent coughing attacks. Astringent properties make it suitable for use in a wash for hemorrhoids and for excessively oily skin. It can also be applied to cuts to stop bleeding and is used as a mouthwash for bleeding gums. Cypress is a circulatory tonic, which can improve poor circulation, relieve fluid retention, and soothe muscular cramp, and can be applied gently to varicose veins. In a foot bath it counteracts excessively sweating and smelly feet. The oil is used to treat PMS, regulate the menstrual cycle, and counteract heavy bleeding. Menopausal symptoms such as hot flashes and irritability can also be alleviated by cypress.

Blends well with juniper, pine, lavender, sandalwood, lemon, mandarin, orange, bergamot, and clary sage.

VARICOSE VEIN TONER

Add 5 drops cypress and 10 drops geranium oil to 5 teaspoons (25ml.) vegetable oil. Starting at the ankle, gently stroke up the legs toward the heart.

CAUTION
Do not use undiluted on the skin.

CYMHOPOGON CITRATUS
LEMONGRASS

Lemongrass is a tall, aromatic grass. It is used as a flavoring in Thai cuisine and has been used in traditional Indian medicine for centuries. The essential oil is distilled from the grass leaves. It has a strong refreshing citrus smell that has many aromatherapy and domestic uses.

PROPERTIES AND USES

Lemongrass has a tonic effect on the nervous system and the body in general. It is also painkilling and antidepressant, good for headaches, lethargy, symptoms of stress, and beneficial for muscular pain and poor muscle tone. It has fever-reducing properties and helps the immune system to fight infections. As a deodorant, lemongrass can be used for excessive perspiration and sweaty feet, and its astringent properties make it an effective skin toner which helps to close open pores. Lemongrass is also an effective flea, lice, and tick repellent. Use it in a vaporizer to keep flies out of the kitchen in the summer and to get rid of pet smells from the home.

Blends well with lavender, orange, geranium, jasmine, rosemary, neroli, basil, sandalwood, and eucalyptus.

GREASY HAIR SHAMPOO

Add 2 drops of lemongrass to a normal dollop of mild, unscented shampoo, rub between your palms, and wash your hair as normal.

CAUTION
Dilute well, as lemongrass may cause skin irritation in some people. Do not use on babies or children. Do not use around the eyes.

CYMHOPOGON MARTINII VAR. MARTINII
PALMAROSA

In Indian Ayurvedic medicine, palmarosa has long been used to combat infectious diseases. Distilled from a fresh scented grass, similar to lemongrass, palmarosa has a gentle floral fragrance like a mix of rose and geranium. In the past it was also known as Indian or Turkish geranium.

PROPERTIES AND USES

Palmarosa is a valuable oil in skin care. The diluted oil applied to the skin rebalances sebum production, thereby hydrating dry skin conditions. It also rejuvenates wrinkled or aging skin by promoting cellular regeneration, and it helps to heal wounds. Palmarosa is beneficial for acne, dermatitis, and skin infections because of its antiseptic properties. It has a stimulatory effect on the circulatory and digestive systems, helping to increase appetite and activate a sluggish digestion. As a bactericide, the oil prevents and treats intestinal infections. Used in a massage blend, palmarosa is good for nervous exhaustion and stress-related problems.

Blends well with sandalwood, lavender, geranium, rosewood, cedarwood, frankincense, lemon, floral, citrus oils, and woody oils.

SKIN REJUVENATOR
Add 6 drops palmarosa, 3 drops rose, 3 drops frankincense to a small bottle containing 5 drops evening primrose and 3 teaspoons (15ml.) apricot kernel oil. Shake well. Gently massage into the face at night.

CYMHOPOGON NARDUS
CITRONELLA

The leaves of this tropical scented grass are valued in many countries for their medicinal properties. The essential oil, which is distilled from the dried leaves, has a strong, fresh, lemony scent. Although it is not widely used in aromatherapy, it is highly valued as a household disinfectant and insecticide.

PROPERTIES AND USES

Refreshing and uplifting, citronella helps to combat headaches, fatigue, and feelings of depression. It has strong deodorant properties, which make it suitable for refreshing tired or sweaty feet, and for treating fungal infections such as athlete's foot. In Eastern cultures it is used to settle digestion and menstrual problems, and as a rub for rheumatic pain. It makes an excellent insect repellent, either used in a room spray, vaporizer, or dropped on to a square of cotton and added to a linen cupboard to keep clothes fresh and free from moths. Cats dislike the smell of citronella, so it can be used to keep them away from areas of the garden.

Blends well with geranium, lemon, orange, cedarwood, cypress, tea tree, bergamot, eucalyptus, and pine.

REFRESHING FOOT SOAK
Add 4 drops citronella, 2 drops tea tree, 3 drops cypress to a foot bath to refresh hot and sweaty feet.

CAUTION
Do not use during pregnancy. Dilute well, as it may cause irritation to some people with sensitive skin.

ELETTARIA CARDAMONUM
CARDAMOM

This spice has been used since antiquity as a food flavoring, but it has also played a part in Indian Ayurvedic medicine for thousands of years. The Greek physician Hippocrates also acknowledged the therapeutic benefits of cardamom. The essential oil distilled from the seeds has a warm, sweet, spicy aroma and a warming quality similar to ginger.

PROPERTIES AND USES

Mainly used as a digestive remedy because of its soothing, antispasmodic, and digestive properties, cardamom is good for indigestion, flatulence, abdominal pain, heartburn, bloating, nausea, and bad breath. It has a diuretic effect which can help to relieve water retention. Cardamom also has a wonderful, stimulating, and tonic effect on mind and body; it makes a refreshing bath which can relieve fatigue and soothe strained nerves, and helps to clear the mind of confusion. In India cardamom is reputed to be an aphrodisiac.

Blends well with bergamot, rose, frankinscense, clove, ylang ylang, neroli, basil, cedarwood, fennel, lemon, and ginger.

MASSAGE OIL FOR STOMACH CRAMPS

Add 1 drop cardamom, 1 drop basil, 2 drops marjoram to 2 teaspoons (10ml.) vegetable oil and massage in a clockwise direction over the stomach and abdominal area.

CAUTION

Do not take internally. Use sparingly, as spicy oils may cause irritation in some people.

EUCALYPTUS GLOBULUS
BLUE GUM EUCALYPTUS

Several of the 700 species of eucalyptus are used to distill medicinal-quality essential oil, but the Australian "blue gum" is by far the most widely used. Eucalyptus is a traditional remedy in Australia and a familiar ingredient in numerous chest rubs and decongestants. The oil also eradicates lice and fleas.

PROPERTIES AND USES

Eucalyptus is a powerful antiseptic and renowned decongestant, used mostly for coughs, colds, chest infections, and sinusitis. It alleviates inflammation generally, and is helpful in treating rheumatism, muscular aches and pains, and fibrositis. It is a diuretic and a deodorant, with strong antiviral and immune-stimulating properties, and is an effective local painkiller, especially for nerve pain. Urinary tract problems such as cystitis respond well to eucalyptus. The oil is also used to reduce fevers and treat skin infections, cuts, and blisters, genital and oral herpes, chicken pox, and shingles. Eucalyptus eases the pain of burns and helps new tissue to form.

Blends well with peppermint, tea tree, rosemary, thyme, lavender, cedarwood, lemon, and pine.

DISINFECTANT WASH FOR INSECT BITES

Add 3 drops eucalyptus, 3 drops thyme, 3 drops lavender to a bowl of clean water. Use cotton wool or a clean cotton cloth to dab repeatedly on the affected area.

CAUTION

Do not take when using homeopathic remedies. Do not use for more than a few days at a time because of the risk of toxicity. Do not use on babies or very young children.

FOENICULUM VULGARE
FENNEL

In folklore fennel was believed to convey courage and strength and contribute to a long life. It also has a history of use as an antidote to poisons. The essential oil, distilled from the crushed seeds, is still valued for its detoxifying properties.

PROPERTIES AND USES

Fennel appears to have a rebalancing effect on hormones, probably due to an estrogen-like plant hormone. As such it helps to stabilize hormone activity during menopause and has traditionally been used to increase milk flow in breast-feeding mothers. It is a good diuretic, antimicrobial, and antiseptic which can help with premenstrual water retention and urinary tract infections. It helps to eliminate toxic wastes from the body, making it valuable in treating arthritis and cellulite. It reduces digestive spasms, calms and tones the stomach and digestive system, and has a slightly laxative effect, benefiting nausea, indigestion, constipation, and stomach cramps. Fennel also makes a good mouthwash for gum disease or infections.

Blends well with lavender, lemon, orange, peppermint, rose, geranium, juniper, sandalwood, and clary sage.

ANTICELLULITE MASSAGE OIL

Add 8 drops fennel, 8 drops juniper, 10 drops grapefruit oil to 5 teaspoons (25ml.) sweet almond oil and 5 drops jojoba oil. Store in a dark glass bottle and massage into the affected area every day after your bath or shower.

CAUTION
Use only sweet fennel (also known as Roman or French fennel), as bitter fennel should not be used on the skin. Do not use during pregnancy. Not suitable for epileptics, or children under six years old. Narcotic in large doses.

HYSSOPUS OFFICINALIS
HYSSOP

Revered as a sacred cleansing herb by the Hebrews and the ancient Greeks, hyssop has also long been valued by herbalists for its medicinal properties. Both the leaves and the small blue or mauve flowers are distilled for their essential oil, which has a strong, spicy, herbaceous scent.

PROPERTIES AND USES

Hyssop is an expectorant with antispasmodic, bactericidal, and antiseptic properties, which can be helpful for coughing, whooping cough, catarrh, sore throats, and chest infections. It can be used in skin care for cuts, bruises, and inflammation. Hyssop has hypertensive properties, making it useful in the treatment of low blood pressure, and has a general tonic effect on circulation.

As an emmenagogue, it can be used for scanty or no menstrual bleeding. The oil can also soothe indigestion and relieve colicky cramps. Hyssop's sedative and tonic properties can benefit stress- or anxiety-related problems. It helps to relieve fatigue, and increase alertness.

Blends well with sandalwood, lavender, ylang ylang, rosemary, clary sage, cypress, lemon, and other citrus oils.

INHALATION FOR CHEST INFECTIONS
Add 2 drops hyssop, 2 drops lavender, 2 drops benzoin to a bowl of steaming water. Cover your head with a towel, bend over the bowl, and inhale.

CAUTION
Dilute well and use for no more than a few days at a time because there is some risk of toxicity. Do not use during pregnancy. Do not use if you are epileptic. For people with high blood pressure, hyssop should only be used as directed by a qualified aromatherapist.

JUNIPERUS COMMUNIS
JUNIPER

Used in ancient Greece and Egypt to combat the spread of disease, juniper was still being used in French hospitals during the First World War. This warm, woody-scented oil can be distilled from juniper berries and twigs, but the best oil is produced by distilling the ripe berries only.

PROPERTIES AND USES

Juniper is physically and emotionally cleansing. It helps to detoxify the body of harmful waste products that contribute to problems such as rheumatoid arthritis and cellulite, and clears the mind of confusion and exhaustion. Juniper is also diuretic, has an affinity with the genitourinary system, and is excellent for treating cystitis. Skin problems, especially weepy eczema and acne, respond well to its toning, astringent, and antiseptic properties. Juniper is also good for hemorrhoids and hair loss, and assists with wound healing. In addition, it stimulates appetite, relieves nervous tension, and is an excellent disinfectant.

Blends well with pine, lavender, cypress, clary sage, sandalwood, vetiver, benzoin, rosemary, fennel, geranium, bergamot, and other citrus oils.

> **CAUTION**
> Do not use during pregnancy. Not suitable for people with kidney disease.

JASMINUM OFFICINALE
JASMINE

It takes huge quantities of jasmine flowers to produce a small amount of this very expensive essential oil. However, very little is needed to produce an effect, and the sensual floral perfume makes it a highly prized oil.

PROPERTIES AND USES

Jasmine has a reputation as an aphrodisiac, benefiting impotence in men and frigidity in women. It is also a uterine tonic which can help with menstrual cramp and disorders of the uterus. Its pain-relieving properties and ability to strengthen contractions make it one of the best oils to use during childbirth. It is also believed to strengthen male sex organs and has been used for prostate problems. Its relaxing and antidepressant effect helps to clear postnatal depression. It is excellent for stress relief and is uplifting during times of lethargy. Jasmine has a soothing, warming, and anti-inflammatory effect on joints and a rejuvenating effect on dry, wrinkled, or aging skin. Its antiseptic and expectorant properties also make it applicable for catarrh, and infections of the chest and throat.

Blends well with lavender, geranium, chamomile, clary sage, sandalwood, rose, neroli, and other citrus oils.

> **CAUTION**
> Jasmine may cause an allergic reaction in rare cases.

LAVENDULA AUGUSTIFOLIA
LAVENDER

Of the several varieties of lavender used medicinally, Lavendula augustifolia is the most important. Lavender is the most versatile, best loved, and most widely therapeutic of all essential oils. Both the flowers and the leaves are highly aromatic, but only the flowers are used to make essential oil.

PROPERTIES AND USES

Lavender is calming, soothing, antidepressant, and emotionally balancing. Its antiseptic, antibacterial, and painkilling properties make it valuable in treating cuts, wounds, burns, bruises, spots, allergies, insect bites, and throat infections. Because it is a decongestant, it is also effective against colds, flu, and catarrhal conditions. Lavender lowers blood pressure, prevents and eases digestive spasms, nausea, and indigestion. It is antirheumatic and a tonic. Tension, depression, insomnia, headaches, stress, and hypertension respond particularly well to its soothing properties.

Blends well with florals such as rose, geranium, ylang ylang, chamomile, jasmine, citrus oils such as orange, lemon, bergamot, and grapefruit, rosemary, marjoram, patchouli, clary sage, cedarwood, clove, and tea tree.

> **BATH OR MASSAGE BLEND FOR IRRITABILITY**
> Add 3 drops lavender, 3 drops chamomile, 2 drops neroli directly to a warm bath and disperse with your hand. Alternatively, add to 3 teaspoons (15ml.) grapeseed or sweet almond oil for a soothing massage.

> **CAUTION**
> Lavender is usually safe for all age groups, but some hay fever or asthma sufferers may be allergic. Dilute well if taking homeopathic remedies.

MELALEUCA ALTERNIFOLIA
TEA TREE

This small tree or shrub is a traditional remedy among the Aboriginal people of Australia. Originally, the leaves were made into a tea, and hence its name. More recently, scientific research has shown that tea tree oil can combat all types of infection.

PROPERTIES AND USES

Primarily an anti-infection oil, tea tree has antifungal, antibacterial, and antiviral properties. It is frequently used for skin problems such as spots, acne, warts, verrucae, athlete's foot, rashes, insect bites, burns, and blisters. It is used to clean cuts and infected wounds, and it helps skin to heal by encouraging the formation of scar tissue. Tea tree is effective against dandruff, cold sores, and urinary or genital infections such as cystitis and thrush. It is an expectorant that also alleviates inflammation and is a valuable immune stimulant. It is an excellent choice when fighting colds, flu, respiratory infections, catarrhal problems, and infectious illnesses. Tea tree is also used to bring down a fever, to kill fleas and lice, and as a deodorant.

Blends well with lavender, geranium, chamomile, myrrh, lemon, rosemary, marjoram, clary sage, pine, and spice oils such as clove and cinnamon.

TREATMENT OIL FOR ACNE

Add 4 drops tea tree, 3 drops bergamot, 3 drops lavender to 2 teaspoons (10ml.) jojoba oil, which is excellent for inflamed or acne-prone skin. Dab onto the affected areas.

CAUTION

People with sensitive skin should introduce the oil with caution. Do not swallow mouthwashes or gargles.

MELALEUCA CAJEPUTI
CAJEPUT

In Malaysia, the Philippines, Indonesia, and Australia, wild cajeput is used extensively for all manner of ills, from colds to toothache. Closely related to tea tree, this oil is distilled from the leaves and buds of cajeput, and has a distinctly medicinal camphorous odor.

PROPERTIES AND USES

Cajeput is antiseptic, antimicrobial, and it clears mucus. It is good to use in steam inhalations for colds, flu, sinusitis, asthma, bronchitis, and other respiratory infections. It has painkilling properties which can ease headaches and sore throats, and can be used to good effect on muscular and arthritic pain. The oil is also a urinary antiseptic. Used with care, it is effective against cystitis and other urinary infections. Cajeput can be used to soothe the stomach, counteract digestive spasms, and kill infections in the gastrointestinal system. It is widely used for minor conditions such as insect bites and spots. Inhalation, which is one of the best ways to use this oil, helps to dispel mental fatigue and apathy.

Blends well with sandalwood, juniper, hyssop, pine, lavender, rosemary, lemon, eucalyptus, and marjoram.

INHALATION FOR COLDS AND FLU

Add 4 drops cajeput, 3 drops rosemary, 2 drops eucalyptus to a bowl of steaming water, cover your head with a towel, bend over the bowl, and inhale for 5–10 minutes.

CAUTION

Dilute well, as cajeput is a skin irritant. Do not use as a gargle or as a vaginal wash as the oil can irritate the mucous membranes. Cajeput is a stimulant, and so is best avoided in the late evening.

MELALEUCA VIRIDIFLORA
NIAOULI

Closely related to cajeput and tea tree, niaouli is distilled from the leaves of a large tree grown in Australia and New Caledonia. It is a much more gentle oil than cajeput, and less likely to irritate the skin or mucous membranes. Niaouli, which has a strong medicinal odor, is sometimes labeled as "gomenol."

PROPERTIES AND USES

Antiseptic and bactericidal, niaouli is good for cystitis and other urinary infections. A few drops added to cooled boiled water also makes a healing antiseptic wash for cleaning minor wounds, cuts, or burns. Niaouli also stimulates the healing of burns and promotes the growth of new tissue. Oily skin, spots, acne, and insect bites can all be treated in this way. Inhalations of niaouli are helpful in all cases of colds, flu, respiratory, and catarrhal conditions. Added to a good chest rub, this oil helps to alleviate infections and stimulate the immune system. Because it is antispasmodic, niaouli can also benefit digestive problems. It has a general balancing and regulatory effect on body functions.

Blends well with frankincense, basil, clary sage, geranium, lavender, neroli, ylang ylang, and other citrus oils.

CHEST RUB FOR COUGHS

Add 3 drops niaouli, 2 drops hyssop, 1 drop myrrh to 3 teaspoons (15ml.) vegetable oil and rub into the chest.

CAUTION
Dilute well, as it may irritate the skin of some people.

MELISSA OFFICINALIS
LEMON BALM

Melissa, also known as "heart's delight," has been used medicinally since the 17th century. The fresh, lemony essential oil is distilled from the leaves and flowering tops. Unfortunately, the plant yields very little essential oil, which is why true melissa is so expensive, and why most commercial melissa oil is adulterated with other lemon oils.

PROPERTIES AND USES

Melissa helps to reduce high blood pressure, and because it also helps to calm palpitations and rapid breathing it is a good remedy for shock. The oil is often used for menstrual problems, as it has a calming and regulating effect on the menstrual cycle, helps to ease menstrual cramps, and alleviates scanty menstruation and amenorrhea. Melissa can be used to reduce digestive spasms in colic, nausea, and indigestion. It can be used to relieve migraine and combat fever. Low dilutions can be beneficial for eczema and other skin problems. Allergies affecting the skin and the respiratory system can benefit from its antihistamine properties. Melissa calms the nervous system, relieves anxiety, and has an uplifting effect on the emotions, dispelling sadness and loss, and counteracting hysteria. It also has a general tonic effect on mind and body.

Blends well with lavender, geranium, patchouli, tea tree, bergamot, rosemary, hyssop, pine, and petitgrain.

MELISSA MIND AND BODY SOOTHER

For frazzled nerves, irritability, and exhaustion, dilute 3 drops melissa, 2 drops chamomile, 2 drops bergamot in 1 teaspoon (5ml.) of sweet almond oil and add to your bath water.

CAUTION
This oil is sometimes adulterated with other lemon oils.

MENTHA PIPERITA
PEPPERMINT

Peppermint is best known as a remedy for digestive problems. It was used as such by the Romans and possibly the ancient Egyptians. Apart from its many therapeutic applications, it is also used as a humane form of pest control. Peppermint grows throughout Europe, but most oil comes from the U.S.

PROPERTIES AND USES

Refreshing and stimulating, peppermint tones and settles the digestive system. It relieves indigestion, flatulence, spasms, diarrhea, nausea, stomach cramps, and travel sickness. It also helps to tone the liver, intestines, and the nervous system. It is a valuable expectorant in the treatment of bronchitis, colds, and flu, and it can reduce fevers by inducing sweating and cooling the body. Peppermint is a painkiller, beneficial for toothache, headaches, and some migraines. It relieves itching, is a useful antiseptic for acne and congested skin, and is an emergency remedy for shock. Muscle and mental fatigue are both relieved by peppermint.

Blends well with lavender, chamomile, rosemary, lemon, eucalyptus, benzoin, sandalwood, and marjoram.

FOOT BATH FOR CHILBLAINS

Add 3 drops peppermint, 3 drops lavender, and 5 drops rosemary to a bowl of lukewarm water and soak the feet for at least 10 minutes.

CAUTION

Do not use during pregnancy. May irritate the skin of sensitive people. Do not use while taking homeopathic remedies. Do not use for long periods of time.

OCIMUM BASILICUM
BASIL

The Greeks considered basil to be a regal plant. It is also valued and widely used in Traditional Chinese and Indian Ayurvedic medicines. There are many varieties of basil, but French basil is the most commonly used in aromatherapy. This uplifting and refreshing oil has a strong spicy-sweet smell that is often most appealing in a blend with other oils.

PROPERTIES AND USES

Basil is a stimulating and antidepressant oil which relieves mental fatigue, clears the mind, and improves concentration. It is expectorant and antiseptic, used for all types of chest infections, also good for congested sinuses, chronic colds, head colds, and whooping cough. The antispasmodic and carminative properties of basil help to relieve abdominal pains, indigestion, and vomiting. It works well on tired muscles, especially in a massage oil used after hard physical work or strenuous exercise; it also eases arthritis and gout. It is reputed to be one of the best nerve tonics among all essential oils.

VAPORIZER BLEND FOR MIGRAINE

Add 3 drops basil, 4 drops lavender, 3 drops peppermint to a vaporizer. Relax in a darkened room and inhale deeply.

CAUTION

Do not use during pregnancy. May irritate people with sensitive skin. Do not use the oil from exotic basil, which is slightly toxic.

ORIGANUM MARJORANA
SWEET MARJORAM

In ancient times marjoram was reputed to promote longevity, a belief that encouraged the ancient Greeks to include it in perfumes, cosmetics, and medicine. In folk tradition marjoram was believed to bring joy to newlyweds and peace to the dead. The essential oil, with its warm, spicy scent, is still used to relieve agitation, dispel grief, and restore calm.

PROPERTIES AND USES

Marjoram is warming and pain-relieving. It also has antispasmodic properties, making it good for muscle spasms and strains. It is a sedative and nerve tonic which works to relieve nervous tension and promote restful sleep. Inhaling marjoram can help to relieve headaches and migraine. Antiviral and bactericidal properties help to fend off colds and infections, and its expectorant properties make it a useful oil to include in a steam inhalation for chest infections. Massaged into the chest or throat, marjoram can also relieve painful coughs. The oil is a vasodilator which is beneficial in treating high blood pressure and improving circulation. It also calms digestion, strengthens intestinal peristalsis, and eases menstrual cramps. Marjoram is a comforting oil that reduces sexual desire.

Blends well with bergamot, chamomile, frankincense, rose, sandalwood, lavender, rosemary, and tea tree.

MARJORAM COLD CURE

Add 4 drops marjoram and 2 drops eucalyptus to a hot bath to relieve cold symptoms, or add 2 drops to 1 teaspoon (5ml.) of vegetable oil and use as a chest rub.

CAUTION

Do not use during pregnancy.

PELARGONIUM GRAVEOLENS
GERANIUM

Potted geraniums have a long history of medicinal use. Over 700 varieties exist, and their essential oils differ depending on where the plant is grown. Fresh and floral in fragrance, geranium was traditionally regarded as a feminine oil, a powerful healer, and a valuable insect repellent.

PROPERTIES AND USES

Geranium is mentally uplifting and refreshing. It has a balancing effect on the nervous system, helping to alleviate apathy, anxiety, stress, hyperactivity, and depression. The anti-inflammatory, soothing, and astringent properties of geranium account for its success in treating arthritis, acne, diaper rash, burns, blisters, eczema, cuts, and congested pores. Antiseptic properties make it useful for cuts and infections, sore throats, and mouth ulcers. It is also a diuretic, used to relieve swollen breasts and fluid retention, and to stimulate sluggish lymph and blood circulation. Geranium helps to stop bleeding, and acts as a tonic for the liver and kidneys. It is used to treat PMS and menopausal problems, and has a balancing effect on mind and body.

Blends well with lavender, bergamot, rose, and rosewood.

MASSAGE BLEND FOR PMS

Add 10 drops geranium, 10 drops clary sage, 10 drops bergamot to a bottle containing 1 fl. oz. (30ml.) or 6 teaspoons vegetable oil and shake well. Put 6–8 drops in your bath and use a little as a body oil to massage around your abdomen, hips, and lower back.

CAUTION

Do not use during the first three months of pregnancy and not at all if there is a history of miscarriage.

PETROSELIMUM SATIVUM
PARSLEY

Common garden parsley is not only rich in vitamins, but also has significant therapeutic properties. The root is used in herbalism for digestive disorders, while the herb and seeds are used mainly for kidney and bladder problems. The essential oil, distilled mainly from the seeds, has a warm, spicy, herbaceous scent.

PROPERTIES AND USES

Used mainly as a diuretic, parsley is good for fluid retention, PMS, and cellulite, and because of its antiseptic effect, it also helps with cystitis. Parsley has a tonic effect on the reproductive system. It is sometimes used during labor and it helps to regulate the menstrual cycle. It has the ability to shrink small blood vessels and is helpful in treating piles, broken or thread veins, and bruising. Parsley is also used to stimulate appetite; it has a laxative effect on sluggish digestion, and it relieves flatulence, stomach cramps, and indigestion. Parsley has antirheumatic properties.

Blends well with geranium, rose, rosemary, lavender, bergamot, lemon, neroli, clary sage, tea tree, and spice oils.

PARSLEY BATH FOR WATER RETENTION

Add 2 drops parsley, 3 drops geranium, 3 drops fennel to a warm bath and swirl through the water with your hand.

CAUTION

Use in moderation, as parsley can be toxic and irritant. Do not use during pregnancy.

PINUS SYLVESTRIS
SCOTCH PINE

Perhaps one of the best-known natural fragrances is the fresh, invigorating aroma of pine. The Arabs, Greeks, and Romans all made use of its medicinal properties, while Native Americans are believed to have used pine to prevent scurvy and infestation with lice and fleas.

PROPERTIES AND USES

Inhalations of pine are wonderful for colds, catarrhal conditions, including hay fever and sore throats. The oil, which is expectorant, antiseptic, and antiviral, helps to clear chest infections, sinuses, and ease breathing. Pine stimulates the circulation and helps to relieve rheumatic and muscular aches, pains, and stiffness. Pine is also deodorizing and insecticidal, good for excessive perspiration, and for clearing lice and scabies. The invigorating, refreshing aroma dispels apathy, relieves mental fatigue, nervous exhaustion, and stress-related problems.

Blends well with lavender, rosemary, cedarwood, eucalyptus, tea tree, juniper, and sandalwood.

INHALATION FOR SINUSITIS AND STUFFY COLDS

Add 2 drops pine, 2 drops eucalyptus, 2 drops peppermint to a bowl of steaming hot water. Bend your head over the bowl and cover with a towel to keep in the steam. Inhale for 5–10 minutes. Do this five or six times a day.

CAUTION

Use only small amounts in the bath or in massage. Do not use if you have an allergic skin condition. Always check the source of your oil, as oils are distilled from several species of pine, some of which are unsuitable for use in aromatherapy.

PIPER NIGRUM
BLACK PEPPER

Best known for its use in cooking, black pepper also has a 4,000-year-old medicinal history. Prized by the Chinese, Romans, and Greeks, pepper was one of the earliest spices ever used. The spicy-scented essential oil is extracted from dried, crushed black peppercorns.

PROPERTIES AND USES

Black pepper stimulates the nervous, digestive, and circulatory systems, which makes it good for poor circulation, constipation, sluggish digestion, and drowsiness. It also has a laxative effect, tones the muscles of the colon, soothes the stomach, helps to prevent food poisoning, and stimulates the appetite. As a rubefacient it helps with rheumatic and arthritic pain, poor muscle tone, and muscular aches and pains. It helps the immune system fight off infections and viruses, warms against chills, and as an expectorant it clear mucus from the chest. Black pepper helps prevent anemia and is credited with aphrodisiac properties.

Blends well with frankincense, lavender, rosemary, marjoram, lavender, lemon, benzoin, cedarwood, parsley, fennel, spice oils, and floral oils.

COMPRESS FOR PAINFUL JOINTS
Add 3 drops black pepper, 2 drops chamomile, 2 drops marjoram to a bowl of hot or cold water and apply to the affected area as directed.

CAUTION
Dilute well when using on the skin. Do not use while taking homeopathic remedies.

POGOSTEMON CABLIN
PATCHOULI

The distinctive exotic and earthy aroma of patchouli is one that you either love or hate. Smell is important to the success of aromatherapy, so only use this oil if you like its scent. Patchouli has many uses, and is especially pleasant when used as part of a blend. It is an intense odor, which improves with age.

PROPERTIES AND USES

An important antidepressant, nervous tonic, and reputedly an aphrodisiac, patchouli is valued in treating depression, anxiety, nervous exhaustion, lack of interest in sex, and stress-related problems. It is astringent, antiviral, antiseptic, and anti-inflammatory, good for chapped or cracked skin and open pores, and is also effective for acne, eczema, and dermatitis. It is one of the best choices for dandruff and fungal infections of the skin. It is a cell regenerator, good for aging skins, and it promotes wound-healing. Patchouli acts as a diuretic. It is often recommended for cellulite and as a general tonic.

Blends well with rose, geranium, bergamot, neroli, ylang ylang, lemon, sandalwood, clary sage, clove, cedarwood, and lavender.

ANTIWRINKLE NIGHT OIL
Add 2 drops patchouli, 3 drops lemon, 5 drops rose to 2 drops evening primrose oil and 1 teaspoon (10ml.) sweet almond or hazelnut oil. Blend well and apply to the face and neck at night.

CAUTION
Keep all essential oils out of the reach of children.

ROSA CENTIFOLIA
ROSA DAMASCENA, ROSE

Most of the rose oil used in aromatherapy is produced from two types of rose. They vary slightly in color and fragrance, but have similar properties and uses. Rose oil is expensive, but you need only use a little of this complex oil to reap the benefits.

PROPERTIES AND USES

A renowned aphrodisiac, sedative, and a tonic with antidepressant properties, rose has an affinity with the female reproductive system, helping to regulate the menstrual cycle and alleviate PMS or post-natal depression. It benefits stress-related conditions such as insomnia and nervous tension, and is a powerful antiseptic against viruses and bacteria. Rose oil acts as a tonic for the heart, circulation, liver, stomach, and uterus, and helps to detoxify the blood and organs. It regulates the appetite, and prevents and relieves digestive spasms, constipation, and nausea. It soothes cracked, chapped, sensitive, dry, inflamed, or allergy-prone skin, stops bleeding, and encourages wound-healing. Broken veins, and aging or wrinkled skin also benefit. Rose is also useful in treating headaches, earache, conjunctivitis, coughs, and hay fever.

Blends well with most oils, especially clary sage, lavender, sandalwood, bergamot, patchouli, and ylang ylang.

COMFORTING MASSAGE BLEND FOR GRIEF

Add 4 drops rose, 2 drops frankincense, 4 drops chamomile to 3 teaspoons (15ml.) sweet almond or grapeseed oil.

CAUTION

Do not use during the first three months of pregnancy and not at all if there is a history of miscarriage.

ROSMARINUS OFFICINALIS
ROSEMARY

Rosemary was one of the first herbs to be used medicinally. Traditionally it was used to ward off evil, to offer protection from the plague, and to preserve and flavor meat. This strong, distinctively scented oil is one of the most valuable of all essential oils.

PROPERTIES AND USES

Refreshing rosemary is a circulation stimulant, excellent for low blood pressure, muscle fatigue, poor circulation, aches, pains, and strains. It acts as a tonic for the nervous system and is antidepressant. It relieves stress-related disorders, mental exhaustion, and promotes mental clarity. It also tones the skin, liver, and gall bladder. It is used for acne, eczema, dandruff, lice, and hair loss. Antiseptic and antibacterial, antifungal, and a diuretic, it is generally cleansing, and useful for fluid retention. It has properties that help to relieve painful menstruation and clear vaginal discharge, flatulence, indigestion, and constipation. Rosemary prevents and reduces digestive spasms, relieves wind, and regulates digestion. It helps to clear catarrh, coughs, colds, and headaches.

Blends well with frankincense, petitgrain, basil, thyme, bergamot, lavender, peppermint, cypress, and spice oils such as cinnamon, clove, ginger, and black pepper.

AFTER-SPORT SHOWER FORMULA

Add 2 drops rosemary, 2 drops pine, 4 drops lemon to a large dollop of a gentle, unscented shower gel. Step into a hot shower and work into a lather using a sponge or flannel.

SALVIA SCLAREA
CLARY SAGE

Affectionately known as "clear eye," clary sage was used in medieval times for clearing foreign bodies from the eyes. It remains popular in aromatherapy because of its gentle action and pleasant nutty fragrance. The oil is extracted from the flowering tops and leaves.

PROPERTIES AND USES

Clary is antidepressant, and sometimes described as euphoric. It helps to regulate the nervous system and is most beneficial in treating anxiety, depression, and stress-related problems. It acts as a powerful muscle relaxant, helping to ease muscular aches and pains, and benefits digestion, relieving indigestion and flatulence. Its astringent properties make it useful for oily skin and scalp conditions. Clary helps to prevent and arrest convulsions. It is antibacterial, and useful for throat and respiratory infections. Clary helps to lower blood pressure. It is recommended for absent or scanty menstruation and PMS, and is a renowned aphrodisiac that can benefit frigidity and impotence.

Blends well with lavender, frankincense, sandalwood, cedarwood, citrus oils, such as lemon, orange, and bergamot, geranium, ylang ylang, juniper, and coriander.

PREMENSTRUAL BATH BLEND

Add 3 drops clary sage, 2 drops chamomile, 2 drops geranium to a warm bath, disperse with your hand, and relax for at least 10 minutes.

CAUTION

Do not use during pregnancy. Do not use when drinking alcohol, as it can make you drunk, drowsy, and can cause nightmares.

SANTALUM ALBUM
SANDALWOOD

The sweet, woody, oriental smell of sandalwood is one of the most appealing fragrances of all essential oils. The best sandalwood oil comes from India, where it has been used for at least 4,000 years for medicinal and religious purposes.

PROPERTIES AND USES

Sandalwood is an antiseptic, especially effective for all urinary disorders—above all cystitis. It is bactericidal, astringent, and a trusted insect repellent. It clears catarrh and is effective for respiratory conditions such as bronchitis, dry coughs, and sore throats. The oil contains constituents that soothe the stomach, reduce digestive spasms, relieve fluid retention, and reduce inflammation. Sandalwood encourages wound-healing, and skin problems such as dry, chapped skin, acne, psoriasis, eczema, and shaving rash can all benefit from its soothing, rehydrating and antiseptic action. It is an antidepressant oil that calms the nervous system. The fragrance can also help to lift depression and banish feelings of anxiety and lack of sexual desire.

Blends well with lavender, rose, ylang ylang, geranium, chamomile, patchouli, bergamot, frankincense, black pepper, benzoin, tea tree, juniper, myrrh, and cypress.

AFTERSHAVE SOOTHER

Add 4 drops sandalwood, 6 drops benzoin, 4 drops chamomile to a bottle containing 4 teaspoons (20ml.) hazelnut oil. Warm a tiny amount in your hands and smooth into the face after shaving.

CAUTION

Do not use undiluted on the skin.

STYRAX BENZOIN
BENZOIN

Benzoin has been used in the East since antiquity as a medicine and as incense. It came into use in the West in the Middle Ages as a remedy for respiratory complaints. The oil, which has a sweet vanilla-like scent, is extracted from the resin of the tropical benzoin tree. It is not strictly an essential oil, but a resinoid dissolved in alcohol.

PROPERTIES AND USES

Warming and decongestant, benzoin is helpful for colds and flu, and for clearing mucus from the system. Inhaled, it can soothe sore throats and help to restore a lost voice. Benzoin blended with cream or oil and rubbed into the skin soothes chapped or irritated skin on the hands, as well as cuts and skin inflammation. As a diuretic and antiseptic, benzoin is good for urinary tract infections. It also stimulates the circulation, and its anti-inflammatory action helps to alleviate arthritis and rheumatism. Benzoin is emotionally calming in a crisis, warming and comforting in times of loneliness, and helps to dispel depression, anxiety, and nervous tension.

Blends well with sandalwood, lemon, rose, juniper, myrrh, frankincense, jasmine, cypress, and spice oils.

WARMING WINTER BATH

Add 2 drops benzoin, 3 drops marjoram, 2 drops clary sage to a warm bath. Disperse with your hand, close the bathroom door to keep in the steam, and soak for at least 10 minutes.

CAUTION
Can cause irritation in some sensitive individuals.

THYMUS VULGARIS
THYME

One of the most useful medicinal herbs in natural healthcare, thyme was also one of the first plants to be used for its healing properties. The oil, distilled from the leaves and tiny purple flowering tops of this sub-shrub, has a fresh green scent.

PROPERTIES AND USES

Thyme is antiseptic and antibiotic, disinfectant, and strongly germicidal. It is valuable for all infections, especially gastric and bladder infections, as it also has digestive and diuretic properties. The oil's antirheumatic and antitoxic properties are beneficial in treating arthritis, gout, and cellulite. Rubefacient and stimulant actions also help with muscle and joint pain, and poor circulation. Thyme stimulates the immune system to effectively fight off colds, flu, and catarrh, and ease coughing. The diluted oil is good for cleaning wounds, burns, bruises, and clearing lice. Used as a mouthwash it helps to soothe and heal abscesses and gum infections. Thyme has an uplifting fragrance, which can relieve depression, headaches, and stress.

ANTISEPTIC MOUTHWASH

Add 10 drops thyme, 15 drops peppermint, 5 drops fennel, and 5 drops myrrh to a bottle containing ½ cup (125ml) of cheap brandy. Shake well and add 2 teaspoons (10ml) of the mix to a glass of warm water. Rinse the mouth thoroughly, but do not swallow.

CAUTION
Dilute well, as thyme may cause irritation and sensitization in some people. Do not use if you have high blood pressure. Avoid during pregnancy. Do not use if you are taking homeopathic remedies.

VETIVERIA ZIZANIOIDES
VETIVER

In India and Sri Lanka, where vetiver grows, the essential oil is known as "the oil of tranquility." The tall grass is also cultivated in other countries, and the essential oil is distilled from the dried roots. The deep, smoky, earthy aroma of vetiver is wonderfully grounding and relaxing.

PROPERTIES AND USES

Valued most for its sedative properties, vetiver is used in massage and in baths to relieve stress, anxiety, nervous tension, and insomnia. It also helps to ground people who live too much in their head, or who need to feel stable after shock or a period of insecurity. Vetiver is a circulation stimulant and rubefacient, so it can provide relief from arthritis or rheumatism, and general muscular aches and pains. It is useful in skin care as an antiseptic, tonic, and detoxifier. It helps to clear acne, and because it promotes skin regeneration and strengthens the connective tissue, it assists with wound-healing and benefits aging skin.

Blends well with jasmine, cedarwood, lavender, sandalwood, rose, ylang ylang, clary sage, petitgrain, and mandarin.

TRANQUILITY BATH OIL

Add 2 drops vetiver, 2 drops lavender, 4 drops rose to 2 teaspoons (10ml.) of sweet almond oil. Add to a running bath and disperse with your hand. Relax for at least 10 minutes.

CAUTION

Keep out of the eyes. Do not take internally. Keep away from children.

ZINGIBER OFFICINALE
GINGER

Originally from India and China, warm, spicy ginger is now grown commercially throughout the tropics. It is a perennial herb with a thick, rhizomatus root. It has been used both to flavor food, and in medicine, for thousands of years, particularly by the Chinese. The essential oil distilled from the root smells similar to fresh root ginger.

PROPERTIES AND USES

Ginger is a rubefacient which can effectively ease painful conditions such as arthritis, rheumatism, or muscle pain, and improve poor circulation. Massaged around the stomach and abdomen, diluted ginger calms the digestion, tones and soothes the stomach, and stimulates the appetite. It helps to alleviate nausea, travel sickness, indigestion, pain, and diarrhea. Ginger is pain-relieving, antiseptic, and antioxidant, valuable for preventing and treating colds, sore throats, and catarrhal congestion. It also eases coughing, and because it promotes sweating, it can be useful for flu. When inhaled, the warming ginger essence eases mental confusion, and helps to relieve fatigue and nervous exhaustion.

Blends well with rose, cedarwood, rosewood, frankincense, vetiver, patchouli, petitgrain, neroli, lime, and other citrus oils.

GINGER THROAT GARGLE

Add 2 drops of ginger oil to 1 teaspoon (5ml.) of vodka and dilute with hot water. When it has cooled sufficiently, use it as a gargle for a sore throat.

CAUTION

Use sparingly, as high concentrations of ginger can cause irritation in sensitive people. Do not use in excessively hot or inflamed conditions.

HOMEOPATHY

OMEOPATHY WORKS BY TREATING a person as a whole, or holistically, so although presenting symptoms will be looked at, the individual person—his or her mental, physical, emotional, and spiritual health—will also be taken into account. Homeopathy is based on the principle that "like cures like," meaning the treatment given is similar in substance to the illness it is helping. Although it has roots that go back many centuries, it began in its present form a mere 200 years ago and today is popular as a safe and effective treatment of many problems.

THE ORIGINS OF HOMEOPATHY

It was the Greek physician Hippocrates, known as the "father of medicine" who, in the 5th century B.C.E., was the first to understand the principle of treating the body with a remedy which will produce similar symptoms to the ailment suffered. He also believed that symptoms specific to an individual, that person's reactions to an ailment, and a person's own powers of healing were important in diagnosing and choosing cure. On this basis, he built up his own medicine chest of homeopathic remedies. But it was the German physician Samuel Hahnemann (1755–1843) who first developed homeopathy as it is known and practiced today. A prominent physician, chemist, and author,

Hahnemann had become increasingly disillusioned with the methods of treatment of the day. These included harsh practices such as blood-letting and purging, and large doses of medicines that were often more debilitating than the illness itself. Yet it was obvious these practices were not working—disease was rampant. Hahnemann was one of the first physicians to advocate the improvement of poor hygiene, both in the home and in public places, and he stressed the importance of a good diet, fresh air, and higher standards of living for all. But disillusionment with the lack of response to his initiatives meant that he eventually decided to give up medical practice. In 1789 he moved to Leipzig, where he became a translator of medical texts. While translating one of these texts in 1790, *A Treatise on Materia Medica*, by Dr. William Cullen of London University, Hahnemann noticed an entry which was to set him on a path which would lead to the founding of homeopathic practice.

Cullen wrote that quinine (an extract of Peruvian bark) was an effective treatment for malaria because of its astringent qualities. As a chemist, Hahnemann knew quinine was effective against the disease, but doubted this was due to its astringency. He decided to explore this further and for days took doses of quinine himself and recorded his reactions. He found that he developed all the symptoms of malaria—palpitating heart, irregular pulse, drowsiness, and thirst—although he did not have the disease. Each time he took a new dose, the symptoms recurred. He speculated that it was the quinine's ability to induce the malarial symptoms that made it effective as a treatment. To back up his theory, he gave doses of quinine to volunteers, whom he called "provings," recorded their reactions, and found similar results.

A PICTURE OF SYMPTOMS AND VITAL FORCE

Hahnemann believed that we all have our own energy, or vital force. The force, which stimulates the body mentally, physically, and emotionally, can be disrupted by poor diet, stress, lack of exercise, pollution, and hereditary problems, weakening it so that illness results. The remedies stimulate the force, enabling the body to heal itself.

He experimented with other substances, as well as quinine, which were used as medicines at the time, such as arsenic, belladonna, and mercury. With each new substance given, he noted that individuals differed in their severity of symptoms and how they healed. Some showed few symptoms, while others suffered badly.

He found that some symptoms were commonly found after giving a substance. He called these first-line, or keynote, symptoms. The less common symptoms he called second-line, and those that were more rare he called third-line symptoms. The combination of all these types of symptoms enabled him to build up a "drug picture" for each substance that he tested.

Following this, Hahnemann went on to develop a "symptoms picture" of his patients. This included a physical examination, questions about their symptoms and general health, what made them feel better or worse, their likes and dislikes, and their lifestyle. He found that the more information he had about the patient, the more accurately he could match up the symptom picture to the remedy picture before prescribing, and therefore the more successful the eventual treatment. Hahnemann believed he had developed a new system of medicine—a system that worked on the principle that a substance and a disease that produce similar symptoms can negate each other, resulting in the full health of the patient. He called his new system "homeopathy," from the Greek words *homios*, meaning, "like," and *pathos*, meaning "suffering."

WHAT IS HOMEOPATHY?

The efficacy of homeopathy is proven by the popularity it has across the world, the number of practitioners and hospitals dedicated to homeopathic care, and the clinical trials that have been undertaken. Even so, it can be difficult to understand exactly how the principles of homeopathy actually work in practice, leading some modern doctors to remain skeptical about its effectiveness.

From Hahnemann's first experiment with quinine, he went on to prove the efficacy of around 100 homeopathic remedies. There are now more than 2000 available, with new ones continually being added. The remedies are made from animal, vegetable, and mineral sources, which are as varied as honey bees (including the sting), snake venom, and poison ivy leaves, onions, coffee beans, and daisies. But the amounts used are so minute that no substance can be tasted or side-effects experienced, however poisonous or toxic the substance might be.

In his "provings," Hahnemann had been worried by some patients who got worse before they got better after taking the substances given to them. To prevent this happening, he developed a new system of diluting the remedies. He diluted each remedy and then "succussed" or shook it. He believed that doing this released the energy of the substance. He found not only that the new system of diluting prevented the worsening of symptoms, but also, to his astonishment, that the more diluted the substance, the better its effects. He called this method "potentization." The process of making the remedies is very precise. Soluble substances such as plant and animal extracts are dissolved in a solution of about 90 percent alcohol and 10 percent distilled water, depending on the substance. The mixture is kept in an airtight container and left to stand for two to four weeks, occasionally being shaken. Insoluble substances, such as gold, are first ground down into a fine powder until they become soluble, and then undergo the same process. The mixture is then strained, and the resulting solution is known as the mother tincture.

The mother tincture is then diluted again to produce the different potencies which make up the homeopathic remedies. The dilution is measured as either decimal (x) or centesimal (c). Decimal remedies are diluted to the ratio 1:10, while the centesimal ratio is 1:100. So to produce a 1c potency, one drop of the mother tincture is added to 99 drops of an alcohol and water solution, and then succussed. To produce a 2c potency, one drop of the 1c solution is mixed with an alcohol and water solution, and then succussed. By the time the remedy reaches a 12c potency, it is unlikely that any of the original substance remains in the solution, and yet it remains effective. This is why some skeptics find it difficult to accept the efficacy of homeopathy. But the therapy's supporters believe that physics is not yet developed enough to explain the phenomenon. However, one theory is that the dilution process triggers an electromagnetic imprint which affects our own electromagnetic field, another is that the method of succussion creates and stores an electrochemical pattern in the solution which then spreads through the patient when taken. Once the solution has been succussed and diluted to a certain level, the potentized remedy is then added to lactose, or milk sugar, in the form of tablets, pilules, granules, or powder, and stored in a dark glass bottle, away from direct sunlight. For treatment purposes, different potencies are prescribed. For an acute illness, a low-potency remedy is recommended, for a chronic disease, a higher potency is more useful.

THE 12 TISSUE SALTS

Biochemic tissue salts are homeopathically prepared ingredients which were introduced at the end of the 19th century by a German physician, Wilhelm Schussler. He believed that many diseases were caused by a deficiency of one or more of 12 vital minerals. A deficiency in each salt would manifest as particular symptoms. Lack of calcarea phosphorica (Calc. phos.), for example, would show up as teething problems or an inability to absorb nutrients properly, while lack of magnesium phosphate (Mag. phos.) would affect nerve endings and muscles. Replacing the missing mineral with a minute dose of the tissue salt can correct the problem. Tissue salts are prepared only from mineral sources such as calcium, iron, and salt, but homeopathic remedies are made from animal, vegetable, and mineral sources. These can be as exotic and deadly as snake's venom or as common as the stinging nettle, but in all cases they are diluted to such an extent that there can be no possible side effects from even the most toxic substances.

Wilhelm Schussler's 12 minerals that he believed

were vital to human health can be taken in the form of homeopathically prepared tissue salts:

- **Calc. phos.** Produced from calcium phosphate
- **Sil.** Produced from silicon dioxide
- **Kali sulf.** Produced from potassium sulfate
- **Nat. mur.** From sodium chloride (common salt)
- **Calc. sulf.** Produced from calcium sulfate
- **Kali mur.** Produced from potassium chloride
- **Mac. phos.** Produced from magnesium phosphate
- **Nat. phos.** Produced from sodium phosphate
- **Ferr. phos.** Produced from iron phosphate
- **Kali phos.** Produced from potassium phosphate
- **Calc. fluor.** Produced from calcium fluoride
- **Nat. sulf.** Produced from sodium sulfate

HOMEOPATHIC TECHNIQUES

Homeopathy's popularity has grown since the first homeopathic hospital opened in 1849. It is widely used in Europe, particularly France and Germany, and in South America. It has spread, too, across continents, to Asia and India, where it is now officially recognized as a branch of medicine. In the U.S. homeopathy is becoming a recognized alternative to conventional healthcare, and homeopathic remedies are widely available in health stores.

HOW HOMEOPATHY WORKS

Homeopathy sees symptoms of disease as a positive outward sign that the body is trying to heal itself. Therefore, it holds that the symptoms should not be suppressed (as they are in allopathic medicine), and remedies are used which will help stimulate and support the healing process. In some cases, the symptoms will worsen before they improve.

A homeopath prescribes remedies for the "whole" person, basing his or her decision on Hahnemann's principles—the law of similars, the principle of minimum dose, and prescribing for the individual.

THE LAW OF SIMILARS Formulated in 1796, it states that a substance that, in large doses, can produce symptoms of illness in a healthy person can cure similar symptoms in a sick person if used in minute doses. Hahnemann believed this was because nature allows for the existence of two similar diseases in the body at the same time. Homeopathic remedies work by introducing a similar artificial disease that negates the original disease, and yet its own effects are so minimal it causes no suffering.

THE MINIMUM DOSE This states that successive dilutions enhance the curative properties of a substance, while eradicating any side-effects. This means only the most minute dose of the substance is needed to help heal.

WHOLE-PERSON PRESCRIBING Homeopaths believe that symptoms, pain, or diseases do not occur in isolation, but are an overall reflection of a person. They therefore do not just look at the problem presented to them, but at the person as a "whole." Each person is treated as an individual, and the homeopath will consider the patient's personality, temperament, emotional and physical state, and likes and dislikes before prescribing a treatment. In this way, a homeopath might see two people with similar symptoms, but would treat them totally differently.

Homeopaths also believe treatment works according to a set of three rules known as the Laws of Cure. These are:

- A remedy starts healing from the top of the body and works downward.
- It starts from within the body, working outward, and from major to minor organs.
- Symptoms clear up in reverse order to their appearance.

Homeopaths also believe that treatment should be prescribed according to a person's constitution, which is made up of inherited and acquired mental, physical, and emotional characteristics. This constitutional profile corresponds to a particular remedy, and a person might therefore be known as a Sepia type, or a Lachesis type.

HOW TO TAKE AND STORE REMEDIES

- Take only one remedy at a time.
- Do not touch the remedies; empty them onto a teaspoon and put under the tongue.
- Take in a "clean mouth" at least 30 minutes after meals. If you need to take them sooner, rinse your mouth out first with water. Avoid alcoholic drinks and cigarettes, spicy or minty foods while taking the remedies.
- Store in a cool dark place in tightly closed bottle away from strong smells. Stored correctly, remedies will keep for around five years.

VISITING A HOMEOPATH

A first visit may last around an hour, as the homeopath asks detailed questions to build up an overall picture of your mental, physical, emotional, spiritual, and general health. Only then will the homeopath prescribe a remedy specifically to suit you. One remedy at a time is usually given, although the prescription may change as your symptoms change. You may not be told which remedy has been prescribed. This is because some people are not happy with the constitutional character type attributed to them. Diet and lifestyle changes may also be recommended.

The remedies should be handled as little as possible, so are usually taken on a spoon and slipped under the tongue to dissolve. Food and drink should be avoided for a half-hour before and afterward. You may also be advised to avoid coffee and peppermints as they may counteract the remedies.

A follow-up appointment will be made for about a month later to assess progress. You may only need two appointments, but chronic conditions tend to take longer. If there is no improvement after around four visits, think about trying alternative treatment. Once symptoms improve, the remedy should be stopped. The remedies are perfectly safe, and although "overdosing" will do no harm, as with any medicine it is best avoided. Treatment can be given alongside conventional medicine, although some drugs may affect the efficacy of homeopathic remedies.

Home use

The remedies can be used at home for simple ailments and first aid, but should not be taken as a substitute for professional care. As a general rule, low potencies (e.g. 6c) are used for chronic conditions, and higher potencies (e.g. 30c) for acute conditions such as a cold. Remedies for acute conditions are usually taken on a half-hourly basis at first, and then the intervals spread out to about 8–12 hours. More chronic conditions may combine both low and high potencies.

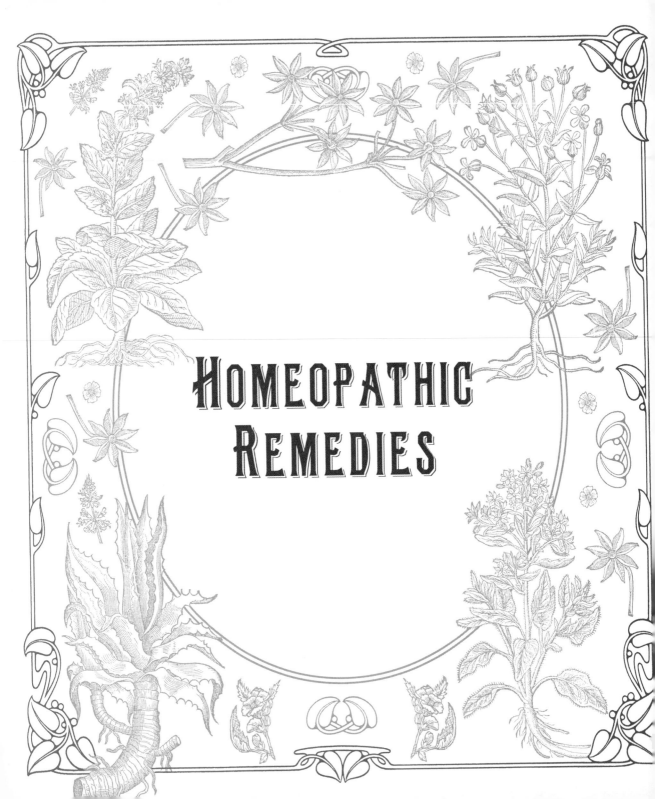

Homeopathic Remedies

ACONITUM NAPELLUS
WOLFSBANE, BLUE MONKSHOOD, ACONITE

This deadly plant has been used for its poison for centuries. Saxon hunters dipped the tips of their arrows into its juice before hunting wolves, giving it one of its common names, wolfsbane—although its original title comes from the Latin word *acon*, meaning "dart." It is grown in the European mountains, and the flowers, root, and leaves are used.

Relieves
- acute conditions which begin suddenly and after shock or exposure to abrupt changes of climate
- skin irritations
- fears

USES
Works well when given in the early stages of infections and inflammation, such as sore throats, coughs, and ear and eye problems and when the skin becomes hot, dry, and burning. Used for complaints which come on suddenly—for instance, after shock or exposure to weather extremes. Also, when restlessness and fear accompany an illness or complaint, resulting in palpitations, panic attacks, or agoraphobia.

Which type of person?
- strong, full-blooded, healthy-looking
- when well, happiest in company, but may be malicious and insensitive to cover a lack of self-esteem
- when ill, avoid company
- do not handle shock well and fear dying, even to the extent of predicting their own time of death

SYMPTOMS
- mainly fears—general anxiety, of crowds, of dying
- infections or inflammation due to injury
- sudden fevers, accompanied by hot, dry skin
- tingling in hands and feet
- thirst

ALLIUM CEPA
RED ONION, ALLIUM

The onion, grown worldwide, has been used across many continents and by many religions for its healing properties. The whole red onion bulb is used, and its potent oil stimulates the tear glands and nasal mucous membranes, causing the eyes and nose to water. In homeopathy it is used to treat any condition which includes these symptoms, such as colds, allergies, and hay fever.

Relieves
- streaming eyes and nose
- headaches, burning pain, and neuralgia
- pains that move from side to side, commonly from left to right

USES
Particularly good for cold and hay fever symptoms—profuse discharge, smarting and swollen eyes, sneezing, sore nose and upper lip from irritation due to streaming. Also for burning or neuralgic pain that moves from side to side. Also, in children, neuralgic pain which accompanies earache, molar toothache which moves around, and headaches behind the forehead. Coughing and the early stages of laryngitis can also be helped.

Which type of person?
- no particular type

SYMPTOMS
- fear of pain
- headache, toothache, earache in children, stuffiness, cough, neuralgia, colic in babies.
- Symptoms improve in fresh, cool air, and worsen in warm, stuffy rooms, and in the cold and damp.

ANACARDIUM ORIENTALE, SEMECARPUS ANACARDIUM
MARKING NUT TREE, ANACARD. OR.

Grown in the East Indies, the Hindus use the acrid black juice of this nut to burn away moles, warts, and other skin complaints. They also use it, mixed with ink, to make markings on linen. The Arabs used the juice for a number of conditions, such as mental illness, memory loss, and paralysis. Homeopathically, cardol, the juice extracted from the pith between the shell and kernel, is used to make the remedy which is given for "tight" feelings of pain.

Relieves
- constricted pain
- plugged ear, nose, or back passage
- inferiority complex

USES
This remedy is useful when there is a feeling of tightness or constricted pain. Other conditions that may be relieved are itchy skin, piles, constipation, indigestion, rheumatism, and duodenal ulcers which feel better immediately after eating, but cause discomfort two hours later. It is particularly beneficial for those who suffer an inferiority complex and who want to prove themselves, for those who feel possessed, or those who just don't quite feel themselves.

Which type of person?
- pale face
- blue rings around the eyes
- strong moral sense, so feel guilt acutely
- easily offended
- lack self-confidence
- like dairy products

SYMPTOMS
- loss of memory, leading to instances of harsh behavior
- obsessive behavior
- fixations
- irritability
- nervous exhaustion
- tight feeling of constriction
- duodenal ulcers
- blocked gut or anus
- Symptoms improve immediately after eating, when lying on the affected part, after rubbing, and worsen around midnight, after washing in hot water and using a compress.

ANTIMONIUM
TARTARICUM, ANTIMONY, POTASSIUM TARTRATE, TARTAR EMETIC, ANT. TART.

Antimony potassium tartrate is a poisonous crystalline salt which has no color or odor and is used as a fix for leather and textiles, and in insecticides. In the past it was used in conventional medicine as an emetic, and as an expectorant. Homeopathically, it is used to treat gastric disorders and chest complaints.

Relieves
- chest conditions
- gastric or bowel complaints

USES
This remedy is particularly good in the very young or very old who are too feeble or weak to help themselves—for instance, by coughing up phlegm. Wet, cold conditions bring on excess thick mucus in the air passages, leading to rattling breathing. Sour food or drink can lead to gastric problems, intense nausea, and lack of thirst. Other symptoms treated include headaches with the feeling that there is a tight band around the head; a face cold to the touch; a thickly coated tongue; fluid retention leading to bloated legs; nausea.

Which type of person?
- pale, sickly looking
- dark rings around the eyes

- cold sweat on face
- look run down
- do not like being fussed over or interfered with when ill
- do not like being disturbed
- babies who whine, moan, or always want to be carried

SYMPTOMS

- irritable and anxious
- despairing
- stomach upsets
- sweats
- build-up of mucus and phlegm
- off food and do not want to drink
- drowsy
- Symptoms improve when sitting up, after vomiting, and in cold air, and worsen in stuffy rooms, if wearing too much, with movement, or when lying down.

APIS MELLIFICA
APIS MELLIFERA, HONEY BEE, APIS

The bee is known for its unique ability to produce honey and for its painful sting. Bee products—honey, beeswax, propolis (resin used in the building of hives), and royal jelly (fed to queen bees)—are used in complementary medicine. In homeopathy, apis is used to treat stinging pain and inflamed, burning skin which has swollen and is painful to touch. The honey bee is commonly found in Europe, Canada, and America. Homeopathically, the whole live bee is used, including the sting, and dissolved in alcohol. The remedy was first "proved" in the U.S., at the Central New York State Homeopathic Society.

Relieves

- hot, stinging pain
- smarting, watery swellings, which are sensitive to the touch
- fever with dry skin
- violent headache
- lack of thirst

USES

Used for complaints such as bites, stings, and urticaria, when the skin becomes swollen, dry, and itchy, or burns and is sensitive to the touch. Also used for urinary tract infections, such as cystitis, and for urine and fluid retention. Allergic reactions which affect the nose, eyes, and throat, such as anaphylactic shock, when watery swelling occurs, and complaints where joints become swollen, such as arthritis, can also be treated. Also good for fever, accompanied by dry skin, sore throat, severe headache, and lack of thirst.

Which type of person?

- protective of own territory, resentful of outsiders
- irritable, agitated, and difficult to please
- love trying to organize other people's lives but have a "sting in the tail" for those who cross them, perhaps leading to the nickname "queen bee"
- spend hours trying to achieve things without making much headway

> **CAUTION**
> During pregnancy, avoid apis below 30c potency.

SYMPTOMS

- restlessness
- jealousy
- irritability
- sensitivity
- depression
- unpredictability
- watery swellings, from stings to edema
- fevers with dry, sensitive skin
- intense headaches
- lack of urination
- Symptoms improve under cool conditions, but worsen when touched, in beat, or during sleep.

ARGENTUM NITRICUM
HELL STONE, DEVIL'S STONE, LUNAR CAUSTIC, ARG. NIT.

Silver nitrate, the source of this remedy, was given the names "hell stone" or "devil's stone" because of its corrosive effect. Silver nitrate is extracted from the mineral acanthite, the main ore of silver, and is produced mainly in the U.S., South America, and Norway. In the past, due to its caustic and antibacterial qualities, it was used in medicine to cauterize wounds after surgery and treat conditions such as warts and eye infections. Although it is safe in small doses, large amounts are poisonous, causing breathing problems and damaging the kidneys, liver, spleen, and aorta, and overdosing affects the skin, turning it permanently blue. It has also long had a less lethal use—for making the backs of mirrors. In homeopathy, the remedy is most often used for nervous and digestive complaints.

SYMPTOMS
- under stress, find it hard to control emotions, leading to irrational thoughts and impulses
- under pressure, and push themselves, because of a fear of failing
- headaches, brought on by overwork, excitement, and sweet foods, will be slow in onset, then disappear
- tension in the neck
- weak areas: nerves, lining of the stomach, the left side of the body.
- Symptoms improve in fresh air and in coolness, and if pressure is applied, but worsen in heat, at night, under stress, and if lying on the left side.

Relieves
- fears, anxiety, phobias
- palpitations, sweating
- mental exhaustion
- digestive complaints brought on by nerves and other tension
- problems due to overconsumption of sweet, sugary foods
- vertigo

USES

Arg. nit. is mainly used for fear and anxiety, usually brought on by stress, and can help with problems such as claustrophobia, dangerous impulses, such as throwing oneself off a bridge, and stage fright. It can also control superstition—the feeling that something awful is about to happen. It is also very useful for digestive problems, such as diarrhea and vomiting, particularly if brought on by nerves; and headaches which begin slowly and are caused by overeating sweet foods. It also helps other conditions such as asthma, colic in babies, epilepsy, warts, and sore throats. During labor, it can help bring relief when bearing down.

Which type of person?
- look fraught and prematurely old, with hollowed features, and an accumulation of wrinkles
- do work where quick thinking, rapid responses, and a good memory are necessary, such as acting, lecturing, or executive positions in business
- outwardly exuberant and happy, inwardly suffer from wild emotions, leading them to laugh, cry, or lose their tempers easily
- when worried and agitated, fret about what may go wrong in the future, even becoming irrational
- may break out in sudden nervous sweats
- prefer salty foods, dislike cold food, and crave sweetness, though this causes stomach upset
- children look older than their years; may be sick through apprehension at the thought of school, and dislike airless rooms; overindulge in sweet or salty foods, leading to diarrhea
- breast-fed babies will suffer diarrhea and colic if the mother eats sweet food

ARNICA MONTANA
LEOPARD'S BANE, MOUNTAIN TOBACCO, SNEEZEWORT, ARNICA

Arnica has been used for its healing properties for centuries. It grows in the mountain regions of Europe and Siberia. In folk remedies it was used for aches and bruises, and in conventional medicine for rheumatism, gout, and dysentery. Homeopathically, the remedy was first "proved" by Hahnemann. The whole fresh plant is used when in flower, externally as a cream for sprains and bruises, and internally for shock, often after the patient has suffered an injury.

Relieves
- bruises, sprains, pain
- shock (from injury or emotional shock)

USES
Arnica is an effective first-aid treatment for sprains, strains, and bruising. Internally, it can help control bleeding and stimulates the healing of damaged tissue. It is also useful for shock, after either an injury or emotional trauma. It can be used for long-term joint and muscle complaints such as osteoarthritis. Internal treatment can aid external conditions such as eczema and boils.

Which type of person?
- morose, morbidly imaginative
- when ill, deny there is a problem, refusing to see a doctor, and preferring to be left alone

> **CAUTION**
> Do not use arnica cream on broken skin.

SYMPTOMS
- hypochondria
- fear of being touched due to pain
- nightmares
- find it hard to concentrate because easily distracted

- impatient, indifferent, and restless, even in bed
- obstinate
- severe fever
- broken capillaries
- sprained joints
- eczema
- Symptoms improve during movement and lying down with the head lower than the feet, and worsen after prolonged movement or rest, under light pressure, in heat.

ARSENICUM ALBUM
ARSENIC TRIOXIDE, ARS. ALB.

Arsenic has long been known as a useful poison for those intent on murder! These days, arsenic poisoning is more likely to be the result of accidental ingestion—for instance, of agricultural pesticides. In large doses, swallowing arsenic leads to severe stomach upset, vomiting, convulsions, diarrhea, and, if not treated, death. In the past, small doses were given to treat syphilis, anthrax, and to improve stamina. Arsenic is contained in the mineral arsenopyrite, found in countries such as England, Canada, Germany, Norway, and Sweden. It is made up of metallic crystals which cannot be destroyed. In homeopathy, a minute compound of arsenic is used, which works beneficially on the sensitive lining of the digestive tract and respiratory system. Arsenic was first "proved" by Hahnemann.

SYMPTOMS
- fear being alone, burgled, dying
- anxiety leads to restlessness and irritability and a need to do everything meticulously
- possessive, hoard
- sensitive to touch, smell, cold
- digestive disorders
- headaches
- dizziness, vomiting
- asthma which is triggered by anxiety
- fluid retention, diarrhea
- cracked lips, mouth ulcers
- Symptoms improve with movement, in warmth, when lying down with the head propped up, and are worse on the right side, in the cold, after cold food and drink.

Relieves
- digestive disorders
- fears and anxiety
- regular, painful headaches
- problems associated with burning pain

USES

Ars. alb. is given to those suffering from fear—fear of going out alone, fear of the dark, fear of failure, and so on—which is caused by underlying feelings of insecurity. It is also useful for problems of the digestive system, such as indigestion, diarrhea, food poisoning, and excessive eating, such as overconsumption of fruit or ice cream, and drinking too much alcohol. Also, for a range of conditions which particularly sting or burn, such as mouth ulcers, sore lips, eye inflammation, vomiting, burning pains in the rectum. Asthma, fatigue, and fluid retention, especially around the ankles, can also be helped.

Which type of person?
- elegant, even dapper, everything in place
- attentive to detail, plan for every contingency as a way of covering up insecurity and lack of confidence
- strong ideas, making them intolerant of others; want everything to be done perfectly their way
- constant planning does nothing to relieve restlessness and worries, so fret about own health and the health of their family
- children are tidy, restless, and have a wild imagination
- prefer warm foods which are fatty, sweet, or sour; warm drinks, alcohol

ATROPA BELLADONNA
DEADLY NIGHTSHADE, BELLADONNA

It was thought during the Middle Ages that deadly nightshade was used in witchcraft. In Italian "Bella donna" means beautiful woman, and Italian women used it in eye drops to enlarge their pupils to make themselves more attractive. In conventional medicine, the plant's alkaloid properties of atropine, hyoscamine, and scopolamine are used to treat spasms and nausea. It is grown throughout Europe, and in homeopathy the fresh leaves and flowers are used. Hahnemann first "proved" the remedy in 1799.

SYMPTOMS
- restless
- excitable behavior
- wild imagination, even hallucinations, nightmares
- fear when approached
- very sensitive to light, touch, and movement
- throbbing headaches
- earache, especially on the right side of the head
- hot, dry face, bright red tongue
- Symptoms improve in warmth, when standing up, with warm compresses, and worsen when cool, on the right side, at night, with movement, noise, light, pressure.

Relieves
- sudden, violent complaints, with flushing and throbbing, due to increased circulation
- ailments which include sensitivity to light, noise, pressure, touch
- fever, with staring eyes, dilated pupils

USES
Commonly used for complaints with sudden onset, inflamed infections, such as fever, tonsillitis, flu, earache—particularly on the right side. Helps severe, pounding headaches jarred by eye movement; boils; labor pain; sore breasts from breast-feeding; fits; cystitis; teething babies.

Which type of person?
- fit, healthy, normally strong in mind and body
- lively and entertaining when well
- agitated, restless, stubborn, and maybe violent when ill
- extremely sensitive to light, touch, movement, and noise

THE HEALING REMEDIES SOURCEBOOK

AURUM METALLICUM
GOLD, AURUM MET.

In the 12th century, gold was used by Arab physicians to treat heart conditions. In the early 20th century, it was used in diagnosing syphilis and treating tuberculosis, and today is used for treating cancer and rheumatoid arthritis. It is found in Canada, the U.S., South Africa, and Australia. Homeopathically, it is given to treat a range of clinical complaints, such as heart disease and depression.

Relieves
- depression
- ailments accompanied by sensitivity to touch, taste, smell, noise
- vascular complaints

USES
Useful for mental conditions such as depression and suicidal tendencies. Also for ailments where an increase in blood circulation leads to congestion in the head, as in pulsating headaches, or other organs. Symptoms of heart disease, such as chest pain and breathlessness, can also be helped. Liver problems and sinusitis can be relieved.

Which type of person?
- workaholics who set themselves high goals
- deep sense of duty
- sensitive to the opinions of others as never feel they have achieved as much as they should
- feelings of failure can lead to depression, and even suicidal thoughts

SYMPTOMS
- depression, even suicidal leanings
- explosive behavior if contradicted
- red flushes when angry
- blood congestion in organs, such as liver and heart
- inflammation of testes in young boys
- Symptoms improve in fresh air and when walking, after washing in cold water and resting, and worsen after mental exertion, when emotionally upset, and at night.

BAPTISIA TINCTORIA
WILD INDIGO, HORSEFLY WEED, RATTLEBUSH, BAPTISIA

Wild indigo is a perennial plant which is native to the U.S. and Canada. Poisonous if ingested in high doses, causing gastrointestinal problems, its medicinal properties were first discovered by Native Americans, who also used it as the basis for indigo dye. It is also used in herbal medicine as a cooling agent, and as an antiseptic and an antibacterial treatment. Homeopathically, the fresh root is used. The remedy was originally "proved" using only seven volunteers, the results being published in the North American Journal of Homeopathy in 1857 and 1859.

CAUTION
A patient needing baptisia is usually severely ill and will need professional medical care.

Relieves
- toxic and septic conditions
- acute feverish illness

USES
This remedy is mainly used for complaints which have quickly deteriorated into a serious condition, such as acute flu and typhoid fever. Symptoms treated include a rambling mind; restlessness; severe aches and tenderness; prostration and falling asleep mid-sentence; inability to sleep because of delirious mind; foul-smelling breath and stools; dry, coated tongue; mouth ulcers; and persistent ear infections.

Which type of person?
- no particular type, but will be very ill, with puffy face and a drugged look

SYMPTOMS
- restlessness
- confused, wandering mind and talk
- fear of poisoning from food
- unable to move around to make themselves more comfortable
- ulcers of the mouth and throat
- foul breath; coated tongue; gum sores
- breathing difficulties
- Symptoms improve in fresh air and worsen in humidity.

BARYTA CARBONICA
BARIUM CARBONATE, WITHERITE, BARYTA CARB.

The source of barium carbonate is barite and witherite, found in the earth's crust in the U.S. and parts of Europe. When heated, it glows and is a useful tool in radiology. Witherite obtains its name from the man who first discovered it in 1783, William Withering. It was given medicinally to treat glandular swellings and tuberculosis. Homeopathically, it was first "proved" by Hahnemann, and the remedy is used mainly for children and the elderly.

Relieves
- enlarged glands
- headaches
- slow development

USES

This is a particularly useful remedy for children, adults who have immature tendencies as if going through a second childhood, and the elderly. Children who are shy, are late in walking and talking, are slow to develop physically. Those who are slow intellectually, physically, and emotionally respond well. As they are susceptible to infection, they suffer recurrent problems such as sore throats. The elderly, suffering from senile dementia or a stroke, also respond well.

Which type of person?
- tend to be overweight
- dry, lined skin
- mentally dull, may be mentally challenged
- forgetful, with a short attention span
- children are timid and slow developers
- like cold food

SYMPTOMS
- fear of strangers, minor things, things that may happen
- memory loss
- tendency to dwell on past problems
- confusion
- lack of self-confidence
- odd sensations such as cobwebs on face or as if inhaling smoke
- recurrent sore throats, accompanied by enlarged glands
- palpitations when lying on the left side
- frequent urination and constipation
- Symptoms improve in the open air, when warmly wrapped, and worsen when thinking about problems, after washing, when lying on the affected side, with exposure to cold or damp.

BRYONIA ALBA
COMMON BRYONY, WHITE BRYONY, WILD HOPS, BRYONIA

The Greek physician Hippocrates was one of the first physicians to use bryony, in the 5th century B.C.E. The Romans also used it to treat paralysis, gout, hysteria, and epilepsy. The plant has a deadly, bitter root which, if eaten, can kill within hours. The homeopathic remedy, in which the fresh root is first pounded to a pulp, was one of the first treatments to be "proved" by Hahnemann, in 1834.

Relieves
- acute complaints with slow onset, painful with movement, thirst
- ailments accompanied by dryness of the mouth, lips, eyes, chest

USES
Often used for coughs, colds, headaches, and flu which develop slowly and are accompanied by dryness—for instance, in the throat, and great thirst. The condition worsens with movement. Also useful for joint inflammation such as rheumatism and osteoarthritis; chest and abdominal inflammation; pleurisy; pneumonia; constipation; mastitis.

Which type of person?
- fear poverty, so materialistic
- worry about financial security, even if well-off; anxious, irritable if security is threatened
- plod, but straightforward, reliable
- meticulous, critical
- usually have dark hair and complexion

SYMPTOMS

- reluctant to speak or to move
- irritable, heavy-headed
- want things, but do not know what, then refuse it when offered
- fears of not getting better, even of dying
- worry about finances and job
- excessive sweating
- dryness, constricted throat, thirst
- stabbing headaches
- heavy eyelids
- cravings
- Symptoms improve after rest, when pressure is applied, and worsen with movement.

CALCAREA CARBONICA
CALCIUM CARBONATE, CALC. CARB.

The source of this remedy is the mother-of-pearl in oyster shells. Mother-of-pearl was commonly used for its beauty to adorn combs and the backs of hairbrushes. In homeopathy, it also has wide-ranging uses, but is most often used for problems relating to the teeth and bones. It is particularly good for broken bones which are slow to heal, backache, and joint pain.

SYMPTOMS

- fear of poverty, illness, and death
- swing from being productive at work to lazy
- fear of the dark, ghosts
- dislike small spaces, thunderstorms, mice
- discuss every detail of each illness to the irritation of others
- sensitive to cold
- often tired and anxious
- excessive, sour-smelling sweat, even after light exertion
- constipated, but feel better for it
- Symptoms improve when lying on the affected side, late morning, and in dry weather, and worsen with sweating, after exertion, in the damp and cold, on waking, and before menstruation.

Relieves

- aches and pains in the bones and joints
- slow development of teeth and bones
- excessive sweating
- fears, anxieties

USES

Used to treat bones and joints which are slow to develop, or slow to heal after injury. Also relieves complaints which may be due to this, such as backache. Also helps slow-growing teeth and pain during teething. Eye infections characterized by redness, particularly in the right eye, and ear infections accompanied by unpleasant-smelling discharge are also treated. Right-sided headaches, premenstrual tension, heavy menstruation, menopause, thrush, eczema, and digestive problems can also be helped by Calc. carb.

Which type of person?

- shy, quiet, sensitive
- seem withdrawn, but are more afraid of making a fool of themselves
- when well, happy and work hard; when ill, slightly depressed and need constant reassurance
- although generally healthy, tend to be overweight, sloth
- prefer sweet, sour, and starchy foods, cold drinks, oysters, and dislike coffee and milk; suffer unusual cravings—chalk, for instance

CALCAREA PHOSPHORICA
CALCIUM PHOSPHATE, CALC. PHOS.

Calcium phosphate is a mineral salt which is the main constituent, along with collagen, of bones and teeth. A natural version is the mineral apatite. For homeopathic use, it is prepared chemically from dilute phosphoric acid and calcium hydroxide, which form fine particles of calcium phosphate. These are then filtered and dried. Calcium phosphate is also used in making porcelain and glass, and as plant food. The remedy is also used as a tissue salt, to treat complaints affecting the bones and teeth.

SYMPTOMS

- restless, dislike routine
- need constant stimulation
- hate getting up in the morning
- growing pains
- slow-healing fractures
- cravings
- weak digestion
- Symptoms improve in dry, warm weather, and worsen in cold, damp weather, when worrying, after excessive sexual activity or other overexertion.

Relieves

- painful teeth and bones
- digestive complaints
- growing pains

USES

Used to treat slow growth and growing pains in children. For instance, a fontanel that is slow to close in a toddler, painful teething, numbness and tingling attributed to growing. Also used to treat bones and joints that are healing slowly; slow recovery after illness due to weakness and fatigue; for digestive problems such as diarrhea and indigestion; recurrent throat infections.

Which type of person?

- thin, with dark hair, long legs
- discontented, unhappy
- friendly, but always complaining
- dislike routine
- babies are irritable, needing constant attention; when older easily bored

CALENDULA OFFICINALIS
MARIGOLD, CALENDULA

The common, or pot, marigold is a hardy annual bush which grows in southern Europe. It should not be confused with the African marigold, tagetes, which is toxic. Calendula has bright orange or yellow daisy-like flowers and narrow pale green leaves, and it grows to a height of about 2ft. (70cm.). The plant has been used for centuries for its healing properties. It is a popular herbal medicine, and is used for its anti-inflammatory and antimicrobial qualities in conditions ranging from skin complaints to cancer. It is a common first-aid treatment for cuts, grazes, and scalds in both herbal and homeopathic medicine. Homeopathically, the fresh leaves and flowers of the plant are used to make the remedy, and a cream for external use.

SYMPTOMS

- none in particular, although patient may be irritable and frightened
- cuts, grazes, scalds
- perineal tears
- bleeding after tooth extraction
- Symptoms improve when lying still or walking, and worsen in damp weather, in draughts, and after eating.

Relieves

- cuts, grazes, minor wounds
- perineal tears, after childbirth
- mouth ulcers

USES

An excellent first-aid treatment for small cuts, grazes, and scalds to help control bleeding, for its cleansing antiseptic qualities, and to promote healing by aiding clotting.

Also, after childbirth it is used by midwives in baths or lotions to aid perineal tears. After tooth extraction profuse bleeding can be controlled by gargling with calendula in cooled boiled water. Other conditions which can be helped by calendula include fever accompanied by agitation; jaundice.

Which type of person?

- no particular type

> **CAUTION**
> Ensure cuts are clean before use so that rapid healing does not close in dirt or germs. Do not use for puncture wounds or deep cuts, as rapid healing may seal the infection inside the wound.

THE HEALING REMEDIES SOURCEBOOK

CANTHARIS VESICATORIA, LYTTA VESICATORIA

SPANISH FLY, BLISTER BEETLE, CANTHARIS

Spanish fly is in fact a bright green beetle which is native to southern Europe and western Asia. It emits a fast-acting irritant, cantharidin, causing blistering, hence its other common name. In the past, it was used as an aphrodisiac, causing sexual frenzy in some cases, and medicinally was used to treat a variety of ailments from warts to rheumatism. It was first "proved" by Hahnemann, and the remedy is made up from the whole beetle, dried, and then powdered. Homeopathically, it is used to treat complaints characterized by a burning sensation.

SYMPTOMS
- irritability
- feels excessive sexual desire
- violent tendencies
- thirst, but no wish to drink
- loss of appetite
- burning sensation in the stomach
- sweating, and palpitations
- rapidly worsening infections
- Symptoms improve in the warmth, with massage, after flatulence or burping, and at night, and worsen with movement, after drinking coffee or cold water, and in the afternoon.

Relieves
- conditions accompanied by stinging or a burning sensation
- rapidly spreading infection
- stings, burns

USES
Ailments characterized by burning or stinging, particularly urinary tract infections such as cystitis, frequent but painful urination, insect bites, burns and scalds, infections, burning abdominal pains, and stinging diarrhea. Also for infections which spread rapidly, or conditions which quickly deteriorate. Other conditions which respond well include great thirst without a desire to drink because of breathlessness; pus-filled eruptions on hands; burning throat; burning soles of the feet; loss of appetite. Mental problems such as rage, agitation leading to violence, excessive sexual desire, and severe anxiety can be relieved by cantharis.

Which type of person?
- have a head full of ideas, but are confused
- maniacal tendencies explosive anger
- strong sexual urges

CARBO VEGITABILIS

CHARCOAL, CARB. VEG.

Charcoal is wood that has been burned without air, forming a hard carbon. It has been used as a fuel, in explosives, for smelting, and as an absorbent. In the past, it was used medicinally for its deodorizing and disinfecting qualities, for septic conditions, and flatulence. Today, it is still used to treat the latter in conventional medicine. In homeopathy, charcoal from beech, poplar, and silver birch trees grown in the northern hemisphere is used, and the remedy was first "proved" by Hahnemann.

SYMPTOMS
- never quite feel well following an ailment
- lack mental energy
- fear of the supernatural
- burping, regurgitating food
- flatulence
- headaches, especially prevalent in the morning and after eating too much
- clammy hands
- indigestion
- poor circulation
- Symptoms improve in cold, fresh air, and are relieved after burping, and worsen in warm, wet air, after fatty, milky foods and wine, and when lying down.

Relieves
- lack of vitality; fatigue
- cold, clamminess externally, heat internally, associated with shock
- excess mucus from digestive system
- poor circulation

USES

Used to aid recovery after an illness, when there is exhaustion and weakness, and for shock that may follow an operation which leaves the patient with cold, pale skin, but feeling hot inside. Also treats poor circulation, when the face, hands, or feet are cold and turn bluish; and bleeding varicose veins. Useful for digestive problems, such as indigestion and flatulence, asthma, whooping cough.

Which type of person?
- complain of never quite recovering after an illness
- prefer day to darkness
- fixed ideas
- mentally and physically tired and sluggish; erratic memory

CAUSTICUM HAHNEMANNI
POTASSIUM HYDRATE, CAUSTICUM

This remedy was invented and "proved" by Samuel Hahnemann himself and is unique to homeopathy. It is made chemically from quicklime (calcium oxide) and potassium bisulfate. He found that it caused a burning taste in the back of the mouth and an acerbic sensation. It is used for a set of symptoms known as the Causticum cough (*see "Uses"*) and for various neuromuscular conditions.

Relieves
- Causticum cough
- progressive weakness leading to paralysis
- burning, bursting pain

USES

Symptoms of the Causticum cough include a raw, tickly throat with dry cough; burning in the throat; hard, racking cough; chest filled with mucus which is difficult to cough up; incontinence with each cough, and coughing which is worse on breathing out. Also helps neuromuscular problems such as weakness; stiffness; neuralgia; tearing pains in the joints, muscles, and bones; cramps, particularly affecting the vocal cords, bladder, larynx, or the right side of the face. Other conditions alleviated include dizziness when bending forward; heartburn in pregnancy; burning rheumatic pain; roaring sounds in the ears; nasal soreness; and tender scars and injury sites.

Which type of person?
- dark hair and eyes, with sallow skin
- often mentally and physically exhausted
- narrow-minded
- hypersensitive, weepy
- dislike the smell of food and feel worse after drinking coffee

SYMPTOMS
- fear of animals, darkness, ghosts, strangers, death
- can be very critical of others
- empathize with the suffering of others
- despair of recovering from illness
- chilly
- prone to warts
- symptoms tend to come on slowly
- tearing, bursting pain in joints, muscles, and bones
- paralytic problems
- contractions of the muscles and tendons
- Symptoms improve in warm, damp weather, after cold drinks and washing, and worsen in dry, cold winds, with movement.

CEPHAELIS IPECACUANHA
IPECACUANHA, IPECAC.

Ipecacuanha is a small, perennial shrub grown in the tropical rainforests of South and Central America. The first recorded medicinal use—for treating vomiting—was around 1600, by a Portuguese friar in Brazil. It was brought to Europe some 70 years later, where it was used as an antidysentery drug in France, as well as for a variety of ailments. It is still used in conventional medicine to induce vomiting in cases of drug overdoses or poisoning, and as an expectorant. Homeopathically, the root is used to treat nausea and vomiting. It is collected when the plant is in flower and then dried.

Relieves
- persistent nausea
- breathing difficulties

USES
Commonly used for nausea and vomiting, and accompanying sweats and clamminess. Also good for stomach complaints accompanied by salivating, lack of thirst, weak pulse, and fainting; conditions causing breathing difficulties, such as asthma and coughing; coughing and vomiting at the same time; persistent nausea.

Which type of person?
- no particular type

SYMPTOMS
- contemptuous
- anxiety, including fear of death
- morose
- breathing difficulties
- constant nausea
- fainting, cold or hot sweats, clamminess
- bleeding
- weak pulse
- Symptoms improve in fresh air, and worsen in warmth, in the winter, when moving or lying down, and when under stress or embarrassed.

CHINA OFFICINALIS
CINCHONA SUCCIRUBRA, PERUVIAN BARK, CINCHONA BARK, JESUITS' BARK, CHINA

The China remedy is made from Peruvian bark—grown in the tropical rainforests of South America, in India, and Southeast Asia—which is stripped and dried. Quinine, an extract of the bark, was the first substance to be tested and "proven" by Hahnemann, in 1790. He used quinine on himself, noting that large doses caused similar symptoms to malaria, while small doses acted as an antidote. Quinine is still used in conventional medicine today as part of the treatment for malaria. Homeopathically, the dried bark of China is used for exhaustion.

Relieves
- nervous exhaustion after incapacitating illness
- weakness after vomiting, diarrhea, or sweating, as a result of loss of body fluids

USES
Aids recovery from nervous exhaustion after debilitating illness and as a result of loss of fluids from vomiting, diarrhea, or sweating. Also for digestive conditions such as gastroenteritis, flatulence, and gall bladder problems; mental upsets such as lack of concentration, indifference, and outbursts that are out of character; also neuralgia, dizziness, tired and twitchy muscles, tinnitus, hemorrhages.

Which type of person?
- sensitive
- intense
- artistic
- idealistic
- their own intensity is tiring, making them lazy, depressed, sometimes violent
- find it difficult to express themselves to others so do so through their creativity
- prefer talking about meaningful issues, not trivia
- imaginative mind, fantasize about heroic deeds

SYMPTOMS

- emotionally fragile
- difficulty in expressing feelings
- lacks concentration
- nervous exhaustion
- headaches, dizziness
- convulsions
- weak muscles
- sallow skin
- indigestion, flatulence, a feeling that food is stuck behind the breastbone
- Symptoms improve in the warmth, when firm pressure is applied to the affected area, and after sleeping, and worsen in the cold or draughts, in the fall.

CIMICIFUGA RACEMOSA
BLACK COHOSH, BUGBANE, BLACK SNAKEROOT, RATTLEROOT, CIMIC.

Grown in the U.S. and Canada, the Native Americans used the rhizome or underground stem of this plant to cure rattlesnake bites, giving it one of its common names, rattleroot, and for rheumatism and gynecological problems. It has also been used for menstrual and labor pain as well as being chewed as a sedative to help with depression. Brewed in a tea which was then sprinkled around a room, it was said to prevent the presence of evil spirits. Homeopathically, it was "proved" in the U.S. The fresh black root is commonly used for treating problems arising during pregnancy and childbirth.

SYMPTOMS

- emotional and highly strung
- sigh repeatedly when sad
- strong fears, such as insanity and death, particularly when menopausal
- cramps and backache when premenstrual
- nausea and vomiting in pregnancy
- depression after childbirth
- faints and flushes during menopause
- Symptoms improve when warm, in fresh air, when

pressure is applied, and with gentle movement, but worsen in cold, damp, draughty conditions, with alcohol or excitement.

Relieves

- menstrual symptoms
- nausea, vomiting in pregnancy
- head, neck aches to woefulness
- to conditions accompanied by chills

USES

Cimic. works well on the nerves and muscles of the uterus, making it useful for menstrual problems such as back cramps and headaches; early miscarriage; pregnancy complaints, such as pain in the uterus, difficulty sleeping, nausea, and vomiting; and postnatal depression and menopausal problems. The upheaval in emotions associated with these problems can also be relieved.

Which type of person?

- mainly women
- often extrovert, talkative, and excitable
- when sad become depressed, often sigh
- experience strong, intense emotions
- fear death

CUCUMIS COLOCYNTHIS
BITTER APPLE, BITTER CUCUMBER, COLOCYNTHIS

Colocynthis, or Coloc., comes from a gourd, Cucumis colocynthis. In the past, the bitter apple, as it is also known, was used by Arab and ancient Greek physicians as a purgative (with radical results), in order to induce abortion, and to treat derangement, lethargy, and dropsy. The seeds alone are harmless, but when the whole fruit is eaten, it causes bowel inflammation and cramping pains, due to the release of a resin called colocynthin. Homeopathically, the fruit—which grows in hot, arid conditions—is dried and powdered, without the seeds. It was first used in 1834, and is given as treatment for digestive complaints and colic.

SYMPTOMS

- upset if contradicted, especially if feel humiliated
- keen for justice to be done
- digestive problems
- neuralgia and headaches
- abdominal pain
- Symptoms improve in the warmth, after flatulence, or drinking coffee, but worsen after eating, when indignant or angry, and in damp, cold weather.

Relieves

- digestive complaints
- neuralgia, headaches, and stomach pains brought on by anger

USES

Mainly used to treat symptoms brought on by anger, particularly suppressed anger, such as neuralgia and abdominal pain; stomach pain, facial neuralgia, and headaches respond well, as does nerve pain in the ovaries or kidneys; gout, sciatica, and rheumatism symptoms can also be helped.

Which type of person?

- tend to be fair-haired and fair-skinned
- reserved
- have a strong sense of right and wrong
- dislike being contradicted
- suffer physical effects when angry or indignant

COFFEA ARABICA
COFFEA CRUDA, COFFEE

Coffee is native to Arabia and Ethiopia, and is thought to have been first drunk in Persia. Now grown in Central America and the West Indies, it has been used widely for medicinal purposes as a diuretic, painkiller, and to ease indigestion. It is also a well-known stimulant. Homeopathically, coffea is made from the raw berries of the coffee tree, and was first "proved" by Hahnemann himself and a handful of volunteers. It is mainly used to treat those who are excitable and mentally overstimulated.

SYMPTOMS

- irritable
- heightened senses
- mind buzzing with ideas
- anxiety leading to restlessness
- insomnia
- guilt
- trembling limbs
- toothache
- headaches
- palpitations
- hypersensitive skin
- Symptoms improve in the warmth, after lying down, and when holding cold water in the mouth. They worsen with extreme emotions such as anger, with touch, smell; or noise, and during cold, windy weather.

Relieves

- excitability
- mental overstimulation
- sleeplessness

USES

Commonly used to treat excessive mental activity when the mind seems to be buzzing; where the person is very excitable and hypersensitive—for instance, with toothache or labor pain; when all the senses are acutely affected, making any noise, smell, or touch seem unbearable; headaches which are so severe it feels like a nail is being driven into the skull; palpitations when excited or angry; and for acute premenstrual symptoms.

Which type of person?

- tall, lean, with a tendency to stoop
- dark complexion
- symptoms may appear after a failed relationship, and with exhaustion or after a trauma
- on a high, but will then descend into despair
- tend to "burn out"

CUPRUM METTALICUM
COPPER, CUPRUM MET

Copper, a red-gold metal, is often found in many tools and weapons. In the past, coppersmiths often suffered toxic poisoning due to working with the metal, falling ill with complaints such as coughs, malnutrition, colicky pain, and sometimes even paralysis and death. In the days when alcohol was often made secretly in home distilleries, poisoning occurred from the copper tubing. Small amounts were also used medicinally to help heal wounds. Homeopathically, it was first "proved" in 1834, and is used to treat respiratory problems and various complaints of the nervous system.

SYMPTOMS
- hide deep emotions
- suppression of feelings leads to physical problems
- cry, becoming morose
- twitches, jerks, convulsions
- erratic breathing
- pale color, sometimes turning blue
- Symptoms improve after sweating and cold drinks, and worsen if emotions are being suppressed, in the heat, when touched, and after vomiting.

Relieves
- muscular spasm, cramp to breathing problems
- tiredness associated with mental exhaustion

USES
Problems of the nervous system are commonly treated. Tics, twitches—particularly those that start in a minor way and spread more deeply—and convulsions can be helped. Epilepsy responds well. Tiredness brought on after much mental activity can be treated, as can respiratory problems when breathing seems to be intermittent, such as with asthma.

Which type of person?
- intensely emotional, but suppress feelings, so may appear reserved
- serious, self-critical
- swing from being headstrong to submissive
- children tend to hold their breath when angry until they go blue, have a destructive mentality, and need their own space; teenagers tend to suppress sexual urges

DROSERA ROTUNDIFOLIA
SUNDEW, MOOR GRASS, RED ROT, YOUTHWORT, DROSERA

The sundew is a carnivorous plant which grows widely in the heaths and boggy areas of Europe, South America, the U.S., China, and India. Insects are attracted by the long, red hairs on the leaves of the plant. Glands on the surface of the leaves, then secrete a fluid which traps and breaks down the insect, digesting it. The juice of the plant is caustic, affecting the respiratory system, and when eaten by sheep, leads to a harsh, spasmodic cough. It was used in the Middle Ages to treat the plague, and 16th-century physicians used it for tuberculosis. Homeopathically, it was "proved" by Hahnemann, and the whole fresh plant is used, mainly to treat coughs.

Relieves
- severe, spasmodic hollow-sounding cough
- breathing difficulties
- retching or the vomiting of mucus
- growing pains

USES
Complaints, such as whooping cough, characterized by a violent, spasmodic, hollow-sounding cough, triggered by a tickling sensation in the throat. The cough worsens after midnight, and at the acute stage is accompanied by retching and vomiting, cold sweats, and nosebleeds, after which the patient becomes talkative. Also helps the uncomfortable tingling sensation associated with growing pains, stiffness, and a hoarse voice.

Which type of person?
- restless, obstinate when ill
- unable to concentrate

- dislike being left alone to fear of ghosts
- worry about being given bad news

SYMPTOMS

- feel persecuted
- difficulty in concentrating
- unable to settle, and become stubborn
- barking cough
- tingling in leg bones
- Symptoms improve when walking, in fresh air, with pressure, when sitting up, and when quiet. They worsen after midnight, after cold food and drinking, when lying down, and if the bed is too warm.

EUPHRASIA OFFICINALIS
EUPHRASIA STRICTA, EYEBRIGHT, EUPHASIA

Grown in Europe and America, eyebright—as its name suggests—has been used for centuries to treat eye problems. It is believed the name comes from one of the Three Graces, Euphrosyne, who was known for her gladness and joy. First mentioned as an eye treatment in 1305, it was used in later centuries as an infusion for eyes, and in the 19th century was also used as a treatment for coughs, headaches, and earaches. It is commonly used in herbal medicine. Homeopathically, the whole fresh plant is used when in flower to make a remedy for sore, irritated eyes and eye injuries.

Relieves

- stinging, watery discharge from the eyes
- inflammation or injury to the eyes
- running eyes associated with hay fever

USES

Any eye irritation or inflammation, such as conjunctivitis, inflammation of the eyelid or iris, small blisters on the cornea. Also for dimmed vision; dislike of bright lights; watery, irritated eyes associated with hay fever sufferers, but accompanied by only bland nasal discharge; colds accompanied by flushed face and runny catarrh; eye injuries; dry eyes associated with menopause. Also useful for constipation, exploding headaches, short painful menstruation, the early stages of measles, and, in men, inflammation of the prostate gland.

Which type of person?

- no particular type

SYMPTOMS

- stinging discharge from the eyes
- watering eyes
- an intolerance of bright light
- hot cheeks
- bursting headaches
- Symptoms improve after lying down in a darkened room and with drinking coffee, and worsen in bright light, in the evening, in enclosed spaces, and during warm, windy weather.

FERRUM PHOSPHORICUM
IRON PHOSPHATE, FERR. PHOS.

The Ferr. phos. remedy is made from iron phosphate, which is a chemical combination of iron sulfate, sodium phosphate, and sodium acetate. It is one of the 12 biochemical tissue salts developed by the German physician Wilhelm Schussler between 1872 and 1898. Schussler believed many complaints were the result of a deficiency of minerals, and that by replacing these minerals, or tissue salts, health could be restored. Schussler found Ferr. phos. particularly useful in the early stages of inflammation, and the homeopathic remedy is used for similar purposes.

SYMPTOMS

- headaches and head colds
- dry, hacking cough, laryngitis, hoarseness
- shooting rheumatic pains
- facial flushing and rapid pulse

- chills starting in the early afternoon
- Symptoms improve with gentle exercise and cold compresses, and worsen in the heat, with movement, when touched, lying on the right side, between 4a.m. and 6a.m., when suppressing sweating.

Relieves
- early stages of inflammation or infection
- coughs and colds which come on slowly

USES

First stages of inflammation or infection, when more blood is flowing to the affected areas, causing congestion, and before the onset of other symptoms. Also slow-starting colds accompanied by nosebleeds and fevers, with hacking cough; headaches which are helped by cool water; rheumatic pain; gastritis including vomiting undigested food; indigestion with sour-tasting burps; hemorrhages; in women, intermittent, painful menstruation; stress incontinence; first stages of dysentery with bloody stools.

Which type of person?
- pale, anemic-looking
- full of ideas
- susceptible to sudden facial flushes
- complaining but good-natured
- dislike milk, meat; crave coffee
- tend to suffer respiratory and gastrointestinal complaints

GELSEMIUM SEMPERVIRENS
YELLOW JASMINE, CAROLINA JASMINE, FALSE JASMINE, GELSEMIUM

This climbing plant, with its fragrant yellow flowers, is native to the southern States of the U.S. and, despite being attractive to look at, is poisonous if eaten. Ingesting large quantities will affect the respiratory system and movement, leading to shaking, inflammation, and paralysis. Historically, its medicinal uses were first noted when a farmer in Mississippi in the 1840s accidentally ate the plant's root and found his fever was cured. It was used as a treatment for fevers in herbalism before being "proven" in homeopathy.

SYMPTOMS
- fears and phobias, accompanied by trembling and need to urinate
- fears such as the dentist, falling or throwing oneself from a height
- dull and lethargic
- nervous and feel inadequate
- headaches causing tightness
- faintness
- facial flushing
- visual disturbances
- muscle pain
- trembling
- Symptoms improve after urinating and perspiring, after alcohol or stimulants, and when bending forward. They worsen after physical exertion, in heat, humidity, damp, or fog, with excitement, worry, or stress about symptoms.

Relieves
- complaints of the nervous system
- fears and phobias
- colds, flu
- visual disturbances

USES

Conditions which affect the nervous system respond well, such as problems of the nerves and muscles. Headaches which worsen with movement or light; muscle pain which accompanies fever; nervous disorders such as multiple sclerosis; nerve inflammation; right eye pain; heavy, drooping eyelids; inflamed tonsils and summer colds can all be helped. Also fevers, including flushing; an unpleasant taste in the mouth; twitchy muscles, and chills. It can help alleviate fears and shock accompanied by shaking or trembling. Visual disturbances and blurred vision can also be treated.

Which type of person?
- dull and heavy-looking, often with a blue tinge to the skin
- intelligence is often below average
- heavy smokers
- cowardly
- mentally weak

GLONOINUM
NITROGLYCERINE, GLYCERYL TRINITRATE, GLON.

Nitroglycerine, a thick, clear, toxic liquid, was discovered by the Italian chemist A. Sobrero in the mid-19th century. Two decades later, Swedish scientist Alfred Nobel used it as the explosive component in dynamite. In conventional medicine, it is used to treat heart disease. Homeopathically, the remedy is made from glycerine, nitric and sulfuric acid. In Victorian times, typesetters and printers who worked under the powerful heat of incandescent gas lamps used it to treat the severe headaches they suffered. The remedy is mainly used for blood and circulation conditions.

Relieves
- heatstroke
- headaches
- hot flashes

USES
This is a useful remedy for heatstroke, when an increase in blood circulation flows to the head, causing flushes of heat and a painful bursting sensation in the head. It is also good for headaches and migraine when the head feels very hot and blood vessels seem to be expanding, the patient feels like vomiting, and pressure on the head is unbearable; dizziness; for headaches which are aggravated by heat or cold; and for the cessation of menstruation and the hot flashes often associated with menopause.

Which type of person?
- no particular type

SYMPTOMS
- quick and violent
- expansive
- strong emotions
- confused
- lacks sense of direction in life
- violent symptoms
- bursting feeling in head and neck
- headaches, migraine

- circulation not particularly good
- hot flashes
- Symptoms improve in fresh air, and worsen in the heat, if in direct sunlight, with any movement of the head.

GRAPHITES
GRAPHITE, PLUMBAGO, BLACK LEAD, GRAPH.

Graphite is a mineral found in marble, granite, and crystalline rocks, and is mined in Sri Lanka, Canada, the U.S., and Mexico. It is a mixture of carbon, iron, and silica, and is contained in products such as batteries, polishes, lubricants, and also pencils—its name comes from the Greek *graphein*, meaning "to write." It was first "proved" by Hahnemann when he discovered that workmen were using black lead to heal cold sores. Homeopathically, graphite is ground to a powder to make the remedy, and is used to treat skin complaints and metabolic imbalances.

Relieves
- skin problems, nail malformation, and obesity, which have been triggered by metabolic imbalances
- menstrual problems
- stomach ulcers
- problems on the left side of the body

USES
Commonly used for skin problems such as eczema, where the skin cracks in places such as the palms of the hands, behind the knees and ears, and a thick discharge oozes out. Skin complaints which have been triggered by a metabolic imbalance, such as psoriasis, where the skin becomes dry and cracked, and nail malformation; cuts and grazes that refuse to heal and become septic; inflamed, itchy scars, and obesity can be treated. Conditions that develop on the soft mucous membranes—for instance, in the mouth or stomach, such as cold sores and ulcers—can also be helped. Other conditions, such as hair loss, cramps in hands and feet, catarrh, swollen glands, and sweating after nosebleeds are responsive.

Which type of person?

- dark-haired, coarse-featured, with pale, dry skin
- overweight, even obese
- only able to concentrate for short periods
- moody, apprehensive, indecisive, slow reactions
- prefer sour and acidic cold drinks, dislike seafood, sweet and salty things
- grumpy on waking and become more irritable throughout the day
- prefer outdoor, manual employment
- children tend to be plump and pale-looking; pessimistic and anxious; prone to carsickness; and tend to have little stamina

SYMPTOMS

- fear of thunderstorms, insanity, death
- anxiety as do not feel mentally alert
- easily startled
- tend to be morose and occasionally depressed
- dry, rough skin
- flaky and crusted scalp
- easily flushed
- no stamina
- headaches if a meal is missed
- ulcers or cold sores
- problems tend to occur on left side
- Symptoms improve in warm, fresh air, after eating or sleeping, and in the dark. They worsen in cold, damp air, in the morning and evening, during menstruation, after eating sweet food or seafood, and if the skin problems are suppressed, for instance with steroids.

HAMAMELIS VIRGINIANA
WITCH HAZEL, SNAPPING HAZELNUT, SPOTTED ALDER, HAMAMELIS

Grown in parts of Canada, the U.S., and Europe, witch hazel, which can come from a number of trees or shrubs in the *Hamamelis* family, has historically been used for its astringent qualities. In conventional medicine, it has been used for treating minor cuts, burns, rashes, and insect bites. In the homeopathic remedy, the outer skin of the root and bark of the twigs are chopped and pounded to a pulp. The remedy was first "proved" in 1850 by Dr. Hering, an American follower of Hahnemann, and is commonly used to treat piles and varicose veins by improving circulation.

SYMPTOMS

- depression, wanting to be left alone
- restlessness and irritability
- demand respect
- big ideas
- piles, varicose veins
- painful bruising
- bloodshot eyes
- headaches, relieved by nosebleeds
- in women, inflammation of the ovaries or uterus, heavy menstrual bleeding, and/or pain at the time of ovulation
- Symptoms improve in fresh air and after thinking about the problem, talking, or reading, and worsen in warm, damp air, and with pressure or movement.

Relieves

- varicose veins, piles
- nosebleeds
- bruises
- depression

USES

Primarily used to treat problems associated with bleeding, such as varicose veins and piles (hemorrhoids), which occur when the veins become weakened and swollen with blood; also when the fragile blood vessels in the nose rupture, causing nosebleeds; bruises and soreness due to injury; bloodshot eyes; phlegm dotted with blood after coughing. It is also used for heavy bleeding during menstruation and pain during ovulation, as well as being given to treat bouts of depression.

Which type of person?

- no particular type

HEPAR SULFURIS CALCAREUM
CALCIUM SULFIDE, HEP. SULF.

Historically, calcium sulfide was used to treat a number of complaints such as rheumatism, gout, and itching. In conventional medicine, it is used for skin conditions such as acne and boils. It was first "proved" by Hahnemann in 1794 and was used to counter the effects of mercury, which was often used to treat illnesses at that time. Homeopathically, the remedy, made from heating the calcareous inner layer of oyster shells with flowers of sulfur, is used to treat skin infections and ailments accompanied by a discharge.

SYMPTOMS
- anxious and irritable
- tendency to be depressed
- sluggish
- sensitive to touch, pain, cold air, noise
- sour-smelling secretions—sweat, urine, stools
- skin moist and sensitive
- low pain threshold
- seeping ailments: ulcers, cold sores, acne, boils
- coughs, colds, sore throats, flu
- Symptoms improve in warmth, after applying warm compresses, and after eating, and worsen in the morning, in the cold, when touching or lying on the affected parts.

Relieves
- pus-producing infections
- skin infections
- conditions accompanied by sensitivity to touch

USES
Commonly treats infections in which there is discharge, such as conjunctivitis, sinusitis, cold sores, and mouth ulcers, as well as general infections such as earache, tonsillitis, phlegm-filled chests, and flu. Also used for infections to aid in expelling pus, such as for acne where the spots are sensitive to touch. Other conditions which it can be used to help include colds accompanied by a tickly cough, and dry, hoarse coughs accompanied by a lot of phlegm.

Which type of person?
- to tend to be flabby or are quite overweight
- pale-looking
- lethargic and listless
- have exaggerated likes and dislikes
- anxious and frequently bad-tempered
- fail to think things through properly
- easily offended

HYOSCYAMUS NIGER
HENBANE, BLACK HENBANE, HOG'S BEAN, STINKING ROGER HYOSCYAMUS

It is believed the Romans first brought this poisonous plant to Europe, although it is also grown in parts of the U.S., Canada, and Asia, thriving on garbage heaps and cemeteries. In conventional medicine, it was used as a painkiller, sedative, and anticonvulsant, and the drug hyoscine is currently given as an antispasmodic. Homeopathically, it was first "proved" by Hahnemann. The remedy is made by extracting juice from the whole fresh plant (which is of the same botanical family as belladonna) when in flower. It is a useful remedy for the elderly due to its gentle approach.

Relieves
- emotional problems
- twitches
- dry coughs

USES
Used when emotions, such as jealousy or paranoia, seem to have taken over, and the sufferer feels that he or she is being watched or poisoned. The patient will be either silent or very talkative, with violent outbursts and foul language. Physical conditions are characterized by confusion and passive stupor, with the patient mumbling and weak; twitching and trembling may occur. Dry, spasmodic coughs that are accompanied by twitching and jerking, and helped by sitting up, also respond.

Which type of person?

- lack of self-expression
- suspicious
- may hallucinate
- urge to count things

SYMPTOMS

- talkative, even obscene
- want to expose body
- may laugh at anything
- fear of animals
- ritual behavior
- agitation
- muscle tremors, involuntary jerking
- cough
- sensitive skin
- urge to urinate, although little and infrequent flow
- Symptoms improve when bending or sitting up, and worsen after emotional upset, when touched, after food, when lying down, and in the evening.

HYPERICUM PERFORATUM
ST. JOHN'S WORT, HYPERICUM

The St. John's wort shrub is native to Asia and Europe, but is now grown worldwide. Its glandular leaves and yellow flowers secrete a blood-red juice, which led it to be used for cuts and wounds in the past. Its name comes from John the Baptist, and the black marks on the leaves were said to be a symbol of his beheading at the insistence of Herod's daughter, Salome. It is commonly used in herbal medicine, where, as in homeopathy, it is valued for its antidepressant action. In homeopathy, the whole fresh plant is used when in flower, and it is most often given to treat nerve pain following injury, due to its effective action on the central nervous system. Hypericum was "proved" by Dr. G. F. Mueller.

SYMPTOMS

- depression
- sleepiness
- neuralgia
- concussion

- toothache
- severe shooting pains that travel upward
- cravings for hot drinks, wine
- Symptoms improve when the head is tilted backward, but worsen in warm, stuffy rooms, in damp, cold, or foggy weather, when touched, or when the affected part is exposed.

Relieves

- nerve pain after injury
- head injuries
- shooting pains

USES

Hypericum works well on any area affected by nerve pain and injury, but particularly on injuries to parts of the body where there are many nerve endings, such as the spine, head, fingers, toes, and lips. It can also help concussion, neuralgia, back pain, pain that shoots upward, pain after dentistry, small wounds such as bites or splinters, nausea, asthma which worsens in fog, painful piles, and rectal nerve pain. In women, headaches associated with late menstruation can also be alleviated.

Which type of person?

- no particular type

IGNATIA AMARA
STRYCHNOS IGNATII,
ST. IGNATIUS' BEAN, IGNATIA

The Ignatia amara tree is found in the Philippines, Indonesia, and China. Its seeds have been used for centuries for healing, and native Filipinos wore them as amulets to ward off disease. The Spanish Jesuits brought the seeds to Europe in the 17th century, naming the tree after the Catholic priest Ignatius Loyola, who founded the Society of Jesus. In conventional medicine, they were used to treat cholera and epilepsy. Homeopathically, the seeds are separated from their pod and powdered. The remedy is used to treat emotional upsets, such as shock and grief, as the strychnine acts on the central nervous system.

Relieves

- emotional traumas
- bereavement
- depression
- headaches
- changeable ailments

USES

Ignatia is commonly used to treat shock, anger, and grief characterized by changes of mood, insomnia, and hysteria. All emotional upsets—mild depression, love traumas, self-pity, tearfulness, nervous headaches, fainting, sweating, choking, or a tickly cough—can be alleviated. Contradictory symptoms—for instance, a sore throat which feels better after eating solids—are helped. In women, lack of menstruation, or uterine spasm during menstruation, constipation, piles, and shooting pain in a prolapsed rectum are all relieved.

Which type of person?

- mainly thin, dark-haired women
- tired, look strained
- emotionally sensitive, artistic, nervous disposition
- unpredictable to high expectations
- prefer sour food, dairy products, bread, coffee; dislike fruit, sweet food, and also alcohol
- children tend to be bright, excitable, highly strung; do not cope well with stress, becoming angry and scared. Suffer nervous headaches; are prone to nervous coughing

SYMPTOMS

- fears emotional hurt
- dislikes losing control, enclosed spaces, crowds
- difficulty in expressing emotions
- often contradictory
- sensitive to pain
- moody, laughs and cries at the same time
- yawns or sighs a lot
- intense headaches, spasmodic cough
- faints in small spaces
- food cravings, constipation
- Symptoms improve after eating, urinating, with firm pressure, or lying on the affected side, with heat. They worsen in the cold, when touched, after emotional upset, when taking coffee or smoking, when exposed to strong odors.

KALI BICHROMICUM
POTASSIUM DICHROMATE, POTASSIUM BICHROMATE, KALI BICH.

Potassium dichromate is an orange-red crystalline substance which has caustic and corrosive effects. It is used in a variety of manufacturing processes such as color dyeing, photography, calico printing, and as a bleaching agent. The homeopathic remedy was first "proved" in 1844, and is commonly given to treat ailments affecting the mucous membranes which lead to mucus and discharge—for example, in the nose, throat, stomach, and vagina.

Relieves

- all forms of mucus or discharge
- pain that moves about

USES

This remedy is useful for any condition which affects the mucous membranes, leading to a stringy, yellow, or white discharge. It can help alleviate problems such as sinusitis; glue ear; coughs and colds accompanied by catarrh, where the affected areas feel congested and under pressure. Vomiting where the cause is a digestive disorder and yellow mucus is ejected can also be helped, as can rheumatic pain in joints when the pain tends to move about and becomes worse in hot weather. Migraines which begin at night, feel worse when bending, but better when pressure is applied to the base of the nose also respond well.

Which type of person?

- down-to-earth, straightforward
- high morals
- self-absorbed
- conservative
- like routine, pay attention to detail
- prefer orderliness

SYMPTOMS

- preoccupied with details
- dislike hot weather
- chilly and sensitive to cold when ill

- discharge from nose, throat, stomach, vagina
- catarrhal coughs
- heavy colds and blocked ears
- migraines
- Symptoms improve in the warmth, after eating, vomiting, or moving. They worsen in cold, wet weather, after drinking, and on waking, between 3a.m. and 5a.m., in summer heat, and when feeling cold.

KALI PHOSPHORICUM
POTASSIUM PHOSPHATE, PHOSPHATE OF POTASH, KALI PHOS.

Potassium is found naturally in almost all foods and is an essential part of our diet. We need it to maintain healthy function of the brain and nerve cells. In conventional medicine, it is given when levels of phosphorus are low—for instance, after gastroenteritis or for those who need to be fed intravenously. Kali phos. is also one of the 12 tissue salts identified by the German physician Wilhelm Schussler. Homeopathically, it is prepared by adding dilute phosphoric acid to a solution of potassium carbonate (also known as potash), and is used to treat conditions affecting the nervous system, and for exhaustion.

SYMPTOMS
- worry
- stressed out
- easily upset on hearing sad news
- easily exhausted by hard work
- sensitive to disturbances and cold
- suffer a discharge from the bladder, vagina, or lungs
- muscular weakness
- Symptoms improve in the warmth, after eating or gentle movement, and in cloudy weather. They worsen in cold, dry conditions, in winter, after cold drinks, after physical exertion or talking, and when exposed to noise.

Relieves
- physical and mental exhaustion
- disorders of the nervous system

USES
Used to treat mental and physical exhaustion, particularly when the nerves become so frayed the patient is on edge, and sensitive to any disturbance or distraction. Sufferers wish to be left alone and become introverted. Conditions such as sensitivity to cold, pus or yellow vaginal discharge, discharge from the lungs or in the stools, muscle fatigue, unwelcome early morning awakening, and chronic fatigue syndrome can all be alleviated.

Which type of person?
- conservative but outgoing
- clear-sighted
- easily upset by bad or distressing news
- stress and overwork tire them out easily

LEDUM PALUSTRE
WILD ROSEMARY, MARSH TEA, LEDUM

It is the fine, woolly hairs on the underside of the rosemary plant which give it its Greek name, *ledos*, meaning woolly robe. Wild rosemary has been used for its antiseptic qualities for centuries, and was used more than 700 years ago by the Finns to deter vermin. In the U.S. colonies, it was first used in 1773 as a substitute for tea when the tea taxes were introduced. It grows in Ireland, Scandinavia, the U.S., and Canada. Homeopathically, ledum is made from the whole fresh plant in flower, which is dried and powdered.

Relieves
- cuts, grazes, stings
- pain that moves about
- prevents wounds becoming infected

USES

Ledum is a useful first-aid remedy and helps prevent infection in cuts and wounds. Complaints that need immediate treatment—such as stings, cuts, grazes, eye injuries, and puncture wounds—respond well, and ledum is effective if there is accompanying bruising and the area becomes painful, swollen, and puffy. It can also help to alleviate rheumatic pain which starts in the feet and moves up; painful or injured joints which may look pale or bluish; and where the affected part feels cold to the touch, but the person feels hot inside.

Which type of person?

- no particular type

SYMPTOMS

- timid, but impatient
- morose and want to be left alone
- get extremely angry
- hate others
- stiff joints
- puffy, bluish skin
- night sweats
- black eyes
- Symptoms improve when cold compresses are applied to the affected part, and if the area is left uncovered, and worsen if warm, touched, when in bed, and at night.

LYCOPODIUM CLAVATUM
CLUB MOSS, WOLF'S CLAW, STAGSHORN MOSS, RUNNING PINE, LYCOPODIUM

This plant has long been used to treat stomach complaints and urinary disorders, and is grown in the mountains and forests of the northern hemisphere. Historically, Arab physicians used it to disperse kidney stones, while 300 years ago its yellow pollen was used to treat urine retention and gout. It flares up when exposed to naked flame and in the past was used in fireworks. It is also water resistant and was used to coat pills to prevent them

from gluing together. Lycopodium was first "proved" by Hahnemann, and for homeopathic use the pollen dust is shaken out of the spikes of the fresh plant.

SYMPTOMS

- fear of being alone, enclosed spaces, crowds, death
- hatred of the thought of failure
- dislike of the dark
- intolerance of weakness in others and illness
- sexual promiscuity
- weakness on right side of body
- sensitive areas include the digestive organs, brain, lungs, skin, liver, kidneys, and bladder
- fatigue
- Symptoms improve when in cool, fresh air, when wearing loose clothing, after hot food and drink, and at night. They are worse on the right side, in stuffy rooms, when wearing tight clothing, after overeating or not eating, between 4a.m. and 5a.m., and between 4p.m. and 5p.m.

Relieves

- stomach disorders
- digestive conditions
- complaints of the bladder and kidney
- problems on the right side
- in men, enlarged prostate, inability to have an erection
- emotional problems and anxiety caused by insecurity

USES

This remedy is commonly used to treat digestive complaints, such as vomiting, indigestion, distended abdomen with flatulence, constipation, bleeding piles, and hunger which turns to discomfort after eating. Other problems that can be alleviated include swelling in the ankles, feet, or hands (edema); burst blood vessels in the eye; chronic catarrh; psoriasis on the hands; and pneumonia. Most problems tend to occur on the right side of the body, and are accompanied by cravings for sweet food. In men, the remedy is helpful for an enlarged prostate; urine which has a reddish tinge and contains a sandy sediment due to kidney stones; increased libido, but without the ability to achieve or sustain an erection.

Which type of person?

- distinguished appearance
- tall and lean in physique, but not physically strong

- deep facial frown lines, may also be prematurely bald or gray
- detached and poised
- hold important positions, e.g. diplomat or lawyer
- deep insecurity leads to gross exaggerations
- dislike change and having to face challenges
- enjoy company but avoid commitment
- prefer shellfish, sweet food, hot food and drink, cabbage, and onions
- children tend to be thin and sallow, are shy and lack confidence, prefer reading to outdoor activities, have a slightly distended abdomen, and although well behaved at school, are bossy at home

MAGNESIA PHOSPHORICA
MAGNESIUM PHOSPHATE, PHOSPHATE OF MAGNESIA, MAG. PHOS.

Magnesium phosphate is one of the homeopathically prepared tissue salts introduced by the German physician Wilhelm Schussler at the end of the 19th century. He believed a deficiency of a mineral salt such as Mag. phos., could lead to disease. In the case of Mag. phos., he found deficiency caused problems associated with muscular nerve endings and tissue. The homeopathic remedy is made chemically from magnesium sulfate and sodium phosphate, and has an antispasmodic effect. Magnesium phosphate is also found naturally in grain cereals like wheat and oats.

SYMPTOMS
- impulsive
- dislike mental effort
- may stammer
- forgetful
- complain of coldness in the spine
- headaches
- dizziness
- jerky movements
- pain on right side of body

- Symptoms improve in the warmth, with pressure, hot compresses, and bending double, and are worse on the right side, when cool, when touched, and at night.

Relieves
- cramps
- neuralgia
- pains on the right side

USES
A useful remedy for any type of cramp from infant colic and abdominal cramp, to menstrual pains and writer's cramp, with the sufferer doubled up in pain. Abdominal cramps are sharp and intense, with the pain jumping from one part to another, and may improve when bending, with heat, and hard pressure, and worsen in the cold, draughts, and at night. Certain types of headache and neuralgia can also be helped—when the head throbs, the face is flushed, and pain suddenly comes and goes—which improve in the warmth and if the head is bound, but worsen in the cold and draughts, and at night. Pains tend to be on the right side of the body.

Which type of person?
- thin, weak
- sensitive, artistic
- intellectual, intense
- restless and nervous

MATRICARIA RECUTITA
GERMAN CHAMOMILE, WILD CHAMOMILE, CHAMOMILLA

Hippocrates was one of the first physicians to understand the medicinal benefits of chamomile. It is extensively used in herbal medicine to treat conditions such as asthma and eczema, and during childbirth to strengthen the uterus. Chamomile tea is a popular, soothing herbal drink. The plant is a member of the daisy family, and the aromatic flowers can be found all over Europe and America. Homeopathically, the juice is extracted from the whole fresh plant when it is in flower in the late spring, and the remedy is given for those who are sensitive and have a low pain threshold, and is particularly good for children.

Relieves
- low pain tolerance
- nervous afflictions
- children's ailments

USES
Chamomilla works well for those who are sensitive to pain and are unable to deal with their discomfort, being impatient, rude, and angry when ill. Often the reaction seems disproportionate to the amount of pain being felt. Even slight pain may cause sweats and fainting in women and children. Children particularly benefit from the remedy. Teething newborns, who are feverish and want to be held all the time, can be soothed; earache when the child is unable to sit still due to the pain and may scream, and toothache which makes one cheek red and hot can also be alleviated. Other conditions treated include heavy, painful menstruation, tinnitus, heartburn, and slimy green diarrhea.

Which type of person?
- low pain tolerance
- whining
- impatient
- never satisfied

SYMPTOMS
- angry, irritable
- spiteful
- sensitive to people and surroundings
- cries in sleep
- restless
- teething
- earache
- toothache
- Symptoms improve in the warmth, in wet weather, for not eating, and if carried (children). They worsen in heat, fresh air, cold winds, when angry, and after drinking coffee.

MERCURIUS SOLUBILIS HAHNEMANNI
MERCURY, QUICKSILVER, MERC. SOL.

In Roman times, Mercury was known as the messenger of the gods. In recent centuries, the substance has been used for various medicinal purposes. Although it is toxic and if given in too large a dose causes salivation and vomiting, it was once used in small amounts to treat conditions such as syphilis and to encourage secretions. Mercury is usually found in cinnabar, a mineral which forms near hot springs and volcanoes. A silvery-white liquid metal, it is dissolved in dilute nitric acid, forming particles which are dried and powdered for homeopathic use. Although there are many Mercurius remedies, Merc. sol. is mainly used to treat conditions associated with foul-smelling secretions.

SYMPTOMS
- restlessness, anxiety
- worry about family becoming ill
- fear of insanity, death
- dislike of thunderstorms
- explosive anger, even murderous feelings if upset
- any complaint which is characterized by a strong-smelling discharge
- burning secretions
- eye complaints
- skin conditions
- aching joints
- weak areas include lining of the stomach and respiratory system, skin, bones and joints, blood, mouth and throat, liver
- Symptoms improve in temperate weather and after rest, and worsen in changeable weather, when lying on the right side, if too hot in bed, when sweating, and at night.

Relieves
- complaints accompanied by strong-smelling secretions
- conditions affecting the mouth and throat
- offensive sweating

USES

Conditions characterized by a smelly discharge are helped by this remedy, including chronic conjunctivitis, pus secretions from the ears, watery catarrh, nasal cold sores, glutinous saliva which stains the pillow during sleep, throat ulcers which make swallowing painful, phlegmy cough which is worse in the warmth and at night, drenching sweats, pus-filled skin eruptions, sores, and, in women, excessive vaginal discharge and green-looking stools flecked with blood. In the mouth and throat, gingivitis, thrush, bad breath, loose teeth in infected gums, swollen tonsils, and ulcers can be helped. Other symptoms which can be alleviated are foul-smelling sweat which chills the skin as it dries, and oily sweats which make other symptoms worse; stinging, watery eyes and swollen lids due to conjunctivitis; burning nasal secretions; and blisters and scalp lesions.

Which type of person?
- fair-haired, with smooth, clear skin
- outwardly detached, yet sensitive to criticism
- inner sense of haste
- insecure, cautious, and suspicious of others
- dislike being contradicted and may react badly
- strong emotional undercurrents
- when ill, become slow, uncomprehending, forgetful, and lack will-power
- prefer cold drinks, lemons, bread and butter, dislike sweet food, alcohol (except beer), meat, salt
- children tend to appear very grown up, flirty, and precocious, but inwardly are cautious and easily upset; may also be shy and introverted with a tendency to stammer; prone to problems with ears, nose, and throat

NATRUM MURIATICUM
ROCK SALT, SODIUM CHLORIDE, HALITE, NAT. MUR.

Salt has long been a valuable commodity. In the past, it was used instead of money for trading purposes and was given as payment to soldiers for services, hence the word salary, which comes from the Latin *salarium*. Many people add salt to food for flavor, but in fact we get more than enough salt, or sodium chloride, naturally from what we eat. In conventional medicine, salt is used in the form of saline solution—for instance, during surgery to replace fluids. Homeopathically, the Nat. mur. remedy is made from rock salt which is formed through the evaporation of salty water, leaving a crusty crystalline solid. The remedy is used to treat a number of conditions resulting from emotional problems and ailments characterized by a discharge. It is also one of the 12 tissue salts identified by Dr. Wilhelm Schussler.

SYMPTOMS
- impatient, easily upset when judged
- mildly depressed on waking
- fear enclosed spaces, crowds, insanity, death
- worry about losing self-control, and being hurt in the emotional sense
- dislike the dark, being late, thunderstorms
- lower lip often has a center crack
- headaches
- conditions accompanied by discharge
- constipation
- feel the cold but dislike heat
- Symptoms improve with fresh air, after sweating, and avoiding food. They worsen in the cold, hot weather, sea air, between 9a.m. and 11a.m., after overexertion, if fussed over.

Relieves
- anxiety and depression from suppressed emotions
- conditions accompanied by secretions or discharge
- skin complaints
- in women, irregular or absent menstruation
- headaches

USES

Nat. mur. works well for emotional problems, such as distress, restlessness, and depression, which tend to occur because of the suppression of other emotions, such as fear and grief. Conditions characterized by secretions or discharge, such as colds, catarrh, vaginismus, mouth ulcers, nasal boils, acne, cold sores, and other skin complaints, such as hangnails, warts, and a cracked lower lip, are alleviated. In women, it helps with erratic menstruation; menstruation which has stopped due to stress, shock, or grief; malaise or swollen ankles before and after menstruation; and a dry or sore vagina. Headaches respond well—those caused by trauma or exercise, explosive headaches, blinding migraines, headaches which feel like the head is being hammered, and are worse between 10a.m. and 11a.m., and those that start on the left side.

Relieves
- mainly women
- usually have a square- or pear-shaped figure
- sandy or dark hair
- greasy, pale, pasty skin
- watery, red-rimmed eyes
- civilized, sensitive
- when hurt, become quiet and introverted
- enjoy the company of others, but tend to be alone
- prefer sour food and beer, like but cannot tolerate starchy food and milk, dislike chicken and also coffee
- love or loathe salty food
- children tend to be slow walkers and talkers, small for their age, flush and sweat easily, are responsible and diligent, but timid and easily upset, although dislike fuss; prone to headaches and hangnails

NATRUM SULFURICUM
SODIUM SULFATE, GLAUBER'S SALT, SAL MIRABILE, NAT. SULF.

Sodium sulfate, a white crystalline compound, is found naturally in spa waters, salt water lakes, and in mineral water. It is also known as Glauber's salt. Sodium sulfate is used in the manufacture of paper, detergents, and glass. It is naturally present in the body and helps to maintain water balance. Homeopathically, it was "proved" by Hahnemann's followers, Nenning and Shieler. It is one of the 12 tissue salts identified by Schussler.

Relieves
- chest problems
- emotional changes after head injury
- headaches

USES
Used to treat chest problems such as asthma, bronchitis, colds, and flu, where there is a build-up of thick yellowish catarrh, which comes from the nose; emotional trauma after an accident in which the head is injured, leading to depression and suicidal thoughts or other emotional changes; headaches which have a vice-like grip at the back of the head and behind the forehead. Other conditions treated include dry mouth, with the tongue having a dirty coating; biliousness; thirst and frequent urination, leading to an inability to deal with damp conditions and sharp liver pains.

Which type of person?
- flabby
- prefer cool weather, dislike damp and humidity
- materialistic
- sometimes sensitive and artistic
- restless
- serious, responsible
- discontented

SYMPTOMS
- sad; sometimes have suicidal thoughts
- more depressed in the morning; brood
- sensitive, sometimes cry on hearing music
- prone to asthma brought on by damp
- tend to have profuse discharges of yellow-green mucus
- chest complaints
- triggered by damp
- Symptoms improve in fresh air, dry atmosphere, and after changing position, and worsen in the morning, late evening, when lying on the back or left side, when listening to music, and in damp weather.

PAPAVER SOMNIFERUM
OPIUM POPPY, OPIUM

The opium poppy has grayish-green leaves and flowers which range from white to various shades of red. It is grown in Indo-China, India, Turkey, and Iran. Opium is a well-known painkiller and tranquilizer, and an addictive narcotic drug. The unripe seed capsules contain alkaloids such as codeine and morphine, derivatives of which are used in conventional medicine as analgesics and hypnotics. The homeopathic remedy is made from the dried milky juice excreted by the seed capsules.

Relieves
- apathy after shock
- excitability after shock

USES
Commonly used as a treatment after a shock, such as bereavement, when the patient may be either listless and indifferent to what is going on, or overexcited, even appearing delirious, and unable to sleep; also the patient may not be aware of pain, is very sleepy, but has no recollection of dreams once awake, and perspires easily. It is also given for slow workings of the bowel and urinary system, which can lead to constipation and water retention. Stroke victims also respond well.

Which type of person?
- no particular type

SYMPTOMS
- apathetic
- uncomprehending
- overexcited
- may be delirious
- panicky
- in shock
- frightened
- loss of appetite
- constipation
- infrequent urination
- stroke
- irregular breathing
- sweaty skin
- Symptoms improve in cool surroundings and with movement, and worsen in the warmth, in heat, during and after sleep.

PHOSPHORUS
PHOSPHORUS, PHOS.

The name phosphorus comes from the Greek, meaning "light-bringing." It is a yellowish-white, nonmetallic element which occurs in phosphates and living matter. Because of its flammable properties, white phosphate, a toxic substance, was used to make matches and fireworks, but this was replaced by the nontoxic red phosphorus. Because of the ease with which it ignites, phosphorus is kept submerged in water. Our bodies need phosphorus for the healthy functioning of our teeth, bones, bodily fluids, and DNA. In conventional medicine, it has been used to treat conditions as diverse as measles and malaria. As a homeopathic treatment, it is mainly given to those suffering from anxiety and digestive disorders.

SYMPTOMS
- mentally alert
- nervous under pressure
- tend to bottle things up
- indifferent to family and friends when ill
- fear illness and death
- weak areas include digestive organs, circulation, nervous system, the left side of the body, liver
- bleeding, such as nosebleeds
- respiratory problems
- headaches
- Symptoms improve in fresh air, after sleeping, when touched, and when lying on the right side.

Relieves
- anxieties, fears
- digestive complaints
- circulatory conditions and those causing bleeding
- respiratory problems

USES
Phosphorus is used to treat symptoms such as exhaustion, insomnia, nerves which are caused by underlying stress, anxiety, and fears—for instance, due to exam pressure—overwork, or fear of dying. Other problems that can be helped include digestive problems such as nausea and vomiting due to coughing, stress, or food poisoning, cravings for certain foods, and pressure in the stomach; poor circulation, such as cold or overheated fingers and

toes; excessive bleeding, such as bleeding gums, nosebleeds, and heavy menstrual bleeding; respiratory problems such as acute bronchitis or asthma, difficulty in breathing, tight chest, pneumonia, dry tickly coughs, and red-tinged phlegm. Other conditions which can be alleviated include headaches which are worse in heat but improve after a cold compress or eating; dry skin; sensitive red eyes; perspiring under stress; fever with alternate sweating and shivering; cramps; unresolved sexual problems.

Which type of person?
- well proportioned, tall, and lean
- fine or dark hair, with reddish tinge
- pale skin, blush easily
- intelligent, outgoing, an eye for clothes, often artistic
- open and affectionate
- enthusiastic, but only in short spurts
- tend to offer more than can deliver
- imagination needs constant stimulation
- tend to crumble when subjected to pressure
- crave attention, particularly when ill
- prefer spicy, salty, sweet foods, carbonated drinks, cheese, and wine, and dislike fruit, fish, and tomatoes
- children tend to be tall for their age, smooth-featured, but blush easily; prefer company but become restless and nervous; perceptive, artistic, and affectionate. They dislike doing homework, the dark, and thunderstorms

PULSATILLA NIGRICANS
ANEMONE PRATENSIS, PASQUE FLOWER, PASCHAL FLOWER, MEADOW ANEMONE, WIND FLOWER, PULSATILLA

The pasque flower is distinguishable from other members of the *Pulsatilla* family by its beautiful, deep-purple flowers. It is found growing in central and northern Europe, Russia, and western Asia. The name passe-fleur was given by the French in the 16th century, meaning "flower that excels." It took its later name, pasque or paschal flower, meaning

Easter flower, because it usually blooms at that time. It has long been used medicinally for a number of ailments such as ulcers, tooth decay, and cataracts. In homeopathy, the whole fresh plant in flower is used to make the remedy, and it is given for a number of conditions, such as digestive disorders, depression, and gynecological problems.

SYMPTOMS
- avoid confronting people
- depressed
- self-conscious
- cry easily
- fear being alone, the dark, insanity, death
- ailments characterized by discharge
- gynecological conditions
- digestive problems
- bad taste in mouth, dry mouth
- aching joints
- Symptoms improve in fresh air, with gentle movement, and with sympathy, and worsen in the heat, on eating rich foods, after lengthy standing, when lying on the left side, and in the evening.

Relieves
- digestive disorders
- gynecological conditions
- emotional traumas
- conditions accompanied by excessive discharge

USES
Pulsatilla can help relieve a number of digestive problems, such as rich food causing lack of sleep, a stomach which is tight on waking in the morning and which reacts badly to rich or fatty food, particularly pork, heaviness under the breastbone after eating, cravings for sweet foods, and a rumbling stomach. In women, it can be used to treat lack of or late menstruation, particularly if due to shock or illness, thick, stinging discharge, and menopausal problems, all of which tend to be accompanied by crying and depression. Moodiness, depression, and fear of being alone can also be treated. Ailments characterized by excessive discharge or secretions, such as conjunctivitis, catarrh with yellow phlegm, sinusitis, and a runny nose, can also be helped. Other troublesome conditions which respond well include headaches above the eyes, backache, rheumatism, varicose veins, corneal ulcers, loose coughs, palpitations, bed-wetting.

Which type of person?
- usually women
- fair skin and fair hair, with blue eyes
- blush easily
- tend to be plump
- good-natured, kind, popular, easily influenced by, and depend on, others
- lack assertiveness, and avoid confrontation
- led by emotions rather than head
- relate to those in distress, including animals
- prefer sweet food, cold food and drink, dislike spicy food
- children tend to be either small and fair with delicate features, easygoing, affectionate yet shy, blushing easily; or darker-haired, small, listless, needing reassurance and attention, but slow in returning it

RUTA GRAVEOLENS
RUE, BITTER HERB, HERB OF GRACE, RUTA GRAV.

In the Middle Ages, rue was used to ward off the plague. In the 16th and 17th centuries, it was scattered over courtroom floors to prevent the spread of typhus, or jail fever, which was carried by the lice which thrived in the squalid jail conditions. It has also been used to treat croup, colic, headaches, and coughs, and was given as an antidote to mushroom poisoning. The homeopathic remedy is made from the juice of the whole plant, which is picked before it flowers. It is given mainly for bruising and restlessness.

Relieves
- bruises, strained ligaments
- restlessness
- eyestrain

USES

The treatment of bruised bones and tendon injuries, aching bones, deep aching pain, rheumatism, sciatica which is worse when lying down, and the restlessness which goes with having to be still. Also good for eyestrain, when the eyes feel hot and sore from overuse or reading small print, and accompanying headaches. Other conditions treated include infection after tooth extraction; weak chest with breathing difficulties; prolapsed rectum; constipation with stools that are either large and difficult to pass or loose, containing blood and mucus.

Which type of person?
- no particular type

SYMPTOMS
- contradict, criticize others
- depressed when ill
- restless
- anxious, troubled
- dissatisfied with self and with others
- painful, aching limbs
- bruises
- headaches due to eyestrain
- Symptoms improve with movement and worsen in the cold and damp, when resting or lying down.

RHUS TOXICODENDRON
RHUS RADICANS, POISON IVY, POISON OAK, RHUS TOX.

Rhus tox. is made from both poison ivy, and a variety of it, poison oak, both of which are native to the U.S. and Canada. Brushing against the leaves can cause a severe skin reaction, as well as headache, swollen glands, and fever, as they contain a poisonous sap. In homeopathy, poison ivy was first "proved" by Hahnemann. The fresh leaves of the plant are collected before it flowers, when the poison is most potent, and pounded to a pulp. The remedy is used for skin conditions and rheumatic pain.

Relieves
- joint and muscle pain, and general stiffness
- red, itchy skin eruptions

USES

It can be used to treat skin complaints characterized by red, itchy, puffy areas which feel like they are burning and which tend to form a scaly surface, such as eczema, herpes, diaper rash, and raised patches of skin where there is a clear demarcation line between the affected and unaffected part. Muscle and joint pain, such as that associated with rheumatism, osteoarthritis, cramps, restless legs, stiffness in the lower back, numbness in arms and legs, and strains can also be alleviated. Other complaints, such as headaches, dizziness, fever, stitch pains made worse by cold and damp, and abdominal pain, can also be relieved. In women, early, heavy, or prolonged menstrual bleeding and accompanying abdominal pain can be treated.

Which type of person?
- lively, extrovert
- diligent workers
- restless
- cry for no reason
- anxious at night
- like milk, always thirsty

SYMPTOMS
- fear being poisoned
- anxious at night
- depressed and may contemplate suicide
- may act compulsively
- headaches after being cold or damp
- eyes are inflamed after being wet
- backache
- blistering skin
- Symptoms improve in the warmth, with movement or after changing position, and after stretching. They worsen during cold, wet weather, with rest, when lying on the back or on the right side, and at night.

SILICEA TERRA
QUARTZ, SILICA, FLINT, ROCK CRYSTAL, SIL.

Silica, the main constituent of rock, is prepared from silicon dioxide, found in flint, quartz, and sandstone. Plants absorb it through their stems and in humans it is essential for the growth of bones, teeth, hair, and nails, and for the maintenance of connective tissue. In homeopathy, it is useful for problems of the digestive and nervous systems, bone and skin conditions, and for its ability to promote the expulsion of foreign bodies such as thorns and splinters. It is also one of the 12 tissue salts identified by Dr. Wilhelm Schussler.

SYMPTOMS
- fear of failure, exertion, sharp objects
- timidity, lack of self-confidence
- worry about future events
- fear of commitment because of being hurt
- feet often sweaty
- chills
- slow healing
- discharges
- cracked lips, brittle nails
- Symptoms improve in heat and when wrapped up, and worsen in draughts, cold, and damp, when lying on the left side, after washing, by suppressing sweat, and in the morning.

Relieves
- conditions caused by low immunity due to being malnourished
- bone and skin conditions
- assists in the expulsion of foreign bodies

USES
Silica is good for complaints which have occurred as a result of low immunity due to lack of nourishment, such as colds, ear infections, catarrh. It can also be used to treat skin and bone conditions, such as acne, weak nails, slow growth, or fontanels which are slow to close in babies, slow-healing fractures; to assist in expelling splinters, glass shards, or thorns from body tissue; and to alleviate problems associated with the nervous system, such as colic and migraines. Other problems alleviated include catarrh with thick, yellow discharge, enlarged lymph nodes, offensive sweat, headaches which start at the back of the head and move over the forehead, glue ear, and restless sleep.

Which type of person?
- slim, small-boned, with lank hair
- neat appearance but prone to cracked lips, and brittle, uneven nails

- appear fragile and lack stamina, but are tenacious
- lack self-confidence, but are strong-willed
- often tired
- worry about new challenges, but take them on anyway
- prefer cold food and dislike milk, meat, cheese
- children tend to be neat, small, but with large sweaty heads, feel the cold easily, are shy but strong-willed, and conscientious but lacking in confidence

SEPIA OFFICINALIS
CUTTLEFISH, SEPIA

Historically, cuttlefish ink has been used medicinally to treat conditions such as kidney stones, hair loss, and gonorrhea. It is also used as a pigment in paint, which is where Hahnemann first came across it. He noticed that an artist he was treating for apathy and depression often sucked his brushes, which had been dipped in sepia paint. He published his findings in 1834 after "proving" the remedy. Today, sepia is most commonly taken by women, and is used to treat complaints such as menstrual problems and hormonal imbalances.

SYMPTOMS
- fear poverty, being alone, insanity
- irritable with family, but good in company
- bottle up anger
- find it hard to conceal thoughts
- sudden weeping
- easily chilled
- dragging sensation in abdomen
- burning or throbbing pains
- Symptoms improve after food, exertion, especially dancing, sleep, and in the warmth, and are worse on the left side, after physical and mental exertion, in the early morning and evening, in thundery weather, and if near tobacco.

Relieves
- menstrual problems
- conditions associated with hormonal imbalance
- complaints accompanied by exhaustion

USES
Useful for women who feel "dragged down," both physically and emotionally. Useful for complaints relating to the vagina, ovaries, and uterus, such as heavy or painful menstruation, PMS, menopausal hot flashes, thrush, conditions associated with pregnancy, and the feeling of a sagging abdomen, where the woman feels the need to cross her legs. Pain during sex, aversion to sex, or exhaustion afterward can also be treated. Also, any situation where the woman is feeling emotionally and physically tired, and lacking in energy. Also useful for headaches with nausea, hair loss, dizziness, offensive sweating, indigestion, skin discoloration, and circulatory problems.

Which type of person?
- mainly women
- tall, slim, dark hair and eyes, yellowish facial skin pigmentation
- dignified and attractive to detached yet emotional
- martyr
- love dancing
- have strong opinions, hating to be contradicted
- resentful of responsibilities
- either career women who appear tough yet are vulnerable, or wives and mothers whose own needs are not met
- prefer sour and sweet foods, alcohol, and dislike milk and pork
- children tend to be sallow, sweaty-skinned, and tire easily; sensitive to weather; moody and negative, dislike parties and being left alone; tendency to constipation

SPONGIA TOSTA
SPONGE, SPONGIA

Sponge was first treasured for its medicinal properties more than 600 years ago, when it was used as a treatment for goiter, the swelling of the thyroid gland, which is brought on by a deficiency of iodine. Although it was not known then, sponge contains useful amounts of iodine and bromine. Homeopathically, the remedy was first "proved" by Hahnemann, and appears in the sixth volume of his *Materia Medica Pura*. The remedy is made by toasting and powdering the sponge, which is harvested from the waters of the Mediterranean.

Relieves
- croup
- coughs
- laryngitis

USES
This remedy works particularly well for children's croup, characterized by sneezing and a hoarse, dry barking cough, with the patient waking in alarm with the feeling of suffocation, later followed by thick mucus which is difficult to bring up. Associated symptoms of coughs, such as hoarseness, dryness of the larynx from a cold, headaches which are worse when lying down, but improve when sitting up, bronchitis, dry mucous membranes, and feelings of heaviness and exhaustion are also alleviated. Laryngitis, where the throat is raw and dry, and feels like it is burning, responds well. Sponge is also good if chest conditions or tuberculosis tend to run in the family.

Which type of person?
- light-haired, blue-eyed
- lean
- dried-up appearance

SYMPTOMS
- anxiety
- fear of suffocation, and death
- waking from sleep, feeling frightened
- congestion of the chest or heart region
- coughs
- palpitations
- laryngitis
- Symptoms improve with warm food and drink, and when sitting up. They worsen when talking, swallowing, consuming sweet food or cold drinks, moving, touching the affected area, lying with the head lower than the feet, and around midnight.

SOLANUM DULCAMARA
WOODY NIGHTSHADE, BITTERSWEET, DULCAMARA

Woody nightshade has been used since Roman times as a remedy to help those suffering from conditions such as asthma, catarrh, rheumatism, and pneumonia resulting from the effects of cold and wet. It is also extensively used in herbal medicine, where it is known as bittersweet, for conditions such as eczema, psoriasis, and ulcers. The remedy, first "proved" by Hahnemann, is made from the green shoots and leaves of the flowering plant, and is given for complaints resulting from exposure to wet weather and temperature changes.

Relieves
- conditions which are triggered by or worsen with temperature changes

USES
Any condition which is brought on by exposure to cold, wet weather, weather changes—for instance, from warm to cold or from cooling down too quickly after sweating—can be alleviated. Patients tend to be worse in the fall and in damp, cold weather. Other problems brought on by weather conditions and helped by the remedy include diarrhea triggered by hot days and cold nights; back and neck pains from the damp; fevers due to exposure to the cold while the body is hot; congested eyes; ulcers; sore throat; frequent urination if chilled; and catarrhal, or dry, hoarse coughs. Skin conditions such as urticaria, crusty facial eruptions, fleshy or flat warts, and ringworm.

Which type of person?
- strong-minded, domineering personality
- possessive
- restless, confused
- keen to keep on the move
- eager for something, indifferent when get it

SYMPTOMS
- susceptible to cold and weather changes, leading to ailments such as conjunctivitis and diarrhea

- prone to colds
- hungry, but do not want food
- drowsy during the day, restless at night
- Symptoms improve in the warmth and with movement, and worsen in the cold and damp, after sweating, in temperature extremes, and with lack of movement.

STRYCHNOS NUX VOMICA
POISON NUT, QUAKER BUTTONS, NUX VOMICA

The poison nut plant, native to Indonesia, contains strychnine, which is extracted from the seeds. In the past, it was a useful poison for murder. Medicinally, in small amounts, it can help relieve digestive problems, but large doses cause muscular spasm and death from respiratory failure. Strychnine was used during the Middle Ages to help treat sufferers of the plague. Homeopathically, it was first "proved" by Hahnemann. To make the remedy, which is mainly used for oversensitivity and digestive problems, the seeds are extracted from the soft, gelatinous pulp of the fruit and are then dried.

SYMPTOMS
- fear insects, failure, crowds, death
- quarrelsome
- critical of others
- fastidious
- prone to hypochondria
- chills
- sensitive to light, smell, noise
- upset by overindulgence in food, alcohol, coffee
- aching, bursting, burning pains
- Symptoms improve when lying down and after sleep, in warmth and humidity, in the evening, after washing, and with pressure. They worsen in cold, windy weather, in the morning, in open air or under the sun, two hours after food, and after mental exhaustion.

Relieves
- digestive upsets to oversensitivity
- chills

USES
Commonly used to treat emotional problems such as irritability and oversensitivity, it works well for those who bottle up their anger, who are never satisfied, are prone to arguments, dislike having to depend on others, and prefer being left alone. Also used for digestive conditions, such as nausea, vomiting, diarrhea, indigestion, constipation, and piles, which may be brought on by overindulgence in certain foods, or due to suppressing the emotions, or from mental overwork. Other problems it can alleviate include flu, retching coughs, colds with a blocked nose at night and runny nose during the day, chills, headaches which are worse after mental exertion; in women, erratic, early, or heavy menstrual bleeding, morning sickness, constant urination, and labor pain.

Which type of person?
- mainly men
- hypersensitive
- strained-looking, lined face, sallow skin
- criticize, but cannot take criticism from others
- competitive, enjoy meeting challenges
- verbally and mentally alert, with quick wit
- intolerant of others, and easily angered
- may use stimulants to enhance performance
- disgruntled when ill
- prefer rich, fatty food, and like, but are upset by, alcohol and spicy foods
- children tend to be hyperactive and easily irritated, dislike being contradicted; prone to tantrums; diligent and competitive, but hate losing; moody on awakening; prone to stomach aches

SULFUR
BRIMSTONE, FLOWERS OF SULFUR, SULFUR

Sulfur is a mineral which is found in rock forms beside hot springs and in volcanic craters. It has been used medicinally for many centuries—in the 16th century flowers of sulfur was used to fumigate rooms where infection had been present. It was also used as a purgative and to treat rheumatism. Children used to be given brimstone and treacle to encourage bowel function. It has also been used in conventional medicine to treat skin problems such as acne. Homeopathically, it was first "proved" by Hahnemann. A fine, yellow powder is extracted from the mineral. The remedy treats digestive and skin disorders.

SYMPTOMS

- selfishness, egotism
- argumentativeness, aggressiveness
- fear of ghosts, height, failure
- lethargic depression
- full of bright ideas which fade away
- burning, itching sensations
- inflammation of affected part
- offensive odors
- thirstiness
- weak areas include left side of the body, circulation, digestive organs, and skin
- Symptoms improve when lying on the right side, in warm, dry, fresh air, after physical activity, and worsen in stuffy atmospheres, in the morning, particularly around 11a.m., and at night, in the damp and cold, and after washing.

Relieves

- inflamed, itchy skin conditions
- digestive complaints
- offensive odor
- women's conditions
- conditions other remedies do not seem to be helping

USES

Sulfur can be used to soothe hot, red, itchy skin associated with problems such as eczema and diaper rash, digestive complaints such as vomiting and diarrhea which occur in the morning, indigestion which is made worse by drinking milk, and hunger pangs. It can also treat offensive odors, such as foul-smelling sweat or discharge; premenstrual symptoms such as irritability and headaches; and menopausal symptoms, such as flushing and dizzy spells. It is also useful when another remedy has not worked as hoped or if the picture remedy is not clear. Other problems, such as lack

of energy, restless sleep, depression, fever, burning pains and eruptions, congestion, and back pain, can be helped.

Which type of person?

- either round and red-faced or lanky with bad posture
- dry, flaky skin, dull hair, unclean-looking
- selfish, self-centered, and egocentric, but can be giving and good-natured
- full of ideas, but unable to carry them out, because of a lack of will-power
- fuss over minor details
- quickly angered, but just as quickly calm down
- sensitive to smell
- prefer sweet, fatty, spicy, and sour foods, alcohol, stimulants, and dislike milk, hot drinks, and eggs
- children tend to be either well built, with thick hair and a rosy complexion, or thin and pale with dry skin; both types eat well, look disheveled, are happy when stimulated, take care of their possessions, and are difficult to get to bed

TARENTULA HISPANICA
LYCOSA TARENTULA, SPANISH SPIDER, WOLF SPIDER, TARENTULA

Tarentula gets its name from the Italian town of Taranto (Latin name *Tarentum*), where the wolf spider is commonly found. It was given the name wolf spider because of the way it chases after its prey rather than lying in wait on a web. The European wolf spider does not harm humans, unlike the bite of the poisonous South American tarantula, which was said to cause maniacal behavior, twitching, and the feeling of suffocating. The homeopathic remedy is made from the whole live spider and is used to treat restless, frantic behavior.

Relieves

- mental and physical restlessness
- mood swings
- heart complaints
- in women, ovarian disease, genital sensitivity

USES

It can be used to treat nervous disorders, such as mental and physical agitation, twitchy, restless legs, numbness, extreme mood swings, and impatience. Angina and heart disease also respond well. In women, sensitivity of the genitalia, which become itchy, heavy menstrual bleeding, and ovarian disease which feels worse on the left side of the body can be alleviated.

Which type of person?
- hyperactive, behave destructively
- extremely impatient to manipulative
- suffer vertigo
- workaholic

SYMPTOMS
- experience extreme mood swings manic laughter
- edgy, restless
- violent outbursts
- weak legs
- constricting pains
- Symptoms improve in the open air, while listening to music, looking at bright colors, and moving from side to side, and worsen with movement, noise, touch, on seeing others in trouble, and at a particular time each year.

THUJA OCCIDENTALIS
ARBOR VITAE, WHITE CEDAR, TREE OF LIFE, THUJA

The name "thuja" comes from the Greek word *thero*, meaning to sacrifice or fumigate. In pagan sacrifices, the tree was burned when victims were executed. The evergreen tree is grown in Canada and the U.S., and Native Americans used its twigs and leaves to treat rheumatism, gout, and malaria. In homeopathy, the scented leaves and twigs are pounded to a pulp to make both the remedy and a cream that is especially useful for rheumatic pain.

Relieves
- inflamed, swollen joints
- skin complaints
- genitourinary infections

USES

Thuja can be used for joints that have become swollen and inflamed, as in rheumatism; for skin complaints, particularly warts, and for pale, greasy skin which sweats when exposed; urinary infections; headaches brought on by stress or fatigue; yellow-green catarrh; foul-smelling perspiration; tooth decay; weak nails; in women, for uterine or vaginal infections, early or scant menstruation, and loss of appetite in the morning; gurgling bowels.

Which type of person?
- greasy, pale skin
- take little interest in physical appearance
- sensitive, weep easily
- prefer tea and dislike meat, potatoes, fat
- children are small, with a slim build, and are slow

SYMPTOMS
- paranoia that others are taking advantage; anxiety
- headaches
- warts
- weak nails
- urinary conditions
- catarrh
- Symptoms improve when warm and with movement, and worsen in cold and damp.

TRIGONOCEPHALUS LACHESIS
LACHESIS MUTA, BUSHMASTER SNAKE, SURUKUKU, LACHESIS

The South American bushmaster snake is extremely poisonous—one bite into a vein can cause immediate death—as the venom affects the heart and central nervous system. A lesser bite will cause bleeding and blood poisoning. The snake gets its other name, surukuku, from the humming sound it makes as it lies in wait for its prey. Homeopathically, it was first "proved" by Dr. Constantine Hering in 1837, who tested the venom on himself while in the Amazonian jungle. The remedy uses fresh venom, and treats wounds that are slow to heal or that bleed profusely.

SYMPTOMS
- disgruntled on waking; short-tempered
- strong ideas and philosophies
- suspicious of people
- jealous
- prone to post-menopausal depression
- bloating
- restlessness
- oversensitivity to touch and noise
- weak areas include the left side of the body, circulation, nervous system, and female reproductive organs
- Symptoms improve after discharges, such as menstruation, nosebleeds, or bowel movements, in fresh air, and after a cold drink, and are worse with sleep, when touched, with motion, in heat, and after hot drinks.

Relieves
- premenstrual and menopausal complaints
- circulatory and vascular problems
- left-sided complaints to slow-healing wounds

USES
Helpful for premenstrual problems such as erratic pain relieved by blood flow, and problems associated with menopause, such as hot flashes and dizziness. It works well for any problems connected with blood flow and circulation, such as varicose veins, irregular pulse, angina, and palpitations. Problems which occur on the left side, for example earache, headaches, and sore throats, can be alleviated; wounds that are not healing well, such as bleeding piles, ulcers, and cuts are helped. Other conditions include nervous disorders such as fainting and petit mal epileptic attacks; blue wounds; purplish, bloated face; fever; sweats; any pulsations or throbbing; waking up with a sensation of choking; and glands which are swollen.

Which type of person?
- tend to be redheaded, freckled, puffy-looking
- egocentric, with no regard for others
- intuitive, creative, aspiring, and strong ideologists
- selfish, devious, jealous
- dislike commitment, blow hot and cold with partners
- may be gloomy and quiet
- creativity is short-lived
- prefer sour and starchy foods and alcohol, and cannot tolerate hot drinks and wheat
- children tend to be hyperactive and difficult to control, prone to jealousy, possessive of friends

URTICA URENS
STINGING NETTLE, URTICA

The stinging nettle, a common weed found in many countries, has been used for centuries for its medicinal properties. The Greek physician Dioscorides used it as a purgative and detoxification. It is commonly used in herbal medicine for conditions such as piles, nosebleeds, stomach conditions, and as a tea. The 16th-century herbalist John Gerard used it as an antidote to poison. The small plant is covered in soft, spiny hairs which secrete a sap that causes itching and inflammation if touched. In homeopathy, it was first "proved" by Hahnemann and is used to treat conditions which are accompanied by stinging or burning. Urtica can be used externally in the form of a cream, as well as taken internally.

Relieves
- stinging, burning conditions of the skin
- rheumatic pain to neuralgia

USES
Used both as an internal remedy and externally as a cream, Urtica is useful for skin conditions, particularly if the skin is stinging or has the sensation of burning. It is good for rashes where the skin is blotchy and blistered, such as urticaria (hives) and bee stings, or when there is an allergic reaction, for instance after eating strawberries. Other conditions which it can be used to alleviate include rheumatism, neuralgia, neuritis, gout, excess uric acid, and, in women, vulval itching and painful breasts when the milk flow is blocked.

Which type of person?
- no particular type

SYMPTOMS
- stinging, burning skin
- rheumatic pain; gout
- cystitis
- Symptoms improve after massaging the affected area. and when lying down, and worsen in cold, damp air, if touched, and with water.

FLOWER REMEDIES

FLOWER ESSENCES, OR FLOWER REMEDIES, as they are more commonly known, are used therapeutically to harmonize the body, mind, and spirit. The essences are said to contain the life force of the flowers used to make them. Thousands of essences are available in health food stores, and they work "vibrationally" on a mental and emotional level, to relieve negative feelings, encourage the healing process, and to balance the energy in the body.

Flower remedies are ideal for home use, being simple to make and use. They are prepared in water and preserved with alcohol. Historically, flower water and the morning dew collected from flower petals were thought to be imbued with magical properties. That flower remedies work is indisputable; but no one knows how, so there is still an element of magic associated with their use—even today, when our understanding of vibrational medicine is growing.

Flower remedies are so simple that they are often dismissed as a placebo. They do not work in any biochemical way, and because no physical part of the plant remains in the remedy, its properties and actions cannot be detected or analyzed as if it were a drug or herbal preparation. Therapists believe the remedies contain the energy, or imprint, of the plant from which it was made and work in a way that is similar to homeopathic remedies. In this way a remedy is believed to provide the stimulus needed to kick-start your own healing mechanism.

DR. BACH

Until recently, the name Dr. Edward Bach was almost synonymous with flower remedies. His set of 38 remedies became the inspiration for the worldwide development of remedies. They are still the cornerstone of flower remedy therapy and easily available. While working in the London Homeopathic Hospital, just after the First World War, he noticed that people with similar attitudes often had similar complaints. He concluded that, independently of other factors, mood and a negative attitude predisposed people toward ill health, and that illness was a manifestation of a deeper disharmony or an indication that the personality was in conflict. Between 1928 and 1932, he identified seven main negative states and found the first 12 of the flower remedies he needed to address them. Over the subsequent few years, he dedicated himself to finding natural remedies from the countryside, and at his death had made 38 separate remedies. His successors at his house in Oxfordshire, Mount Vernon, continue to make his remedies today, and they are sold under the name Bach Flower Remedies.

OTHER REMEDIES

The Bach Flower Remedies are made from the trees and flowers Dr. Bach saw on his travels, which are native to England, with the exceptions of Olive and Vine. In the last 20 years, remedies from the U.S. and Australia have been made. Sometimes they are called flower essences (do not confuse them with essential oils), but they are said to work in the same way as the original flower remedies. They address the emotional self, unlocking repressions, liberating negativity, and encouraging positive well-being.

THE BACH FLOWER REMEDIES: A QUICK GUIDE

AGRIMONY For those who hide their feelings behind humor and put on a brave face.

ASPEN For fear of the unknown; vague, unsettling fears which cannot be explained.

BEECH For the perfectionist who tends to be intolerant of other people's methods and experience.

CENTAURY For those who find it impossible to say no to the demands of others and thus exhaust themselves by doing too much.

CERATO For those who lack confidence in themselves and are constantly seeking the advice of others to make up their mind.

CHERRY PLUM For the fear of losing one's mind, and for irrational thoughts or behavior.

CHESTNUT BUD For those who find it hard to learn from life and keep making the same mistakes.

CHICORY For the self-obsessed, mothering type who is overprotective and possessive.

CLEMATIS For the absent-minded daydreamer who needs to be awake and focus the mind on the here and now.

CRAB APPLE For those who feel unclean or polluted on any level, either physically, emotionally, or spiritually; Crab Apple is for those who feel they need purification.

ELM For those who suffer temporary feelings of inadequacy brought on by all the responsibilities they have taken on.

GENTIAN For despondency, and for those who are easily discouraged by a setback in life.

GORSE For those who suffer feelings of hopelessness and despair, and who are stuck in a negative pattern; pessimism.

HEATHER For those who like to be listened to when they talk constantly about themselves; for poor listeners and those who are self-obsessed.

HOLLY For those who suffer dissipating bouts of hatred, jealousy, envy, and suspicion.

HONEYSUCKLE For those who suffer from nostalgia or who dwell on the events of the past instead of living in the present.

HORNBEAM For those who are stuck in a rut and feel tired, so that work which used to be fulfilling is now tiresome.

IMPATIENS For impatience and irritability; Impatiens helps those for whom life is always a rush and who are too busy to slow down.

LARCH For those who feel worthless and are suffering from lack of confidence or low self-esteem.

MIMULUS For the fear of known things; for the strength to face everyday fears and all fears which can be named.

MUSTARD For depression without cause, those who feel they are under a dark gloomy cloud for no apparent reason.

OAK For the fighter who never gives in and is exhausting himself or herself by being too persistent in the same old fight.

OLIVE For those who are exhausted on all levels, fatigued, and drained of further optimism and spirit after a long struggle or effort.

PINE For those who suffer self-reproach and guilt; for those who say sorry even when things are not their fault.

RED CHESTNUT For those who are overanxious about the welfare of family or friends; for those who fear that something awful may happen to their loved ones.

ROCK ROSE For those who feel helpless and experience extreme terror or panic, when there may or may not be a reason but the feeling is real.

ROCK WATER For perfectionists who are hard on themselves and demand perfection in all things.

SCLERANTHUS For those who suffer from indecision and who cannot make up their mind.

STAR OF BETHLEHEM For shocks of all kinds, accidents, bad news, sudden startling noise, and trauma.

SWEET CHESTNUT For utter despair and hopelessness; for when there seems no way out.

VERVAIN For enthusiasts and those with a strong sense of justice; those who never rest in their pursuit of an aim.

VINE For the overstrong and dominating leader who may tend toward tyranny; for bullying.

WALNUT For change; for breaking links so that life may develop without hindrance.

WATER VIOLET For people who are aloof, self-reliant, and self-contained; to relax the reserved and enable sharing.

WHITE CHESTNUT For tiresome mental chatter and the overactive mind, full of persistent and unwanted patterns of thought.

WILD OAT For those who need help in deciding on the path and purpose of their life.

WILD ROSE For those who drift through life resigned to accept any eventuality; for fatalists and people too apathetic to try.

WILLOW For those who feel they have been treated unfairly; for resentment and self-pity.

THE FUTURE

The world is more complex than it was in 1920, more is demanded, and people have to delve deeper to find the reserves to cope. Human nature has not changed, however, so the same 38 remedies Dr. Bach found still form a complete system that can address all human emotions. Nevertheless, many people have started to make new essences, and remedies are available now from all corners of the world.

United Kingdom It was in the U.K. that Dr. Edward Bach first identified and began to harness the healing power of flowers.

United States American flower essence makers have developed remedies according to the needs of late 20th-century society.

Australia Flower essence makers in Australia have used the natural fauna of their own country to create Australian Bush remedies.

USING FLOWER REMEDIES

Flower remedies are simple and effective, and they can be used:

- to support in times of crisis.
- to treat the emotional outlook produced by illness.
- to address a particular recurring emotional or behavioral pattern.
- to give strength during a temporary emotional setback.
- as a preventive remedy when things start to go out of balance.
- Remedies act swiftly for passing moods and there should be an improvement very quickly, although it may take months to start to change a long-standing pattern.

The flower remedies or essences bought in a store are sold in stock bottles. They can be used straight from the bottle, but it is better to make a personal remedy mix. Sometimes a single flower remedy is needed, but in most cases two or more are combined.

ARE THEY SAFE?

The remedies are not addictive or dangerous, nor do they interfere with any other form of treatment. They are suitable for people of all ages. Pregnant women and children can take them with confidence. Flower remedies are safe for young babies, should they need them, and they can also be given to animals and plants.

WHICH PROBLEMS CAN THEY HELP?

All types of mental or emotional problems.

CHILDREN

- Flower remedies are ideal for children. Treat them as soon as you notice that something is "not quite right."
- Physical symptoms must be professionally treated. Consult a physician if in doubt.
- Listen and do not trivialize children's emotional lives. Be calm and methodical. Notice the mood or address a previously known pattern. Give the remedy for a day or two, then reassess. Moods in children may change rapidly.
- If worried about a child (or other family member), take Red Chestnut, Rescue Remedy, or any other remedy which seems relevant, to settle yourself before deciding on treatment.
- If the child is of breast-feeding age, give the remedy to the mother. It may also be put in the bath: for example, use Impatiens to treat the hot and restless frustration of a teething baby.
- Support the parents. If home nursing, give Mimulus to minimize known fears. Give Rescue Remedy and Walnut if the child is hospitalized. Other remedies may be applicable.
- Treat the parents. Their emotional problems (even if suppressed) may be the root of a child's distress.

TO MAKE A PERSONAL REMEDY

You'll need:
- 1fl. oz. (30ml.) amber glass dropper bottle
- 1fl. oz. (30ml.) spring water; or 1 teaspoon brandy and 5 teaspoons (25ml.) spring water
- Decide on the remedies which are most applicable. Usually between one and six is enough. If you think you need several, simplify to a maximum of seven covering immediate issues, and check again in a few weeks.
- Put 2 drops of each remedy into a clean 6 teaspoons (30ml.) amber glass dropper bottle. This is the standard amount, but read the label, as occasionally some of the newer essences suggest you use 4 or 7 drops.
- If the remedies are to be used within a week, fill the bottle with clean spring water.
- If the remedies are to be taken for a prolonged period, add 1 teaspoonful (5ml.) of brandy to the bottle and then fill with spring water.
- Label the bottle with your name and the date.
- Give the remedy a title or a few words to remind you of the purpose. Would an affirmation be useful?
- Keep remedies, like other medicines, out of the reach of children.

To use
- The standard dose is 4 drops, on or under the tongue, 4 times a day.
- At times of crisis, 2 drops from the stock bottle can be put into a glass of water (or, in an emergency, any drink) and sipped as needed.
- If for any reason it is impossible to take anything by mouth, put the drops on the skin or in washing water.

ATTITUDE AND AFFIRMATIONS

Flower remedies should not be taken without thought and due care.

Ask these questions:
- Why is it needed?
- What do I expect? There should be a clear reason for taking a herb or remedy and a positive treatment aim or goal.

Some people recommend the use of affirmations, suggesting that an appropriate affirmation is written down several times a day for a week while taking the remedy. An example of a positive affirmation for the Clematis daydreamer would be: "I am awake (or becoming awake) and open to the experience of here and now."

REMEDIES AND ALCOHOL

Flower remedies and essences are preserved in alcohol. The amount of alcohol in a personal remedy made solely with water is minute, but it is enough to upset those who are alcohol intolerant or recovering from alcoholism. Always check the status of those to whom you give a remedy. Thoughtlessness can do untold damage.

It is possible to remove the alcohol by putting the diluted drops of remedy in a boiling hot drink—the steam will evaporate the alcohol. Leave the remedy to cool before taking. Sip throughout the day.

NEGATIVITY CONTRIBUTES TO ILL HEALTH

Negative emotions depress the mind and immune system, repress activity, and contribute to ill health. All are rooted in one or more of the following, which are headings under which Dr. Bach grouped his 38 remedies:

- fear
- uncertainty
- insufficient interest in
- present circumstances
- loneliness
- oversensitivity to influences and ideas
- despondency or despair
- over-care for the welfare of others
- By learning the healing capacity of peace, hope, joy, faith, certainty, wisdom, and love it is possible to develop a positive outlook and a sense of well-being.

HOW TO MAKE FLOWER REMEDIES

Flower remedies are simple to make, and rewarding and effective to use. Remedies are made in two ways: the sun method and the boiling method. Whatever the method, there are a few basic rules:

CORRECT IDENTIFICATION Find the plant and site well before the day of picking. Make sure that it is legal to pick it or that you have the landowner's permission.

PREPARATION Collect essentials. Absolute cleanliness is essential. Wash your hands and rinse them several times. Utensils can be cleaned by boiling in spring or rain water for 20 minutes and then allowing them to drain dry. Wrap them in a clean cloth to keep them ready for a suitable day.

THE RIGHT DAY For sun method remedies, choose a warm, sunny day with no clouds. For boiling method remedies any bright, sunny day is good.

ON THE DAY Pick with respect. Remember that you are making a remedy and what the remedy is designed to treat. Pick flowers that you are drawn to. Pick from all sides of the plant, from the top and bottom branches of trees, or from a wide area with meadow plants. Work quickly so there is only a little time between picking the flowers and putting them into the water to make the remedy. If you need to carry the flowers, cover your palm with a large leaf (preferably from the plant being picked) to prevent the heat and oils from the hand contaminating the blossoms. Use a twig to stir and remove the flowers.

LABELING When you have finished, label and date your remedy clearly. Keep it in a cool, dark place, away from direct sunlight.

THE SUN METHOD

Pick when the flowers are coming into full bloom. This will depend on the climate and the type of season, but the following can serve as a general guide:

EARLY SPRING: oak, gorse, olive, vine.
LATE SPRING: white chestnut, water violet.
SUMMER: rock water, mimulus, agrimony, rock rose, centaury.

LATE SUMMER: scleranthus, wild oat, impatiens, chicory, vervain, clematis, heather.
FALL: cerato, gentian. A 3fl. oz. (100ml.) bottle of mother tincture will last the average family many years. The recipe can make more, up to six bottles. If you wish to make more for family or friends, prepare more bottles. Each 3fl.oz. (100ml.] should contain 1½fl. oz. (50ml.) of brandy and be made up as outlined below:

You'll need:

- bottle of spring or mineral water
- plain glass bowl
- 3fl. oz. (100ml.) amber bottle(s)
- 1½fl. oz. (50ml.) brandy
- natural and unbleached filter paper
- pen and label

- Decide beforehand on the plants, where to pick from, and where to place the bowl, then wait for a suitable sunny day.
- The bowl should be placed in a clear open place, as close to the plants as possible, but away from shadows and possible contamination.
- The best time of the day for harvesting the plants is between 9a.m. and noon. The flowers are dry from the dew, but not yet exhausted by the sun.
- Pick the flowers and put in the water as quickly as possible.
- Float the flowers on the water until the whole surface is covered. Use a twig or leaf to arrange them, not your fingers.
- Leave the bowl out in the open where it will receive direct sunshine for three hours.
- After 3 hours, remove the flowers with a twig and filter the liquid.
- Pour 1 ½fl. oz. (50ml.) of the water into the bottle with the brandy. Shake and label with the name, "flower essence mother tincture," and date. This mother tincture will be used to prepare stock bottles and it will keep for many years. To prepare a stock bottle, put 2 drops of mother tincture into a 1fl. oz. (30ml.) dropper bottle, and top up with brandy. Then, from the stock bottle, use 2 drops to make up the treatment bottle as already described.

THE BOILING METHOD

The boiling method is mainly used for the flowers of trees. In any case, more than just the flower are picked— in addition, it is necessary to collect twigs that have a few leaves on them.

Pick when the flowers are at their best:

EARLY SPRING: cherry plum.
SPRING: elm, aspen.
LATE SPRING: beech, chestnut bud, hornbeam, larch, walnut, and Star of Bethlehem.
LATE SPRING: holly, crab apple, willow.
EARLY SUMMER: red chestnut, pine, mustard.
SUMMER: honeysuckle, sweet chestnut, wild rose.
Again, cleanliness is vital to avoid contamination. Sterilize utensils.

You'll need:
- 3-quart (3l.) saucepan with lid (use an enamel, glass, or stainless steel pan; avoid copper, aluminum, and Teflon-coated pans)
- a glass measuring jug
- 4 cups (1l.) of cold water (rain water or mineral water)
- 3fl.oz. (100ml.) amber glass bottle(s) (up to six)
- 1½fl. oz. (50ml.) of brandy natural and unbleached filter paper pen and label

- Decide on the plants beforehand; prepare and clean the utensils. If you are going to boil the remedy outside, check your camping stove and equipment. Wait for the perfect day.
- Take everything into the field between 9a.m. and 11a.m. on a sunny day.
- Touch as little as possible. Pick twigs or flowers until the saucepan is three-quarters full; put on the lid and take to the heat source as quickly as possible.
- When the pan is on the heat source, cover the flowers and twigs with the cold water and bring to the boil.
- Once it has reached boiling point, simmer for a half-hour. Use a twig from the tree to push the twigs under the water.
- After a half-hour, remove the pan from the heat, put the lid on it, and stand it outside to cool.

- When cool, remove the twigs, then carefully filter the water into the jug.
- Put 1 ½fl. oz. (50ml.) of the flower water into the 3fl. oz. (100ml.) bottle(s) with the brandy. Label with the name, "flower essence mother tincture," and date.
- This is the mother tincture from which a stock bottle is made. It will keep for many years, and is used to make up personal remedies as previously described.

SEEING A PROFESSIONAL

Flower remedies were created to be so simple to use that people could treat themselves. However, many practitioners of other disciplines—such as herbalism, homeopathy, and aromatherapy—use flower remedies to complement their own remedies, and a few flower essence therapists use the remedies exclusively.

Most therapists have their own ways of working. But every consultation should begin with an interview between you and the therapist. This can last from as little as 15 minutes to over an hour. During this time, the therapist will explain the system to you if you do not already know how it works. He or she will ask why you have come to see a therapist and will listen while you talk about yourself and your worries. The therapist will observe your posture and appearance, and will listen to the tone of your voice and the way you say things, as these can be as revealing as what you say. While you chat, the therapist may take notes and ask questions to work out, by a process of elimination, which remedies would be best for you. He or she might ask questions about your fears, how you feel about your children or other family members, or how easily you give up when something you attempt does not work out. It is not enough for the therapist to know that you have a problem at home or at work.

At the end of the consultation the therapist will help you select the remedies. The number of remedies prescribed depends on the individual, but it is unlikely to be more than six, and will often be much fewer. Most people feel at least a little better at the end of the consultation because they have been able to talk through their problems.

The Dr. Edward Bach Foundation maintains an international register of qualified practitioners in the Bach Flower Remedies.

FLOWER ESSENCES

USING THE REMEDIES

Successful treatment depends on accurate diagnosis. Get to know the different essences available and then aim to match the remedies to the individual character.

For yourself

If you find it hard to decide on a remedy, make a note of the one you think you need and then ask yourself the same questions you would ask anyone for whom you were prescribing:

- How do you feel?
- Why are you feeling like that?
- How do the symptoms affect you?
- What could have caused the problem?

For children

Children show their nature in their behavior and play. Try to match the behavior of the child to the remedy:

- Is the child always active like Vervain?
- Timid and shy like Mimulus?
- Gentle and obedient like Centaury?
- Bossy like Vine?
- Or sulky like Willow?

For animals

You need to know the animal's nature and note how differently it behaves when ill. For example, a dog which looks sorry for itself needs Willow; an aggressive one needs Holly or Vine; and cats often need Water Violet for their pride and independence. Add 4 drops to a small animal's drinking water, and 10 drops for large animals such as horses and cows. Add more drops whenever the water is replaced.

AESCULUS CARNEA
RED CHESTNUT

This essence is extracted from the pink-flowered chestnut tree, which is frequently grown for ornamental decoration in parks.

Use

Red Chestnut is for those who suffer fear and anxiety for others. They may have forsaken worrying about themselves, but project their fear onto their loved ones. They often anticipate that some unfortunate accident or illness (the worst scenario) will befall friends and relations, and ceaselessly worry. This inappropriate fear limits the social interactions of both the sufferer and his or her loved ones. Red Chestnut helps us realize that the anxiety is a projection of personal fear. It brings the calm necessary to be sensitive to the real problems and concerns of our loved ones, and to give empathetic support.

Method

The boiling method (*see page 207*)

GOAL—Sensitivity to others

- People who need Red Chestnut fear that something awful may happen to their loved ones.
- They experience unnecessary fear, overworry, even hypochondria on another person's behalf.
- Red Chestnut encourages calm and rationality, a response based on sensitivity to others, to replace the projected fear.

AESCULUS HIPPOCASTANUM WHITE CHESTNUT

The common horse chestnut tree has distinctive, upright clusters of white flowers and divided spatulate leaves.

Use

When the mind is full of unwanted thoughts, ideas, or persistent and worrying mental arguments—overactive and exhausting mental chatter going around and around in a never-ending circle.

Method

The sun method (*see page 206*)

GOAL—Clear mind, clarity

- For people who suffer from constant mental chatter, persistent thoughts, and worries.
- For sleeplessness due to worry.
- White Chestnut switches off unwanted thoughts so that it is possible to find peace and mental clarity.
- Other remedies might be needed to address the root cause.

AESCULUS HIPPOCASTANUM
CHESTNUT BUD

The white chestnut tree is used to make two remedies: White Chestnut and Chestnut Bud. The large leaf buds, called "sticky buds," are picked when they are just about to open to make this particular essence.

Use

For those who make the same mistake over and over again, and who are thus slow to learn from experience. Chestnut Bud is for people who find themselves stuck in the same repeating pattern, who regretfully do not seem able to learn the lessons of past experience, events, and relationships.

Method

The boiling method (*see page 207*)

GOAL—Vision

- The person who needs Chestnut Bud may suffer poor health, chronic conditions may continually "flare up," or they may suffer from preventable illness.

- If the same pattern is continually repeated, they are stuck in the energy of that moment.
- Chestnut Bud helps focus the mind and enable us to see our path with greater objectivity.

AGRIMONIA EUPATORIA
AGRIMONY

A wild plant with small yellow flowers on tapering spikes like church spires, sometimes known as "church steeples." The seed vessels are covered in hooked hairs and cling to animals coming into contact with them.

GOAL—Self-acceptance

- People who need Agrimony will put on a brave face of cheerfulness. Laughter hides things as well as being distracting, other distractions may be drink, drugs, or dangerous or thrill-seeking hobbies or occupations.
- They may be restless sleepers or unable to sleep without help.
- Agrimony helps us to love ourselves as we are, and to put aside the mask. It helps us cope with the difficult sides of our nature and use humor appropriately.

Use

For those who hide their problems and inner selves behind a cheerful face, masking real feelings of unhappiness and unworthiness. They are the life and soul of a party, and will make jokes, perhaps even inappropriately. The person who needs Agrimony finds it hard to deal with the darker, less pleasant parts of life and extreme emotions. They are reluctant to burden others and dread arguments, pursuing peace at all costs. This can lead to an inner anguish that is often masked by alcohol or drugs.

Method

The sun method (*see page 206*)

THE HEALING REMEDIES SOURCEBOOK

ANIGOZANTHOS MANGLESII
KANGAROO PAW

This large Australian perennial is one of the first plants to recolonize after bush fires. It is so named because the flowers at the end of the long stems resemble a kangaroo's front paw.

GOAL—**Kindness and sensitivity**
- For people who are inexperienced, socially inept, or embarrassed.
- Associated symptoms include clumsiness, nervousness, stuttering or stammering, blushing and embarrassment, shyness and timidity.
- Kangaroo Paw encourages sensitivity and empathy, and gives us the courage to just be, to accept, and be kind to ourselves and others. It allows us to experience true two-way communication.

Use

For people who have poor social skills, and difficulties relating to and communicating with others, who are so self-conscious and self-aware that they feel "out of place" at work, at meetings, gatherings, or parties. This may be noticed by others and become a joke. Interactions feel like competitions, and they find it impossible to find the space to think before acting, or to be aware of other people's feelings. Kangaroo Paw makes it possible for them to relax and get in tune with themselves and others, and to become aware of their surroundings. It encourages sensitive and appropriate social interaction.

Method
The sun method (*see page 206*); pick the whole cluster (or paw) of flowers

BROMUS RAMOSUS
WILD OAT

An elegant woodland grass, wild oat stands between 2 and 5 ft. (½–1 ½m.) high. The common name is hairy or wood brome grass, because of the soft, hairy leaves.

GOAL—**Meaningful purpose, a positive direction**
- Wild Oat is for uncertainty and frustration with current activities, when a person has the desire to find a purpose, yet is aimless, drifting from one job or relationship to another.
- Wild Oat helps us listen to our calling, find our true vocation, and gives the strength of character to act on this.

Use

Wild Oat is for capable people who have ambition to do something meaningful in their lives but have not yet found their true calling. They may have several choices or directions they could follow and may be working hard on a given path, but fundamentally they are dissatisfied and frustrated. Somewhere deep down they know that they have not found their vocation in life, and are emotionally or spiritually unsatisfied. Wild Oat helps to tune the heart to what will bring true meaning and purpose. It helps us to make choices, sometimes difficult, which unite all aspirations.

Method
The sun method (*see page 206*)

CALLUNA VULGARIS
HEATHER

This common plant is often found in Alpine areas, on heaths, and waste ground. Calluna prefers acid soil. According to variety, flowers are produced from summer to fall.

Use

For people who are caught up with themselves and their own interests, who are the center of the universe. They are poor listeners and do not like to be alone. It is hard for them to share. They may be concentrating on fulfiling personal needs in order to avoid loneliness.

Method

The sun method (*see page 206*)

GOAL—**Love with space to share; to listen: A useful affirmation might be: "I am listening and letting the love of the world nourish my heart."**

- People who need Heather can be self-centered and self-obsessed. They may intrude into other people's personal space, cling, or be aggressively talkative.
- They can be weepy and hypochondriac.
- They may be lonely, as friends may avoid them because they demand too much.
- We should love and nurture ourselves. Heather helps us to look after ourselves without being obsessed with our own personal needs. It gives us the space to listen to others, and experience genuine love and companionship.

CARPINUS BETULUS
HORNBEAM

A medium-sized, deciduous tree common in woods. It grows well in a sunny or lightly shaded position, and its leaves turn a rich yellow-orange in the fall.

Use

Hornbeam is for those who feel that they do not possess enough strength to fulfill the responsibilities of daily life, for the "Monday morning blues." This feeling often comes from boredom or some basic dissatisfaction with the work they are doing. These people might feel that they are in the wrong job, or in some way not fully expressing their creative potential. Hornbeam restores confidence and optimism, and helps us find the satisfaction in the mundane "nine-to-five" aspects of our lives.

Method

The boiling method (*see page 207*)

GOAL—**Strength to carry out daily tasks**

- People who need Hornbeam feel exhausted at the thought of working. They may feel stuck in a rut.
- Procrastination is a common avoidance stratagem.
- Hornbeam is usually for a temporary feeling. If the weakness is a regular occurrence, the person may be exhausting himself or herself in the wrong direction, and other remedies may be needed.

CASTANEA SATIVA
SWEET CHESTNUT

This chestnut tree produces edible fruit after its creamy flowers. The tree grows to 100ft. (30m.) and is deciduous.

GOAL—**Transformation, to widen the boundaries**

- Hornbeam is for the feeling Dr. Bach called the "dark night of the soul," when it feels that annihilation is all that will be left.
- Associated symptoms may include sleep disturbance, hopelessness, and perhaps hidden despair.

Use

Sweet Chestnut is for those moments when anguish is so great as to seem unbearable, when people feel that they have "come to the end of their tether," reached their limit, and are being stretched beyond endurance. When this happens things have to change. Sweet Chestnut helps to bring out hidden reserves, opening boundaries and expanding limits, which gives people the strength to grow.

Method

The boiling method (*see page 207*)

THE HEALING REMEDIES SOURCEBOOK

CENTAURIUM ERYTHRAEA
CENTAURY

A small pink flower of chalky soil. It is named after a centaur in Greek mythology, who used it to cure himself from a poisoned arrow wound.

Use
Centaury is for people who have an excessive desire to please and a willingness to serve. They can be taken for granted and exploited. Their will to help others is so strong that it undermines their individuality and they find it hard to say "no." They can become servants rather than helpers, and end up doing more than their fair share. This leads to frustration and a loss of self-confidence, appreciation, and expression.

Method
The sun method (*see page 206*)

GOAL—**Service, in the widest sense**
- People who need Centaury lack will-power; they may be tired and exhausted. Inner frustration and anger may sap their inner strength.
- The "weaker" partner in a codependent relationship may benefit from Centaury.
- Centaury helps balance the desire to serve by strengthening our will power and appreciation of ourselves. It helps us make a choice, to say "yes" or "no" from the heart.

CERATOSTIGMA WILLMOTTIANA
CERATO

A small shrub with bright blue flowers which is often grown in gardens. It originally came from China and the Himalayas. Cerato is the only Bach Flower Remedy to be made from a cultivated plant.

GOAL—**Inner confidence; to trust intuition**
- People who need Cerato may appear weak-willed and silly. They lack constancy, and may imitate others or become an ever-changing "fashion victim."
- They may join cults or take up fads.
- Cerato helps us to listen to advice from within, restores confidence, and strengthens our trust in ourselves to follow our path even if it runs contrary to the expectations of others.

Use
Cerato is for lack of trust in our own abilities and judgment. People who need Cerato are intelligent and curious, but they lack confidence in themselves, distrust their own intuition, and constantly seek the advice and approval of other people. They like to be seen to be doing the "right thing."

Method
The sun method (*see page 206*)

CHICORIUM INTYBUS
CHICORY

A wayside plant with bright blue flowers. It is cultivated as a vegetable and blanched as a bitter plant to add to salads. The flowers close in the afternoon and open again in the morning.

GOAL—**Love, free-flowing and without strings**
- Those who need Chicory may be possessive and selfish. They may be fussy, nagging, and manipulative. They may be prone to illness if not "loved," or to hypochondria.
- Chicory helps us to see love as a universal force, to give love selflessly and freely so that it may freely return to us.

Use
Chicory is for those who see love as a transaction incurring duty, and as a method of control. They give love in order

to receive it. Chicory types love and care publicly, even melodramatically, building up a stock of good works which they expect to be reciprocated, but love still does not flow their way.

Method
The sun method (*see page 206*)

CLEMATIS VITALBA
CLEMATIS

The wild clematis is a rambling, perennial climber of woods and country hedges. Its common name is travelers' joy, and it bursts forth with a mass of beautiful flowers.

Use
For those who are dreamy and not fully awake. Sometimes they daydream or fantasize about a Utopian future. Clematis people prefer to live in the mind or the spirit, rather than deal with contemporary issues and the mundane functions of everyday life. They tend to be airy and impractical individuals, drifting off into their own ideas, the typical "mad professor." They sometimes lead a sedentary life, are pale, and lack vitality and ambition. They are sensitive and sometimes need lots of sleep.

Method
The sun method (*see page 206*)

GOAL—**Being awake and grounded in the body and in the present**
- People who need Clematis are dreamy, absent-minded, and lack interest in the present. They sometimes have a poor will to live. They may forget to eat, experience faintness and tiredness.
- If children resort to daydreaming as an escape, Clematis may be useful, although the child should be questioned to find the underlying cause.

EPACRIS LONGIFLORA
BUSH FUCHSIA

A low, straggly shrub, bush fuschia flowers throughout the year with bright red, elongated, bell-like flowers hanging in a row from the stem. The leaves are small and heart-shaped. The plant needs full sun.

GOAL—**Mental balance and clarity; to read or speak clearly**
- People who need Bush Fuchsia may be nervous and stammer. Although intelligent, they are slow to learn. They may avoid situations which highlight this, or become shy.
- They have difficulties with determining left and right, up and down.
- Bush Fuchsia is specific for children with dyslexia or learning difficulties.
- Bush Fuchsia aids concentration and confidence.
- It is also useful when we are "stuck" in one mode of thinking, releasing energy to rebalance the mind.

Use
Bush Fuchsia is used to balance the hemispheres of the brain so that the rational left side and creative right side can be expressed with confidence. It is useful for all problems with learning difficulties, or translating marks from the page (words, symbols, music) into physical action. It boosts confidence when performing or speaking in public. Dyslexia and other learning disabilities, if not understood and addressed, can seriously affect self-worth and hinder the development of social skills.

Method
The sun method (*see page 206*)

FAGUS SYLVATICA
BEECH

The common beech tree grows to a majestic 100ft. (30m.), with a spread of 80ft. (25m.) The leaves take on rich yellow and orange hues in the fall.

Use

Beech is for those who are being overcritical and intolerant, and according to Dr Bach, "for those who need to see beauty in all that surrounds them." Beech types have their own "way" and are very proud that they can cope. They think problems can be solved in their way, and are intolerant of those who cannot do this. They do not understand that everyone has different strengths and experiences. They think "cannot" means "will not," and therefore become irritable and short-tempered with others. They may also feel unappreciated.

Method

The boiling method (*see page 207*)

GOAL—Tolerance and empathy

- People who need Beech may be lonely and isolated. Lack of understanding leads to narrow views.
- Beech fills hearts with empathy and opens eyes to see beauty without judgment. It shows that we are individuals, with different ways of dealing with the world.

GENTIANELLA AMARELLA
GENTIAN

Gentianella amerella flowers from late summer onward, with rich blue, violet to purple flowers. It likes dry, well-drained conditions, and sandy or chalky soils.

GOAL—Courage to accept what is; encouragement to face the future positively

- Gentian helps us to put setbacks and disappointments into perspective, and to once again display a positive attitude.

Use

For despondency and mild depression due to circumstances. Gentian people are easily discouraged. When everything is going well they are happy, but they can be easily disheartened, and can slip back into a negative outlook. Doubt and lack of faith are important elements. Gentian restores the courage to recognize that life is not a competition and that there is no failure when trying our best.

Method

The sun method (*see page 206*)

GREVILLEA BUXIFOLIA
GRAY SPIDER FLOWER

A common Australian evergreen, this shrub flowers for most of the year. It prefers acid soil and full sun.

Use

Aspen and Mimulus are both for fear, but Gray Spider Flower is for extreme and intense feelings of terror, a blind panic which is immobilizing. The fear may be known or unknown, and it is associated with physical symptoms of inner terror which freeze the mind and body, and prevent thoughts moving forward. Gray Spider Flower frees the body and the mind to move, bringing faith that the terror will pass.

Method

The sun method (*see page 206*); pick the whole flower head at the end of the branch

GOAL—Faith

- For extreme, immobilizing terror of day or night; nightmares, disturbed sleep, or fear of sleep.
- For shivering, pallor, palpitations, depression, and feelings of being psychically drained and exhausted.
- Gray Spider Flower brings lightness, courage, and faith, the certainty that we are loved by the world.
- It is ideal for children terrorized by bad dreams.
- Take with Fringed Violet Flower for protection from fear of the supernatural and of psychic attack.

GOSSYPIUM STURTIANUM
STURT DESERT ROSE

Sturt desert rose is a small shrub with mauve, hibiscus-like flowers which likes dry, stony ground. The flower remedy is good for feelings of worthlessness.

Use

People who need Sturt Desert Rose are always apologizing for themselves and their actions. They blame themselves for everything, for things they should or should not have done, and feel guilt and remorse. They may have an acute sense of obligation and duty which is hard (or impossible) to live up to. Guilt and shame are both disabling emotions. Sturt Desert Rose enables self-acceptance, the understanding that we do what we can and must take responsibility (not blame) for the consequences. It enables reconciliation, allowing us to accept, forgive, and move on to pastures new.

Method

The sun method (*see page 206*)

GOAL—**Self-acceptance, conciliation, communication, true to self**

- For guilt, regret, remorse. People who need Sturt Desert Rose feel useless. They have low self-esteem and a sense of shame. They are characterized by self-criticism. Associated symptoms include anxiety dreams, depression, especially of old hidden guilt.
- Sturt Desert Rose facilitates self-acceptance, allowing forgiveness and healing.

HELIANTHEMUM NUMMULARIUM
ROCK ROSE

A low-growing, yellow-flowered plant found on chalky or gravely soils. Some varieties of rock rose are cultivated in rock gardens, but these are not suitable for use as flower remedies.

Use

Rock Rose is one of the main ingredients of Rescue Remedy. It is to be taken in all cases of extreme fear, terror, panic, urgency, or danger. Rock Rose gives the courage to face life and death, frees the mind to act, bringing faith that the terror or panic will soon pass.

Method

The sun method (*see page 206*)

GOAL—**Personal courage**

- The person who needs Rock Rose experiences feelings of helplessness, terror, and blind panic.
- Fear may cause palpitations, heart jitters, or panic attacks.
- Rock Rose should be given for any perceived threat to the person, their self-image, or personal integrity.

HIBBERTIA PENDUNCULATA
HIBBERTIA

A low, trailing plant of the open bush. The large, bright, and gleaming yellow flowers bloom in spring. It is frost-tender. The flower essence is good for those with a love of learning.

Use

People who need Hibbertia love ideas and pursue knowledge at all costs. They may repress or deny their body and its needs, or have a rigid or dogmatic lifestyle. They continually read, attend lectures, courses, and workshops to improve themselves and gain status. They want to "know it all." They look deep within books, but never around at their surroundings. Their head is in the air and they are ungrounded. The search is ultimately unsatisfactory; knowledge grows from within and they must find themselves before they can change.

Method

The sun method (*see page 206*)

GOAL—Wisdom

- For those who are intelligent, the "constant student," characterized by continual pursuit of knowledge for self-improvement or status, and love of "hidden knowledge." Such people may be fanatical or cult followers.
- They may be neglectful of their body, or suffer sedentary and stress-related illnesses, indigestion, skin rashes, wasting or stiffness of muscles and joints.
- Hibbertia encourages confidence and contentment. It links external knowledge with personal observations and physical needs, producing wisdom.

HOTTONIA PALUSTRIS
WATER VIOLET

This is a delicate perennial plant with pale violet flowers and feathery leaves which is often found in ditches, as it grows submerged in water. The flowers appear above the water in the summer.

Use

Water Violet is for self-reliant people with an aloof, "live-and-let-live" attitude. They are quiet and spend much time alone, keeping others at a distance. When ill, they keep to themselves and do not wish to be any "trouble" to those around them. They find it hard to share. In their isolation they may feel special, or chosen, a sensation which can distort their sense of belonging and self-worth. Water Violet gives the confidence to share—the strengths and weaknesses, the ups and downs, all of life's rich tapestry.

Method

The sun method (*see page 206*)

GOAL—Communication; sharing

- The person needing Water Violet is reserved and self-contained. This can be seen as standoffish aloofness and pride, and thus lead to loneliness.

- He or she may be solitary yet proud.
- Water Violet allows us to acknowledge the inner self as a starting point from which to expand, communicate with the world, and share from the heart.

ILEX AQUIFOLIUM
HOLLY

Holly is a common evergreen tree, with spiky leaves and red berries. It is a powerful symbol of winter and is used in Christmas decorations. To produce berries on a female plant, a male plant needs to be grown nearby.

GOAL—Unconditional expression of affection and love. A useful affirmation might be: "I am opening my heart to express my love."

The negative emotions of the person who needs Holly may be spiteful and nagging, with intense feeling and outbursts of temper. They may be suspicious or mildly paranoid. Useful for the "no!" negative states and temper tantrums of two-year-olds.

Holly allows us to recognize that these feelings are the negative expression of our caring interaction with others. It gives us the strength to open our hearts to the full flow of love.

Use

Holly is for those who are attacked by feelings of hatred, envy, jealousy, suspicion, and revenge. The person who needs Holly has intense negative feelings. They also have other intense emotions, but they are too frightened to express these fully. The free flow of emotion and love is then blocked or expressed unclearly. This leads to tension, unclear communication, frustration, anger, and emotional outbursts.

Method

The boiling method (*see page 207*)

JUGLANS REGIA
WALNUT

A large, handsome, deciduous tree which is easily recognized by its popular edible nuts, walnut grows to about 50ft. (15m.) tall and is wide-spreading.

Use

Walnut is for people who need to find constancy and protection from outside forces, those who need to move on and break links and old patterns with people and things. Walnut frees the person from interference, and gives protection so that it is possible to break inappropriate ties and pursue personal freedom. Walnut is useful for people on the brink of some major decision or change—for example, children leaving home, menopause, marriage, or having babies.

Method

The boiling method (*see page 207*)

GOAL—Protection, sanctuary

- Walnut is useful at any of the milestones of life: puberty, marriage, leaving home, change of job or country, etc.
- People who have moved on but find old habits persistent can take Walnut to break links with the past.
- Walnut is also useful for temporary distraction, or for domination by enthusiasm, or strong opinions of others.

IMPATIENS GLANDULIFERA
IMPATIENS

A tall annual with large mauve flowers and exploding seed pods, Impatiens is common in damp places. It is sometimes called "touch me not," as the tightly coiled seed pods are apt to explode at the slightest touch.

GOAL—Patience

- Impatiens is for impatience and irritability at slowness, the desire to do everything quickly.
- People who need Impatiens may fidget, find it hard to sit still, and therefore suffer from indigestion and nervous tension.
- People who have learned the lesson of Impatiens have patience, they are capable and decisive, knowing how to get things done and turn the pace of life to advantage.

Use

For those who are quick in thought and action, and who are always on the go. They know their mind and want things to be done at speed. They become irritable at hindrance, hesitation, and delay, and impatiently blame others. They can alienate people by being brusque and unsympathetic, speaking their mind quickly and without thought. They refuse to slow down even when illness overtakes them. They are truly in the "rat race." Impatiens restores acceptance of the natural pace of life, rather than fighting against it.

Method

The sun method (*see page 206*)

LARIX DECIDUA
LARCH

Larch is a tall conifer with needle-like leaves that are shed in the fall. Male and female flowers appear on the same tree in spring. It can grow to 100ft. (30m.) high, and the cones are small and erect.

GOAL—Confidence

- Larch can be used for any lack of confidence and self-esteem, for passivity and fear of trying, and for poor self-image and feelings of inferiority.
- It is suitable for children starting a new school, and who feel they will not be as clever as the other children and so fear failure.

THE HEALING REMEDIES SOURCEBOOK

- Feelings of worthlessness may hide deeper problems or a pattern of abuse. Other remedies may also be useful.
- Larch strengthens confidence, and helps us appreciate our real worth and value our personal contribution to the planet.

Use

Larch is for those who lack confidence in themselves and fear failure, those who feel that they are not as capable as those around them. At times, lack of confidence may completely immobilize them and prevent them from even trying. They do not think that they are capable, or worthy of success. Feelings of total uselessness also can lead to great unhappiness, despair, and isolation. Larch increases confidence and strengthens personal will.

Method
The boiling method (*see page 207*)

LONICERA CAPRIFOLIUM
HONEYSUCKLE

Lonicera caprifolium is a strongly scented climber found in woods. The fragrance is sweet and long-lasting. The flowers are tubular and form a spreading head.

Use

Honeysuckle is for those who dwell too much on memories of the past, on the "good old days," and who do not expect to experience such happiness and companionship again. The past seems rosy and familiar; the future seems dark, bleak, forbidding, and unknown. For nostalgia, a faraway sense of regret or loss, often tinged with pessimism. Nostalgia may be a temporary sensation, a fleeting regret, or it may be a pattern which prevents further joy and expression. Honeysuckle is appropriate for both.

Method
The boiling method (*see page 207*)

GOAL—**To be completely "here"**
- A useful affirmation might be: "I am here and now, growing from my past into a positive future."
- Honeysuckle is for people who are not grounded in the present, who (for many reasons) are stuck in the past.
- It is for homesickness or regrets.
- It is also useful for grief and bereavement where these cause the person to dwell on the past.
- Honeysuckle integrates past experiences and gives strength to face new challenges.

MALUS SYLVESTRIS
CRAB APPLE

The fruit yielded by this plant are small, yellow, and very acid. It grows in hedges and on waste ground. The crab apples make a piquant preserve. Malus provides a good show of color in the fall.

GOAL—**Cleaning and purification**
- Crab Apple is for people who feel unclean on any level. They may feel self-disgust or self-loathing and may hurt, punish, cut, or otherwise abuse themselves. They may have phobias or rituals around purity or cleanliness.
- Crab Apple is also useful for spots and rashes on the face, so that they can be faced and the self accepted.
- This remedy is a cleanser on all levels: physical, emotional, and spiritual.
- It is also used to cleanse the body and spirit after contact with anything contagious or which feels unclean.
- It may be added to baths or to skin creams.

Use

Crab Apple is a bitter acid fruit, useful for those who feel self-condemnation and disgust, in need of cleaning or detoxification. This may be a temporary feeling brought on by shame or remorse, or guilt over some act of which they are ashamed, or thoughts which are felt to be unclean. Crab Apple is also useful to encourage acceptance of spots or physical blemishes, and for a deep phobia or cleanliness fetish. It cleanses both the mind and body.

Method
The boiling method (*see page 207*)

MIMULUS GUTTATUS
MIMULUS

A pretty, water-loving plant common in damp places, mimulus has rich yellow flowers in midsummer that resemble the snapdragon. It grows to 2ft. (60cm.)

Use
Mimulus is for fear which can be identified, of known or worldly things. (Aspen is also for fear, but for unknown fears.) Mimulus should be taken for the everyday fears of pain, accidents, poverty, being alone, and misfortune. These understandable fears dominate responses, either prodding people into hasty action or freezing them into inaction. They are easily identified and faced, but underneath they are fed by insecurity and a negative attitude toward past experience. Mimulus is also for shy, timid people who tend to avoid social occasions and large crowds of people.

Method
The sun method (*see page 206*)

GOAL—**Freedom, freedom from fear**
- For any fear which can be named. A trivial fear or phobia, if it can be named, will respond to Mimulus.
- Fear can lead to stammering, palpitations, indigestion, sleeplessness, and troubled dreams.
- Mimulus liberates us from fear and helps us to understand the rhythms and balances of everyday life, to grow beyond the limits set by fear, and to have the courage and freedom to respond in appropriate ways.

ORNITHOGALUM UMBELLATUM
STAR OF BETHLEHEM

The delicate flowers of this wild lily are like six-pointed stars and bloom in the late spring. Ornithogalum umbellatum is a spring-flowering bulb.

Use
Star of Bethlehem is used in Rescue Remedy to ameliorate the effects of shock—the shock of bad news, of loss, of an accident, even of being born. People "jump" with shock; waves ripple outward through the body, affecting every cell and tissue. Time is needed for everything to settle, to be comfortable in the body, but sometimes the trauma may be so extreme, or the shock unrealized or repressed, that the effects continue to resonate years later. Star of Bethlehem neutralizes the effects so that the body is able to harmonize.

Method
The boiling method (*see page 207*)

GOAL—**Peace and comfort**
- For shock, and its physical and emotional effects.
- Long-repressed shock or trauma may lead to psychosomatic symptoms.
- Star of Bethlehem neutralizes the effects of shock, so that the body and mind can again find equilibrium and comfort.

OLEA EUROPEA
OLIVE

Olive is a small evergreen common in southern Europe. The fruit yield olive oil.

GOAL—**Renewal and regeneration**
- For all exhaustion, physical, and mental tiredness after some effort or struggle.

- Exhaustion can be so profound that life loses its interest and spark.
- Olive helps restore vitality by helping people to relax and take a more balanced attitude toward life, making sure they allow themselves "quality" time for unwinding, rest, and spiritual renewal.

Use

For extreme fatigue of mind, body, or spirit after effort. People in need of Olive feel totally exhausted in every way. They feel that life is hard and without pleasure, that they have no more strength, and at times hardly know how they manage to keep going. They burn the candle at both ends, and become too tired even to think. They may depend on others for help. Olive helps people relax and switch off, so that the simple things of life—a warm bath, a walk in the sunshine, watching children, or sharing with friends—can refresh the spirit.

Method

The sun method (*see page 206*)

PINUS SYLVESTRIS
PINE

The Scotch pine is an evergreen tree often depicted in painting and song as the "lonesome pine." It has blue-green leaves and gray or reddish cones.

Use

Pine is a very specific remedy for those who blame themselves and are suffering from self-reproach. Even when successful they are never content, and always feel that they could have done better. They blame themselves even when the fault is someone else's.

Method

The boiling method (*see page 207*)

GOAL—Appropriate response; responsibility
- For self-reproach and guilt, frequently groundless.

- People who need Pine may carry the blame for the actions of others, and may apologize frequently and often needlessly.
- Pine helps us understand that "responsibility" is the ability to respond. If we respond honestly and freely, there is no need for blame and we can move on.

PRUNUS CERASUS
CHERRY PLUM

A small tree with red or yellow fruit, cherry plum is often grown as hedging and windbreaks. It flowers from early spring, with delicate pale pink flowers.

GOAL—Release; to let go of fear and to regain control of the emotions
- People who need Cherry Plum may feel desperate, and fear they may hurt themselves and others. They may have bouts of hysteria.
- Cherry Plum is useful for uncontrolled tantrums in children, when they are frightened by their own loss of temper.
- Cherry Plum restores control and trust of the mind and emotions.

Use

Cherry Plum is for the fear of letting go or of losing control. The fearful thoughts may be of a suicidal, compulsive, or destructive nature. This mental pain and turmoil may happen during a period of great emotional or physical change, when the person is worn and stressed. Dr. Bach says it is "for fear of the mind being overstrained, of reason giving way, of doing fearful and dreaded things, not wished and known wrong, yet there comes the thought and impulse to do them."

Method

The boiling method (*see page 207*)

POPULUS TREMULA
ASPEN

Aspen is a slender, silver-barked, deciduous tree. It grows to 30ft. (10m.), its almost circular leaves trembling in the slightest breeze.

GOAL—**Courage to face the unknown**
- The person who needs Aspen may feel frightened, a sense of dread, and that something awful may happen. This may be extreme enough to affect appetite, produce palpitations, and interrupt sleep patterns, bringing nightmares.
- Aspen is suitable for the fears and nightmares of children where they cannot describe what they are frightened of.
- Aspen brings reassurance that there is nothing to fear. It helps us to face the unknown with courage and trust.

Use
Dr. Bach says it is for "vague fear, for which there is no explanation or reason." The fear can be so deep that it is too frightening to express, and the sufferer feels burdened by doom, and inexplicable terror.

Method
The boiling method (*see page 207*)

PTILOTUS ATRIPICFOLIUS
MULLA MULLA

A small plant from desert regions, mulla mulla responds to the weather, and sends out clusters of pink, long-lasting flowers when conditions are favorable. All but one of the many species of Ptilotus are exclusive to Australia.

Use
For those suffering the effects of fire, heat, or radiation. In reality and symbolically, fire is profoundly powerful. In most traditions fire was a gift from the gods and had to be used with wisdom. Do we understand fire and use it wisely? Burning fossil fuels adds to the greenhouse effect and to the depletion of the ozone layer. Mulla Mulla helps the body recover from damage and protects it from harmful rays.

Method
The sun method (*see page 206*)

GOAL—**Rejuvenation**
- People who need Mulla Mulla may have obvious burns, sunburn, or hot rashes. They may be suffering exhaustion from heat, or from working in overhot conditions, or a hot climate.
- Mulla Mulla helps them to be comfortable with the inner and outer manifestations of fire.
- Mulla Mulla also protects from the damaging effects of heat—for example, in laser treatment.

QUERCUS ROBUR
OAK

Quercus robur is the common oak. Most people recognize the acorns, but the flowers are less familiar. Male and female flowers are borne on the same tree and appear from April onward.

Use
Oak people are strong and brave fighters. They struggle through events and physical illnesses even when there is no hope, never thinking of surrender. Their strength may sometimes be inappropriate, and they can exhaust themselves by pushing blindly on in one narrow direction. Strength is a virtue, but it is pointless pushing against an immovable object. Oak helps us surrender, step back, look around, and consider different answers.

Method

The sun method (*see page 206*); pick the small, female catkins only

GOAL—Adaptability and flexibility

- Oak is for those who struggle on, never giving up.
- People who need Oak may overwork, and drive themselves relentlessly.
- They can be obstinate, and, unless they rest or find another strategy, may exhaust themselves and break down.
- Oak restores the true inner strength, which is flexible and adaptable.

RICINOCARPUS PINIFOLIUS
WEDDING BUSH

Ricinocarpus pinifolius is a small bush with abundant, six-petaled white flowers. Male and female flowers grow on the same bush. The flowers were traditionally used for wedding decorations, giving the bush its name.

Use

Wedding Bush is like the glue which holds people together through thick and thin. It is for those who doubt their ability to commit or accept the responsibility of deep caring; for those with a pattern of starting but not finishing, moving on, and running away from the self in all aspects of life; for those who are an "emotional rolling stone." They may be in love with love (or the newness of love) and move from one affair to another, or they may have one job after another. Commitment is not just about long-term endurance; it is an attitude of mind involving self-worth. Wedding Bush reminds us of the privilege of being, and of our commitment to life.

Method

The sun method (*see page 206*); pick both male and female flowers

GOAL—Commitment and dedication

- For those who find commitment difficult and suffer indecision and procrastination.
- For those with a pattern of starting but not finishing.
- Wedding Bush encourages the confidence to commit, to feel the comfort rather than the burden of responsibility, to make a long-term dedication to life and its purpose.
- Wedding Bush can also help us to carry through short-term jobs or commitments to a satisfying conclusion.

ROSA CANINA
WILD ROSE

The common wild rose, Rosa canina can be seen rambling over country hedges. The flowers appear in early summer, and vary in color from almost white to deep pink. The fruit, or rosehip, is a striking scarlet.

Use

Dr. Bach recommends Wild Rose for those who have become resigned to all that happens, for the fatalist. This person glides through life passively, taking it as it is, without motivation or expectation. He or she is apathetic about change and asks, "What is the use?" Such a person has given away his or her power and interest in life. Wild Rose stimulates this interest and an appreciation of life's color and joy. The remedy encourages action, and a purposeful pleasure in being and doing.

Method

The boiling method (*see page 207*)

GOAL—Interest in life; participation and action

- People who need Wild Rose are fatalistic, resigned to events, and apathetic about change.
- Wild Rose helps us to interact with all aspects of life and make an impact by creating our own unique and dynamic reality.

SALIX ALBA VAR. VITELLINA
WILLOW

The willow is an attractive tree with thin, bright yellow twigs and long, narrow leaves. It is also known as the golden osier. The tree is often cut back hard to encourage the growth of strong, young shoots.

GOAL—Maturity and natural balance
- People who need Willow may be sulky and selfish, embittered with self-pity, and ungrateful for help.
- They may experience psychosomatic illness, and tearfulness.
- Willow helps us see that we create our own reality by focusing on different elements of our life. It encourages a more positive and mature attitude.
- Willow may also be taken for a brief embitterment.

Use
Willow is for people who find the bad things that happen to them hard to accept and are embittered. They take problems personally, and feel life has become a personal trial to endure, without hope or happiness. They blame the world when things go wrong. "It's not fair," they say, like a two-year-old child. Willow helps them see that with this self-pitying outlook they are creating their own oppression by continual negative thoughts.

Method
The boiling method (*see page 207*)

SCLERANTHUS ANNUUS
SCLERANTHUS

Scleranthus is a small, bushy, spreading plant with green flowers which grows to 4in. (10cm.) on sandy soils and in cornfields. The green flowers have no petals and grow at the forks and end of the stems.

Use
For those who are unable to decide and who suffer much from hesitation and uncertainty. For confusion. People who need Scleranthus tend to be quiet and are not inclined to discuss their options with others. They need to learn to decide for themselves; it is important that they do so, but they cannot. Scleranthus gives the stability to listen to the inner self, and integrate the emotional and intellectual extremes (which sometimes seem contradictory) into balanced and sustained action.

Method
The sun method (*see page 206*)

GOAL—Stability and balance
- For people who are unable to decide between two things.
- They are uncertain, indecisive, vacillate, and subject to erratic mood swings.
- Scleranthus brings harmony, stability, and balance, allowing us to act decisively.

SYNAPS ARVENSIS
MUSTARD

The common wild mustard found growing in hedges and on waste ground has large yellow flowers that appear in early summer. This annual plant grows to about 2ft. (60cm.) and self-seeds readily.

GOAL—Hope and hopefulness
- Mustard is for depression with no known cause, and for melancholia.
- It is for people whose thoughts turn inward and whose life lacks light and pleasure.
- Although these bouts of depression seem to come from nowhere, there may be a deeply hidden reason. If it happens frequently, look for a cause; if there is a physiological or psychological root, seek professional assistance.

- Mustard lightens our mood, giving us the faith and hope to carry on.

Use

Mustard is used for dark clouds of gloom or deep, black depression that seems to come from nowhere. It is for the feeling of being under a cloud which blocks out the warming rays and optimism of the sun. It may lift just as suddenly as it arrived. While a person is under the dark cloud, it is hard for him or her to muster any feeling of happiness or hope. All clouds pass and Mustard restores hope and a sense of pleasure in living.

Method

The boiling method (*see page 207*)

TELOPEA SPECIOSISSIMA
WARATAH

Waratah is the Aboriginal word for beautiful. It is a shrub with magnificent red flowers packed together into a globe measuring 5in. (12cm.) across. It is a very striking plant.

GOAL—To have the courage to be courageous
- Waratah should be taken in times of crisis, emotional or physical. People who need it may feel unable to go on, trapped in a dark night of despair, even suicidal.
- Physical signs may be exhaustion, interrupted or prolonged sleep, loss of the ability or interest to care for oneself.
- Waratah reunites all aspects of the personality.
- It also helps maintain personal integrity for coping with everyday challenges.

Use

Waratah is a very powerful and fast-acting remedy. It should be taken for despair, deep distress, and any emotional or physical crisis. The image of the globe of the flowers reflects how the remedy of Waratah brings everything in the personality together: strength, old and forgotten skills and lessons, trust, and love. It gives us the faith and confidence to hold our head up in all weathers, to stand erect and just be ourselves—blooming, obvious, and beautiful.

Method

The sun method (*see page 206*)

TETRATHECA ERICIFOLIA
BLACK-EYED SUSAN

This small scrubby plant of the Australian woodland is called "black-eyed" as the drooping, bell-like flowers have a core of black pollen-covered stamens surrounded by four mauve petals.

GOAL—The "stand and stare" remedy; inner peace
- People who need Black-eyed Susan are always "on the go." They hate waiting or delay, as they rush to accomplish things quickly.
- Accompanying physical symptoms are irritability, poor digestion, restless sleep, and general tension and stress. They may also have nervous rashes.
- Black-eyed Susan releases stress and helps us slow down and find the inner peace to "stand and stare," as in the lines of the poem, "What is this life if full of care/We have no time to stand and stare."

Use

Black-eyed Susan is for people who are always rushing and striving, for the workaholic who does not have time for himself or herself or the people around, and is expending all his or her energy at a fast rate. The flowers' petals protect the black center, so the remedy helps us turn inward, slow down, and pay attention to our inner rhythm.

Method

The sun method (*see page 206*)

FLOWER ESSENCES

ULEX EUROPAEUS
GORSE

Gorse is a bushy shrub with pea-like yellow flowers, which is abundant on poor, stony soils and heaths. It is almost leafless, but its green, spiny stems give it an evergreen appearance.

Use
Gorse is for strong feelings of hopelessness and despair. People who need Gorse may seek help in order to please others, but underneath feel that nothing more can be done for them. They have lost the will to strive, perhaps in response to a life event, an accident, a medical diagnosis, or to a long-standing illness or fear. They are caught up in negativity, unwilling to try new avenues, and unwilling to hope. Gorse gives them the courage to try, building renewed hope, and giving the will to continue the fight toward recovery.

Method
The sun method (*see page 206*)

GOAL—Anything is possible; positive possibilities
- Gorse is for hopelessness and despair when the person has decided to give up.
- Gorse can help give people the heart to stay with a course of treatment. It is useful when a long period of retraining is necessary—for example, after a stroke, loss of limbs, or a major accident, when the person feels that there is no use in trying.
- Gorse helps open a door to possibilities, encourages an objective attitude, and strengthens the heart to face them.

ULMUS PROCERA
ELM

The magnificent English elm, once common in hedgerows and fields, is now sadly rare due to Dutch elm disease. It grows to a towering 120ft. (35m.) and spreads to 50ft. (15m.).

GOAL—Restores confidence
- People who need Elm are usually confident and capable, but are temporarily overwhelmed with the scope, weight, and burden of their work. They may be tired or feel exhausted, which can lead to mild depression.
- Elm gives the strength to balance responsibilities with the practical needs of everyday reality and carry on. (*See also Larch.*)

Use
Elm is for temporary feelings of inadequacy. People who benefit from Elm do good work and are proud of themselves and their calling. They hope to do something important, and to be of service and benefit to all of humanity. They seek and aim for perfection. When this goal seems unattainable, they can become overwhelmed. Elm is for brief faltering moments of despair and lack of confidence, when the task seems too much. Elm restores faith in ability, so that we do not strive for unattainable perfection, but instead appreciate the worth of our own actions.

Method
The boiling method (*see page 207*)

VERBENA OFFICINALIS
VERVAIN

A common wayside perennial found in meadows, on the roadside, and in dry, sunny places, vervain bears many small, unscented lilac flowers.

Use

Vervain people have fixed ideas and principles. They are strong-willed and rarely change their views; they think they are right and obstinately maintain a stance, or fight on when others would have conceded. They are great doers and wish to convert all those around them. They strive with mental energy and will power, but the effort of trying to persuade others is extremely stressful, even exhausting. Vervain brings calm and the ability to relax a little and see the other point of view.

Method

The sun method (*see page 206*)

GOAL—**Will; to relax and hear the will of the world**

- People who need Vervain are those whose activity is self-driven, often with overcommitment.
- They may be overworked and experience stress-related illnesses, including anxiety, indigestion, insomnia, and sleep disorders.
- Vervain brings calm and a space for reflection. It relieves stress and helps to bring the personal will into harmony with the world.

VITIS VINIFERA
VINE

The grapevine is a thick-trunked shrub which climbs by means of tendrils. The flower clusters are small and green, and give way to the well-known fruit—green or purple berries.

GOAL—**Power and natural authority; leadership by consent not through fear**

- Those who need Vine are dominating and bullying.
- They can be cruel and callous through thoughtlessness.
- They may also experience stress-related illnesses.
- Vine allows us to stand back and let others express themselves, to respect the absolute authority of each person over their own inner life, and to acknowledge their personal choices.

Use

Vine is for capable, confident, and successful people; for those who would be "king" (or "queen"). They believe they know best and that others would be happier if they followed. They can bully and dominate, disempowering others, and gaining authority at the expense of their confidence. Even in illness, from the sickbed, they can be ruthless and dominating, ordering their carers around. Vine encourages equality, and the respect each of us, as a fellow human being, is due.

Method

The sun method (*see page 206*)

WAHLENBERGIA SPP.
BLUEBELL

This is a small perennial bluebell that is native to Australia. The small, blue, bell-like flowers appear in the spring. Wahlenbergia thrives best in partial shade, and prefers well-drained soil.

Use

Bluebell is a remedy for the heart—it opens the heart to the flow of the universe. The heart may be closed through hurt, fear, or loneliness. People who need Bluebell are emotionally closed and fearful. They fear that love will run out and they will be left with nothing. They may be possessive and greedy, with objects representing love.

Method

The sun method (*see page 206*)

GOAL—**Wholehearted abundance of love; sharing**

- People who need Bluebell are emotionally closed, and find it hard to share without keeping mental tally of all emotional transactions.
- They are possessive, greedy, and possibly house-proud. Children will not share.
- They may also have congestive and containing symptoms such as indigestion, cramps, constipation, or hemorrhoids.

- Bluebell helps us own ourselves. The heart is like the magic wine flask in the fairy tale; it never runs out. Each morning it is refilled to overflowing abundance.

WISTERIA SINENSIS
WISTERIA

Wisteria is a large, woody vine, originally from China. The flowers come before the leaves in the spring, and hang in large drooping plumes of pale lilac and mauve. This climber can grow to 100ft. (30m).

Use

In Western culture, sex and gender issues are sometimes seen as a matter of power and control. The term "war of the sexes" expresses this. Rape and sexual abuse frequently confirm this role and attitude to power. Wisteria helps people to overcome the inhibitions, blocks, and emotional conflicts produced by this dualistic attitude. It can help them to transcend the roles and to be comfortable with their sexuality. Wisteria can enable them to be open, express themselves, and experience the intimate power and passivity of the orgasm.

Method

The sun method (*see page 206*)

GOAL—To be comfortable with own sexuality; intimacy and trust

- Women who need Wisteria may be frigid, cold, have a touch taboo, or not enjoy sex. They cannot "lose control" or give themselves.
- Men who need Wisteria may be equally fearful and "role-bound," being macho or a "New Man," when they should let go and be themselves.
- Associated symptoms may be genital herpes, warts, or pelvic congestion linked to a pattern or history of abuse, as well as very painful menstruation. If there is a history of abuse (in either sex), give other appropriate remedies.

- Wisteria helps us experience intimacy and mutual trust.

ROCK WATER

Water taken from a natural well or spring, preferably one with a traditional reputation for healing. There are many half-forgotten springs and wells. The water should be open and free-flowing. Choose a well or spring which is open to the air and sunshine, and is as natural as possible. Do not use water from a well dedicated to a saint, or within a church or shrine.

GOAL—Harmony and discipline

- People who need Rock Water may be rigid, narrow-minded, and very strict with themselves, to the point of self-denial.
- They are perfectionists with exaggerated ideals, but unlike Vervain people they do not try to convert others. They are content to make themselves perfect.
- Rock Water encourages flexibility in reaching goals which harmonize with the natural order of the world

Use

Rock Water is for people who are very strict with themselves and unforgiving—like the rock. They practice self-discipline and deny themselves anything which might distract them from their goal. They have high ideals and are hard on themselves. True self-discipline does not involve denial. Denial is only necessary when the person is not acting from the heart and has a narrow view of his or her goal. Rock Water gives the flexibility of water, a pure spring flowing toward the sea.

Method

The sun method (*see page 206*)

RESCUE REMEDY

Rescue Remedy can be bought as a liquid or as a cream. It is made from equal amounts of the five following essences:

CHERRY PLUM—for feelings of desperation
ROCK ROSE—to ease terror, fear, or panic
IMPATIENS—to soothe irritability and agitation
CLEMATIS—to counteract the tendency to drift away
   from the present
STAR OF BETHLEHEM—to address the mental and
   physical symptoms of shock

Together, these flower essences make a safe mental sanctuary in which to recover. Carry Rescue Remedy with you for all emergencies.

Use

Rescue Remedy rebalances the body after any emotional or physical upset. It should be taken when a person feels in need of rescue, is unsettled, or is not quite in step with himself or herself. This may be after a shock, an accident, an argument, a trying event like a divorce or separation, or any circumstance which has demanded supreme nervous effort. Rescue must take place before salvage and restoration. Rescue Remedy speeds healing after surgery. Use Rescue Remedy cream after sunburn, cuts, bruises, or damage from accidents.

Rescue Remedy can be added to any skin wash, douche, or compress if some element of rescue is needed. This method is also useful if nothing is allowed by mouth.

Rescue Remedy can also be given before a trying event, examination, court appearance, operation, hospital test, etc., to minimize the trauma. It is for all emergencies; always carry a small bottle with you.

GOAL—Rescue or salvation

- Rescue Remedy is the only Bach Flower Remedy that is usually taken neat, straight from the stock bottle. Put 4 drops directly onto or under the tongue. Repeat dosage as often as needed.
- Put 4 drops into a glass of water and sip throughout the day until you feel more settled.
- Rescue Remedy is ideal for children and animals, and can be dropped into food or drinking water. A startled infant or baby can be reassured by putting 4 drops into the evening bath.
- It can be given to plants and seedlings with success.
- It is never too late to take Rescue Remedy. It will help overcome old and unspoken trauma if these are still upsetting you. But it is not a panacea, so once the immediate emotional crisis has calmed, look at the other remedies with a view to creating your own personal combination.

VITAMINS AND MINERALS

OUR UNDERSTANDING OF VITAMINS and minerals—and other micronutrients, compounds, and elements—and their role in our body has improved dramatically over the last decades. We now know that "micronutrition" or the vitamins, minerals, and other health-giving components of our food, such as amino acids, fiber, enzymes, and lipids—is crucial to life, and that by manipulating our nutritional intake, we can not only ensure good health and address ailments, but prevent illness and some of the degenerative effects of aging. Exciting new discoveries related to the nutrient components of our food mean that more than half of us are now taking supplementation in one form or another, convinced that diet itself—bearing in mind the stresses on our body and the polluted world in which we live—is inadequate to supply us with our nutritional needs.

VITAMINS

Vitamins are a group of unrelated organic nutrients which are essential to regulate the chemical processes that go on in the body—such as releasing the energy from food, maintaining strong bones, and controlling our hormonal activity. Ideally, vitamins are present in roughly the same quantity in various foods.

MINERALS

Minerals are inorganic chemical elements, necessary for many of the biochemical and physiological processes. Inorganic substances required in amounts greater than 100mg. per day are called minerals; those required in amounts less than 100mg. per day are called trace elements. Minerals are not necessarily present in foods—the quality of the soil and the geological conditions of the area they were grown play an important part in determining the mineral content. Even a balanced diet may be lacking in essential minerals or trace elements because of the soil in which the various foodstuffs were grown.

There is evidence that "sub-clinical" deficiencies—a deficiency which is not extensive enough to be life-threatening or to produce large-scale symptoms—may be the cause of certain forms of cancer, heart disease, weight and skin problems, and a host of other health conditions.

AMINO ACIDS

An amino acid is any compound that contains an amino group and an acidic function. There are 20 amino acids necessary for the synthesis of proteins, which are essential for life. These 20 amino acids form the building blocks of all proteins and are involved in important biological processes, such as the formation of neurotransmitters in the brain. There are eight essential amino acids, which are:

- phenylalanine
- valine
- threonine
- tryptophan
- isoleucine
- methionine
- lysine
- leucine

The remaining 12 are called "nonessential," which means that they can usually be made by the body from other substances. In some conditions, however, nonessential amino acids are necessary—for example, in cases of extreme illness or a very poor diet.

LIPIDS AND DERIVATIVES

Lipids are commonly called "fats," and while many fats are now known to be unhealthy, there are many that are essential to body processes and actually work to prevent the effects of "unhealthy" fats in our bodies. Many lipids and their derivatives are used to unclog arteries, work to retard the effects of aging, and to discourage heart disease and the build-up of cholesterol.

OTHER SUPPLEMENTS

There are a number of other food supplements that do not fall strictly within the definitions of vitamins, minerals, lipids, and amino acids. These include various elements that either have healing properties or are now known to be crucial to health.

WHAT DO VITAMINS, MINERALS, AND OTHER ELEMENTS DO?

Vitamins, minerals, and other elements work together within the body to ensure that all processes can be carried out. When even one element is missing, the body becomes unbalanced and unable to work at its optimum level.

WHEN SHOULD SUPPLEMENTS BE TAKEN?

The best time for taking most supplements is after meals, on a full stomach, although some vitamins and minerals work best on an empty stomach. Read the label on any supplement you plan to take to find out the best time to take it.

Time-release formulas need to be taken with food, as their nutrients are slowly released over a number of hours. If there is not enough food to slow their passage through the body, they can pass the sites where they are normally absorbed before they have had a chance to release their nutrients.

Take supplements at even intervals throughout the day for best effect.

WHEN TO SEE A PRACTITIONER

Most supplements can be taken safely without input from a nutritionist, but if you suffer from chronic health problems, or a specific ailment, it is best to seek expert advice. Amino acids and other elements should only be taken with the advice of a professional. A nutritionist will make sure that you are taking a balanced combination of nutrients that will work together to make you healthy. Remember that everyone's needs are different, based on overall health, diet, whether or not you smoke or drink, are pregnant, and other influences. It is sensible to ensure that you receive advice that is tailored specifically to your individual needs.

CHILDREN

Children need far lower doses than adults, and a healthy, organic diet should offer a large proportion of their nutritional needs. A good vitamin and mineral supplement will provide anything extra that is required, but if you feel your child needs further supplements, see a practitioner. If you are buying products yourself, read the label to ensure that the product is safe for children, and follow the advice carefully.

PREGNANCY

A growing baby puts heavy demands on your body when you are pregnant, and it is more important than ever to ensure that you have a good diet. Research has now proved that we need extra folic acid and iron during pregnancy, and a good multivitamin and mineral supplement is often suggested. Do not take vitamin A supplements while pregnant (see page 234).

SHOULD YOU TAKE SUPPLEMENTS?

Supplements are not a replacement for food, and most cannot be ingested without food. They cannot be taken in place of a good diet, but their beneficial effects will be optimized if combined with a balanced intake of nutritious foods. People suffering from chronic conditions or who smoke or drink regularly may need to take supplements to ensure optimum health.

Micronutrients work in conjunction with one another, and taking large doses of any one supplement can upset the balance within the body. A good vitamin

A HEALTHY DIET

Our diet should be made up of complex carbohydrates (5–9 portions per day), fruits and vegetables (4–9 portions), proteins (3–5 portions), and fat (under 30g. per day is recommended for a healthy diet). But eating the right foods doesn't necessarily mean that you are getting enough nutrients. Refining and processing foods takes out much of the nutritional value, and pesticides and other agents used in the growing process place extra demands on our bodies. Before our food ever reaches the grocery store it may be nutritionally deficient. Therefore, take extra steps to preserve the nutritional content of your food whenever possible:

- Eat the skins of vegetables.
- Don't cut, wash, or soak fruit and vegetables until you are ready to eat them. Exposing their cut surfaces to air destroys many nutrients.
- Choose fresh fruit and vegetables first, but remember that nutritional value decreases with age. Frozen is a better option if you aren't going to eat the food immediately.
- Eat raw whenever possible; if cooking, use as little water as possible.
- If you do boil fruit or vegetables, use the water remaining after cooking in your sauces or gravy.
- Eat organic food whenever possible. It may be more expensive, but you can be sure that the food you are eating has not been processed, and has been grown without the use of pesticides and other chemicals.
- Eat brown, unpolished rice and whole grains.

Fresh Fruit and Vegetables

Choose your daily dietary requirements from different groups of food—complex carbohydrates, fruit and vegetables, and fats and proteins.
Pears, Oranges, Apples, Kumquats, Runner Beans, Carrots, White Cabbage, Broccoli

Complex Carbohydrates

Wholemeal Bread, Oats, Potatoes, Pasta, Black beans, Haricot beans, Lentils

Fats and Proteins

Cheese, Vegetable Spread, Yogurt, Chicken, Fish

---

and mineral supplement will ensure that you are getting the correct amounts of each, according to the relationships between them. Extra supplements should only be taken on the advice of a registered nutritionist or medical practitioner. Where supplements are taken to discourage the course of illness—for example, vitamin C for colds or flu—it is safe to take larger doses than usual. Read the packet for further information.

SUPPLEMENT FORMS

Most supplements come in a variety of forms, to allow for individual needs. They are also prepared with different quantities of the active ingredients, so read the label carefully to ensure that you are getting the correct quantity for your needs.

WHICH SUPPLEMENT?

Powders Many supplements come in powder form, which will usually provide you with extra potency, with no binders or additives. This is useful for people with allergies, or those who find it difficult to swallow a tablet. Powders are particularly useful for children—sprinkle a little powder in their breakfast juice, or stir it into some yogurt or dessert.

Capsules are convenient to take and easy to keep. Fat-soluble vitamins are normally taken in capsule form, but many contain vitamin and mineral powders which allow a higher potency. Garlic and evening primrose oil are commonly available as capsules, and the capsules can be broken apart and applied externally as necessary.

Liquids are appropriate for people who have difficulty swallowing tablets or capsules. Many children's formulas come in liquid form for easy administration. Liquids can be mixed with food or stirred into drinks. Liquid supplements can also be applied externally.

Tablets Many supplements come in tablet form and these are the most practical for many people because they can be easily stored and they will keep for a long time. Check the label to see what is added to your tablets in the form of binders or fillers, which are added to preserve or bulk out the active ingredient.

Reading the Label

Supplements work in different ways, and you will need to understand some of the key words that appear on the labels in order to choose which are most suitable for you.

Chelated is a term which appears on mineral supplements, and it means that the mineral is combined with amino acids to make assimilation more efficient. Most nutritionists recommend taking chelated minerals because they are 3 to 5 times more effective.

Time-release formulas are created with a process that allows them to be released into the body over an 8–10-hour period. These are particularly useful for water-soluble vitamins, any excess of which is excreted within 2 or 3 hours of taking the supplement. Time-release formulas are reputed to provide stable blood levels during the day and night.

A HISTORY OF NUTRITION

Prehistory

From the very earliest days of civilization, nutrition has formed the backbone of healthcare. Obtaining and eating food consumed most of early humans' time, and food and herbs were our first medicine, used to treat a large number of conditions ranging from wounds and insect bites to infection. It became clear that food had powerful healing effects, and that a varied diet, rich in natural ingredients, was a prerequisite for good health. From that time, diet became a fundamental part of most therapies, and an integral element in almost all of the others.

18th century

In the 18th century, English sailors were given lime or lemon juice in order to prevent scurvy, a disease caused by lack of vitamin C, which occurred as a result of long periods of time away at sea without fresh fruit or vegetables.

19th century

In the late 19th century, naturopaths drew attention to the use of food and its nutritional elements as medicine, a concept that was not new, but which had not been acknowledged as a therapy in its own right until that time. Naturopaths used nutrition and fasting to cleanse the body, and to encourage its ability to heal itself. As knowledge about food, its makeup, and the effects it has on our body became greater with the development of biochemistry, the first nutritional specialists undertook to treat specific ailments and symptoms with the components of food.

Nutrition today

By the middle of the 20th century, scientists had put together a profile of proteins, carbohydrates, and fats, as well as vitamins and minerals, which were essential to life and to health. More than 40 nutrients were uncovered, including 13 vitamins. It was discovered that minerals were needed for body functions, and a new understanding of the body and its biochemistry fed the growing interest in the subject. In the 1960s, physicians began to treat patients with special diets and supplements, prescribed according to individual symptoms, problems, and needs, but while conventional medical physicians still discussed nutrition in terms of basic food groups, nutritionists were prescribing vitamins in megadoses. Other elements and compounds were soon identified as necessary to human life, and we are now able to purchase and take substances like amino acids; bee pollen; lipids, such as evening primrose oil and cod liver oil; and seaweeds, acidophilus (healthy bacteria), and dietary enzymes.

ANTIOXIDANTS

Much of the cell damage that occurs in disease is caused by highly destructive chemical groups known as free radicals. These are the products of oxidation, a process which occurs naturally in our body as we breathe. Today, because of the other elements in the air, there are more free radicals than ever. In small quantities free radicals can fight bacteria and viruses; in larger quantities they encourage the aging process and cause damage to our cells.

Fortunately, these can be combated by antioxidants—the ACE vitamins (vitamin A in the form of beta carotene, vitamin C, and vitamin E), the minerals selenium and zinc, and to a lesser extent manganese and copper. Antioxidants protect other substances from oxidation. Many trials have shown that additional antioxidant vitamins—such as 2,000mg. of C and 400mg. of E daily—can significantly reduce the incidence of heart attacks, strokes, cataracts, and other diseases, and slow down the process of aging.

RDA AND SUPPLEMENTS

Governments around the world have provided guidelines for how much of each vitamin or mineral we need in our diets. These are called RDAs (recommended daily allowance) or RDIs (recommended daily intake) and they apply to healthy individuals with a good, balanced diet. These levels are an "adequate" intake, and do not reflect new thinking on nutrition for optimal health and longevity. In other words, they are not therapeutic levels and they do not take into account the varying needs of the population. People with illnesses, a stressful lifestyle, or who are on medication, or eat a highly refined diet may need much more than the RDA.

VITAMIN A

U.S. RDA: 3mg. E.U. RDA: 800mcg.

Vitamin A is a fat-soluble vitamin that comes in two forms: retinol, which is found in animal products such as liver, eggs, butter, and cod liver oil; and beta-carotene, which our body converts into vitamin A when we need more. Beta-carotene is found in any brightly-colored fruit and vegetables.

Vitamin A was for many years called a "miracle" vitamin because of its effect on the immune system and growth. It is necessary for healthy skin and eyes, and allows us to see in the dark. Beta-carotene is an antioxidant (*see left*), and it has anticarcinogenic properties.

Best Sources

Vitamin A: cod liver oil, liver, kidney, eggs, dairy produce. Beta-carotene: carrots, tomatoes, watercress, broccoli, spinach, cantaloupe, apricots.

PROPERTIES
- Anticarcinogenic.
- Prevents and treats skin disorders and aging of skin.
- Improves vision and prevents night blindness.
- Improves the body's ability to heal.
- Promotes the growth of strong bones, hair, teeth, skin, and gums.
- May help in the treatment of hyperthyroidism.

Dosage

The RDA is very much a minimum, and people with special needs (following illness, suffering from infections, with diabetes, for example) should have a higher level.

Taken as vitamin A, up to 6,000mcg. is permissible if you are not pregnant.

Taken as beta-carotene, 15mg. can be taken as a preventative measure against illness.

CAUTION
Vitamin A as retinol is toxic and should not be taken at all as a supplement by pregnant women, as it can cause birth defects in the unborn child.

B1 (THIAMINE)

U.S. RDA: 1.2–1.5 mg. E.U. RDA: 1.4mg.

Thiamine is involved in all key metabolic processes in the nervous system, the heart, the blood cells, and the muscles. It is useful in the treatment of nervous disorders, and can protect against imbalances caused by alcoholism.

There are more cases of vitamin B1 deficiency than of any other nutritional element—this has been said to be due to a growth in alcoholism. Thiamine is found in all plant and animal foods, but good sources are whole grains, brown rice, seafood, and pulses.

PROPERTIES

- Protects against imbalances caused by alcohol consumption.
- B1 may be useful in treating heart disease.
- May be beneficial in the treatment of neurological disease (particularly when caused by B1 deficiency).
- May help to treat anemia.
- May improve people's mental agility.
- May help to control diabetes which has been linked to deficiency.
- Useful in the treatment of herpes and infections.
- Helps to convert sugar to energy, in the muscles and the bones.

Best Sources

Pork, milk, eggs, whole grains, organ meats, brown rice, barley, seafood.

Dosage

Heavy drinkers, smokers, pregnant women, or those taking the pill should increase normal dosage to up to 100–300mg. per day.

Increase intake in stressful conditions. Will be most effective as part of a good B-complex supplement.

CAUTION

Thiamine is nontoxic, but it is recommended that you do not take more than 400mg. daily.

B2 (RIBOFLAVIN)

U.S. RDA: 1.7mg. E.U. RDA: 1.6mg.

Riboflavin is a water-soluble member of the B-complex family of vitamins. It is crucial to the production of body energy and has antioxidant qualities. Riboflavin is not stored in any significant amount in the body, and deficiency is common.

Riboflavin is necessary for healthy skin, hair, and nails. Because it is destroyed by sunlight, it is recommended that you keep foods containing this vitamin in a dark, cool place. In particular, milk loses its riboflavin content after only two hours' exposure to the sun.

PROPERTIES

- Works with enzymes to metabolize fats, protein, and carbohydrates.
- Aids vision.
- Promotes healthy skin, hair, and nails.
- Promotes healthy growth and reproductive function.
- Boosts athletic performance.
- Protects against cancer.
- Protects against anemia.

Best Sources

Milk, eggs, cheese, fortified breads and cereals, green leafy vegetables, fish.

Dosage

Pregnancy, breast-feeding, taking the pill, and heavy drinking all call for an increased intake.

Take as part of a B-complex supplement, and increase dosage in stressful situations. 100–300mg. per day is commonly suggested.

CAUTION

Riboflavin is nontoxic in most doses, but it is recommended that you do not take in excess of 400mg. per day unless supervised by a registered practitioner.

B3 (NIACIN)

U.S. RDA: 13–18mg. adults, 5–6mg. infants, 9–13mg. children under 10. E.U. RDA: 15–18mg.

Niacin is one of the water-soluble B-complex vitamins, and it is essential for the synthesis of sex hormones and a healthy nervous system. Niacin may also be valuable in helping to prevent and treat schizophrenia, and in acting as a detoxicant, ridding the body of toxins, pollutants, and drugs. Niacin takes the form of nicotinic acid and nicotinamide, and is a fairly recent addition to the family of B-complex vitamins, named as a vitamin only in 1937. Niacin has been shown to lower blood cholesterol and other body fats, and is useful in the prevention of heart disease. It may help to prevent diabetes.

PROPERTIES

- Prevents and treats schizophrenia.
- Aids in cell respiration.
- Produces energy from sugar, fat, and protein.
- Maintains clear, healthy skin, nerves, tongue, and good digestion.
- May lower cholesterol and therefore protect against heart disease.
- Believed to be antioxidant.
- May help prevent migraine headaches.
- Reduces blood pressure.
- May alleviate arthritis.

Best Sources

Meat, fish, wholegrain cereals, eggs, milk, cheese.

Dosage

Large doses may be used therapeutically, but should be taken under the supervision of a physician or health practitioner.

Doses of 20–100mg. of niacin, taken daily, may be beneficial. Best taken as part of a B-complex supplement.

B5 (PANTOTHENIC ACID)

U.S. RDA: 10mg. E.U. RDA: 6mg.

Pantothenic acid is a water-soluble member of the B-complex family of vitamins that helps maintain normal growth and the health of the nervous system. Pantothenic acid has become a popular supplement over the past decade for its ability to boost energy levels and improve immune response.

There is also evidence that pantothenic acid can lower cholesterol and protect against heart disease. Pantothenic acid is useful in reducing the effects of stress on the body, and is needed to convert choline into acetylcholine, which is necessary for brain functioning.

Best Sources

Yeast, organ meats, eggs, brown rice, wholegrain cereals, molasses.

PROPERTIES

- B5 encourages the healing of wounds.
- Helps the body in the production of energy.
- Reduces stress levels.
- Controls the metabolism of fat.
- Encourages functioning of the immune system.
- Prevents fatigue.
- Lowers cholesterol levels and so protects against heart disease.
- Prevents arthritis, and also treats it.

Dosage

Best taken in B-complex formulas, up to 300mg. per day for therapeutic use.

The normal dosage, which should help to prevent disease, is about 100mg. per day.

CAUTION
No known toxicity, although doses of over 300mg. per day should be supervised by a practitioner. Some people report stomach upsets at doses higher than 10g.

B6 (PYRIDOXINE)

U.S. RDA: 2mg. E.U. RDA: 1.6–2mg.

Pyridoxine is a water-soluble B-complex vitamin which is necessary for the production of antibodies and white blood cells. B6 is necessary for the absorption of vitamin B12. B6 is required for the functioning of more than 60 enzymes in the body and also for protein synthesis.

Of all the B vitamins, B6 is the most important for a healthy immune system, and it is thought to protect the body against some cancers. B6 is widely used for relieving the symptoms of PMS and menopause, and may cure some forms of infertility. This vitamin is also used to prevent skin inflammation, and maintain healthy teeth and gums.

PROPERTIES
- Boosts immunity.
- Helps to control diabetes.
- B6 assimilates proteins and fats.
- Helps prevent skin and nervous disorders.
- Alleviates nausea.
- Treats symptoms of PMS and menopause.
- Reduces muscle cramps and spasms.
- Acts as a natural diuretic.
- Protects against cancer.

Best Sources
Meat, fish, milk, eggs, wholegrain cereals, fresh vegetables.

Dosage
Should always be taken as part of a B-complex supplement, and in equal amounts with B1 and B2.

Time-release formulas are best because it lasts for only eight hours in the body.

CAUTION
Vitamin B6 is toxic in high doses, causing serious nerve damage when taken at quantities of more than 2g. per day. Some people report side-effects with doses as low as 100mg.

B9 (FOLIC ACID)

U.S. RDA: 400mcg. E.U. RDA: 200–360mcg.

Folic acid is a water-soluble vitamin that forms part of the B-complex family. It is also known as vitamin Bc or vitamin B9. Low levels of folic acid may lead to anemia. Folic acid is essential for the division of body cells, and it is also necessary for the utilization of sugar and amino acids.

Recent findings indicate that folic acid can prevent some types of cancer and birth defects, and it is helpful in the treatment of heart disease. Most folic acid deficiency is the result of a poor diet, because it is abundant in foods such as leafy green vegetables, yeast, and liver. Taken from just before conception, and particularly in the first trimester of pregnancy, folic acid can help to prevent spina bifida.

PROPERTIES
- Improves lactation.
- Improves skin condition.
- Natural analgesic.
- Increases appetite in debilitated patients.
- Needed for metabolism of RNA and DNA.
- Helps form blood.
- Builds up babies' resistance to infection.
- Prevents spina bifida.

Best Sources
Green leafy vegetables, wheat germ, nuts, eggs, bananas, oranges, organ meats.

Dosage
There are many people at risk of deficiency, including heavy drinkers, pregnant women, the elderly, and those on low-fat diets. Supplementation at 400–800mcg. is recommended for those at risk.

It is best taken with a good multivitamin and mineral supplement.

CAUTION
Folic acid is toxic in large doses and can cause severe neurological problems. High doses can cause insomnia and interfere with the absorption of zinc in the body.

B12 (COBALAMIN)

U.S. RDA: 3mcg. E.U. RDA: 2mcg.

Cobalamin is a water-soluble member of the B-complex vitamin family, and it is the only vitamin that contains essential minerals. B12 is essential for the healthy metabolism of nerve tissue, and deficiencies can cause brain damage and neurological disorders.

Vitamin B12 was once considered to be a "wonder drug" and was given by injection to rejuvenate. B12 may also reduce the risk of cancer and the severity of allergies, as well as boosting energy levels. Low levels of this vitamin result in anemia.

PROPERTIES

- Needed for maintenance of the nervous system.
- Improves memory and concentration.
- Required to utilize fats, carbohydrates, and proteins.
- Increases energy.
- Promotes healthy growth in children.
- May protect against cancer.
- Protects against allergens and toxic elements.

Best Sources

Liver, beef, pork, eggs, cheese, fish, milk.

CAUTION

Although vitamin B12 is not considered to be toxic, it is recommended that you do not take more than 200mg. daily unless you are under the supervision of a registered practitioner.

Dosage

Dosages of 5–50mcg. should be adequate for most people; higher dosages should be supervised.

Best taken as part of a B-complex supplement.

VITAMIN C

U.S. RDA: 60mg. E.U. RDA: 60mg.

Vitamin C is water soluble, which means that it is not stored by the body and we need to ensure that we get adequate amounts in our daily diet. More people take vitamin C than any other supplement, and yet studies show that a large percentage of the population have deficiencies.

Vitamin C is also known as ascorbic acid, and it is one of the most versatile of the vitamins we need to sustain life. It is one of the antioxidant vitamins (*see page 234*) and is believed to boost immunity, and to fight cancer and infection.

PROPERTIES

- Reduces cholesterol and helps prevent heart disease.
- Speeds up the healing of wounds.
- Maintains healthy bones, teeth, and sex organs.
- Acts as a natural antihistamine.
- May help to overcome male infertility.
- Boosts immunity and reduces the duration of colds and other viruses.
- Helps maintenance of good vision.
- Antioxidant.

Best Sources

Rosehips, blackcurrants, broccoli, citrus fruit, all fresh fruit and vegetables.

Dosage

At least 60mg. per day is necessary for health, but more is required by smokers (25mg. is depleted with every cigarette), and people who are under stress, taking antibiotics, suffering from an infection, drink heavily, as well as after an accident or injury. Daily dosages of up to 1,500mg. per day appear to be safe, but take this in three doses, preferably with meals, and use a time-release formula.

CAUTION

Vitamin C may cause kidney stones and gout in some individuals. Some people suffer from diarrhea and cramps at high dosages, although the vitamin is considered to be nontoxic at even very high levels.

VITAMIN D

U.S. RDA: 10mcg. E.U. RDA: 5mcg.

Vitamin D is a fat-soluble vitamin that is found in foods of animal origin and is known as the "sunshine" vitamin. Vitamin D can be produced in the skin from the energy of the sun, and it is not found in rich supply in any food.

Vitamin D is important for calcium and phosphorus absorption, and helps to regulate calcium metabolism. Deficiency is caused by inadequate exposure to sunlight, and low consumption of foods containing vitamin D.

PROPERTIES
- Protects against osteoporosis.
- Boosts immune system.
- Necessary for strong teeth and bones.

Best Sources
Animal produce, such as dairy, eggs, oily fish, cod liver oil.

Dosage
Supplementation between 5–10mcg. is suggested.

> **CAUTION**
> Vitamin D is the most toxic of all the vitamins, causing nausea, vomiting, headache, and depression, among other problems. Do not take excess of 10mcg. daily.

PROPERTIES
- Antioxidant, so helps to slow the process of aging.
- Protects against neurological disorders.
- Boosts immunity.
- Protects against cardiovascular disease.
- Alleviates fatigue.
- Accelerates healing, particularly of burns.
- Reduces the various symptoms of PMS.
- Treats skin problems and baldness.
- Helps prevent miscarriage.
- Acts as a natural diuretic.
- Prevents formation of thickened scars.

Best Sources
Wheatgerm (fresh), soybeans, vegetable oils, broccoli, leafy green vegetables, whole grains, peanuts, eggs.

Dosage
Available in many forms (the dry form is best for people with skin problems or oil intolerance).

Daily dosage may be from 250–280mg., but you may be advised to take higher doses in some cases.

> **CAUTION**
> Vitamin E is nontoxic even in high doses, but it is suggested that you do not take in excess of 350mg. unless you are supervised by a registered practitioner.

VITAMIN E

U.S. RDA: 20mg. E.U. RDA: 10mg.

Vitamin E is fat soluble and one of the key antioxidant vitamins. Its key function is as an anticoagulant, but its role in boosting the immune system and protecting against cardiovascular disease is becoming increasingly clear.

Apart from its crucial antioxidant value, vitamin E is important for the production of energy and the maintenance of health at every level. Unlike most fat-soluble vitamins, vitamin E is stored in the body for only a short period of time, and up to 75 percent of a daily dose is excreted in the feces.

BIOTIN (VITAMIN H)

U.S. RDA: 300mcg. E.U. RDA: 0.15mg.

Biotin is not a true vitamin, but it works with B-complex vitamins and is often called vitamin H, or co-enzyme R. Biotin is water soluble and is found in many common foods. It is essential for breaking down and metabolizing fats in the body.

Biotin is depleted in the body by alcohol, cooking or refining food, antibiotics, and when taken with raw egg whites, which contain avidin, a protein that prevents biotin absorption. Biotin works more effectively with vitamins B2, B6, B3, and A.

Best Sources

Nuts, fruit, beef liver, egg yolks, milk, kidneys, unpolished rice, brewer's yeast.

Dosage

Biotin is normally included in most readily-available B-complex supplements.

> **CAUTION**
> Biotin is nontoxic, but it is suggested that you do not take an excess of 300mcg. unless supervised by a registered practitioner.

VITAMIN K

U.S. RDA: none. E.U. RDA: none

The K vitamins are fat soluble, and are necessary for normal blood clotting. They are often used to treat the toxic effects of anticoagulant drops, such as Warfarin, and in people who have a poor ability to absorb fats.

Vitamin K occurs naturally in foods as vitamin K1, and is produced by intestinal bacteria as vitamin K2. Synthetic vitamin K is known as K3. Vitamin K1 injections are routinely given to newborn babies to prevent hemorrhage, but since a recent scare linked the vitamin with childhood leukemia it is now more often given as oral drops.

PROPERTIES

- Controls blood clotting.

Best Sources

Cauliflower, spinach, peas, wholegrain cereals.

Dosage

We need an estimated 500–1,000mcg. of vitamin K per day.

> **CAUTION**
> There are reports of toxicity, and because of the possibility injected vitamin K may be related to childhood leukemia, oral drops are suggested.

VITAMIN B (BORON)

U.S. RDA: none. E.U. RDA: none

Boron is a trace mineral found in most plants, and it is essential for human health. Recent research has reported that boron added to the diet of post-menopausal women prevents calcium loss and bone demineralization—a revolutionary discovery for sufferers of osteoporosis.

It is also claimed that boron will raise testosterone levels and build muscle in, and boron is therefore often used by athletes and bodybuilders. Boron is found in most fruit and vegetables. Boron supplements are usually taken in the form of sodium borate.

PROPERTIES

- Assists in the external treatment of bacterial and fungal infections.
- Prevents osteoporosis.
- Used to build muscles.

Best Sources

Root vegetables grown in soil that is rich in boron.

Dosage

No RDA, but it is suggested that 3mg. should be taken daily to prevent osteoporosis.

> **CAUTION**
> Boron can be toxic, with symptoms including a red rash, vomiting, diarrhea, shock, and then coma. A fatal dose is 15–20g., 3–6g. in children. Symptoms appear at about 100mg.

Ca CALCIUM

U.S. RDA: 800–1,200mg. E.U. RDA: 800mg.

Calcium is an important mineral, and recent research shows that we get only about one-third of what we need for good health. Calcium is essential for human life—it makes up bones and teeth, and is crucial in the process of conducting messages along nerves. It ensures that our muscles contract, and that our hearts beat, and it is extremely important in the maintenance of the immune system, among other things.

There are many groups at risk of calcium deficiency—in particular the elderly—and because it is so important to body processes our bodies take what they need from our bones, which causes them to become thin and brittle. It is used therapeutically for allergies, depression, panic attacks, insomnia, and hyperactivity, and extra should be taken during pregnancy and while breast-feeding.

PROPERTIES
- Prevents osteoporosis, and helps to treat the condition.
- Useful in the treatment of high blood pressure.
- Prevents heart disease.
- Useful in treating arthritis.
- Helps to keep skin healthy.
- Encourages regular beating of the heart.
- Helps the body to metabolize iron.

Best Sources

Milk, cheese, dairy produce, leafy green vegetables, hard tap water, salmon, tinned fish, eggs, beans, nuts, tofu.

Dosage

Experts recommend that calcium be taken in a good multivitamin and mineral supplement. More calcium is needed by women after menopause, and while pregnant or breast-feeding.

CAUTION
Doses over 2,000mg. per day may cause hypercalcemia (calcium deposits in the kidneys), but since excess calcium is excreted, it is unlikely to occur unless you are also taking excess quantities of vitamin D.

Co COBALT

U.S. RDA: none. E.U. RDA: none

Cobalt is an essential trace mineral. It is a constituent of vitamin B12. The amount of cobalt in the body is dependent on the amount of cobalt in the soil, and therefore in the food we eat. Most of us are not deficient in cobalt, although deficiency is much more common in vegetarians.

PROPERTIES
Cobalt is able, with vitamin B12, to:
- Prevent pernicious anemia.
- Help in the production of red blood cells.
- Aid in the synthesis of DNA and choline.
- Encourage a healthy nervous system.
- Reduce blood pressure.
- Maintain myelin, the fatty sheath protecting the nerves.

Best Sources

Fresh leafy green vegetables, meat, liver, milk, oysters, clams.

Dosage

Cobalt is rarely found in supplement form, but forms part of a good multivitamin and mineral supplement with the B-complex vitamins. An intake of 8mcg. daily appears to be adequate.

CAUTION
When used therapeutically, side-effects occur at doses above 30mg.; these include goiter, hyperthyroidism, and heart failure.

Cu COPPER

U.S. RDA: 1.5–3mg. E.U. RDA: 1.2mg.

Copper is an essential trace mineral, and is necessary for respiration—iron and copper are required for oxygen to be synthesized in red blood cells. Copper is also important for the production of collagen, which is responsible for the health of our bones, cartilage, and skin. Copper is also one of the antioxidant minerals (*see page 234*), which protect against free-radical damage. Arthritis sufferers report that copper bracelets reduce pain and inflammation associated with the condition, probably because traces of the mineral are absorbed by the skin and enter the bloodstream.

PROPERTIES
- May prevent cancer.
- Protects against cardiovascular disease.
- Useful mineral in the treatment of arthritis.
- Boosts the immune system.
- Acts as an antioxidant.

Best Sources
Animal livers, shellfish, nuts, fruit, oysters, kidneys, legumes.

Dosage
Copper appears in good multivitamin and mineral supplements, and can be taken alone up to 3mg. daily.

Excess intake can cause vomiting, diarrhea, muscular pain, and dementia.

Cr CHROMIUM

U.S. RDA: none. E.U. RDA: none

Chromium is a trace mineral that was discovered in the body in the 1950s. It is an important regulator of blood sugar, and has been used successfully in the control and treatment of diabetes. It is involved in the metabolism of carbohydrates and fats, and is used in the production of insulin in the body.

High levels of sugars in the diet cause chromium to be excreted through the kidneys, so it is important to get enough in your diet if you eat sugary foods. The incidence of diabetes and heart disease decreases with increased levels of chromium in the body.

PROPERTIES
- Aids in the control and production of insulin.
- Aids in the metabolism of carbohydrates and fats.
- Controls levels of cholesterol in the blood.
- Stimulates the synthesis of proteins in the body.
- Increases general resistance to infection.
- Suppresses hunger pains.

Best Sources
Wholegrain cereals, meat, cheese, brewer's yeast, molasses, egg yolk.

Dosage
There is no RDA, but it is suggested that 25mcg. per day is adequate.

If necessary, supplements of up to 200mcg. per day can be taken.

CAUTION
There is no evidence that chromium is toxic, even in high doses, since any excess is excreted. However, it is suggested that you do not take more than 200mcg. daily unless supervised by a registered practitioner.

F FLUORINE

U.S. RDA: 1mg. fluoride, 3.6mg. sodium fluoride. E.U. RDA: none

Fluorine is a trace mineral found naturally in soil, water, plants, and animal tissues. Its electrically charged form is "fluoride," which is how we usually refer to it. Although it has not yet been officially recognized as an essential nutrient, studies show that it is important in many processes, and may play a major role in the prevention of many 20th-century killers, like heart disease.

The major source of fluorine is drinking water, which is sometimes fluoridated, or has enough naturally occurring fluoride to make fluoridation unnecessary. Fluoride supplements should always be taken with calcium.

PROPERTIES
- Fluorine protects against dental caries.
- Protects against, and also treats, osteoporosis.
- It may help to prevent heart disease.
- May help to prevent calcification of organs and musculoskeletal structures.

Best Sources
Seafood, animal meat, fluoridated drinking water, tea.

Dosage
The major source is drinking water, and typical daily intake is 1–2mg.

Tablets and drops are available from pharmacies, but should be limited to 1mg. daily in adults, and 0.25–0.5mg. for children.

CAUTION
An excess of fluoride causes fluorosis, characterized by irregular patches on tooth enamel, and depresses the appetite. Eventually, the spine calcifies. Fluorosis is rare and occurs at levels far above 10mg. per day. Do not supplement fluoride without the advice of your dentist.

Fe IRON

U.S. RDA: 10–18mg., pregnant women 30mg. E.U. RDA: 14mg.

Iron is a trace mineral which is essential for human health. Iron-deficiency anemia, which is the condition most commonly associated with deficiency, was described by Egyptian physicists as long ago as 1500 B.C.E. Today, 10 percent of all women in the Western world suffer from iron-deficiency anemia.

We now know that iron is present in our bodies as hemoglobin, which is the red pigment of blood. Iron is required for muscle protein and is stored in the liver, spleen, bone marrow, and muscles. Efficient absorption of iron is highest in childhood, and reduces as we age. Our bodies need vitamin C in order to assimilate iron in an effective fashion.

PROPERTIES
- Improves physical performance.
- Anticarcinogenic.
- Prevents learning problems in children.
- Improves immunity.
- Boosts energy levels.
- Encourages restful sleep and maintains energy levels.

Best Sources
Shellfish, brewer's yeast, wheat bran, offal, cocoa powder, dried fruit, cereals.

Dosage
Pregnant, breast-feeding, and menstruating women, infants, children, athletes, and vegetarians may require increased levels of iron. Your general physician will prescribe iron supplements if they are necessary.

Maximum dosage is around 15mg. daily, unless under medical supervision.

CAUTION
Excess iron can cause constipation, diarrhea, and, rarely, in high doses, death. Be very cautious when giving children iron supplements—even doses as little as 3g. can cause death.

Ge GERMANIUM

U.S. RDA: none. E.U. RDA: none

Germanium is a mineral which is abundant in the surface of the Earth. Almost all foods commonly eaten contain some germanium. Some conditions have been reported to respond favorably to germanium given at therapeutic doses, including arthritis, angina, stroke, Raynaud's disease, burns, and pain associated with cancer.

Germanium is believed to function by boosting the action of oxygen in generating energy. Because it maintains an equilibrium within the body, germanium is said to reduce high blood pressure, lower cholesterol levels, and generally to exert a good effect on the immune system. Germanium is now considered to be one of the antioxidant minerals (*see page 234*).

PROPERTIES

- Maintains the homeostasis in the body, and therefore may reduce high blood pressure and cholesterol levels.
- Germanium boosts the immune system.
- May be analgesic.
- May have antiviral, antibacterial, and antitumor activity.
- Useful as part of a cancer treatment program.

Best Sources

Bran, wholewheat flour, vegetables, seeds, meats, dairy products.

Dosage

Germanium supplementation is not recommended without a physician's supervision.

CAUTION

Germanium is safe up to quite a high level, although skin eruptions and diarrhea have been reported in some patients taking therapeutic doses. Only use the supplement under the supervision of a physician or nutritionist.

I IODINE

U.S. RDA: 80–150mcg. E.U. RDA: 150mcg.

Iodine is a mineral, which was first discovered in 1812 in kelp. Iodine was extracted and given its name because of its violet color. It occurs naturally and is a crucial constituent of the thyroid hormones, which monitor our energy levels.

Iodine deficiency is one of the key world health problems, and at least 200 million people suffer from conditions linked to inadequate iodine in the diet. Lack of iodine can cause goiter, underactive thyroid, cretinism, and can eventually lead to myxedema.

PROPERTIES

- Determines the level of metabolism and energy in the body.
- Relieves the pain of fibrocystic breasts.
- Protects against the toxic effects of exposure to radioactive materials.
- Prevents goiter.
- Prevents thyroid disorders.
- Loosens mucus in the respiratory tract.
- Natural antiseptic.

Best Sources

Seafood and seaweed. Most table salt is fortified with iodine.

Dosage

Iodine is best taken as potassium iodide.

Take under the supervision of your physician or nutritionist.

150mcg. RDA iodine is adequate.

CAUTION

Iodine is toxic in high doses and may aggravate or cause acne. Large doses may interfere with hormone activity. Cruciferous foods like cabbage, Brussels sprouts, cauliflower, and broccoli contain substances which can cause hypothyroidism by antagonizing iodine. Anyone who eats large quantities of these vegetables should consider an iodine supplement.

K POTASSIUM

U.S. RDA: 3,500mg. E.U. RDA: 3,500mg.

Potassium is one of the most important minerals in our body, working with sodium and chloride to form "electrolytes," the essential body salts that make up our body fluids. Potassium is crucial in order for the body to function. It plays a role in nerve conduction, the beating of the heart, energy production, the synthesis of nucleic acids and proteins, and the contraction of muscles.

Sweating can cause a loss of potassium, as do chronic diarrhea and diuretics. People taking certain drugs, including corticosteroids, high-dose penicillin, and laxatives may suffer from potassium deficiency. Symptoms of this can include vomiting, abdominal distension, muscular weakness, loss of appetite, low blood pressure, and intense thirst.

PROPERTIES

- Activates enzymes which control energy production.
- Prevents and treats high blood pressure.
- May help to protect against stroke.
- Improves athletic performance.
- May help treat and prevent cancer.
- Maintains water balance within cells.
- Stabilizes the internal structure of cells.
- Acts with sodium to conduct nerve impulses.

Best Sources

Fresh fruit and vegetables, particularly bananas.

Dosage

Eat more fresh fruit and vegetables to increase potassium intake. Diuretic users and those in a hot climate may need up to 1.5g. in supplementary potassium daily.

Take with zinc and magnesium for best effect.

Mg MAGNESIUM

U.S. RDA: 300–400mg. E.U. RDA: 300mg.

Magnesium is a mineral that is absolutely essential for every biochemical process taking place in our bodies, including metabolism and the synthesis of nucleic acids and protein.

Magnesium deficiency is very common, particularly in the elderly, heavy drinkers, pregnant women, and regular, strenuous exercisers, and it has been proved that even a very slight deficiency can cause a disruption of the heartbeat. Other symptoms of magnesium deficiency include weakness, fatigue, vertigo, nervousness, muscle cramps, and hyperactivity in children.

PROPERTIES

- Magnesium is necessary for many body functions, including energy production and cell replication.
- Essential for transmission of nerve impulses.
- Helps to prevent kidney stones and gallstones.
- Useful in the treatment of prostate problems.
- Repairs and maintains body cells.
- Required for hormonal activity.
- Required for most body processes, including production of energy.
- Useful in the treatment of high blood pressure.
- Protects against cardiovascular disease.
- Helps to treat the symptoms of PMS.

Best Sources

Brown rice, soybeans, nuts, brewer's yeast, whole wheat flour, legumes.

Dosage

Dietary intake is thought to be inadequate in the average Western diet; supplements of 200–400mg. are recommended daily.

CAUTION

Magnesium is toxic to people with renal problems or atrioventricular blocks. High doses are believed to cause flushing of the skin, thirst, low blood pressure, and loss of reflexes in some people, although this is rare.

Mn MANGANESE

U.S. RDA: 2.5–7mg. E.U. RDA: none

Manganese is an essential trace element that is necessary for the normal functioning of the brain, and effective in the treatment of many nervous disorders, including Alzheimer's disease and schizophrenia. Deficiency is usually related to a poor diet -particularly one where there is a high intake of foods that are processed and refined.

Our understanding of manganese is still incomplete, but it may prove to be one of the most important nutrients in human pathology. It appears likely that manganese is one of the antioxidant minerals (*see page 234*). There is some evidence that diseases such as diabetes, heart disease, and schizophrenia are linked to manganese deficiency.

PROPERTIES

- Manganese maintains the healthy functioning of the nervous system.
- Necessary for female sex hormones.
- Necessary for the synthesis of the structural proteins of body cells.
- Necessary for normal bone structure.
- Important in the formation of thyroxin in the thyroid gland.
- Necessary for the functioning of the brain.
- Used in the treatment of some nervous disorders.
- Necessary for metabolism of glucose.

Best Sources

Cereals, tea, green leaf vegetables, wholewheat bread, legumes, nuts.

Dosage

2–5 mg. is adequate, but doses up to 10mg. are thought to be safe.

CAUTION

Toxic levels are usually quite rare, but symptoms of excess manganese may include lethargy, involuntary movements, posture problems, and coma.

Mo MOLYBDENUM

U.S. RDA: 150–500mcg. E.U. RDA: none

Molybdenum is an essential trace element, and a vital part of the enzyme which is responsible for the utilization of iron in our bodies. Molybdenum may also be an antioxidant, and recent research indicates that it is necessary for optimum health.

Molybdenum can help to prevent anemia and is known to promote a feeling of well-being. A deficiency may result in dental caries, sexual impotence in men, and cancer of the gullet. Deficiency is usually the result of eating foods from molybdenum-deficient soils, or a diet that is high in refined and processed foods.

PROPERTIES

- For utilization of iron, fats, carbohydrates; excretion of uric acid.
- Prevents impotence.
- Protects against cancer, anemia, dental caries.

Best Sources

Wheat, canned beans, wheat germ, liver, legumes, whole grains, offal, eggs.

Dosage

Optimal intake is not decided; 0.075–0.25mg. per day is adequate, and experts suggest 50–100mcg. per day as a preventive measure. Toxic in doses higher than 10–15mg., causing gout.

CAUTION

Molybdenum is toxic in doses higher than 10–15mg. which cause gout (a build-up of uric acid around the joints).

P PHOSPHORUS

U.S. RDA: 800–1,200mg. E.U. RDA: 800mg.

Phosphorus is a mineral that is essential to the structure and function of the body. It is present in the body as phosphates, and in this form aids the process of bone mineralization and helps to create the structure of the bone.

Phosphorus is also essential for communication between cells, and for energy production. Phosphorus appears in many foods and deficiency is rare. Because of its role in strengthening our bones, we should eat twice as much calcium as phosphorus.

PROPERTIES
- Forms bones and teeth.
- Produces energy.
- Cofactor for many enzymes and activates B-complex vitamins.
- Increases endurance, and fights fatigue.
- Forms RNA and DMA.

Best Sources

Yeast, dried milk and milk products, wheat germ, hard cheeses, canned fish, nuts, cereals, eggs.

Dosage

Phosphorus deficiency usually accompanies deficiency in potassium, magnesium, and zinc, so take a supplement containing all four.

Take under medical supervision only.

CAUTION
Phosphorus can be toxic at dosages or intake above 200mg. per day, in some cases causing diarrhea, the calcification of organs and soft tissues, and making the body unable to absorb iron, calcium, magnesium, and zinc.

Se SELENIUM

U.S. RDA: 50–100mcg. E.U. RDA: 10-75mcg.

Selenium is an essential trace element that has recently been recognized as one of the most important nutrients in our diet. It is an antioxidant (*see page 234*) and is vitally important in human metabolism. Selenium has been proved to provide protection against a number of cancers, and other diseases.

Selenium is necessary for the body's manufacture of proteins, and helps the liver to function efficiently. It also forms part of the male sperm, which means that deficiency can be linked to infertility in men. Other symptoms of deficiency include reduced immune activity, hair loss, and chest pains.

PROPERTIES
- Maintains healthy eyes and eyesight.
- Maintains good skin and healthy hair.
- Stimulates immune system.
- Increases male potency and sex drive.
- Alleviates hot flashes and symptoms of menopause.

Best Sources

Selenium is found in wheat germ, bran, tuna fish, onions, tomatoes, broccoli, kidneys, wholewheat bread.

Dosage

There is no RDA, but it has been suggested that men take 75mcg. of supplementary selenium and women take 60mcg.

Selenium supplementation should be taken with 9–120mcg. of vitamin E to ensure that selenium works most efficiently.

Dosages of 400–1,000mcg. have been used for immune stimulation, and for anticarcinogenic effects, but it is recommended that 50–200mcg. should be adequate to experience benefits.

CAUTION
Selenium can be toxic in very small doses. Symptoms of excess include blackened fingernails and a garlic-like odor on the breath and skin. Take no more than 500mcg. daily unless supervised by a registered practitioner.

S₁ SILICON

U.S. RDA: none. E.U. RDA: none

Silicon is a trace element which is only just starting to be understood. It has been proved to be essential to animals, and it is thought that it is crucial to human life as well. Scientists believe that silicon plays some part in the make-up of our connective tissues, bones, skin, and fingernails.

Silicon is also known to play a role in preventing osteoporosis, by assisting the utilization of calcium within the bones. It also improves the strength of hair and nails by improving the production of keratin and collagen. Silicon is available as a supplement in the form of silicon dioxide. Silicea is a homeopathic remedy for disorders of the bones, joints, and skin.

PROPERTIES

- Helps guard against certain heart and circulatory diseases.
- Helps to prevent osteoporosis.
- Believed to help prevent hair falling out.
- Involved in maintaining the health of bones, skin, and fingernails.

Best Sources

Found in whole grains, vegetables, hard drinking water, seafood.

Dosage

There is no official RDA, but we need 20–30mg. each day. Most of us get about 200mg. in our diet.

> ### CAUTION
> Excess silicon can cause kidney stones, but only at very high doses.

V VANADIUM

U.S. RDA: none. E.U. RDA: none

Vanadium is a trace mineral that has only recently been proved necessary for human life. At the turn of the 20th century, French physicians believed that vanadium was a miracle cure for a variety of illnesses, but it proved to be toxic at the levels they were prescribing, and it became less popular.

Today, it is believed that elevated levels of vanadium may cause manic depression, which is perhaps a clue to a little-understood disease. Normal doses are thought to reduce appetite, and to reduce blood fat and cholesterol levels.

PROPERTIES

- Reduces high blood sugar by mimicking the effect of insulin on the cells.
- Prevents dental caries.
- Aids in the production of red blood cells.
- Encourages normal tissue growth and fat metabolism.
- Slows down cholesterol formation in blood vessels.
- Prevents heart disease and heart attacks.

Best Sources

Found in fish, parsley, radishes, strawberries, lettuce, cucumber.

Dosage

Vanadium supplements are not available, although some newer multivitamin and mineral supplements may contain low levels of it.

> ### CAUTION
> Vanadium is very toxic and is linked to manic depression in high quantities. Excess vitamin C can cause deficiency in some individuals.

Zn ZINC

U.S. RDA: 15mg. E.U. RDA: 15mg.

Zinc is one of the most important trace elements in our diet, and it is required for more than 200 enzyme activities within the body. It is the principal protector of the immune system, and is crucial for regulating our genetic information. Zinc is also vital for the structure and function of cell membranes.

Zinc is an antioxidant (*see page 234*) and can help to detoxify the body. A zinc deficiency can cause growth failure, infertility, impotence, and, in some cases, an impaired sense of taste. Eczema is commonly linked to zinc deficiency, and new research points to the fact that postnatal illness may be attributable to insufficient zinc in the diet. A weakened immune system and a poor ability to heal may also indicate deficiency.

PROPERTIES

- Boosts the immune system.
- Prevents cancer.
- Prevents and treats colds.
- Maintains senses of taste, smell, and sight.
- May help to prevent age-related degenerative effects.
- Prevents hair loss.
- Treats acne and various other skin problems.
- Useful in treatment of rheumatoid arthritis.
- Prevents blindness associated with aging.
- Increases male potency and sex drive.
- Used to treat infertility.

Best Sources

Offal, meat, mushrooms, oysters, eggs, wholegrain products, brewer's yeast.

Dosage

Take 15–30mg. daily, and increase copper and selenium intake if taking more zinc.

CAUTION

Very high doses (above 150mg. per day) may cause some nausea, vomiting, and diarrhea.

AMINO ACIDS

L-ARGININE

L-arginine is one of the most important and most useful of the amino acids, with a significant role to play in the function of the muscles, growth, and healing, helping to regulate and support key components of the immune system. It is also extremely important for male fertility.

For adults, L-arginine is a nonessential amino acid, which means that it is capable of being synthesized in the body and it is therefore not essential that we get additional amounts in our daily diet. For children, however, L-arginine is essential.

PROPERTIES

- Boosts immunity.
- Inhibits the growth of a number of tumors.
- Builds muscle and burns fat, by stimulating the pituitary glands to increase growth hormone secretion.
- Helps to promote the healing of burns and other wounds.
- Helps to protect the liver and to detoxify harmful substances.
- Increases sperm count in men with a low count.

Best Sources

Raw cereals, chocolate, nuts.

Dosage

The optimal intake is unknown, but doses up to 1.5g. appear to be safe. Take L-arginine with lysine, which inhibits herpes attacks in carriers.

CAUTION

Take on an empty stomach, and do not take in excess. This could cause mental and metabolic disturbances, as well as nausea and diarrhea. Prolonged high doses may be dangerous to children, and to anyone with liver or kidney problems.

L-ASPARTIC ACID

L-aspartic acid is a nonessential amino acid which has been used for many years in the treatment of chronic fatigue. Studies confirm the efficiency of this amino acid in raising energy levels, and in helping to overcome the side-effects of drug withdrawal.

PROPERTIES
- Disposes of ammonia, helping to protect the central nervous system.
- Helps treat fatigue.
- May improve stamina and endurance.

Dosage
Supplements are available in 250–500mg. tablets; take three times daily with juice or water.

CAUTION
Do not take with protein, such as milk. Do not take more than 1g. without the supervision of your physician.

L-CYSTEINE

L-cysteine contains sulfur, which is said to work as an antioxidant, protecting and preserving the cells in the body. It is also believed to protect the body against pollutants, but much work has still to be done to understand the effects of this amino acid.

Best Sources
Eggs, meat, dairy products, some cereals.

Dosage
Take with vitamin C for best effect (three times as much vitamin C as L-cysteine). Doses up to 1g. are considered to be safe, but consult your physician first.

PROPERTIES
- May protect against copper toxicity.
- Protects the body against damage by free radicals (*see page 234*)
- May help to reverse damage done by smoking and alcohol abuse.
- Offers protection against X-rays and nuclear radiation.
- May help to treat arthritis.
- Helps to repair DNA, thereby preventing the effects of aging.

CAUTION
Diabetics should not take L-cysteine supplements unless supervised by a physician. L-cysteine may also cause kidney stones, but a high vitamin C intake should prevent this from occuring.

L-GLUTAMINE

L-glutamine is a derivative of glutamic acid, which is believed to help reduce cravings for alcohol. Studies are inconclusive as to the real benefits of taking this amino acid, and it is recommended that you do not take more than 1g. daily unless you are supervised by your physician.

PROPERTIES
- Believed to help reduce craving for alcohol.
- May help to speed the healing of peptic ulcers.
- May help to counter attacks of depression.
- May energize the mind.
- May help to treat and prevent colitis.

Dosage
Up to 1g. daily is believed to be safe, but supplement only under the supervision of your physician.

L-HISTADINE

L-histadine is one of the lesser-known amino acids, and its role in our bodies is not yet fully understood. Research is ongoing into the possible effects of histadine supplementation.

PROPERTIES
- Used in the treatment of arthritis sufferers, who have an abnormally low level of this amino acid.

Dosage
Do not take more than 150mg. daily unless supervised by your physician.

GLYCINE

Glycine is considered to be the simplest of the amino acids, with a variety of properties which are still being studied by scientists.

PROPERTIES
- May help to treat low pituitary gland function.
- May be used in the treatment of spastic movement—particularly in patients suffering from MS.
- May help treat progressive muscular dystrophy.
- Used in the treatment of hypoglycemia, since it stimulates the release of glucagon, which mobilizes glycogen, which can then be released into the bloodstream as glucose.

Dosage
Doses below 1g. are thought to be safe, but research is ongoing.

> **CAUTION**
> It is recommended that you do not take this amino acid as a supplement unless supervised by your physician.

L-LYSINE

L-lysine is an essential amino acid, which means that it is necessary for life. It is needed for growth, tissue repair, and for the production of antibodies, hormones, and enzymes. Lysine should be obtained from eating foods such as fish, milk, cheese, and eggs, although it is possible to purchase lysine supplements.

PROPERTIES
- Inhibits herpes—high doses are now believed to be effective in reducing the recurrence of outbreaks.
- May assist in building muscle mass.
- Helps to prevent fertility problems.
- Improves concentration.

Best Sources
Found in fish, milk, lima beans, meat, cheese, yeast, eggs, all proteins.

Dosage
Up to 500mg. daily is believed to be safe.

Some experts recommend 1,000mg. daily at mealtimes.

It is usually advised that amino acids are taken on an empty stomach, with some juice or water.

Take L-lysine with an equal quantity of L-arginine if an increase in muscle mass is the desired goal.

> **CAUTION**
> Not suitable for children.

L-METHIONINE

L-methionine is a sulfur-containing amino acid that is very important in numerous processes in the body. Research shows that it may help to prevent clogging of the arteries by eliminating fatty substances.

PROPERTIES

- May help to eliminate fatty substances from the blood, lowering the risk of heart attack.
- May help to regulate the nervous system.
- In conjunction with choline and folic acid, it may prevent some tumors.
- Necessary for the biosynthesis of taurine and cysteine.

Best Sources
Eggs, milk, liver, fish.

CAUTION
Supplementation is not advised, although some physicians may suggest it in specific circumstances.

DL-PHENYLALANINE (DLPA)

DLPA is a form of the amino acid phenylalanine created from equal parts of D (synthetic) phenylalanine and L (natural) phenylalanine. DLPA has a unique role of activating and producing endorphins, which are the body's natural painkillers. Many people who do not respond to conventional painkillers respond successfully to DLPA, and its painkilling action increases over time. Do not confuse DLPA with L-phenylalanine.

PROPERTIES

- A natural painkiller, useful for chronic pain.
- Antidepressant.

Dosage
Tablets are generally available in 375mg. doses, and can be taken up to six times daily (a maximum dose of 1.5g.).

Higher doses should only be taken under the supervision of your physician. Take two or three times daily, before meals.

CAUTION
Not suitable for pregnant women or for those who suffer from Phenylketonuria (PKU). It may elevate blood pressure, so check with your physician if you suffer from any circulatory disorder.

L-PHENYLALANINE

L-phenylalanine is an essential amino acid that is necessary for a number of biochemical processes, including the synthesis of neurotransmitters in the brain. It is said to promote sexual arousal and to release hormones that help to control appetite.

PROPERTIES

- May help to alleviate a bout of depression.
- May help to control addictive behavior.
- Encourages mental alertness.
- Promotes sexual arousal.
- Reduces hunger and cravings for food.

Best Sources
Found in proteins, cheese, almonds, peanuts, sesame seeds, soybeans.

Dosage
L-phenylalanine is usually available in 500mg. doses. Take on an empty stomach for best effect, and do not take with protein.

L-TYROSINE

L-tyrosine is not an essential amino acid, which means that it is synthesized in the body. Tyrosine is involved with important neurotransmitters in the brain, and it is said to energize and help to relieve the effects of stress.

PROPERTIES

- Helps to relieve stress, and encourages alertness and fewer physical symptoms of tension and stress.
- May act as an antidepressant.
- May be used to treat the emotional symptoms of PMS.
- May help to aid in the treatment of addiction to and withdrawal from cocaine and other addictive drugs.

Dosage

Take with juice or water on an empty stomach (do not take with proteins, such as milk).

Some experts suggest that it is more effective when taken in conjunction with up to 25mg. of vitamin B6.

L-TRYPTOPHAN

This essential amino acid is used by the brain, along with several vitamins and minerals, to produce serotonin, a neurotransmitter. Serotonin, which regulates and induces sleep, is also said to reduce sensitivity to pain. It was one of the first amino acids to be produced for sale as a supplement, and it is useful as a natural sleeping aid.

PROPERTIES

- May help to encourage sleep and to prevent jet lag.
- Reduces sensitivity to pain.
- Lessens a craving for alcohol.
- Natural antidepressant, and may help to reduce anxiety and panic attacks.

Best Sources

Cottage cheese, milk, meat, fish, turkey, bananas, protein sources.

Dosage

Used to prevent panic attacks and depression, L-tryptophan should be taken between meals with juice or water (no proteins).

To help induce sleep, take 500mg. along with vitamin B6, niacinamide, and magnesium an hour or so before bedtime.

LIPIDS AND DERIVATIVES

FISH OILS

Fish oils contain two long-chain fatty acids called eicosopentaenoic acid (EPA) and docosahexaenoic acid (DHA) that affect the synthesis of prostaglandins, which have a regulatory effect on the body. There are numerous claims for fish oils, which are now believed to improve overall health and treat many health conditions.

PROPERTIES

- May be useful in the treatment of kidney disease, and can counteract the effects of some immuno-suppressive drugs.
- May help to prevent cancer, in particular the onset of breast cancer.
- Stops progression of arthritis symptoms.
- May help to protect against high blood pressure.
- Helps to prevent cardiovascular disease.
- May help to prevent and treat psoriasis.

Best Sources
Fish; in particular herring, salmon, tuna, cod, prawns.

Dosage
People suffering from arthritis or psoriasis can take up to 4g. daily, but for most people it is more appropriate to increase your intake of fish and seafood in order to achieve the benefits of the fish oils in their natural form.

The maximum suggested dosage for supplements, taken without the supervision of your physician, is 900mg. per day.

CAUTION
Fish oils may be harmful in diabetics, causing increases in blood sugar and a decline in insulin secretion.

EVENING PRIMROSE (GLA)

Native Americans were the first to recognize the potential of evening primrose oil as a healer, and they decocted (boiled) the seeds to make a liquid for healing wounds. Evening primrose oil is a rich source of gamma-linoleic acid, which is better known as GLA. The body makes GLA from essential fatty acids (EFAs). EFAs have numerous functions in the body, one of which is to manufacture hormone-like substances called "prostaglandins," which have very important effects on the body, such as toning blood vessels, balancing our water levels, and improving the action of the digestive system, and brain functioning. Prostaglandins also have a beneficial effect on the immune system.

Evening primrose oil is most often taken in the form of capsules, but it is also available as an oil (sometimes flavored), and it can be applied to the skin to treat skin conditions.

PROPERTIES

- Reduces scaling and redness, prevents itching, and encourages healing in cases of eczema. Also used in the treatment of psoriasis.
- Discourages dry skin, and ensures that the cellular membranes that make up the skin are stable and strong. There is some evidence that the oil retards the aging process.
- Evening primrose oil may help to prevent MS, and appears to be particularly useful for children suffering from the condition.
- May help in cases of liver damage caused by alcohol (cirrhosis of the liver), hyperactivity in children, and cystic fibrosis.
- May have a stimulating effect on the body, encouraging it to convert fat into energy, which would make it an excellent treatment for obesity.
- Hormonal imbalances, perhaps causing conditions like PMS, and symptoms of menopause may be eased by evening primrose oil, reducing symptoms of bloating, water retention, irritability, and depression.
- Reduces the inflammation of rheumatoid arthritis.
- Evening primrose may have an immuno-suppressive effect on the body.

Take 500mg. each day for two months, and then for the 10 days preceding menstruation if you suffer from PMS. During menopause, 2,000–4,000mg. should be taken daily for four weeks, and then 500–1,000mg. daily thereafter.

For asthma, take two 500mg. tablets three times daily for three to four months; then one tablet three times daily. If you are taking steroids, this treatment will not work because steroids interfere with evening primrose oil's action.

> **CAUTION**
> Do not use if you suffer from temporal-lobe epilepsy or manic depression.

INOSITOL

Inositol is not a true vitamin, as it can be synthesized by the body, but it forms part of the B-complex family of vitamins, and is present in cereals and vegetables as phytic acid. There is a high concentration in the brain, stomach, spleen, liver, and heart.

PROPERTIES
- Helps to dissolve fat.
- Ensures healthy hair and strong nails.
- Controls levels of cholesterol in the blood.
- Helps to encourage natural sleep.
- May help to treat schizophrenia.

Best Sources
Lethicin, liver, wheat germ, brown rice, citrus fruits, nuts, cereals.

Dosage
Natural sources are best, but if you are prescribed supplements, take in the form of myo-inositol to a maximum of 1,000mg. daily.

> **CAUTION**
> Diabetics should only take inositol under the supervision of their physician.

LECITHIN

Lecithin has for some time been a popular supplement, used for a variety of health conditions. It is comprised of choline, inositol, fatty acids, and phosphorus, and is available as a liquid or as dry granules. It is widely used in foods to maintain consistency, and is probably one of the few nutritious food additives.

PROPERTIES
- Protects against cardiovascular disease.
- Helps to reduce high blood pressure.
- Used to treat memory loss and conditions of the nervous system such as dementia and Alzheimer's.
- May help in the treatment of mental disorders such as manic depression.
- Lecithin has some action against viruses.
- May prevent and also treat gallstones.
- May help to treat viral hepatitis, repairing the membranes of the liver cells.

Best Sources
Found in egg yolks, soybeans, liver, meats, fish, cauliflower, cabbage.

Dosage
Doses of up to 1g. daily are acceptable, but see your physician to discuss your individual needs.

Lecithin appears in a wide range of foods, and it is probably best to increase your intake of these rather than supplementing.

> **CAUTION**
> In some people (in large quantities), lecithin may cause depression. Very high doses may cause nausea, vomiting, and dizziness.

OTHER SUPPLEMENTS

ACIDOPHILUS

Acidophilus (also known as *lactobacillus acidophilus*) is a source of friendly intestinal bacteria (flora). Healthy bacteria play an important role in our bodies, and unless they are continually supplied with some form of lactic acid or lactose (such as acidophilus) they can die, causing a host of health problems. Many physicians and health practitioners recommend taking acidophilus alongside oral antibiotics which can cause diarrhea, destroy the healthy flora of the intestines, and lead to fungal infections. Acidophilus may also help to ensure vaginal health.

PROPERTIES
- Keeps the intestines clean.
- Prevents yeast infections of the vagina.
- Aids the absorption of nutrients in food.
- Can eliminate bad breath (which has been caused by intestinal putrefaction).
- Can relieve and prevent constipation and flatulence.
- Can aid the treatment of acne and other skin troubles.
- Maintains intestinal health.

Best Sources
Natural, unflavored, "live" yogurt, sometimes known as "bio yogurt."

Dosage
Acidophilus is not toxic and can be taken daily, with food, in unlimited amounts.

CAUTION
Keep the tablets in the refrigerator.

BEE AND FLOWER POLLEN

In flowering plants the pollen-producing spores are located in the stamens of flowers. Flower pollen is said to be purer than bee pollen. Bee pollen is found in the hives themselves. It is rich in protein and amino acids, and forms, with honey, the basic diet of all the bees in the hive, except for the queen (*see royal jelly, page 260*). Pollen has been used as medicine around the world for thousands of years.

PROPERTIES
- Rich in both amino acids and protein.
- Helps to suppress appetite and cravings.
- May help to improve skin problems and retard the aging process.
- May help to treat problems of the prostate.
- Energizes the body.
- Regulates the bowels.
- May boost immunity and diminish allergies.

Best Sources
Unpasteurized honey contains small amounts of bee pollen.

Dosage
400mg. doses, taken daily with food, appear to be safe.

CAUTION
If you suffer from hay fever or an allergy to bee stings, see your physician before taking this supplement.

BIOFLAVONOIDS

Bioflavonoids were originally called vitamin P, and are also known as flavones. They accompany vitamin C in natural foods, and are responsible for the color in the leaves, flowers, and stems of food plants. Their primary job in the body is to protect the capillaries, to keep them strong, and to prevent bleeding. Bioflavonoids are also anti-inflammatory. Many of the medicinally active substances contained in herbs are bioflavonoids.

PROPERTIES

- Protect capillaries.
- Protect against cerebral and other hemorrhaging.
- Reduce bleeding during menstruation.
- Antioxidant (*see page 234*), and encourage the antioxidant qualities of vitamin C.
- Antiviral activity.
- Anti-inflammatory.
- Antiallergy.

Best Sources

Citrus fruits, apricots, cherries, green peppers, broccoli; the central white core of citrus fruits is the richest source.

Dosage

Bioflavonoids are not toxic, and should be taken together with vitamin C for best effect.

BREWER'S YEAST

Brewer's yeast is the same type of yeast that is used in the brewing process, and is quite different from the yeast that causes thrush. It is a rich source of B-vitamins and amino acids, as well as some minerals, in particular chromium and selenium. It also contains naturally occurring nucleic acids (DNA and RNA), which are said to enhance the immune system, among other things.

PROPERTIES

- May reduce wrinkling and help treat skin problems.
- Works as an effective wound-healing agent.
- Encourages the healing of burns.
- Rich source of B-vitamins, which can help to relieve stress and nervous disorders.
- Encourages the activity of the immune system.
- Increases energy.
- Used externally, to detoxify skin.

Dosage

Brewer's yeast comes in tablets, or as a powder that can be sprinkled on food or drink.

CAUTION

Brewer's yeast is not toxic and can be taken daily without any side-effects. Some experts suggest that it may cause yeast infections and chronic fatigue syndrome, but this has largely been disclaimed.

CHARCOAL

Charcoal is a porous, solid product obtained when materials such as cellulose, wood, peat, bituminous coal, or bone are partially burned in the absence of air. Charcoal has always been popular for dealing with flatulence, bloating, and irritable bowel syndrome, by soaking up gas. Charcoal can also be useful in the long-term management of kidney patients.

PROPERTIES

- Reduces cholesterol in the blood.
- Reduces the risk of atherosclerosis.
- Absorbs gas and so acts as an antacid.
- Binds with cholesterol, toxins, and waste in the intestine, which has a cleansing effect.

Dosage

Charcoal is available in tablet, powder, and capsule form. High doses (more than 50g. per day) should be supplemented with a well-balanced vitamin and mineral supplement.

CAUTION

Activated charcoal can bind with and inactivate some therapeutic drugs and supplemental nutrients, and should be taken at least one hour before or after drugs or supplements are taken. If you are on prescription drugs, take charcoal only with your physician's advice.

CO-ENZYME Q10

Co-enzyme Q10 is a vitamin-like substance found in all cells of the body. It is biologically important, since it forms part of the system across which electrons flow in the cells during the process of energy production. When there is a Q10 deficiency, the cell cannot function effectively, and the rate at which the muscle cells work is adversely affected.

PROPERTIES
- Enhances immunity.
- May help to prevent coronary inefficiency.
- Anti-aging.
- Necessary for healthy functioning of the nervous system and the brain cells.

Best Sources
Meat (it is also made within the body).

Dosage
10mg., taken three times a day is suggested.

CAUTION
Co-enzyme Q10 may be toxic in high doses.

DHEA

Dehydroepiandrosterone (DHEA) is a hormone which we produce in our adrenal glands, and which also occurs naturally in the Mexican wild yam (potato). DHEA was for many years considered to be a cure-all, and indeed research has proved that it has invaluable therapeutic benefits, particularly in the prevention and treatment of cancer, but it is still very much under investigation and its many qualities have yet to be proven. It should be taken only if you have a known deficiency (less than 130mg/dl. in women and less than 180mg/dl. in men).

Best Source
Mexican wild yam.

PROPERTIES
- Inhibits weight gain.
- DHEA is thought to have anti-aging effects.
- Works to reduce stress.
- Improves immunity.

Dosage
See a registered practitioner for advice on supplementation.

CAUTION
Many supplements have no DHEA in them, so exercise caution when choosing a supplement.

DIETARY FIBER

Dietary fiber, also known as bulk and roughage, is an essential element in the diet, though it provides no nutrients. It consists of plant cellulose and other indigestible materials in foods, along with pectin and gum. The chewing it requires stimulates saliva flow, and the bulk it adds in the stomach and intestines during digestion provides more time for absorption of nutrients. A diet with sufficient fiber helps to promote bowel regularity and avoid constipation.

PROPERTIES
- Reduces the production of cholesterol in the body.
- Helps to control diabetes.
- Helps to control weight.
- Can be used to treat certain intestinal disorders.
- Protects against cancers of the colon.

Best Sources
Fruit and vegetables, wholegrain breads and cereals, products made from nuts and legumes.

Dosage
An intake of 20–60g. per day is ideal, and can be taken in the form of food, or as "soluble fiber" – which is less likely to cause loose bowel movements.

GLANDULARS

Glandulars are concentrates of hormonal glands, and have, in the past decade, been hailed as a wonder drug. The premise is that failing or aging glands can be rejuvenated by supplementation, but many experts now discourage their use.

PROPERTIES

- May improve sexual performance and libido.
- May help to build muscle.
- May be used in the treatment of asthma.

Dosage

Consult a registered practitioner before taking.

Do not take them at night, as they will cause insomnia.

CAUTION

Glandulars may contain many of the toxins livestock are exposed to, such as antibiotics, growth hormones, pesticides, herbicides, and fertilizers. Only take this supplement on the advice of a physician.

PABA

Para-aminobenzoic acid (PABA) is often grouped with the B-vitamins, and although it is water soluble, it is stored in the tissues and can be toxic at high doses. Freckles can sometimes be minimized by the use of sunscreen lotions containing para-aminobenzoic acid (PABA). PABA can be synthesized in the body, helps to form folic acid, and is important in the efficient utilization of protein.

PROPERTIES

- Shields the skin from the damage of UV rays.
- May rejuvenate skin.
- Keeps skin healthy and smooth, and helps to delay wrinkles (used externally).
- PABA is used in the treatment of eczema.

Best Sources

Liver, brewer's yeast, kidney, whole grains, rice, bran.

Dosage

Available in 30–1,000mg. strengths, and should be taken three times daily for best effect.

Experts suggest that you do not take more than 30mg. daily because of side-effects (*see Caution*).

Best taken in a good multivitamin supplement.

Ointments are available for external use, and PABA is included in many sunscreen preparations.

CAUTION

High doses can cause nausea, fever, and diarrhea. PABA may prove toxic to the liver in high doses. Do not take if you are using any sulfonamide antibiotics.

PROPOLIS

Propolis is a sticky material collected by bees from buds or tree bark and used to seal the inside of the hive. It is a mixture of wax, resin, balsam oil, and pollen. It is said to act as an antibiotic and bactericide, and may be used to help wounds to heal. Propolis is rich in bioflavonoids.

PROPERTIES

- Enhances immunity.
- Boosts energy.
- A natural anesthetic and antibiotic.
- Reduces cholesterol levels in the blood.

Dosage

Propolis does not appear to have any toxic levels.

See your practitioner for details of suitable dosage.

> **CAUTION**
> Because this product contains pollen, it may cause an allergic reaction in susceptible individuals.

ROYAL JELLY

Royal jelly has been used for centuries for its health-giving and rejuvenating properties, and it is rich in vitamins, amino acids, and minerals. It is also the prime source of fatty acid, which is said to increase alertness and act as a natural tranquilizer (when necessary). Royal jelly is secreted by the salivary glands of the worker bees to feed and stimulate the growth and development of the queen bee.

PROPERTIES
- Antibacterial.
- Has a yeast-inhibiting function, preventing conditions such as thrush and athlete's foot.
- Contains the male sex hormone testosterone, which may increase libido.
- Used to treat subfertility.
- May be useful in the treatment of ME and MD.
- Helps to reduce allergies.

Dosage

Most tablets contain 100–500mg. of royal jelly.
Optimum dosage is about 150mg. per day.
Fresh is better, although more expensive.

SEAWEEDS

Seaweeds are part of the Protista kingdom, better known as "algae." Seaweeds appear in many foods, medicines, and cosmetics, and have been used therapeutically for thousands of years.

PROPERTIES
- Antiviral activity.
- Used in the prevention and treatment of goiter.
- May help to reduce the effects of carcinogens.
- Natural antacid.
- Used in the treatment of intestinal disorders.

Best Sources

Take seaweeds in their natural form, available from health food stores and many grocery stores.

Dosage

Consult a registered practitioner.

SPIRULINA

Spirulina are blue-green bacteria or algae which are rich in GLA (*gammalinoleic acid, see page 254*) and a wide variety of nutrients, including beta-carotene, inositol, calcium, vitamin E, magnesium, and phosphorus. In ancient times, spirulina was used as a staple food by the Aztecs of Mexico. It is now marketed in health food stores as a high-protein food supplement.

PROPERTIES
- Rich in nutrients and high in protein (particularly useful for vegetarians).
- May suppress appetite.
- Maintains skin health and treats skin disorders.
- May contribute to healthy functioning of the intestines.
- Many spirulina have anti-cancer properties.

Best Sources

Fresh or freeze-dried spirulina.

Dosage

There is no recommended dosage for spirulina—consult a registered practitioner.

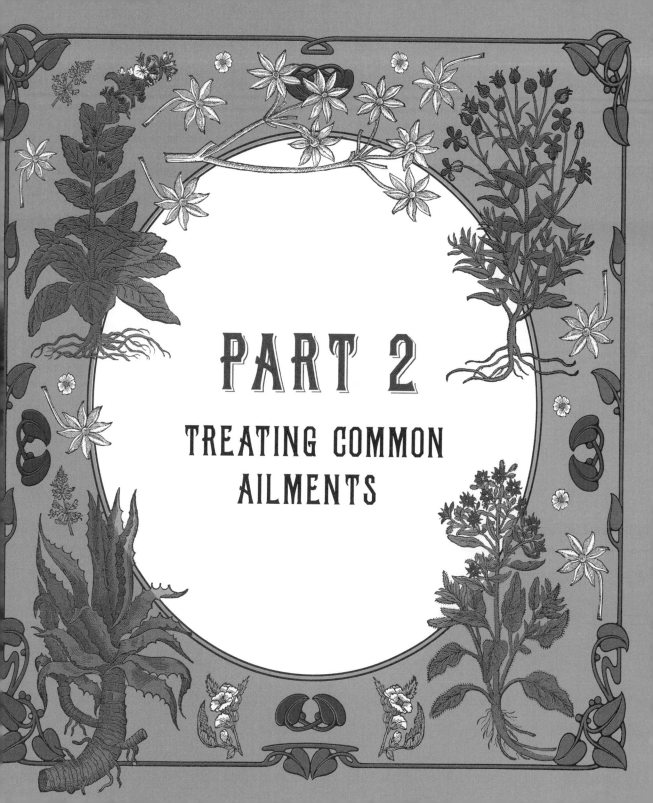

PART 2

TREATING COMMON AILMENTS

DISORDERS OF THE MIND AND EMOTIONS

ADDICTIONS

An addiction is an overwhelming craving for or dependence on a substance, usually a drug, alcohol, or nicotine. The addiction may be limited to mental dependence, but it can become physiological if the way in which the body functions has changed through prolonged use of a substance. In such cases the addict will experience physical "withdrawal" symptoms without the substance in question.

Symptoms

- loss of control over use of the drug or other substance
- mood swings and irrational behavior
- in drug addiction: sore or red eyes with dilated or constricted pupils, irregular breathing, trembling hands, itchy or runny nose, nausea
- drug withdrawal symptoms may include craving, depression, sweating, abdominal pain, vomiting, diarrhea, loss of appetite, and suffering from gooseflesh

Drugs with potential for misuse are narcotics, including morphine, opium, heroin, and methadone; depressants such as alcohol, barbiturates, and sedatives; stimulants such as cocaine and amphetamines; hallucinogenic drugs; and marijuana.

Nicotine and caffeine can also be abused, and anabolic steroids and human growth hormone are often misused by athletes and bodybuilders seeking to increase muscle mass.

True physical addiction is known to occur with the narcotics and depressants; psychological dependence, with or without physical symptoms, can develop from using many other prescription drugs, such as tranquilizers.

Studies show that 50–80 percent of all alcoholics have a close relative who is an alcoholic. Some researchers therefore suggest that some alcoholics have an inherited physical predisposition to alcohol addiction.

Alcoholism and alcohol abuse in the U.S. cost an estimated $98 billion and take 100,000 lives per year, according to the National Institute on Alcohol Abuse and Alcoholism.

One-half of all traffic fatalities and one-third of all traffic injuries are related to the abuse of alcohol.

One-third of all suicides and one-third of all mental health disorders are estimated to be associated with serious alcohol abuse.

The relaxation smokers feel is because tobacco contains nicotine, an addictive alkaloid. A number of diseases have been directly linked to smoking, and in the U.S. alone tobacco use kills about 420,000 smokers each year.

Every day about 3,500 Americans successfully quit smoking.

> **CAUTION**
> Addictions to physical substances should always be treated by a registered practitioner. Do not discontinue any prescription drugs unless you are under supervision.

TREATMENT

Ayurveda
This has proved very successful in treating addictions of all types, which it sees as fundamental imbalance within the body. Treatment will be tailored to your specific constitution and personal characteristics. (*See page 9.*)

Chinese Herbalism
For alcoholism, heat would be cleared from the lung and liver, with watermelon or kudzu vine to detoxify blood.

Treatment would be specific for various other types of addiction.

Strong green tea is used to cool the liver.

Herbalism
Oats will calm you down and help to strengthen your willpower. (*See page 102.*)

Other herbs to calm the nervous system and reduce symptoms when you wish to withdraw from your addiction include skullcap and valerian. Drink daily as a tea. (*See pages 118 and 123.*)

Cramp bark helps nervous tension and jitters. (*See page 125.*)

Aromatherapy

Antidepressant oils include chamomile, clary sage, and ylang ylang. Use in the bath, and in a vaporizer by your bedside. A few drops on your clothing during the day will allow the effect to be maintained. (*See pages 133-157.*)

Massage with aromatherapy oil is extremely rewarding and a positive treatment. Try detoxifying oils such as juniper. (*See page 146.*)

Aromatherapists suggest changing the oils used at regular intervals; although it is almost impossible to become physically addicted to an essential oil, you may come to regard it as a prop. (*See pages 133-157.*)

Bergamot seems to be extremely useful in cases of food addiction. (*See page 140.*)

Homeopathy

Homeopathic treatment would be constitutional, or tailored to your individual needs. Some useful addiction treatments are:
- Nux vomica, which helps to overcome a craving for smoking. (*See page 198.*)
- Kali phos., which strengthens the nervous system and may make it easier for a person to give up an addiction. (*See page 186.*)
- Arsenicum, for great anxiety, restlessness and fear of being alone. (*See page 167.*)
- Absinthium, when you feel depressed, disoriented, and dizzy.

Flower Essences
- Crab Apple, for anyone who needs purification. (*See page 219.*)
- Gorse, when you are stuck in a negative pattern. (*See page 226.*)
- Mustard, for depression for no apparent reason. (*See page 224.*)
- Olive is particularly good for the recovery period. (*See page 220.*)

Vitamins and Minerals

Treatment would ensure that there are no small nutritional deficiencies making you crave certain substances, and that deficiencies caused by addictions (such as vitamin B in alcoholics) are righted. Some amino acids may be used to create a specific physical effect, or act as a natural tranquilizer, which may help. Alcoholics are often deficient in GLA (gammalinolenic acid), and it is recommended that you take evening primrose (a rich source) to help prevent mood swings. (*See page 254.*)

OBSESSIONS AND COMPULSIONS

An obsession is a persistent, recurring thought or idea, while a compulsion is an overwhelming drive to perform a particular act. When a person becomes dominated by these intrusions, despite knowing that they are irrational, he or she is said to be suffering from an obsessive-compulsive disorder. This may take the form of a hand-washing ritual, for example, or repeated checking that doors and windows are locked. The problem is often triggered by a stressful life event, but can also be due to subtle brain damage (usually the result of illnesses affecting the brain), especially when due to encephalitis. Obsessive-compulsive disorder is rare, although minor obsessional symptoms probably occur in about 15 percent of the population. At least two-thirds of all people who have obsessive-compulsive disorder respond well to therapy. Symptoms may recur under stress but can usually be controlled.

Symptoms
- fear of contamination
- dermatitis caused by repeated washing
- inefficiency caused by repeated and meticulous checking
- aggressive thoughts and behavior
- possible depression

TREATMENT
Herbalism
Drink certain infused herbs which act on the nervous system, including hops, valerian, vervain, chamomile, and passiflora. Taken on a regular basis, these herbs may help to ease tension and restrict various behavioral problems. (*See pages 104, 123, and 125.*)

Aromatherapy

Relaxing oils, such as Roman chamomile or marjoram may help to achieve balance. Use regularly in the bath or on a burner in your room. (*See pages 137 and 151.*)

Ylang ylang and clary sage may also help. (*See pages 136 and 155.*)

Homeopathy

Aurum is useful for feelings of worthlessness and overwhelming thoughts of death and dying. (*See page 169.*)

Silicea for unshakable feelings of inadequacy, and an overwhelming urge to count small objects. (*See page 195.*)

Take Anacardium when you feel that your mind is not your own and is being controlled by an external force. (*See page 164.*)

Flower Essences

Cherry Plum, for the fear of losing your mind, and to deal with irrational thoughts or behavior. (*See page 221.*)

Crab Apple, for those who feel unclean or polluted on any level. (*See page 219.*)

Vervain, for those who are strong-willed and need space for reflection. (*See page 226.*)

White Chestnut, for an overactive mind, full of unwanted patterns of thought. (*See page 209.*)

PHOBIAS

A phobia is an irrational fear which the sufferer finds impossible to overcome. Some of the most common fears are claustrophobia (fear of enclosed spaces), agoraphobia (fear of open spaces), and acrophobia (fear of heights). A phobia can, however, relate to just about any object, person, or situation, and is probably caused by a subconscious reflex to avoid repeating an unpleasant experience. For the sufferer it may cause little more than mild embarrassment, or it may be totally debilitating and disruptive to everyday life. An estimated 10 percent of people in the U.K., and slightly more in the U.S., suffer from phobias of some description. Recent research indicates that most sufferers can cure themselves.

Symptoms

- rapid pulse
- profuse sweating
- high blood pressure
- trembling
- nausea

TREATMENT

Ayurveda

Lemon or lime may be suggested for dizziness, and individual treatment would be prescribed according to your specific needs. (*See page 9.*)

Chinese Herbalism

A herbalist may suggest cooling herbs, and Gui Pi Wan, which addresses emotional problems.

Ginseng, Chinese angelica and senega root may also be useful. (*See pages 54, 41, 56.*)

Herbalism

Valerian tea can help to reduce tension. Drink an infusion as required. (*See page 123.*)

Aromatherapy

Essential oils can be very useful in the treatment of phobias. The effect of certain smells can help to release tension and induce a feeling of calm. Some of the best oils to try are: bergamot, chamomile, clary sage, geranium, jasmine, juniper, lavender, marjoram, melissa, and ylang ylang, which are sedative. They can be used in the bath, in massage with a light carrier oil (such as sweet almond), or in a vaporizer. Carry a bottle of diluted oils with you—perhaps in a small sprayer—and apply them to the temples or pulse points in times of fear. (*See page 129.*)

Homeopathy

There are dozens of homeopathic remedies which can be used to treat phobias, but they will be prescribed constitutionally, that is, the treatment would be tailored to your exact needs. Some to try may be:

- Arg. nit., for fear of heights. (*See page 166.*)
- Phosphorus, for fear of the dark. (*See page 192.*)
- Gelsemium, for fear of performing in public, when you feel weak at the knees. (*See page 180.*)

- Aconite, for agoraphobia, when you are terrified of dying or collapsing if you go out. (*See page 163.*)
- Arnica, for fears that are brought on by an accident. (*See page 167.*)
- Sulfur, when you need help and no other remedy seems to be indicated. (*See page 198.*)

Flower Essences

Treatment would be based on your individual state of mind, but some of the following may help:
- Mimulus, for the everyday fears of known things, spiders, being late for work, flying, and being ill. (*See page 220.*)
- Aspen is for unknown fears, the vague and dark fears which hover and play on the imagination. (*See page 222.*)
- Rock Rose should be added when the fear is turning into terror and perhaps even panic. (*See page 216.*)
- Cherry Plum is for the fear that everything will fall apart. (*See page 221.*)
- Red Chestnut is for fear for another's safety. (*See page 209.*)

The most important Bach Flower Remedy for fear, anxiety, and phobias, Rescue Remedy, is made up of five essences: Cherry Plum, Rock Rose, Impatiens, Clematis, and Star of Bethlehem. It works to treat fear, loneliness, despondency, and loss of focus. It rebalances the sufferer after an emotional upset and is particularly useful in panic attacks. Apply a few drops of the remedy to your tongue or pulse points. (*See page 229.*)

Vitamins and Minerals

Vitamin B-complex and C are important for nerve functioning. Ensure that you eat regular meals, since low blood sugar can exacerbate the problem.

DEPRESSION

Depression is a prolonged feeling of unhappiness and despondency, often magnified by a major life event such as bereavement, divorce, or retirement. Many women experience depression after childbirth. Clinical depression is a genuine illness which overwhelms the sufferer so that he or she feels a hopelessness, dejection, and fear out of all proportion to any cause. Someone who is depressed may contemplate or attempt suicide.

Symptoms
- slow speech
- poor concentration
- confusion and irritability
- self-accusation and loss of self-esteem
- insomnia and early-morning waking
- a feeling of emptiness and despair
- loss of appetite
- loss of sexual drive

Major depressions occur in 10–20 percent of the world's population in the course of a lifetime.

Women are more often affected than men, by a 2:1 ratio.

Relatives of patients with major depressive illnesses seem to be at some higher risk of becoming depressed, and about 2 percent of the population may have a chronic disorder known as a depressive personality.

Unipolar depression consists of episodes that can recur several times in a person's life.

Manic depression, or bipolar disorder, is a severe mental disorder involving manic episodes (characterized by an abnormally elevated or irritable mood, grandiosity, sleeplessness, extravagance, and a tendency toward irrational judgment) that are usually accompanied by episodes of depression (possibly including lethargy, a sense of worthlessness, lack of concentration, and guilt). Manic depression occurs in males and females equally, and is found more frequently in close relatives of people with the disorder.

More than 8 billion people in the U.S. consult their general physician about treatment for depression.

Up to 50 percent of people who suffer have a hereditary tendency.

Seasonal affective disorder (SAD) is thought to be caused by a deficiency of corticotropin-releasing hormone.

Cases of SAD are on the increase, and are thought to be partly due to increased stress levels.

TREATMENT

Ayurveda

Detoxification treatment would be followed by specific oral medication to balance the three doshas. Treatment is always individual. (*See page 9.*)

Chinese Herbalism

Depression is believed to be caused by stagnation of the Liver qi, and may be treated with angelica, peony root, licorice, and thorowax root. (*See pages 41, 53, 50.*)

Herbalism

The best antidepressant and nervine (with a specific action for nerves) herbs include: balm, borage, limeflower, oats, rosemary, and vervain. These can be taken as herbal teas, added to the bath, or taken as tablets, or in tincture form (herbs suspended in alcohol).

Aromatherapy

There are a number of antidepressant oils, which can be used in the bath, in a vaporizer, on a light bulb and in massage. They include: neroli, jasmine, geranium, melissa, and rose.

Ylang ylang, lavender, clary sage, and chamomile are sedative and antidepressant.

Homeopathy

It will be necessary to see a homeopath to receive treatment that is suited to you, and which addresses the cause of your depression. Specific remedies include:

- Aurum, for feelings of worthlessness, suicidal feelings, and self-disgust. (*See page 169.*)
- Pulsatilla, for bursting into tears at the smallest hurt. (*See page 193.*)
- Arsenicum, if you feel chilly, tired, restless, and obsessively tidy. (*See page 167.*)
- Ignatia, if depression has an external cause, such as bereavement. (*See page 104.*)

Flower Essences

Cherry Plum, for "fear of the mind being over strained, of doing dreaded things," and of being violent to oneself or others. (*See page 221.*)

Agrimony, for deeply held emotional tensions which are hidden from others. (*See page 210.*)

Gorse helps to combat feelings of hopelessness. (*See page 226.*)

Gentian will help to improve a mild depression and despondency caused by a setback. (*See page 215.*)

Mustard is for blacker and deeper feelings when there is no apparent cause. (*See page 224.*)

Sweet Chestnut should be taken if you feel anguished and stretched beyond endurance. (*See page 212.*)

Vitamins and Minerals

Depression which occurs just before menstruation (PMS) may be caused by a vitamin B6 deficiency; post-natal depression may be caused by a deficiency of vitamin B12, and folic acid. Nutritional supplements and allergy tests may be suggested by a practitioner. Ensure you have an adequate intake of vitamin C. Some therapists may recommend supplementing the amino acid tryptophan. (*See page 253.*)

STRESS

Each individual is able to cope with a different amount of stress in life, and while some seem to draw on endless reserves to keep going, others succumb. A certain amount of stress provides stimulation, but prolonged stress can cause mental and physical damage.

Most of us think of tense situations and worries as being the cause of stress. In reality, stresses are wide-ranging. They include environmental stresses, such as pollution, noise, housing problems, cold, or overheating; physical stresses, such as illnesses, injuries, an inadequate diet; and mental stresses, such as relationship problems, financial strains, bereavement; and job difficulties. All these factors affect the body, causing it to make a series of rapid physiological changes, called "adaptive responses," to deal with threatening or demanding situations. In the first stage of stress, hormones are poured into the bloodstream. The pulse quickens, the lungs take in more oxygen to fuel the muscles, blood sugar increases to supply added energy, digestion slows, and perspiration increases. In the second stage of stress, the body begins to repair the damage caused by the first stage. If the stressful situation is resolved, the stress symptoms vanish. If the situation continues, however, exhaustion sets in, and the body's energy gives out. This stage may continue until vital organs are affected, and then disease or even death can result.

THE HEALING REMEDIES SOURCEBOOK

Symptoms

- the increase in hormones such as adrenaline, noradrenaline, and corticosteroids in response to stress may cause the following: increased breathing and heart rate, nausea, tense muscles
- in the long term it is thought that stress can lead to insomnia, depression, high blood pressure, hair loss, allergies, ulcers, heart disease, digestive disorders, menstrual problems, palpitations, impotence, and premature ejaculation

Psychological stress results from perceived or anticipated threats. The stress may be acute, as in response to immediate danger, or chronic, as when an individual is experiencing an unhappy life situation. In either case, the body mechanisms are similar.

Chronic physical illness is almost always accompanied by significant psychological effects.

Long-lasting psychological stress, in turn, often leads to debilitating changes.

Medical scientists divide people's behavior into two types, depending on their reactions to stress. People with type-A behavior react to stress with aggressiveness, competitiveness, and self-imposed pressure to get things done. Type-A behavior has been linked to increased rates of heart attack and other diseases. People with type-B behavior may be equally serious in their intentions, but are more patient, easygoing, and relaxed.

Stress is a major factor in diseases whose physical symptoms are induced or aggravated by mental or emotional problems.

Stress-related disorders comprise 50–80 percent of all illnesses, though stress may not be the only cause.

TREATMENT

Ayurveda

An Ayurvedic practitioner would prescribe supportive herbs, and use a balancing treatment specific to your needs. (*See page 9.*)

Chinese Herbalism

Chinese medicine takes the view that it is not stress that causes illness, but how we deal with it. Herbs would be prescribed according to your specific needs, in order to support you throughout stressful periods, and tonify. (*See page 35.*)

Treatment may be aimed particularly at the kidneys, which have become exhausted through overwork, and to support the blood and qi, which need to circulate harmoniously in the body. (*See page 35.*)

Traditional Folk and Home Remedies

Pumpkin seeds, which contain high quantities of zinc, iron, and calcium, as well as B vitamins and proteins, which are necessary for brain function, will help you to deal with the effects of stress.

Oats are vital for a healthy nervous system. In periods of stress, start the day with oatmeal, which will help to keep you calm, and prevent depression and general debility. (*See page 72.*)

Herbalism

Herbs that encourage relaxation and act as a tonic to the nervous system include balm, lavender, chamomile, passiflora, and oats. These can be drunk as an infusion—as often as necessary when in a stressful situation. (*See page 94.*)

Ginseng is an excellent "adaptogenic" herb, which means that it lifts you when you are tired and relaxes you when you are stressed. It also works on the immune system and energizes. Some therapists recommend a daily dose at stressful times. (*See page 112.*)

Aromatherapy

Essential oils are excellent for stress reduction because many of them work on the nervous system and the brain to relax and soothe. (*See pages 133–157.*)

Other oils are uplifting, which can be invaluable in times of serious stress. (*See pages 133–157.*)

Massage with aromatherapy oils is very comforting—particularly the physical element of touch—and a few drops of essential oil in the bath can offer an opportunity to "wash away" the problems of the day while experiencing the benefits of the oil. Suitable oils include basil, chamomile, geranium, lavender, neroli, and rose. (*See pages 133–157.*)

Oils which strengthen the adrenal system, which is weakened by stress, include rosemary, ginger, and lemongrass. (*See pages 133–157.*)

Vitamins and Minerals

Eating a good, balanced diet will make your body stronger and able to cope more efficiently with stress. B-vitamins are often depleted by stress, so ensure that you are getting enough in your diet, or take a good supplement. There is some evidence that bee and flower pollen, available in tablets or in grains, can boost immunity and energize the body. Do not eat this if you are allergic to honey or bee stings. An amino acid called L-tyrosine appears to energize and relieve stress, and studies show that people taking this supplement react better to stressful situations, staying more alert, less anxious, more efficient, and have fewer complaints about physical discomforts. Vitamin C is a great stress reliever, and boosts immunity, making you fitter and more healthy. (*See page 238.*)

ANXIETY

Anxiety is a state of fear or apprehension in the face of threat or danger. It is a natural, healthy response since it allows the body to prepare itself (through adrenaline) to cope with the danger. Anxiety can, however, take a person over—a condition known as anxiety neurosis—and the person is then said to be in an anxiety state. This may be chronic anxiety, with a constant feeling of worry, associated with depression, or an acute anxiety attack, when the sufferer will be suddenly overwhelmed by fear and feelings of dread.

When we are faced with a frightening or threatening situation, our body goes into a "fight or flight" response, when adrenaline pours into the system and the body prepares itself for action. When no action follows, and nervous energy is not discharged, there is physiological confusion—otherwise known as a panic attack. Symptoms may include dizziness, visual disturbance, clammy hands, racing heart, dry mouth, and overbreathing.

Up to 70 percent of people who have panic attacks end up seeing as many as ten physicians before being correctly diagnosed.

Anxiety appears to affect twice as many women as men.

Evidence exists that some people may be biochemically vulnerable to panic attacks.

The National Center for Health Statistics reports that drugs for anxiety disorders are among the 20 drugs most frequently prescribed.

In the U.K., a report by the Royal College of Psychiatrists stated that more than 9 million Britons will suffer from abnormal anxiety and fears at some point in their lives.

Anxiety is an element of many psychological disorders, including phobias, panic attacks, obsessive-compulsive disorders, and post-traumatic stress disorder.

Symptoms
- dry mouth
- sweaty palms
- rapid pulse and palpitations
- in anxiety neurosis: breathlessness, headaches, general weakness, and fatigue, feeling of tightness in the chest, high blood pressure, abdominal pain and diarrhea, insomnia, loss of appetite

TREATMENT

Ayurveda

An Ayurvedic medical practitioner would balance the tri-doshas, and use panchakarma for balancing the vátha. (*See page 10.*)

Chinese Herbalism

A Chinese herbalist might suggest ginseng, Chinese angelica, and white peony root with thorowax root for relaxation. Treatment would be designed to strengthen the Spleen and enliven Liver qi. (*See pages 41 and 54.*)

Traditional Folk and Home Remedies

Oats contain thiamin and pantothenic acid, which act as gentle nerve tonics (*See page 72.*)

Herbalism

Herbal remedies would be used to calm the nervous system and to generally relax you.

Skullcap and valerian are useful herbs, blended together for best effect. Drink this as a tea three times daily while suffering anxiety symptoms. (*See pages 118 and 123.*)

Lady's slipper and lime blossom may also work to ease anxiety and tension. (*See page 121.*)

THE HEALING REMEDIES SOURCEBOOK

Aromatherapy

A relaxing blend of essential oils of lavender, geranium, and bergamot in sweet almond oil or peach kernel oil may be used in the bath at times at great stress and anxiety. (*See pages 133–157.*)

Homeopathy

Constitutional treatment will be appropriate for chronic conditions, and there are a number of remedies which will prove useful for relieving acute attacks. These include:

- Aconite, for dispelling a sudden panic attack. (*See page 163.*)
- Arsenicum may be useful if you feel insecure, restless, tired, and tend to fight anxiety by being obsessively tidy or really well organized. (*See page 167.*)
- Nat. mur. may be useful if you have a tendency to dwell on morbid topics and generally hate fuss. (*See page 190.*)
- Calcarea, if you fear for your sanity, forget things, and feel the cold. (*See page 171.*)
- Ignatia, if your anxiety follows the loss of a loved one or a specific, distressing event. (*See page 184.*)

Flower Essences

Remedies are prescribed according to the personal characteristics of the sufferer, and the cause and the nature of the anxiety.

Try Elm for anxiety accompanying a feeling of being unable to cope, or Red Chestnut for anxiety over the welfare of others. (*See pages 209 and 226.*)

Aspen, for anxiety for no apparent reason. (*See page 222.*)

Rescue Remedy or Emergency Essence are useful during attacks. (*See page 229.*)

Vitamins and Minerals

Increase your intake of B-vitamins, which work on the nervous system, and avoid caffeine in any form. (*See pages 235–238.*)

INSECURITY

Insecurity is a feeling that affects everybody at one time or another. It can be triggered by physical, social, financial, or emotional factors, and can often induce anxiety and its associated symptoms. Whatever the initial cause, when a person feels insecure that person's entire perception of his or her own competence and self-worth are thrown into question. Chronic insecurity, which can manifest itself as depression, shyness, lack of confidence, or an inability to form stable relationships, has less to do with external events than with unrealistic expectations and a poor self-image.

Symptoms
- dry mouth
- sweaty palms
- rapid pulse and palpitations
- in anxiety neurosis: breathlessness, headaches, general weakness, and fatigue, feeling of tightness in the chest, high blood pressure, abdominal pain and diarrhea, insomnia, loss of appetite

TREATMENT

Chinese Herbalism

Try herbs which work to balance the nervous system, including fleeceflower stem, poria, and wild jujube seeds. (*See pages 57 and 62.*)

Herbalism

Uplifting herbs such as rosemary, lavender, ginseng, damiana, or valerian. They can be drunk as infusions 3 times daily. (*See pages 114, 112, 122, and 123.*)

Aromatherapy

Jasmine lifts the spirits and improves mental outlook—add a few drops to a vaporizer or your bath (not at bedtime). (*See page 147.*)

Marjoram and thyme are cheering and can boost self-image. (*See pages 151 and 156.*)

Homeopathy

Aconite, for insecurity brought on by a traumatic experience. (*See page 163.*)

Ignatia, for insecurity stemming from a particular cause, for example a bereavement. (*See page 184.*)

Pulsatilla, if you feel tearful, worse for heat, and longing for company. (*See page 193.*)

Flower Essences
Mimulus is appropriate for fear, timidity, and shyness. (*See page 220.*)

Crab Apple, for poor self-image. (*See page 219.*)

Elm, for those who are usually confident but are experiencing a temporary crisis of confidence because they are overwhelmed by responsibility. (*See page 226.*)

MEMORY LOSS

A total or partial loss of memory is known as amnesia. It occurs as a result of either physical or mental disease (such as senile dementia), or physical trauma (such as a blow to the head or a fractured skull). The latter may induce a state of retrograde amnesia where the sufferer has no memory of the events immediately before the injury as well as those after. The period of amnesia in such cases is usually in proportion to the severity of the injury. Amnesia is caused by damage to, or disease of, brain regions concerned with memory function, and can also occur in some forms of psychiatric illness in which there is no apparent physical damage to the brain. Amnesia can very often be a complication of alcoholism, and can result from depression, anxiety, stress, poor nutrition, inadequate sleep, or lack of stimulation.

TREATMENT
Chinese Herbalism
Herbs to aid memory include fleeceflower root and black ginger seed. (*See page 57.*)

Memory loss caused by stress or fatigue may be treated with Chinese wolfberry. (*See page 52.*) (*See also Anxiety, page 268.*)

Herbalism
Ginseng powder can act as a memory aid and general stimulant. (*See page 112.*)

Add a small amount of gotu kola to your food or drink for several days, to revive your memory.

Rosemary is said to comfort the brain and refresh the memory, and sage is also useful. (*See page 114.*)

Homeopathy
Treatment would be constitutional, but the following may be of use:

Anacardium when you are absent-minded because of an inner conflict. (*See page 164.*)

Sulfur, for difficulty remembering words and names. (*See page 198.*)

Calcarea, for wandering attention, particularly in the elderly. (*See page 171.*)

Ignatia, for memory loss caused by a traumatic event or bereavement. (*See page 184.*)

Flower Essences
Star of Bethlehem, when memory is affected by an accident, bad news, or trauma. (*See page 220.*)

Vitamins and Minerals
Your diet should be rich in B-vitamins and protein, for amino acids are necessary for the brain to function efficiently. An amino acid supplement (containing all 22 acids) may be useful. Acetylcholine, which is formed in the body from lecithin, may help. Increase your intake of lecithin (found in sunflower oil and eggs) or take it as a supplement. (*See page 255.*)

INSOMNIA

A common complaint, insomnia is the inability to sleep or the disturbance of normal sleep patterns. It is difficult to qualify, because everyone has different sleep requirements, and sleeplessness is, in fact, a natural feature of aging. Insomnia is often caused by worry, emotional stress, and exhaustion. Other causes include pain; excess caffeine, alcohol and drugs; food allergy; or sleeping in a stuffy room. Insomnia can also be a symptom of depression.

In recent years, sleep-disorder medicine has become virtually a new branch of medicine, with centers for diagnosis and treatment now located throughout the U.S.

- 15–17 percent of the population suffer from sleep problems at some point.
- 50 percent of people who take sleeping pills for insomnia find the condition worsens.
- 200,000–400,000 car accidents each year are caused by drowsiness.

Roughly speaking, 80 percent of our sleep is NREAA (non-rapid eye movement) and 20 percent is REM (rapid eye movement). If you feel tired all the next day, you have probably not had enough NREAA sleep; if you have problems with your memory, then inadequate REM sleep is to blame.

Some 66 percent of people sleep for anything between 6.5 and 8.5 hours each night on a regular basis. Around 16 percent sleep for more than 8.5 hours every night and 18 percent for under 6.5 hours.

Fatigue doesn't necessarily relate to the amount of sleep you have had. Doctors report that one of the most common problems they see in their surgeries on a daily basis is chronic fatigue —or TAT, tired all the time.

Research now shows that some 80 percent of people complaining of being tired all the time (TAT) get adequate sleep, and that the problem lies in nutritional deficiencies which can be cleared up by improving the diet and taking a good multivitamin and mineral supplement.

Symptoms

- overactive mind causing difficulty in falling asleep
- nervousness and restlessness
- nightmares once asleep
- irritability
- mood swings involving hysterical behavior

TREATMENT

Ayurveda
Specific herbs to treat insomnia may include henbane, which is sedative.

Chinese Herbalism
Useful herbs include hoelen, fleeceflower stem, and wild jujube. (*See pages 57 and 62.*)

The herbalist may suggest that you sleep on a gypsum pillow.

Traditional Folk and Home Remedies
A hot foot-bath before bed helps relaxation by drawing blood away from the head. Add a little mustard powder to the water to increase the effect. (*See page 84.*)

Lettuce is said to encourage sleep. Eat a large leaf about half an hour before bedtime.

Herbalism
A warm bath with an infusion of chamomile, catnip, lavender, or limeflowers may be recommended. (*See pages 104 and 121.*)

A cup of warm herb tea just before bed will soothe and help you to relax. Try chamomile, catnip, lemon balm, and limeflowers. (*See pages 104 and 121.*)

Make a lavender pillow and place it under your usual pillow.

Aromatherapy
A few drops of chamomile oil, clary sage, or lavender can be added to the bath. (*See pages 137, 155, and 147.*)

Try a gentle massage just before bedtime, with a few drops of chamomile, lavender, rose, or neroli blended into a light carrier oil. (*See pages 137, 147, 144, and 139.*)

Place a few drops of lavender oil on your bedroom light bulb, just before bed, or place a few drops on a handkerchief and tie it to the bed. (*See page 147.*)

Homeopathy
Remedies can be taken an hour before going to bed, for up to 14 days. Repeat the dose if you wake in the night and cannot get back to sleep. Insomnia is usually treated "constitutionally," so you may need to consult a registered homeopath for treatment. The following remedies may be helpful:

- Coffea, when your mind is overactive, and you are unable to switch off. (*See page 177.*)
- Nux vomica, when your sleeplessness is exacerbated by food or alcohol; you wake around 3 or 4a.m., then fall asleep just as it is time to get up; and consequently are irritable during the day. (*See page 198.*)

- Pulsatilla, when you are restless in the early hours of sleep, feeling uncomfortable, hot and then cold, are not thirsty and sleep with your arms above your head. (*See page 193.*)
- Arnica, when the bed feels too hard, and you are overtired, fidgety, and dream of being chased by animals. (*See page 167.*)
- Lycopodium, when your mind is active at bedtime, going over and over work done that day; you dream a lot, talk and laugh in your sleep, and then wake up at around 4a.m. (*See page 187.*)
- Arsenicum, for when you tend to wake between midnight and 2a.m., feeling restless, worried, and apprehensive. (*See page 167.*)
- Rhus tox., when you cannot sleep, are irritable, restless, and feel a need to walk about; especially if in pain. (*See page 194.*)
- Aurum, when you have dreams about dying, hunger, or problems at work, and consequently become depressed. (*See page 169.*)
- Aconite, when sleep problems are worse after shock or trauma; there is restlessness, nightmares, and fear of dying. (*See page 163.*)
- Chamomilla, when you are feeling irritable at bedtime. (*See page 188.*)

Flower Essences

Worrying thoughts and mental arguments might respond to White Chestnut. (*See page 209.*)

Indecision can be treated with Scleranthus. (*See page 224.*)

Stress, strain, frustration, and inability to relax might respond to Vervain or Rock Water, Vine, Elm, Beech, or Impatiens could apply. (*See pages 226, 227, and 215.*)

Vitamins and Minerals

Increase your intake of vitamins B, C, folic acid, zinc, and calcium. Try a calcium supplement just before bedtime. (*See page 241.*)

DISORDERS OF THE BRAIN AND NERVES

SHINGLES

Shingles is an extremely painful disease caused by the herpes zoster virus (which is also the chickenpox virus). Following an attack of chickenpox the virus remains dormant in the body. Many years later a drop in the efficiency of the immune system may cause reactivation of the virus, this time in the form of shingles, causing acute inflammation in the ganglia near the spinal cord.

- Occurs most often in people over the age of 50 and may be activated through surgery or X-ray therapy.
- In younger people, it is often associated with a weakening of the immune system.
- The pain, which can be disabling, may continue for a few months after the blisters heal.
- Shingles strikes 850,000 Americans each year.

> **CAUTION**
> Shingles of the face may affect the eyes and should receive appropriate specialist medical attention.

Symptoms
- the first sign of shingles is sensitivity in the area to be affected, then pain
- fever; sickness
- a rash of small blisters develops on the fourth or fifth day; these turn yellow within a few days, form scabs, then drop off, sometimes leaving scars
- in some cases there may be persistent pain for months

TREATMENT

For treating the spots which develop, apply allspice paste. Grind cinnamon, cloves, and nutmeg in a pestle and mortar. Add water to make a thick paste. Apply to spots to numb the pain. (You can also buy allspice as a pre-ground powder.)

Herbalism

Make an infusion of the following nervine herbs and drink three times daily: oats, skullcap, St. John's wort, and vervain. (*See pages 102, 118, and 110.*)

Diluted tinctures or cold infusion of marigold, plantain, and St. John's wort can be used to bathe the affected area.

Aromatheraphy

Essential oils can combine analgesics with antiviral properties, and can be applied as a compress, added to the bath, or massaged into the skin. Try combining two or more of bergamot, chamomile, geranium, eucalyptus, melissa, lavender, and tea tree. (*See pages 133–157.*)

Dab the sores with lemon or geranium oil diluted in a little water. (*See pages 140 and 151.*)

Chinese Herbalism

Treatment would address gall bladder heat and damp. Useful herbs include gentian and Oriental wormwood.

Traditional Home and Folk Remedies

Grind allspice and make a paste, then apply to the spots to relieve pain.

Celery juice or celery tea can alleviate the pain and help to tone up the nervous system.

Apply bruised juniper berries to the spots for effective pain relief.

Fresh lemon can be cut and applied to the affected areas to relieve the pain.

Homeopathy

The following remedies can be taken every two hours for up to ten doses:

- Arsenicum, for burning pains which are worse between midnight and 2a.m., accompanied by skin eruptions and feeling restless, chilly, and anxious. (*See page 167.*)
- Lachesis, when the left side of the body is affected by swelling. (*See page 200.*)
- Rhus tox., for red, blistered, and itching skin which is improved with movement and warmth. (*See page 194.*)
- Fanunculus, for nerve pains and itching which are made worse by movement and eating.
- Sponge the blisters with a blend of Hypericum and Calendula tinctures, added to a little hot water.

Vitamins and Minerals

Eat plenty of foods that are rich in the B-complex vitamins, to aid nervous health. (*See pages 235–238.*)

Increase your intake of vitamin C, and take a supplement of 1g. up to four times daily. (*See page 238.*)

Supplementation with vitamin E is now known to reduce the long-term symptoms associated with shingles. Take up to 1mg. daily, broken into three doses, with food.

Vitamin E oil, applied directly to the sores, will encourage healing. (*See page 239.*)

Shingles is a sign of debility. Treatments suggested for stress (*see page 266*) will help to tone up the system.

NEURALGIA

Neuralgia is the term used to describe any pain originating in a nerve. If there is damage at any point along the route of a nerve, pain will then be referred to the area served by the affected nerve. Infection causing inflammation in a nerve can also cause neuralgia. The pain may be intermittent or continuous. Neuralgia has different causes, which give rise to certain specific types of neuralgic pain—trigeminal neuralgia, sciatica, post-herpetic neuralgia, and glossopharyngeal neuralgia.

Specific types of neuralgia include:

- trigeminal neuralgia, in which the facial nerve is affected, causing severe one-sided facial pain
- sciatica, causing pain of varying severity in the back, sometimes extending down to the foot
- post-herpetic neuralgia, which causes a burning pain at the site of a previous attack of shingles.
- glossopharyngeal neuralgia, in which pain is felt in the ear, the throat, and at the back of the tongue

TREATMENT

Chinese Herbalism

Treatment would be aimed at addressing Wind, Damp and Heat which may have entered the meridians and are causing the illness. (*See page 35.*)

Gentian and oriental wormwood may be useful.

Traditional Home and Folk Remedies

Celery juice or celery tea will help to ease the pain of neuralgia. (*See page 71.*)

Warm chamomile compresses applied to the affected area will ease inflammation and pain.

Rub lemons on the affected area for pain relief. (*See page 74.*)

Rub peppermint oil into the affected area.

Clove oil can be used where pain is experienced inside the mouth. (*See page 74.*)

Aromatherapy

Massage essential oil of eucalyptus, lavender, or chamomile into the affected area, or add the infused herbs to the bath. (*See pages 133–157.*)

A compress of rosemary essential oil will improve the circulation in that area, which will encourage healing. (*See page 154.*)

Blend one drop of mustard and pepper oils in some grapeseed oil, and massage into the affected area. (*See pages 133–157.*)

Homeopathy

Treatment should be constitutional, and supervised by an experienced homeopath. Some of the following remedies may be helpful:

Arsenicum, for an attack brought on by dry cold. You feel chilly, tired, restless, and have burning pains. (*See page 167.*)

Lachesis, for pain that is worse after sleep. (*See page 200.*)

Mag. phos., for pain that is relieved by applying heat and pressure. (*See page 188.*)

Aconite, when symptoms come on suddenly, particularly after exposure to cold; the body feels congested and numb. (*See page 163.*)

Colocynthis, for a neuralgia attack brought on by cold or damp, and which feels better for heat. (*See page 176.*)

Vitamins and Minerals

Vitamins B1, B2, and biotin help nerve health. (*See pages 235 and 239.*)

Take both extra vitamin E and chromium. (*See pages 239 and 242.*)

MIGRAINE

The classic feature of a migraine is a throbbing headache, usually on one side of the head only. This is caused by the narrowing and dilating of the blood vessels in a part of one side of the brain. An attack may last for up to two days. There are two main types of migraine: common and the comparatively rare classical. Migraine can be hereditary, and may be triggered by many factors, including stress, hormonal changes (around menopause, menstruation, and occasionally pregnancy), oral contraceptives, and food that contains tyramine, an amino acid which affects the blood vessels. Foods rich in tyramine include bananas, cheese, chocolate, eggs, oranges, spinach, tomatoes, and wine. Migraine occurs in about 10 percent of the population, and is more common in women. Children may suffer from migraine, but this often manifests itself as an abdominal pain rather than a headache.

Symptoms

Common migraine: slowly developing severe headache, lasting from a few hours to two days—made worse by the smallest movement or noise—nausea and sometimes vomiting.

Classical migraine: headache preceded by an aura which generally takes the form a visual disturbance—this may consist of temporary loss of vision, focusing problems, blind spots, and flashing lights, possible speech problems, occasional weakness or temporary paralysis of the limbs or extremities, nausea and vomiting, sensitivity to light.

Some 16–18 million Americans suffer from migraine. Studies suggest that people who feel compelled to excel are especially susceptible to migraine.

About 60 percent of all migraine sufferers are women, and most patients first develop symptoms between the ages of 10 and 30.

TREATMENT

Ayurveda

Treatment would be aimed at Ayurvedic oral formulas, and panchakarma shirovirechana. (*See page 11.*)

Vilwadi lehya can help with nausea.

Chinese Herbalism

The cause is believed to be excess Liver qi stagnation, weakness in the stomach, and an imbalance of stomach and liver. Useful herbs include cassia tora and chrysanthemum.

Herbalism

Feverfew is an effective remedy for reducing the frequency of migraine. Take two or three small leaves between a little fresh bread, daily. Feverfew tablets are also available. (*See page 120.*)

The following herbs can be infused for treating a mild attack of neuralgia: balm, meadowsweet, rosemary, and skullcap. (*See pages 106, 114, and 118.*)

Apply a warm compress with Jamaican dogwood to the temples and forehead during an attack.

Aromatherapy

Peppermint and lavender oils, applied to a cool compress, will help to relieve symptoms. (*See pages 150 and 147.*)

Inhalations, baths, or massage of melissa, rosemary, or sweet marjoram can relieve the pain and shorten the duration of attacks. Used regularly, these methods can be preventive. (*See pages 133–157.*)

A dab of lavender oil at the base of the nostrils can be used at the first signs of an attack. (*See page 147.*)

Homeopathy

Treatment is constitutional, but the following remedies may be helpful in the event of an attack:

Pulsatilla, for headache which is worse in the evening or during menstruation, and aggravated by rich, fatty foods; also for tearfulness. (*See page 193.*)

Thuja, for a left-sided headache with the sensation of a nail being drilled into the skull. (*See page 200.*)

Silicea, for pain that begins in the back of the head, settling above an eye. This is alleviated by wrapping the head. (*See page 195.*)

Lycopodium, for pain that is worse on the right side of the body, painful temples and dizziness. (*See page 187.*)

Nat. mur., for a headache which is blinding and throbs, and which is worsened by warmth and movement, and where the attack is preceded by numbness around the mouth and nose. (*See page 190.*)

Vitamins and Minerals

Take extra vitamins B5, C, and E, and also evening primrose oil. Add fresh root ginger to food.

HEADACHE

Headaches are an extremely common complaint, and for the most part are due to muscular tension in the head, neck, or shoulders, or to congestion of the blood vessels supplying blood to the brain and muscles. In some cases a headache may be a symptom of a more serious underlying disorder, but often headaches are caused by stress, tiredness, poor posture, caffeine, alcohol, drugs, food allergy, eye strain, sinusitis, or low blood sugar. They can also be the result of a head injury. There are many different types of headache and the degree and intensity of pain vary accordingly. It may occur in any part of the head, usually worsening towards the end of the day.

Almost 90 percent of all people seeking medical help for headaches suffer from tension-type headaches.

Cluster headaches produce short, severe attacks of pain centered over one eye. They are so called because they occur in clusters, many times a day, for several months. Spontaneous remissions often take place, but the pain usually returns some months or years later.

Cluster headaches are suffered most often by males.

Researchers suspect that cluster headaches may be caused by a disorder in histamine metabolism, since they are usually accompanied by allergy symptoms such as tearing, nasal congestion, and a runny nose.

> **CAUTION**
> Headaches with associated features such as double vision, projectile vomiting, weakness, paralysis, vertigo, or one-sided deafness require urgent medical attention.

Symptoms

- sensation of a tight band around the head
- a feeling of pressure at the top of the head
- bursting or throbbing sensation
- eye and neck pain
- dizziness

TREATMENT

An Ayurvedic treatment for sinus-related headaches is the steam inhalation of coriander seeds. Put the coriander seeds into a small bowl, pour on some boiling water, drape a towel over your head and the bowl, and inhale the steam. Coriander's active ingredient is a volatile oil.

Ayurveda

For headaches, heat 3 tablespoons of mustard oil, soak a cloth in the solution and apply to the forehead as required. (*See page 19.*)

Coriander seeds, steeped for several minutes in boiling water, can be inhaled under a towel to relieve sinus-related headaches. (*See page 24.*) Asna vilwadi thaila is an oil, for external use, which relieves headaches.

Chinese Herbalism

Traditional Chinese herbal medicine recommends ginger for headaches. Eat a small piece of fresh ginger root or make ginger tea from the fresh root or tea bags. If you prefer, mix a large pinch of powdered ginger into a glass of cool water and drink it, or try powdered ginger in capsules, available from health food stores.

Ginseng is another favorite Chinese herbal remedy for headaches. (*See page 54.*)

Traditional Home and Folk Remedies

A ginger foot bath may ease the pain and warm the body.

Chamomile tea soothes headache symptoms.

A mustard foot bath is a traditional headache remedy. (*See page 84.*)

A few grains of cayenne pepper, added to tea, ease a headache. (*See page 103.*)

Fresh garlic bulbs, eaten in a salad, will clear headaches which have a feeling of congestion. (*See page 70.*)

Parsley and peppermint teas will clear the head.

Herbalism

Sitting down with a relaxing cup of mild herbal tea is often good for a tension headache. Good choices are peppermint, spearmint, chamomile, rose hip, meadowsweet, or lemon balm. (*See pages 111, 104, and 106.*)

Valerian root tea can also be helpful, but it may induce sleep—use it with caution. (*See page 223.*)

Researchers are studying the benefits of the herb feverfew for treating chronic headaches and migraines. The leaves of this plant contain a substance that relaxes the blood vessels in your brain. Studies suggest that patients who eat a few fresh feverfew leaves or take an extract of the leaves every day have fewer and less severe migraines; the herb has no unpleasant side-effects. (*See page 120.*)

Aromatherapy

The relaxing qualities of lavender oil make it a good treatment for a tension headache. This essential oil is very gentle, so you can massage a few drops of neat oil into your temples and the base of your neck. (*See page 147.*)

Try mixing a drop or two of peppermint oil in a bowl of hot water and inhaling the steam, then lie down with a warm compress soaked in sweet marjoram oil on your forehead. (*See pages 150 and 151.*)

Place a few drops of lavender oil at the base of your nostrils for almost instant pain relief. (*See page 147.*)

Try taking a bath with relaxing oils such as chamomile or ylang ylang to soothe and relieve pain.

Homeopathy

Most headaches would be dealt with constitutionally, that is, the treatment would be tailored to your individual needs. Other remedies to try include:

- Ignatia, for headaches caused by emotional stress. (*See page 184.*)
- Nux vomica, for headaches caused by overindulgence or stress. (*See page 198.*)
- Cimicifuga may be useful for pain caused by nervous muscular tension in the shoulders and neck.
- Nux vomica or Pulsatilla are both useful in many cases of migraine. (*See pages 198 and 193.*)
- Aconite, for a sudden headache which feels worse for cold and is characterized by a tight band around the head. (*See page 163.*)
- Apis, for stinging, stabbing or burning headaches; when the body feels tender and sore. (*See page 165.*)
- Belladonna, for throbbing, drumming headaches with a flushed face. (*See page 168.*)
- Bryonia, for sharp, stabbing pain when the eyes are moved. (*See page 170.*)

- Hypericum, for a bursting, aching headache with a sensitive scalp. (*See page 184.*)
- Ruta, for a pressing headache caused by fatigue, and made worse by reading. (*See page 194.*)

Vitamins and Minerals

Frequent headaches could be a signal that you are low on some important vitamins and minerals. Low levels of niacin and vitamin B6 can cause headaches, for example, and all the B vitamins are needed to help combat stress and avoid tension headaches. Protein-rich foods such as chicken, fish, beans and peas, milk, cheese, nuts, and peanut butter are all good dietary sources of both niacin and vitamin B6. (*See pages 236 and 237.*)

The minerals calcium and magnesium work together to help prevent headaches, especially those related to a woman's menstrual cycle. Good sources of calcium are dairy products, tofu, dark green leafy vegetables such as kale or broccoli, and beans and peas. Magnesium is found in dark green leafy vegetables, nuts, bananas, wheat germ, seafood, and beans and peas. (*See pages 245 and 241.*)

If you can't eat some of these foods because they are headache triggers for you, taking a good daily multivitamin with minerals should provide enough of all the nutrients you need to help prevent headaches.

FAINTING

Fainting (or a vasovagal attack) is a brief loss of consciousness, usually brought on by strong emotion, shock, distress, or pain, and is most likely to occur in warm, crowded places. It is caused by a temporary shortage of blood supply to the brain, and there is also a slowing of the heart rate. A fainting episode acts, in fact, as a type of safety mechanism in that the fall restores the blood supply to the brain by gravity.

Symptoms

The characteristic loss of consciousness may be preceded by:
- yawning
- sweating
- nausea

- deep, rapid breathing and a weak pulse
- impaired vision
- ringing in the ears
- weakness and confusion

Fainting often occurs as a result of a vasovagal attack, in which overstimulation of the vagus nerve causes slowing of the heartbeat and a fall in blood pressure—which reduces the flow of blood to the brain. These attacks are commonly caused by pain, stress, shock, fear, or in a room with little oxygen. Other causes include prolonged coughing, straining to defecate or urinate, or blowing an instrument.

Fainting may also result from postural hypotension (*see page 278*), which may occur when a person stands still for a long time, or suddenly stands up. This is common in the elderly, in sufferers of diabetes, and people taking high blood pressure medication or vasodilator drugs.

TREATMENT

Ayurveda

The following Ayurvedic preparations will help to cure the condition: Aswagandharishta, an oral tonic; Chandanadi thaila, an external oil; Kalyanaka ghritha, oral ghee. (*See page 10.*)

Chinese Herbalism

Fresh ginger, cinnamon, twigs, and peppermint would be useful, taken internally as an infusion or decoction, as required.

Traditional Home and Folk Remedies

Eat fresh or grated apple when you start to feel faint; it is both restorative and calming. (*See page 80.*)

Chew dried cloves, which are stimulating and can improve circulation. (*See page 76.*)

Herbalism

Small sips of ginger tea, or root ginger chewed, will help to restore, and prevent an attack. (*See page 112.*)

Rosemary is stimulating, and taken regularly can prevent fainting spells. (*See page 114.*)

A hot drink of honey and peppermint will help to prevent loss of consciousness. Drink when you first start to feel faint. (*See page 111.*)

Aromatherapy

Hold a tissue with a few drops of peppermint or neroli oil, which can help when you feel faint or are in a state of shock.

A few drops of rosemary oil, massaged into the temples, prevents loss of consciousness. (*See page 154.*)

Homeopathy

Constitutional treatment is necessary if the condition is chronic, but specific remedies which can be taken every 5 minutes after or immediately before fainting (when the sensation of fainting begins) include:

Veratrum, for fainting caused by anger.

Coffea, for fainting brought on by excitement.

Ignatia, for fainting caused by an emotional shock or trauma. (*See page 184.*)

Aconite, for fainting caused by fright and characterized by tension and pale, clammy skin. (*See page 163.*)

Cocculus, for fainting caused by lack of sleep.

Gelsemium, when you feel weak and shaky.

Flower Essences

Rescue Remedy or Emergency Essence placed on the tongue or temples may help to prevent fainting. If you are prone to fainting, carry a bottle at all times and take at the first signs of weakness. (*See page 229.*)

Clematis can be taken for the "far away" feeling that comes before an attack, to bring the mind back to reality.

DIZZINESS

Dizziness is the sensation that everything around the sufferer is spinning, or that the brain is moving within the skull. In severe cases the sufferer may lose his or her balance and fall to the ground. Dizziness can be caused by a fault in the inner ear's balancing mechanism, or it may be due to a neurological disturbance. It can also be brought on by travel sickness, hyperventilation, anxiety, alcohol, drugs, and standing up suddenly from a sitting or lying position (postural hypotension). Postural hypotension is more common in the elderly and in people taking antihypertensive (high blood pressure) drugs.

Symptoms

- spinning sensation
- cold sweats
- nausea
- vomiting
- pallor

TREATMENT

Ayurveda

Add the juice of a lime or lemon to half a glass of soda water and sip in small doses.

Chinese Herbalism

Fresh ginger, cinnamon, and peppermint may help.

Mulberry can be used to nourish the blood.

Herbalism

Small sips of fresh ginger tea, made with root ginger, will help to ease the symptoms. (*See page 112.*)

Teas of rock rose flowers or wild rose flowers, with a little honey, will be helpful.

Homeopathy

Gelsemium, for dizziness accompanied by a fit of trembling. (*See page 180.*)

Nux vom., for when symptoms are made worse by flickering lights.

Calcarea, when symptoms become worse after looking up.

Borax, for symptoms made worse by downward motion.

Conium, when you feel worse lying down.

Flower Essences

If dizziness is associated with panic, stress, or anxiety, Emergency Essence or Rescue Remedy will be calming and restorative; take as required. (*See page 229.*)

Vitamins and Minerals

Take vitamins B2 and B3, and extra salt if you are sweating a great deal. (*See pages 235 and 236.*)

> **CAUTION**
> Severe or prolonged dizziness should be reported to your physician.

SKIN AND HAIR PROBLEMS

DERMATITIS

Dermatitis is a very loose term (often used interchangeably with eczema) used to describe an inflammation of the skin from any cause. Exogenous dermatitis is caused by external factors (irritants such as washing powder), and tends to occur around infected wounds or ulcers. Endogenous forms are due to internal problems, including metabolic disorders. Scratching always aggravates dermatitis and may also cause infection. Types of dermatitis include: diaper rash, caused by the ammonia in urine; atopic dermatitis, complicated by allergies such as hay fever; infantile eczema; seborrheic dermatitis (*see Dandruff, page 285*); dermatitis artefacta, caused by unnecessary scratching (it is self-inflicted and usually indicates an underlying emotional problem). The symptoms of dermatitis vary in severity and appearance according to the cause.

Symptoms
- redness and blistering
- swelling, weeping, and crusting of skin
- itching with a strong impulse to scratch
- burning sensation

Skin-contact dermatitis includes primary irritant dermatitis, allergic dermatitis, and photochemical dermatitis.

Primary irritant dermatitis is the most common type and is caused by the direct toxicity of certain chemicals that come in contact with the skin.

Allergic dermatitis involves the immune mechanism and requires prior sensitization of an individual to agents such as cosmetics, chemicals, plants, drugs, or costume jewelry.

Photochemical dermatitis occurs when an individual with photosensitizing chemicals on their skin is exposed to light.

Atopic dermatitis, or eczema, is a chronic inflammation that runs in families with a history of asthma and hay fever.

Dermatitis can occur in single episodes, or may be chronic. Up to 90 percent of the U.S. population will suffer from dermatitis during their lifetime.

TREATMENT

Chinese Herbalism
Dittany bark and puncture vine fruit may help with itching.

Traditional Home and Folk Remedies
For dermatitis on the hands, rub them with the cold wet coffee grounds left after you have brewed a pot of coffee, to soothe.

Herbalism
Apply compresses of verbena or thyme tea to the area to soothe and cool. (*See pages 125 and 122.*)

Aromatherapy
Dilute and massage a few drops of aspic, cedarwood, niaouli, or chamomile into the affected area to ease itching. (*See pages 135–157.*)

For contact dermatitis, calendula or chamomile oil. (*See pages 135 and 137.*)

Homeopathy
Sulfur, for when the skin feels as if it is burning, and becomes red, hot, and itchy. (*See page 198.*)

Graphites, when the skin appears infected. (*See page 181.*)

Petroleum, when there are deep cracks with a watery discharge.

Urtica urens, for a nettle rash-type itchiness. (*See page 201.*)

Rhus tox., for blisters that are worse at night and improve with warmth. (*See page 194.*)

Flower Essences
Crab Apple is the cleansing remedy. It works well when added to water for washing and baths. (*See page 219.*)

Impatiens is very useful for people whose rashes are associated with feelings of irritability and impatience. Take internally or mix into a neutral cream. (*See page 218.*)

Rescue Remedy, taken internally or used externally in a cream or wash, is useful for treating most skin problems. (*See page 229.*)

ECZEMA

Eczema (also called dermatitis) is an inflammation of the skin that causes itching and redness. It is a feature of many different skin disorders arising from many different causes. It can also be hereditary. Eczema is only infectious if it becomes secondarily infected. Types of eczema include: contact eczema (caused by allergens such as plants, metals, detergents, and chemical irritants); atopic eczema (associated with allergies such as hay fever); pomphylox eczema (triggered by emotional stress); and varicose eczema (occurring in the region of varicose veins).

Symptoms
- red, scaly, cracked patches of skin, particularly on the bands, ears, feet, and legs
- burning and itching with a strong urge to scratch, possibly leading to infection, particularly in children
- small fluid-filled blisters which may burst to form sores

A person may contract eczema at any age and at any place on the body, but the ailment occurs chiefly on the ears, hands, feet, and legs.

In infants, eczema is often caused by allergy to certain proteins in wheat, milk, and eggs.

Emotional problems and severe mental stress are suspected of causing eczema in adults.

Often, a family history of eczema exists, implying that heredity is also involved in some way.

TREATMENT

Ayurveda
Cassia pods and aloe vera may be used. (*See pages 20 and 17.*)

Treatment might consist of a number of related therapies, including herbalism, diet and lifestyle changes, cleansing routines, and treatment to balance the body systems so that they work more efficiently. (*See page 10.*)

Chinese Herbalism
Chinese herbs will be prescribed according to the specific cause and symptoms of your eczema, but some possible herbs are: wormwood, peony root, and Chinese gentian.

Dittany bark and puncture vine fruit may help itching.

Traditional Home and Folk Remedies
An oatmeal bath will soothe irritation and reduce annoying itching. (*See page 72.*)

Bathe sore patches with an infusion of witch hazel diluted in some warm water. (*See page 78.*)

Herbalism
Try drinking an infusion of burdock, chamomile, heartsease, marigold, and red clover, all of which are anti-inflammatory herbs. (*See pages 100, 104 and 102.*)

Chickweed ointment can be applied directly to the affected area, and calendula oil may also be useful.

Blackberry leaf tea can be used topically.

Aloe vera gel, from the leaf of the plant, will encourage healing. (*See page 99.*)

Aromatherapy
A gentle massage with a blend of chamomile, lavender, and/or melissa essential oil in a little carrier oil can be used to treat eczema. (*See pages 133–157.*)

Massage the affected areas with essential oils of chamomile, sage, geranium, and lavender, all blended together with a little carrier oil. (*See pages 133–157.*)

Homeopathy
Eczema requires constitutional treatment, which means that treatment is tailored to your specific needs. The following remedies may be useful in the meantime:
- Sulfur, when the skin is burning, red, hot, and itchy. (*See page 198.*)
- Graphites, when the skin appears infected. (*See page 181.*)
- Petroleum, when there are deep cracks with a watery discharge.
- Urtica urens, for a nettle rash-type itchiness. (*See page 201.*)
- Rhus tox., for blisters which are worse at night and improve with warmth. (*See page 194.*)

Flower Essences
Impatiens is very useful for people whose rashes are associated with feelings of irritability and impatience. Take internally or mix into a neutral cream.

Rescue Remedy, taken internally or used externally in a cream or wash, is useful for skin troubles.

Vitamins and Minerals

Increase your intake of vitamin A, found in liver, eggs, butter, milk, and red and orange vegetables.

Take a B-complex supplement each day, and make sure your tablet contains good levels of niacin (B3), which is also found naturally in peanuts, meat, fish, and pulses.

Vitamin C and bioflavonoids (which are often contained in a good vitamin C supplement) act as a natural antihistamine. (*See pages 254–256.*)

Evening primrose oil has been used successfully in the treatment of eczema, reducing itching and encouraging healing. (*See page 254.*)

PSORIASIS

Psoriasis is a common skin disorder which may affect any part of the body, but most often the elbows, knees, shins, scalp, and lower back. The characteristic bright pink or red plaques covered with silvery scaling are caused by a thickening of the outer skin layers. Psoriasis tends to run in families and usually begins in adolescence. Cold damp conditions, stress, anxiety, or an acute illness (such as tonsillitis) may all be triggers. There is also an association with arthritis of the fingers or toes. Psoriasis does not usually cause itching, nor is it contagious.

Symptoms

- pain (rather than itching), with cracks appearing in the dry areas of the hands and feet
- pustules on the palms of the hands or soles of the feet
- glazed but not scaly plaques in moist areas of the body (flexural psoriasis)
- distortion and pitting of the nails in some cases

TREATMENT

Chinese Herbalism

Dittany bark and puncture vine fruit may help with itching.

Traditional Home and Folk Remedies

Take at least 1 tablespoonful of olive oil a day and at least one raw vegetable salad. (*See page 81.*)

Garlic is cleansing, and may ease the symptoms and prevent attacks. (*See page 70.*)

Herbalism

Licorice, for the inflammation of psoriasis. (*See page 108.*)

Yarrow used twice weekly in bath water has proved beneficial in some cases. (*See page 97.*)

Nettle tea and products based on nettles may be helpful. (*See page 124.*)

Aromatherapy

Sedative and antidepressant oils such as lavender and chamomile can help to reduce the stress that exacerbates the condition. Use in the bath, massage, and skin creams. (*See pages 147 and 137.*)

Bergamot essential oil, cajeput, and Roman chamomile can all be used as a beneficial massage oil. They may also be added to a bath, or placed in a vaporizer. (*See pages 133–157.*)

Homeopathy

Kali ars., for scaly skin aggravated by warmth.

Arsenicum, for burning, hot areas, and feeling chilly and restless. (*See page 167.*)

Graphites, for psoriasis that is worse behind the ears and weeping. (*See page 181.*)

Sulfur, for patches that become worse after a bath and in heat. (*See page 198.*)

Petroleum, when the condition is worse in winter.

Flower Essences

Impatiens is very useful for people whose rashes are associated with feelings of irritability and impatience. Take internally or mix into a neutral cream. (*See page 218.*)

Rescue Remedy, taken internally or used externally in a cream or wash, treats most skin troubles. (*See page 229.*)

Crab Apple is the cleansing remedy. It works well when added to water for washing and baths. (*See page 219.*)

Vitamins and Minerals

Increase your intake of vitamin A (as beta carotene), vitamin C, vitamin E, selenium, B-complex vitamins as part of a good multivitamin and mineral supplement, and also protein. (*See pages 235–239 and 247.*)

URTICARIA

Urticaria is an allergic condition also known as hives or nettle rash. The rash of raised, whitish-yellow areas of skin surrounded by red inflammation is caused by the release of histamine into the tissues in response to triggers which may include heat, cold, sunlight, scabies, bites and stings, contact with plants, food additives, sensitivity to certain foods, and stress or anxiety. Acute urticaria typically develops very quickly, and usually disappears just as quickly; chronic urticaria is more persistent.

Symptoms
- rash of weals, especially on limbs and trunk
- intense itching
- swelling of the tongue and larynx may occur, possibly interfering with breathing
- a feverish feeling
- possibly nausea

TREATMENT
Ayurveda
Aloe vera can be used topically to soothe the rash. (*See page 17.*)

Chinese Herbalism
The source of urticaria is considered to be Heat and Wind when red; and Heat, Cold and Wind for a cold white rash. Treatment may include chizomeotea or ledebouriella. (*See page 51.*)

Traditional Home and Folk Remedies
Add a few tablespoons of baking soda to the bath to relieve itching. (*See page 86.*)

An oatmeal bath will soothe the rash. (*See page 72.*)

Add a cupful of vinegar to the bath water to restore the balance of the skin. (*See page 87.*)

Herbalism
An infusion of chickweed and chamomile can be used to bathe the affected area. (*See page 104.*)

Balm and heartsease can be drunk three times daily to soothe and reduce inflammation.

For urticaria brought on by anxiety and stress, drink an infusion of valerian twice daily. (*See page 123.*)

Urtica urens cream will soothe and promote healing.

Aromatherapy
A warm bath with essential oil of chamomile or melissa will soothe the skin and help to prevent stress-related attacks.

Homeopathy
Apis, for burning and swelling, particularly of the lips and eyelids. (*See page 165.*)

Urtica, for a rash that feels like stinging nettles, and is worse when touched or after it has been scratched.

Nat. mur., for chronic urticaria exacerbated by stress.

Rhus tox., for burning, itching, and blisters.

Sulfur, for relief of red, itchy, puffy skin, which is made worse by heat. (*See page 198.*)

Arsenicum, for symptoms accompanied by restlessness and anxiety. (*See page 167.*)

Flower Essences
Impatiens is very useful for people whose rashes are associated with feelings of irritability and impatience. Take internally or mix into a neutral cream. (*See page 218.*)

PRICKLY HEAT

Prickly heat, or heat rash, occurs as a result of sweat duct blockage (probably due to excessive dampness of the skin) in particularly hot and humid weather. It produces a rash of red spots on the face and/or body, which usually disappears within hours of the sufferer moving into the shade, or his or her acclimatization. Occasionally, however, it may develop into patches of eczema. Children, the elderly and the obese are all particularly susceptible.

TREATMENT
Herbalism
Chickweed infusions can be made into cool compresses and applied to the affected area. Chickweed ointment can be applied as needed.

Aromatherapy
Add a few drops of lavender and sandalwood oils to a little calendula oil, and massage into the affected area. (*See pages 133–157.*)

Homeopathy
Apis, taken every 2 hours for up to 10 doses. (*See page 165.*)

Merc. Sol. can be used as a preventive measure. (*See page 189.*)

Flower Essences
Impatiens is very useful for itching. Take internally or mix into a neutral cream. (*See page 218.*)

Rescue Remedy, taken internally or applied externally in a cream or wash, helps most skin troubles. (*See page 229.*)

Vitamins and Minerals
Take plenty of vitamin C, which will help to discourage itching and the rash. (*See page 238.*)

Symptoms
- a constant prickling or itching sensation
- tiny blisters may form in severe cases as a result of salt crystals forming in the sweat gland ducts

PERSPIRATION

Perspiration is generally stimulated by heat and is the body's way of regulating temperature. Excessive sweating (or hyperhidrosis) is caused by overactive sweat glands. It may be confined to specific areas such as the palms of the hands, armpits, groin and feet, or it may occur all over the body. When perspiration exceeds the bounds of what is considered normal, it may be due to an overactive thyroid gland, the menopause, prolonged fever, or stress or other psychological factors.

Symptoms
- an unpleasant body odor may occur if perspiration comes into contact with bacteria on the skin
- in severe cases the skin in affected areas may become damp and damaged

TREATMENT
Chinese Herbalism
Excess sweating is thought to be caused by a deficiency of qi or yin. (*See page 35.*)

For yin deficiency, use gray lily turf root, cork tree bark, and peony. (*See pages 55 and 53.*)

Try ledebouriella and astragalus for deficient qi. (*See pages 51 and 42.*)

Herbalism
Marigold infusion can be drunk to produce a perspiration increase, when necessary. (*See page 102.*)

A herbal deodorant would include cloves, myrrh, coriander seeds, cassia, lavender flowers, and thyme, in equal amounts and ground into a powder. Use in the bath, or under the arms. This may cause a rash in sensitive people.

Aromatherapy
Cypress oil is astringent and refreshing, and can be massaged into the feet for excess perspiration, or combined with lavender oil in a light massage oil and massaged under the arms. (*See page 143.*)

Oils with deodorizing properties are bergamot, clary sage, eucalyptus, lavender, neroli, petitgrain, and rosewood. (*See pages 133–157.*)

Detoxifying oils include fennel, garlic, juniper, and rose.

Basil, chamomile, juniper, peppermint, and tea tree oils promote sweating, if there is a lack of it.

Homeopathy
Constitutional treatment is most appropriate, but the following may help:

Lycopodium, for smelly perspiration, worse on feet and under arms. (*See page 187.*)

Mercurius, for smelly sweat. (*See page 189.*)

Sulfur, for sweating on the head, with morning diarrhea. (*See page 198.*)

Calcarea, for sour sweat. The sufferer is likely to be overweight, and feels cold and clammy. (*See page 171.*)

Silicea, for sweaty, smelly feet in a thin person. (*See page 195.*)

Aethusa, for insufficient perspiration production.

SUNBURN

Sunburn occurs on exposure to bright sunlight and is caused by the effects of ultraviolet light. It is most likely to affect people with pale complexions or those who are unused to being in the sun.

Symptoms
- redness and extreme soreness in affected areas
- a sensation of heat in burned areas
- blistering in severe cases

TREATMENT

Ayurveda
Aloe vera can be used on burned areas to soothe and to heal.

Herbalism
Urtica urens ointment eases the pain and helps to prevent skin damage.

Aromatherapy
Add a few drops of lavender and chamomile oils to a tub of live yogurt, and apply to affected areas to soothe, encourage healing, and reduce inflammation. (*See pages 147 and 137.*)

Homeopathy
Merc. Sol. can be used to prevent and treat sunburn.

Flower Essences
Rescue Remedy cream heals damaged tissue.

Vitamins and Minerals
Rub a little vitamin E oil into the affected area, soon after the burning, to help the healing process and prevent peels and scarring. (*See page 239.*)

WARTS

A wart is a small, hard growth, usually brown or flesh-colored, on the skin. It may be caused by any one of 30 strains of the human papilloma virus. Warts are highly contagious, but not dangerous, and can occur more frequently when the immune system is compromised.

> **CAUTION**
> Genital warts must be treated in an STD or GU (Genitourinary) clinic, and treatment can be complemented by healing remedies, but only under the care of a registered practitioner.

TREATMENT

Traditional Home and Folk Remedies
Rub fresh lemon into the wart daily, and keep moist (with a plaster), paring back any hardened skin. (*See page 74.*)

Rub fresh garlic into the wart to fight the fungal infection, and eat lots of garlic to boost immunity. (*See page 70.*)

Mix castor oil and baking powder into a paste, and apply at night with a plaster, leaving it exposed during the day.

Herbalism
Squeeze the fresh sap of a dandelion stalk on to the wart every day until it disappears. (*See page 121.*)

Milkwort can be mashed and applied directly to the wart.

Aromatherapy
Apply a little lemon oil directly to the wart; continue treatment until the wart disappears. (*See page 140.*)

When the wart disappears, add a few drops of lavender oil to vitamin E oil and apply to the area for a week, to encourage healing and prevent scarring and further infection. (*See page 147.*)

Overall body massage with rosemary, juniper, or geranium will help to strengthen the immune system.

Homeopathy
Thuja, for soft, fleshy warts that ooze and bleed.

Causticum, for warts on the face or fingertips, and painful verrucas. (*See page 174.*)

Dulcamara, for hard, smooth, fleshy warts on the back of hands. (*See page 197.*)

Kali mur., for warts growing on the hands.

Nat. carb., for weeping warts on the toes.

Antimonium, for horny warts caused by or associated with a callus. (*See page 164.*)

The common wart, verruca vulgaris, may occur anywhere on the body.

Verruca plana is a round, yellowish, flat-topped wart found mainly on the backs of the hands.

Verruca filiformis is a long, thin wart found on the eyelids, armpits, and neck.

The venereal wart, a pink, cauliflower-like growth, is found on the genitals (sexually transmitted).

The plantar wart (or verruca) is a flat wart on the sole of the foot which may be forced into the thick skin of that area.

DANDRUFF

Dandruff occurs when the fine cells of the outer layer of skin on the scalp are shed at a faster rate than normal, causing the characteristic flakes of dead skin. This is caused by a disorder of the sebaceous glands. If too little sebum is secreted the hair is dry and dandruff appears as white flakes; if too much sebum is produced the hair is greasy, and the dandruff yellow. The flakes are usually most obvious after brushing or combing the hair, which loosens them. Certain types of seborrheic dermatitis are also responsible for dandruff, which will cause inflammation and itchiness in addition to flaking.

TREATMENT

Herbalism
Improve circulation to the scalp. Rosemary is the herb of choice, taken internally as a tea and used as an application.

For dry hair, rub rosemary-infused oil into the scalp before washing. (*See page 114.*)

For greasy hair, add rosemary vinegar or a few drops of rosemary essential oil to the rinsing water.

Take a combination of the herbs burdock, kelp, and heartsease internally to improve the general condition of the scalp. (*See page 100.*)

Aromatherapy
Rosemary, cedarwood, tea tree, or patchouli can be massaged into the scalp, added to unscented shampoos, and used in the final rinse when washing your hair.

Dilute lavender oil in a little almond or coconut oil and massage into the scalp to eliminate dandruff. (*See page 147.*)

Homeopathy
Constitutional treatment may be useful, but the following remedies may help:
- Arsenicum, for a dry, sensitive, hot scalp with bare patches of skin. (*See page 167.*)
- Nat. mur., for a white crust around the hairline, and greasy hair. (*See page 190.*)
- Fluoric acid, for flaky scalp and hair loss.
- Graphites, for a moist scalp with smelly crusting. (*See page 181.*)
- Sulfur, for thick dandruff which is itchier at night.
- Sepia, for moist, greasy scalp, which is sensitive around the ears. (*See page 196.*)

Vitamins and Minerals
Increase your intake of selenium, vitamin E, vitamin C, B-complex vitamins, and zinc. (*See pages 247, 235–239, and 249.*)

HAIR LOSS

It is normal to shed about 150 hairs a day, but sometimes this number may be increased by various stresses on the body. Hereditary hair loss is known as alopecia. It affects men far more than women and tends to be a feature of aging, starting with a receding at the temples or forehead, which gradually progresses (though rarely ending in total baldness). Other causes of hair loss include severe illness with high fever, pregnancy and childbirth, shock, stress, damage to the skin (from burns, infection, radiation, chemical injury), skin cancer, chemotherapy, excess of vitamin A, hypothyroidism, and syphilis.

Baldness, or alopecia, is total or partial loss of scalp hair. The condition may be temporary or permanent.

The most common type of alopecia is pattern baldness, a hereditary trait that is expressed more often in males than in females because it depends on the influence of the male hormone testosterone.

Pattern baldness in males extends until only a sparse growth of hair remains on the back and sides of the head. Up to 86 percent of men in the U.S. will experience some pattern balding.

In women, baldness usually extends until only a sparse growth remains across the crown.

Premature baldness may partly result from an imbalance of sex hormones.

Sudden temporary hair loss sometimes occurs as a result of typhoid fever, flu, pneumonia, or stress.

Gradual thinning of the hair may be caused by severe nutritional deficiency, tuberculosis, cancer, and disorders of the thyroid gland or pituitary gland.

Temporary baldness may also be caused by exposure to nuclear radiation or X-rays, or by the internal use of certain anticancer drugs.

Chinese Herbalism
Shou Wu Pian nourishes Liver, Blood, Kidney qi and jing. It is commonly used in China to keep hair from graying.

Hair loss is attributed to Deficient Liver and Kidneys, and specific herbs to address this include wolfberry, mulberry, and fleeceflower root.

Traditional Home and Folk Remedies
Sage tea, drunk and applied externally, will stimulate hair growth.

Nettle tea helps to cleanse the system, and encourages the growth of hair.

Herbalism
Improve circulation to the head with a daily intake of rosemary tea and shoulder stands. (*See page 114.*)

Massage the scalp with infused oil of fenugreek or ginger. (*See page 126.*)

Rinse with nettle vinegar. (*See page 124.*)

Aromatherapy
Lavender, rosemary, sage, cedarwood, patchouli, or ylang ylang can be massaged into the scalp and added to mild unfragranced shampoos. (*See pages 133–157.*)

Homeopathy
Lycopodium, for hair loss after childbirth. (*See page 187.*)

Aurum, for hair loss with headaches and boils breaking out on the scalp. (*See page 169.*)

Phosphoric acid, for hair loss after grief, and with exhaustion.

Arnica, for hair loss starting after injury. (*See page 167.*)

Selenium, for painful scalp and loss of body hair along with hair on head.

Sepia, for hair loss related to menopause and childbirth. (*See page 196.*)

Vitamins and Minerals
Increase your intake of vitamin B-complex (high-dosage tablet, twice daily), choline, inositol, calcium, magnesium, vitamins and minerals in a good supplement. (*See pages 235–238, 255, 241, and 245.*)

BOILS

A boil is a swollen, pus-filled area occurring on the site of an infected hair follicle. The staphylococcus bacterium is usually responsible, but other causes may include eczema, scabies, diabetes, poor personal hygiene, or obesity. A boil begins as a painful red lump, then hardens and forms a yellow head. The most common areas for boils to appear are the back of the neck, the groin, and the armpits. A boil on an eyelash is known as a stye, and where a group of adjacent hair follicles are affected the resultant boil is known as a carbuncle.

Symptoms
- burning, throbbing sensation in and around the affected area
- sensitivity to the slightest touch once pus has formed

TREATMENT
Traditional Home and Folk Remedies
Apply a warm poultice made with figs or honey to the affected area. (*See pages 77 and 87.*)

Soak a sterile cloth with hot thyme tea and hold it over the boil for a time.

A hot cabbage leaf poultice, applied to the area, will help to draw out the infection. (*See page 73.*)

Eat plenty of garlic if you are prone to boils; garlic is cleansing and chronic boils indicate that you may have a high level of toxins in your body. (*See page 70.*)

Herbalism

Drink infusions of thyme or red clover three times daily during attacks. (*See page 122.*)

Drink echinacea two or three times daily to boost the immune system and purify the blood. (*See page 105.*)

Aromatherapy

A warm compress with essential oil of chamomile, lemon, lavender, or thyme will help to bring the boil out.

Homeopathy

Belladonna, for red, tender, new boils. (*See page 168.*)

Hep. sulf., for boils that are sensitive and weep easily. This will also bring the boil to a head. (*See page 183.*)

Gunpowder, for weeping but not painful boils.

Arsenicum, for burning skin aggravated by heat.

COLD SORES

Cold sores are painful fluid-filled blisters which crust over after bursting. They usually appear on the mouth and around the lips or nose, sometimes in clusters. They are caused by viral infection (herpes simplex). The virus is harbored by most people, most of the time, but is most likely to cause problems when the immune system is compromised, dealing with other viral infections (such as a cold), or when one is run down. Cold sores are highly contagious.

> **CAUTION**
> Cold sores are infectious—wash hands carefully after applying any lotion, and use a personal towel.

Symptoms
- pain and soreness from the characteristic crusting blister
- cracking and weeping may occur, particularly if sores are in the comers of the mouth

TREATMENT
Herbalism
St. John's wort tincture, applied immediately, should prevent development of a sore. (*See page 110.*)

Once the cold sore is established, myrrh tincture can be applied sparingly to help dry it up.

Aromatherapy
Bergamot, eucalyptus, and tea tree oils will help to treat the blisters, and should be applied at the first sign of a sore.

Lavender oil will help to heal blisters that erupt.

Homeopathy
Constitutional treatment is best, but the following remedies may help:
- Nat. mur., for deep cracks in the lower lip, dry mouth, and puffy burning cold sores. (*See page 190.*)
- Rhus tox., for mouth and chin sores, and ulcers at the corner of the mouth. (*See page 194.*)
- Sempervivum, for ulcers in the mouth, and bleeding gums; and when the condition is worse at night.
- Capsicum, for cracks at the corners of the mouth.

Vitamins and Minerals
Cold sores tend to crop up when you feel run down, so it is important that you eat healthily and ensure that you get plenty of the following nutrients, which boost immunity:

Wholegrain cereals like brown rice and wholewheat bread, fruit, pulses (beans and lentils), a few nuts and seeds for their vital oils.

A daily multivitamin and multimineral preparation—especially one containing high amounts of the antioxidant nutrients—acts to boost immune activity. (*See page 234.*)

Vitamin C stimulates immunity and is antiviral as well as being anti-fungal. (*See page 238.*)

Acidophilus will encourage the healthy bacteria in your gut, which will help to fight off infections and infestations.

Zinc stimulates the immune system, and acts as an antiviral and antifungal agent. (*See page 249.*)

ABSCESS

An abscess is a pocket of pus which may occur in any bacterially infected area of the body. White blood cells are sent by the body's defense system to attack the bacteria in question and they do so by engulfing them, thereby creating the pus-filled swelling. Dental abscesses (usually around the root of a tooth) are particularly common—and very painful.

Symptoms
- swelling, pain, and discomfort in the affected area
- the abscess and surrounding area may feel hot to the touch
- fever
- nausea
- sweating

TREATMENT

Ayurveda
Kalanchoe may be useful.

Chinese Herbalism
Treatment would address Heat and Fire poison in the Blood.

Externally, use peony flowers or rhubarb ointment. (*See pages 53 and 60.*)

Internally, violet, wild chrysanthemum, dandelion, and golden thread are useful. (*See page 47.*)

Traditional Home and Folk Remedies
Apply a warm fig or honey poultice to the abscess.

Soak a sterile cloth with hot thyme tea and apply.

A hot poultice, made with cabbage leaves, will help to draw out infection. (*See page 73.*)

Herbalism
Drink infusions of thyme or red clover three times daily during attacks. (*See page 122.*)

Drink echinacea two or three times daily to boost the immune system and purify the blood. (*See page 105.*)

Aromatherapy
A warm compress with essential oil of chamomile, lemon, lavender, or thyme will help to bring the abscess out.

Homeopathy
Hep. sulf., for an abscess which is tender, causing sharp pain. (*See page 183.*)

Belladonna, for early stages, where there is tenderness and throbbing pain. (*See page 168.*)

Silicea, for a slow-forming abscess, with swelling, which does not appear to come to a head. (*See page 195.*)

Mercurius, for the early stages, if perspiration is smelly and you are irritable. (*See page 189.*)

To make a warm fig poultice, you can use either lightly roasted fresh figs, or dried figs. Split the fig and mash up the soft, pulpy interior. This can be warmed by adding a little boiling water. Place the mixture on a clean piece of cloth. Use either linen, gauze, or cotton. The whole compress can then be warmed by placing on a hot water bottle. (This is also useful to warm it up again after it cools.) Apply to the skin.

ACNE

Acne is a skin disorder most common among adolescents. It is caused by the hormonal changes at puberty, which lead to an increase in the activity of the sebaceous (oil-producing) glands. Sebaceous glands secrete through pores and hair follicles—which are most abundant on the face and scalp—a fatty lubricant known as sebum. Acne occurs when the pores become clogged with sebum. Blackheads—external plugs formed of sebum and dead cells—may be invaded by bacteria, which cause pus-filled inflammations, or pimples. The overlying skin may become stretched to the point of rupture, resulting in lesions and, in prolonged severe cases, eventual scarring. Sweating can aggravate acne, as do some oral contraceptives, lack of sunlight, poor skin hygiene, face creams, cosmetics, and exercise.

Symptoms
- red spots
- spots may become inflamed and infected, in which case they are extremely painful

Males are more often affected than females, and the condition is not confined to adolescence.

The exact cause of acne is not known, but it is believed to be related both to genetic predisposition and to the increased hormonal activity that occurs during puberty.

In a reaction comparable to allergy, certain foods may increase irritation in susceptible persons.

TREATMENT

Chinese Herbalism

Cai Feng Zhen Zhu an Chuang Wan/Margarite acne pills. This is an excellent remedy for acne. It contains Pearl.

Treatments to clear excess Heat in the Blood and Stomach include chrysanthemum, dandelion, and honeysuckle, with cucumber and watermelon juice applied externally. (*See page 52.*)

Herbalism

A facial steam with chickweed, elderflower, and marigold may be useful for soothing and drawing out infection. (*See pages 116 and 102.*)

Take echinacea, burdock root, cleavers, or yellow dock, sipped three times daily as a decoction, to cleanse the system and fight infection. (*See pages 105, 100, and 115.*)

Massage comfrey ointment into any old spots to reduce scarring. (*See page 119.*)

Homeopathy

Treatment should be constitutional, but the following remedies may help:

- Silicea, when there is scarring. (*See page 195.*)
- Ant. tart., for pus-filled pimples. (*See page 164.*)
- Sulfur, for chronic acne, with rough hard skin, and proneness to diarrhea. (*See page 198.*)
- Kali brom., for itchy spots, accompanied by bad dreams.
- Hep. sulf., for large spots resembling boils. (*See page 183.*)
- Pulsatilla, when the spots are aggravated by rich, fatty foods; and if the sufferer dislikes stuffy rooms and is often tearful. (*See page 193.*)

Flower Essences

Gorse is useful for people who have given up hope of finding a cure. (*See page 226.*)

Vitamins and Minerals

Try a multivitamin and mineral supplement which is low in iodine. (*See page 244.*)

Increase intake of vitamin E, vitamin A (as retinol, *see* Vitamin A, caution, *page 234*), zinc. Eliminate processed foods.

IMPETIGO

Impetigo is a highly contagious skin infection caused by bacteria such as streptococci and staphylococci. Infection may follow a break in the skin or occur secondarily to dermatitis, insect bites, and fungus infections. The skin reddens and small, fluid-filled blisters appear on the surface. The blisters tend to burst, leaving moist, weeping areas underneath. The released fluid dries to leave honey-colored crusts on the skin. The infected area may spread at the edges, or another patch may develop nearby. In severe cases there may be swelling of the lymph nodes in the face or neck, accompanied by fever. Itching is common and scratching can spread the infection. It usually first appears around the mouth and nose, but can spread rapidly if other parts of the body are touched after touching a blister. It can be passed on to others by direct contact or by sharing towels. Impetigo occurs most commonly (although not exclusively) in children, particularly in hot, humid climates. Severe attacks are often attributed to poor standards of personal hygiene.

Symptoms

- reddening of affected areas
- small fluid-filled blisters which often burst and weep, then dry out to form a yellow crust
- itching
- very rarely, a kidney inflammation or blood poisoning may develop

TREATMENT

Traditional Home and Folk Remedies

Dab the area with cider vinegar, as often as possible throughout the day. (*See page 87.*)

Clean the area with fresh cabbage juice two or three times daily. (*See page 73.*)

Honey is a strong antibiotic and can be applied directly to the sores, and taken internally to boost the immune system. (*See page 87.*)

Herbalism

Heartsease can be taken internally or used as a wash to treat impetigo; it is both softening and drying, and can soothe the skin.

Aromatherapy
A few drops of tea tree oil, applied neat to the affected area, will encourage healing and prevent the infection from spreading; it also has immuno-stimulant properties to help your body fight infection. (*See page 148.*)

Homeopathy
Antimonium, for blisters cropping up around the nostrils and mouth. (*See page 164.*)

Arsenicum, for blisters and feelings of exhaustion.

Croton, for blisters around the scrotum.

Vitamins and Minerals
Vitamin A is necessary for healthy skin. (*See page 234.*)

Ensure that you get enough of the B-complex vitamins in your diet. (*See pages 235–238.*)

Vitamin C will help the body to fight infection.

NAIL PROBLEMS

The nail forms a shield at the end of the fingers and toes. The nail itself is transparent, but appears pink because of the blood vessels lying under the skin. The end of the nail is white because of air beneath it. The crescent, also called the lunule, appears white because it does not firmly adhere to the connective tissue. The nail plate consists of dead, cornified cells. Nails grow from between 1/500–1/20in. (0.05–1.2mm.) per week. Fingernails grow faster than toenails, and nails of individual fingers of the same hand grow at different rates. Growth increases during the summer, and is slower in cold climates, and sometimes during illness.

Onycholysis—detachment of the nail from its bed. This may occur as a result of a collection of blood (a hematoma) forming underneath it, most commonly caused by injury. Other possible causes of onycholysis include psoriasis, thyrotoxicosis, and fungus infection. Complete shedding of the nail can lead to a cessation of nail growth.

Paronychia—an infection of the soft tissue around the nail. It is usually the result of repeated minor injury, causing pain, swelling, and inflammation.

Horizontal ridges—these usually indicate an infection in the skin around the nail.

Nail thickening—a feature of psoriasis and fungus infection.

Nail-biting—an anxiety- or boredom-related habit which, in severe cases, may cause damage to the cuticles and even infection.

TREATMENT

Chinese Herbalism
Brittle nails are attributed to the kidneys, and watermelon and nori (seaweed) would be advised.

Aromatherapy
Add a little rosemary oil to a light carrier oil and massage into the base of the finger and toenails to improve circulation to the area. (*See page 154.*)

Use tea tree oil on the affected area for bacterial or fungal infections. (*See page 148.*)

Homeopathy
Antimonium, for brittle, horny nails. (*See page 164.*)

Thuja, for brittle nails with a red base. Also for ingrown toenails. (*See page 200.*)

Graphites, for thick, deformed, brittle, painful, or crumbling nails. (*See page 181.*)

Belladonna, for the early stages of infection (yeast or bacterial). (*See page 168.*)

Vitamins and Minerals
Take zinc, vitamin C, and vitamin B-complex for fungal infections. (*See pages 249, 235–238.*)

White spots are often a sign of a deficiency of zinc or vitamin A. (*See pages 249 and 234.*)

Deformed nails can be caused by deficiency of vitamins A, B-complex, and C, calcium, magnesium, zinc, and essential fatty acids. (*See pages 234–238, 241, 245, and 249.*)

Iron deficiency can lead to nail problems; increase your iron intake. (*See page 243.*)

Fungal infections can be improved by eating live yogurt each day, or taking acidophilus supplements. (*See page 256.*)

EDEMA

Edema is swelling or puffiness of tissues due to fluid retention. It is an obvious physical symptom of a number of disorders including kidney disease, heart failure, and cirrhosis of the liver. Edema may also occur as a result of injury (where the injured blood vessels are made more water-permeable) and changes in hormonal levels (before menstruation, during pregnancy, or through the use of oral contraceptives).

Symptoms
- edema may be accompanied by weight gain and breathing difficulties

TREATMENT

Ayurveda
Hollyhock is a diuretic, and may help ease the condition.

Chinese Herbalism
The problem is thought to be due to excess water and Kidney Deficiency; useful herbs for treatment include ginseng, water plantain, poria, cinnamon twigs, and ephedra. (*See pages 54 and 44.*)

Wu Ling San pills tonify the spleen to move water and resolve edema, particularly edema of the lower abdomen.

Jin Gui Shen Qi Wan tonifies the Kidney Yang to resolve edema, particularly of the lower legs.

In practice, the latter two may be applicable in any particular case.

Traditional Home and Folk Remedies
Evening primrose oil, taken in capsule form daily, can help to prevent water retention.

Swelling can be relieved by eating plenty of fresh apples. (*See page 80.*)

Celery is also a good diuretic, and acts on the kidneys to encourage their action. (*See page 71.*)

Eat fresh grapes to prevent bloating.

Herbalism
Yarrow, dandelion, and uva ursi are natural diuretics, and they can be drunk three times daily, as required.

Aromatherapy
Essential oils of rosemary, lavender, and geranium will help to reduce bloating and discourage depression.

Rub a little cedarwood, fennel, rosemary, or sandalwood oils, blended in a light carrier oil, into the areas most affected, or in a whole body massage to have an overall diuretic effect. (*See pages 133–157.*)

Homeopathy
Arsenicum, when the feet and ankles are swollen, and you feel restless and chilly. (*See page 167.*)

Apis, for swelling accompanying inflammation, with stinging pains that become worse in heat.

Nat. mur., for swelling in hot weather or in hot rooms.

SCABIES

Scabies is an infestation of the skin by the mite Sarcoptes scabiei, or itch mite. The mites burrow in the skin to lay eggs, particularly in the sides of the fingers, the elbows, groin, buttocks, nipples, and penis. The newly hatched mites reach adulthood within 14 days, and they, in turn, mate on the skin, thus perpetuating the infestation. Scabies is extremely infectious and can be transmitted by direct or indirect contact.

Symptoms
- intense itching, particularly at night
- a rash, which may become infected as a result of scratching

TREATMENT

Aromatherapy
Use tea tree or lavender oil on the sores, to heal and prevent itching and inflammation. (*See pages 148 and 147.*)

Rub the whole body with neat lavender oil, and then make a solution of lavender, aspic, and juniper in 4 teaspoons of vodka, and use that daily until symptoms improve.

Homeopathy
Sulfur, given every 10 hours for three or four days, for

the infected or anyone who has been in contact with someone infected.

Psorinum, derived from the scabies mite, may be useful.

> **CAUTION**
> Do not give sulfur to anyone suffering from eczema without the supervision of a homeopath.

CELLULITE

Cellulite, believed to be accumulations of fat under the skin, is recognizable by its characteristic orange peel look. The uneven appearance results from the thickened fat cells, fluids, and toxins. It is far more prevalent among women than men, and is thought to have some links with female hormones. Possible triggers are poor circulation, alcohol, refined sugars, and caffeine, which contribute to the build-up of toxins in the body. Cellulite is not generally recognized as a medical condition by many doctors. Persistent, unsightly fat is often a deposit for toxins, either environmental or dietary. Exercise, skin brushing, massage, and eating as many organic and as few processed foods as possible may help.

Symptoms
- areas of skin with a dimpled orange peel appearance which may be slightly tender
- these patches occur predominantly on the buttocks, hips, thighs, and upper arms

TREATMENT
Traditional Home and Folk Remedies
Eat fresh parsley, which is a good detoxificant and diuretic.

Herbalism
Massage with juniper-infused oil and take a cleansing tea with herbs such as marigold. (*See page 102.*)

Fresh ginger improves circulation in the body; drink an infusion, or chew fresh ginger daily to help reduce the condition. (*See page 126.*)

Juniper berries are cleansing and detoxifying, and chewing them can help prevent and treat cellulite.

Aromatherapy
A blend of geranium and rosemary or grapefruit, juniper or cypress used in massage and skin lotion, or add to the bath and use a loofa to stimulate the tissues.

Rose oil soothes tissues, and affects the liver function, to encourage cleansing. It also strengthen the veins, which helps circulation. Add a little to the bath, or massage some into the area. (*See page 154.*)

Vitamins and Minerals
Avoid cigarettes, caffeine, alcohol, and other toxins, which are believed to build up in the body, and drink plenty of fresh water to flush the system.

> **CAUTION**
> Do not use juniper berries in herbal preparations if you have diabetes, for they lower the blood sugar. Do not eat fresh parsley in pregnancy.

CORNS AND CALLUSES

A callus is a hardened and thickened area of skin occurring as a result of constant friction. The skin cells respond to the friction by reproducing, which results in the characteristic hardening of skin. Calluses generally appear on the fingers and toes, knees, palms of the hands, and soles of the feet. When a callus on a toe joint becomes painful, it is known as a corn. The pain is caused by pressure on nerve endings. Soft corns can appear between the toes. Manual laborers are prone to calluses, which can be permanent, while ill-fitting shoes and high heels can be responsible for calluses on the feet or corns.

TREATMENT
Ayurveda
Place your feet in a basin with 4 tablespoons of mustard seeds and some boiling water to soothe. (*See page 19.*)

Traditional Home and Folk Remedies

Corns can be softened and treated by painting them with fresh lemon juice or vinegar. (*See pages 74 and 87.*)

Apply compresses of fresh garlic to the area.

Aromatherapy

Tea tree is a good oil for skin problems, and has mild analgesic and anti-inflammatory properties, which will help to ease the discomfort of corns and calluses. (*See page 148.*)

Pare the thickening skin away, and apply an emollient cream with rose oil. (*See page 154.*)

Homeopathy

Antimonium is the most effective remedy. (*See page 164.*)

Vitamins and Minerals

Increased intake of vitamins A and E can help to encourage the health of the skin. (*See pages 234 and 239.*)

ATHLETE'S FOOT

Athlete's foot (or tinea pedis) is a fungal infection which attacks the warm, moist areas between the toes, most commonly between the fourth and fifth toes. It is highly infectious, spreading through close physical contact, notoriously in the changing facilities at public swimming baths. Once acquired, athlete's foot is very persistent. It usually affects people with particularly sweaty feet, and those whose personal hygiene is inadequate.

Symptoms

- discomfort and itching in the affected area
- painful cracks in the skin
- peeling skin
- dry and scaly or damp and blistered skin
- unpleasant odor
- in severe cases the toenails may crumble

TREATMENT

Herbalism

Echinacea, marigold, and myrrh tinctures, which are antifungal, can be dabbed on the affected area as often as required. (*See pages 105 and 87.*)

Aromatherapy

A foot bath with tea tree oil, eucalyptus, patchouli, myrrh, and/or lavender is effective as all the oils are soothing and antifungal. Also add to unscented skin lotion.

Homeopathy

Treatment would be constitutional to boost the immune system, but Silicea might be useful. (*See page 195.*)

Vitamins and Minerals

Take extra vitamin C and zinc, to boost immune activity and help fight infection. (*See pages 238 and 249.*)

Apply a little live yogurt to the area daily, for its antifungal properties.

Take acidophilus tablets daily to help restore natural bacteria in the body which help to fight fungal infections.

CHILBLAINS

A chilblain is a circular, raised, red swelling appearing on the fingers or toes during cold weather. It is caused by the narrowing of small arteries in the cold, which restricts the flow of blood. This leads to tissue damage in the area concerned from shortage of oxygen and glucose fuel, and bacteria may also accumulate there.

Symptoms

- pain and itching in the area of skin affected
- swelling and redness

TREATMENT

Chinese Herbalism

Treatment would be aimed at Deficient Yang qi, and useful herbs include cinnamon twigs, red sage, angelica, dried ginger, and aconite root.

Traditional Home and Folk Remedies

Ginger, taken internally as a tea, or chewed (the root), or externally (in the bath) will warm the body, and both prevent and treat chilblains.

A roasted onion poultice can be applied to chilblains to draw the heat to the surface and encourage healing.

A poultice of mustard can be applied to chilblains to warm the area. (*See page 84.*)

Herbalism

Nettle tea, and creams and ointments can be applied to the affected area. Drink an. infusion of nettle. (*See page 124.*)

Improve the general circulation of the body by taking rosemary tea with a pinch of cayenne. (*See pages 114 and 103.*)

Rub a hot oil made with cayenne, pepper or mustard over the chilblain. Do not apply this if the skin is broken; use marigold ointment instead.

When chilblains have caused the skin to break, apply calendula ointment to promote healing. (*See page 102.*)

Aromatherapy

Lemon, lavender, chamomile, cypress, peppermint, or black pepper essential oil can be used in massage, in a bath or foot bath, or dabbed on the affected area.

Homeopathy

Agaricus, for chilblains that burn and itch and are not relieved by cold compresses.

Petroleum, for burning, itching chilblains worsened by damp.

Calcarea, when the chilblains are worse in cold weather, and the patient feels chilly and prone to head sweats. (*See page 171.*)

Pulsatilla, for chilblains that are most painful when the limbs hang down, and which are worsened by warmth. (*See page 193.*)

Vitamins and Minerals

Eat plenty of garlic, and brewer's yeast, which will encourage the healthy functioning of the circulatory system.

Increase your intake of oily fish.

Vitamins C and E will encourage the healthy functioning of the circulatory system.

Vitamin E oil, applied to burst chilblains, will help prevent scarring and encourage healing. (*See page 239.*)

EYE PROBLEMS
GLAUCOMA

Glaucoma results from the pressure of fluid in the eyeball becoming too high. This causes compression and obstruction of the blood vessels which feed the optic nerve, resulting in optic nerve fiber damage and visual disturbances. Untreated, glaucoma leads to blindness, but is usually only found if looked for, say through routine checks. It tends to run in families, and its incidence increases with age.

Symptoms

- acute glaucoma: painful, red eye, hard and tender to touch, possibly with dilated pupil; misting of vision, then severe visual impairment; nausea and/or vomiting; possibly abdominal pain
- a warning sign of acute glaucoma may be a sub-acute attack, usually at night. There will be: visual disturbances such as seeing concentric rings around lights, fogginess of vision, dull aching pain in the eye
- chronic simple glaucoma: slow but progressive loss of peripheral vision which can go unnoticed until the damage is irreversible; loss of central vision follows

TREATMENT

Homeopathy

Belladonna is the prime remedy, and it can be taken every 15 minutes, for up to 10 or 12 doses, as soon as you experience symptoms. This is suitable for chronic simple glaucoma only. (*See page 168.*)

Flower Essences

When symptoms begin, take Rescue Remedy or Emergency Essence, which will calm you and help you to deal with the pain. (*See page 229.*)

Vitamins and Minerals

Avoid excessive quantities of protein in your diet, which can exacerbate or contribute to glaucoma.

Ensure you have an adequate intake of vitamins A, Bl, B12, C, and the minerals chromium and zinc, which can contribute to the health of the eyes.

CATARACT

A cataract is an opacification of the edges of the lens of the
eye which has spread inward to reach the part of the lens
that is directly behind the pupil. It is caused by a coagulation
of the proteins of the lens. Cataracts are often hereditary
or a part of aging, but may also be a feature of Down's
syndrome, diabetes, nutritional deficiencies, severe skin
problems, or long-term use of steroids. Radiation or injury
to the eye can also cause cataracts, and they may be present
at birth as a result of German measles during pregnancy.

Symptoms

- loss of image clarity and blurring, with progressively less
  and less perception of detail; a person with a fully formed
  cataract may only be able to distinguish the presence of
  light and the direction from which it is coming
- a change in the perception of colors
- scattering of light rays caused by the opacity of the
  lens, which can make night driving difficult or even
  dangerous

TREATMENT

Chinese Herbalism

Treatment would address weak Liver and Kidneys
resulting from Deficient Blood. Herbal remedies
might include wolfberry, chrysanthemum flowers,
dendronbrum, rumania.

Homeopathy

See a homeopath for constitutional treatment, or if the
following remedies fail to work after about two months.
Specific remedies, which can be taken three times daily
for up to a week, and then twice daily thereafter include:

Silicea, if your cataract has begun to affect your sight.
(*See page 195.*)

Phosphorus, for a misting sensation. (*See page 192.*)

Calcarea, when circular lines are evident on the lens.
(*See page 171.*)

Vitamins and Minerals

Increase your intake of antioxidants, including vitamins A,
C, and E, and also selenium, which prevent the growth
of cataracts in the eyes. (*See pages 234, 238, 239, and 247.*)

Bioflavonoids will also help in prevention and treatment,
and these can be taken separately or in conjunction with
vitamin C. (*See pages 256 and 238.*)

BLACK EYE

A "black eye" (known medically as a periorbital
hematoma) is the result of blood being released from
veins in the eyelids and surrounding area into the
tissues around the eye. This produces the characteristic
blackish-blue bruising. It is usually caused by a blow to
the eye. The bruising can last from a few days to a month,
and will go through several color changes, usually ending
in pale yellow before fading completely.

Symptoms

- soreness in and around the eye
- pain on pressure
- in severe cases there could be swelling, which may
  make it difficult to open the eye

TREATMENT

Herbalism

Make an infusion of fresh lavender leaves, and wrap it in
a fine handkerchief. Place it on the bruised area when the
leaves have cooled.

Traditional Home and Folk Remedies

Bruise caraway seeds, and heat them with hot, soft bread.
Cool slightly and apply to the bruised area.

A cool witch hazel compress can be applied to the area
to encourage healing. (*See page 78.*)

Place a cold compress on the area, which will
reduce swelling and allow fluid to circulate, which will
facilitate healing.

Aromatherapy

A few drops of calendula, lavender, and marjoram oil can be placed on a cool cloth and applied to the bruise. Avoid the eyelids and the corner of the eye. (*See pages 133–157.*)

Homeopathy

Arnica should be taken as soon as possible after the injury, and continued until the bruising disappears. Follow this with Ledum, which will disperse the swelling. (*See page 186.*)

Aconite is useful in the initial stages, following the blow or trauma to the area. (*See page 163.*)

Flower Essences

Use Rescue Remedy or Emergency Essence cream and lightly dab over the affected area to help the healing process. (*See page 229.*)

Rescue Remedy or Emergency Essence can also be taken internally after the trauma to help you cope with pain and encourage healing. (*See page 229.*)

CONJUNCTIVITIS

Conjunctivitis is an inflammation of the conjunctiva (the mucous membrane that covers the outer layer of the eyeball and lines the eyelids). It is generally caused by either viral or bacterial infection, or by an allergic reaction to substances such as pollen, cosmetics, and solutions used for contact lenses. Either one or both eyes may be affected. Viral conjunctivitis is a common ailment which sometimes occurs in epidemic proportions, spreading rapidly.

Symptoms

- redness and soreness with irritation, dryness, and grittiness of the eyes
- possibly slightly blurred vision
- bacterial conjunctivitis produces a yellow discharge which hardens during sleep, causing stickiness in and around the eye
- viral conjunctivitis produces only minimal discharge
- swollen and puffy eyelids in allergic conjunctivitis, but no discharge

TREATMENT

Ayurveda

Treatment would consist of panchakarma treatment (detoxification), and nasya, together with inhalations and an eyewash. Treatment would be specific to your needs. (*See page 10.*)

Chinese Herbalism

The source of the problem is believed to be Wind Heat in the Liver meridians, and herbal treatment might include bamboo leaves, violets, and chrysanthemum flowers. Boil these together, strain, and use the cool water to bathe the eyes.

Traditional Home and Folk Remedies

Apply cold bread to closed eyes to reduce the inflammation of conjunctivitis, and soothe itching. (*See page 86.*)

Boil fennel seeds to make an eyewash for conjunctivitis and sore, inflamed eyes.

Honey water can be used to cleanse the eye; it acts to destroy any infection, soothe, and encourage healing. (*See page 87.*)

Herbalism

Infusions of the following herbs can be taken internally to ease the condition: echinacea (which boosts the immune system and acts as a natural antibiotic), eyebright, golden seal, sage. (*See pages 105 and 116.*)

Infusions of chamomile, elderflower, eyebright, and golden seal can be applied externally. A tincture of some of these herbs can also be used to make an eyewash. (*See page 116.*)

Aromatherapy

Make a warm compress with a few drops of lavender, chamomile, or rose oil, and apply to the affected area to encourage healing and draw out infection. (*See pages 133–157.*)

Homeopathy

Euphrasia is suitable for burning, itchy eyes. (*See page 179.*)

One or two drops of Euphrasia tincture can also be used to bathe the eyes. (*See page 179.*)

Pulsatilla can be used when there is mucus collecting in the corner of the eyes. (*See page 193.*)

Hep. sulf. will be useful to draw out infection.

STYE

A stye is an abscess occurring around the root of an eyelash, usually caused by staphylococcal bacteria. A collection of pus at the base of the eyelash produces the characteristic small, yellow head. Styes usually last for around seven days, but the infection may spread to adjacent follicles. They tend to occur when general resistance is low.

Symptoms
- redness, soreness, and swelling
- pain and sometimes irritation

TREATMENT

Chinese Herbalism
Anti-inflammatory herbs, and herbs to detoxify and boost the immune system will be appropriate, including the preparation Jin Yin Hua, which acts as an antibiotic to help fight the bacterial infection. (*See page 52.*)

Traditional Home and Folk Remedies
A warm bread poultice applied directly to the stye will help bring out the infection. (*See page 86.*)

Herbalism
Echinacea and poke root will boost the immune system, which is particularly useful if you suffer from recurrent styes. (*See page 105.*)

Chamomile or eyebright can help to reduce swelling. (*See page 116.*)

Marigold tincture can be applied directly to the stye, and taken internally to boost the immune system.

Aromatherapy
A drop of lavender or tea tree oil, on a cotton swab, can be dabbed at the base of the stye. Take care not to let it enter your eyes. (*See pages 147 and 148.*)

Homeopathy
Recurrent styes should be treated constitutionally, and your homeopath will take steps to improve your overall immune response.

Pulsatilla, in the first instance. (*See page 193.*)

If this does not work, try Staphisagria, every hour, for up to 10 doses.

> **CAUTION**
> Recurrent episodes of styes may be an indication of diabetes and should therefore be investigated.

EYESTRAIN

Eyestrain is used to describe any discomfort or distress related to the eyes or seeing. It is not, however, a medical term. The body's response to visual difficulty is to contract the muscles around the eye, and it is this that may cause the sensation of strain. Prolonged and constant use of a VDU system, intense periods of reading, wearing incorrectly prescribed glasses, and working in bad light can all lead to eyestrain, but these things do not necessarily damage the eyes, as is popularly believed.

Symptoms
- feeling of tightness around the eyes
- focusing difficulties
- recurrent headaches, particularly across the forehead and behind the eyes

TREATMENT

Traditional Folk and Home Remedies
A slice of cucumber over tired, strained eyes is invigorating and soothing. (*See page 75.*)

Drink fresh lemon juice, which is restorative. (*See page 74.*)

Roast an apple and apply the pulp to the eye area to relieve inflamed or tired eyes. (*See page 80.*)

The ancient Greeks used fresh white cabbage juice, mixed with a small amount of honey, to relieve sore or inflamed eyes. (*See page 73.*)

Chinese Herbalism

Chinese practitioners believe that eye problems may be due to exhausted Blood, and the following herbs may be useful: wolfberry, mulberry, chrysanthemum flowers, and cassia seed.

Herbalism

Cool compresses of chickweed, eyebright, or marigold should be placed over the eyes and left for 10–15 minutes.

Aromatherapy

A few drops of fennel oil, on a cool compress laid over the eye area, will soothe puffy, inflamed eyes. (*See page 145.*)

Add 1 drop of lemon or rose aromatherapy oil to 2 tablespoons of carrier oil, and massage into the temples and the bony areas around the eyes (avoid the immediate eye area). (*See pages 140 and 154.*)

Homeopathy

The following remedies can be taken up to four times per day for a week. If the symptoms persist, see your homeopath.

Ruta, when eyes feel strained after reading for long periods; also good for a burning sensation. (*See page 194.*)

Arnica, for tired eyes resulting from long periods of driving and looking into the distance. (*See page 167.*)

Nat. mur, when eyes are painful on looking up, down, or sideways. (*See page 190.*)

Vitamins and Minerals

Vitamin A and vitamin B12 are useful if you suffer from periodic or chronic eyestrain. (*See pages 234 and 238.*)

SQUINT

A squint (or strabismus) is a condition in which only one eye focuses on an object of interest. In a divergent squint the other eye looks outward, while in a convergent squint it looks inward. A squint in children may be caused by congenital hypermetropia (long-sightedness), or physical defects in the cornea, lens, retina, nerves, and muscles of the eye. Acquired in adulthood, a squint is usually indicative of an underlying disease elsewhere in the body (possibly encephalitis, meningitis, septicemia, syphilis, or various brain disorders).

Symptoms

- in addition to the characteristic squint appearance adults may also experience double vision

---

CAUTION
If you begin to experience double vision, see your physician.

TREATMENT

Ayurveda

A practitioner would address any imbalances resulting in eye problems, and treatment would be specific to your needs. Balancing the three doshas through herbs and other treatments would be a likely course of treatment. (*See page 10.*)

Homeopathy

Constitutional homeopathic treatment would be accompanied by exercise for the eye.

Specific remedies, to be taken three times daily for up to 14 days, include Gelsemium. (*See page 180.*) If this does not work, try Alumina.

TWITCHING EYELIDS

Twitching (fasciculation) of the eyelids is caused by a brief, involuntary contraction of the flat muscle around the eye. It is a very common phenomenon and is only a cause for concern if it is very persistent, as it may then be an indication of nerve disease. A twitch or tic commonly affecting adults is blepharospasm, in which there is spasmodic closure of one or both eyes. This is usually a feature of psychological disturbance and may be associated with other bodily tics.

TREATMENT

Traditional Home and Folk Remedies

Place a slice of cucumber on the eyes to soothe and reduce irritation. (*See page 75.*)

Herbalism

Because most twitches are caused by tension or tiredness, relaxing herbs would be prescribed, including chamomile, lavender, and vervain. Drink as infusions.

Aromatherapy

A few drops of lavender or marjoram oil added to the bath will relax and rejuvenate. (*See pages 147 and 151.*)

Try a few drops of chamomile or rose oil on a cool compress, placed over the eye area, and massage a drop in a light carrier oil into the muscles surrounding the eye area. Avoid the immediate eye area. (*See pages 137 and 154.*)

Homeopathy

Constitutional treatment would be most appropriate, but the following remedies can be taken every 4 hours for up to six doses:

Pulsatilla, for twitching accompanied by inflammation of the eye. (*See page 193.*)

Codeinum, for twitching eyelids.

Flower Essences

Vervain is useful for those whose overenthusiasm is putting them under stress. (*See page 226.*)

Hornbeam, for exhaustion and the feeling of being in a rut. (*See page 212.*)

Impatiens, for irritability and a rushed lifestyle. (*See page 218.*)

EAR PROBLEMS

TINNITUS

Tinnitus is a hissing, buzzing, whistling, or ringing sound experienced in the ear (one or both). It is usually continuous, but the sufferer's awareness of it is intermittent.

Tinnitus is related to damage to the hair cells of the inner ear. Persistent tinnitus is usually associated with a degree of hearing loss, and can be triggered by explosions or prolonged loud noise. It may also be a symptom of colds and flu, ear infections and excessive ear wax, brain or head injuries, Ménière's disease, and otosclerosis.

The ringing, roaring, clicking, or hissing sounds heard with tinnitus are actually warning signs of such things as infection, Ménière's disease, and otosclerosis. They may also be caused by hard masses of wax in the ear; a stuffy nose; such drugs as quinine, antibiotics, aspirin, and alcohol; and excessive smoking.

Sensorineural hearing loss is often accompanied by ear noise, or tinnitus. Because the inner ear has no pain fibers, damage is not accompanied by pain.

More people lose hearing today than in past years; the average pop concert or stereo headset can impair hearing in less than a half-hour.

About 30 percent of adults over 65 have hearing loss, and as much as one-third of cases are associated with exposure to loud noise.

TREATMENT

Chinese Herbalism

A herbalist might treat a Blood Deficiency, and use the following herbs: Shu di Huang and Tu Su Zi, which are commonly used in the treatment of tinnitus. (*See page 48.*)

Herbalism

For tinnitus caused by blood congestion or pressure in the head, try black cohosh. Use 10–30 drops of tincture diluted in water, and drink it as often as necessary.

Feverfew is effective for tinnitus, and taken daily may prevent attacks. (*See page 120.*)

Tinnitus caused by poor circulation or high blood pressure may respond to treatment with hawthorn. (*See page 104.*)

Aromatherapy

Use oils which increase the circulation, including rosemary, cypress, lemon, and rose. Massage of the head, neck, and chest using these oils may help, as will one or more in a blend heated in a vaporizer or burner. (*See pages 133–157.*)

Homeopathy
Treatment should be constitutional, but some remedies which may help include:

Salicylic acid, for roaring in the ears, dizziness, and deafness.

China sulf., for any buzzing, hissing, or singing sounds in the ears.

Kali iod., for ringing in the ears and no other obvious symptoms.

Vitamins and Minerals
Try increasing the following nutrients in your diet: magnesium, potassium, and manganese. Deficiency of these has been linked with tinnitus. (*See pages 245–246.*)

Eat plenty of food rich in vitamins A and C, and bioflavonoids, which are very good for circulation. (*See pages 234 and 238.*)

MIDDLE EAR INFECTION (OTITIS MEDIA)

The most common ear infections are middle ear infections (otitis media). The middle ear is located behind the eardrum and connected to the throat by the Eustachian tube. Bacteria may therefore travel to the middle ear from the throat when infections occur there, or they may also enter through a perforation in the eardrum. The eardrum may be perforated, or ruptured, by shattering blasts or sharp objects, as well as by infection. Very loud noises, a change in pressure (such as when flying), and violent sneezing while suffering an ear infection may also, in some cases, cause perforation.

Young children, with shorter and straighter Eustachian tubes than adults, are especially prone to middle ear infections. The tendency is also apparently inherited. Chronic infections may also be associated with allergies, tuberculosis, measles, and other diseases.

Symptoms
- intense pain
- fever
- in severe cases pressure in the middle ear builds up to such an extent that the eardrum perforates in order to release the discharge, this may lead to external ear infection and a degree of temporary or permanent hearing loss

> **CAUTION**
> Always consult your physician if the ear drum "bursts" or perforates, as it can lead to serious complications, including deafness and, in some cases, meningitis.

TREATMENT
Ayurveda
Purified and concentrated extracts of garlic might be used to control and treat infection. (*See page 16.*)

Panchakarma would be appropriate. (*See page 11.*)

Traditional Home and Folk Remedies
Peel the skin from a bud of garlic, and cut to fit the outside of the ear canal. Wrap in a piece of gauze, heat gently, and insert into the canal. (*See page 70.*)

Herbalism
Mullein oil is a traditional herbal treatment. Place a few drops on a cotton ball and gently place in the ear canal. (*See page 124.*)

Anti-inflammatory and antibacterial herbs include chamomile, echinacea, golden rod, and golden seal, and they can be taken internally or infused and dropped into the ear canal. (*See pages 104 and 105*)

Steep yarrow and pour the warm liquid into the ear canal to soothe and reduce infection. (*See page 97.*)

Aromatherapy
Massage a blend of anti-infectious oils around the ear and down the neck. Suitable oils include lavender, chamomile, and tea tree. (*See pages 147, 137, and 148.*)

Mix a drop of clove oil in a little grapeseed carrier oil and massage around the neck and ear.

Homeopathy

Chronic ear infections should be treated constitutionally. Acute attacks may respond to the following, taken every half-hour for up to 10 doses.

Hep. sulf. may be useful for infection accompanied by sharp pain. (*See page 183.*)

Belladonna, for a throbbing earache with redness around the ear, accompanied by fever. (*See page 168.*)

Aconite, for an attack which comes on suddenly, particularly after exposure to cold. (*See page 163.*)

Pulsatilla, when there is pain, as if the eardrum is being pushed out. (*See page 193.*)

OUTER EAR INFECTION (OTITIS EXTERNA)

An inflammation or infection of the outer ear can cause severe pain, possibly a discharge, and impaired hearing. Such symptoms may be due to a number of factors, such as infection by fungi or bacteria, or a foreign body in the ear. Boils or abscesses lead to a build-up of pus which causes severe pain in the ear.

Reasons for infection include:

Boils often result from infection by staphylococcus bacteria. Infection often occurs through a break in the skin caused by scratching an itch, or may enter the ear from polluted water. Boils are painful, the ear may swell, and infection may spread to the inner ear.

Fungus infections are sometimes called "swimmer's ear" because dampness is favorable to fungal growth.

Damage from constant probing of the ear may lead to bacterial or fungal infection or inflammation.

An allergic reaction to a foreign body can cause an ear infection.

TREATMENT

Traditional Home and Folk Remedies

A roasted onion can be applied to the outer ear canal (hot) to draw out infection and to ease the pain. (*See page 70.*)

A bread poultice (*see Earache, page 303*) will reduce inflammation and pain. (*See page 86.*)

Warm a little garlic oil, saturate a cotton bud, and place in the ear canal to draw out infection. (*See page 70.*)

Herbalism

Mullein oil will reduce external pain and encourage healing. St. John's wort oil exerts a similar beneficial effect. (*See pages 124 and 110.*)

Wash the ear canal with a warm infusion of herbs such as chamomile, elderflower, or golden seal, which are antiseptic. (*See pages 104 and 116.*)

Aromatherapy

Apply a little tea tree oil to the end of a cotton bud and gently swab the outer ear canal, and the ear itself. (*See page 148.*)

Warm some marjoram oil in grapeseed oil, massage around the ear and dab a few drops into the ear canal. Apply a little more to a cotton ball and insert into the ear and leave overnight. This will reduce pain and encourage healing. (*See page 151.*)

Homeopathy

Belladonna, for pain and redness. (*See page 168.*)

Mercurius, when there is a smelly discharge. (*See page 189.*)

Aconite, for an acute infection characterized by sharp shooting pains. (*See page 163.*)

Flower Essences

Take Rescue Remedy or Emergency Essence to ease symptoms and induce calm. (*See page 229.*)

LABYRINTHITIS (OTITIS INTERNA)

Labyrinthitis (otitis interna) is an inflammation of the part of the inner ear responsible for balance (the labyrinth). A viral infection is usually the cause of labyrinthitis (possibly in the course of mumps or flu), although it may be the result of infection spreading through the bone from middle ear infection. Infection may also reach the inner ear (via the bloodstream) from somewhere else in the body. Less commonly, a bacterial labyrinthitis results from a head injury. In labyrinthitis, inflammation of the fluid-filled chambers (labyrinth) of the inner ear causes disruption of the individual's sense of balance. As well as vertigo, labyrinthitis may cause nausea, vomiting, nystagmus (abnormal, jerky movements of the eyes), tinnitus, and hearing loss.

> **CAUTION**
> Untreated bacterial labyrinthitis may lead to permanent deafness, or spread to cause meningitis.

Symptoms
• a spinning sensation
• unsteadiness, faintness, and possibly falling
• partial deafness
• ringing or hissing in the ears (see Tinnitus, page 299)

TREATMENT
Chinese Herbalism
Fresh ginger, cinnamon twigs, and peppermint will help with the dizziness. (See page 44.)
Mulberry can be taken to nourish the Blood.

Herbalism
Treatment to boost the immune system, including echinacea, would be appropriate. (See page 105.)
Ginger root, candied or chewed raw, will help to ease the nausea. (See page 126.)
Try Chinese angelica, which can restore energy, stimulate white blood cells and the formation of antibodies to fight infection. (See page 100.)
Licorice helps recovery, stimulating formation and efficiency of white blood cells and antibodies.

Homeopathy
Conium, for dizziness which worsens when lying down.
Belladonna, for a feeling of fullness in the ear, worsened by moving around. (See page 168.)

Nat. mur., for symptoms accompanied by a headache and sometimes by constipation. (See page 190.)
Phosphorus, when dizziness is made worse by looking down. (See page 192.)
Gelsemium, when you feel weak and trembling.
Calcarea, when an attack of dizziness is made worse by looking up. (See page 171.)

GLUE EAR

Glue ear is a persistent condition in children in which there is a build-up of sticky fluid in the middle ear. It may be caused by chronic nose or throat infection, but can also be due to allergies or exposure to draughts. It may also be associated with chronically enlarged tonsils and adenoids, causing Eustachian tube obstruction. Glue ear does not cause any pain but does impair normal hearing. This in turn can lead to other problems, such as falling behind in class, since hearing is essential for speech development and learning.

> **CAUTION**
> Severe inattention among children under two years could well be due to partial deafness caused by glue ear. It is essential that this is investigated in order to avoid long-term speech, comprehension, and intellectual impairment.

Symptoms
• hearing impairment

TREATMENT
Chinese Herbalism
Herbs to reduce inflammation and mucus (phlegm) would be Sheng di Huang or Chinese senega root/Polygala. (See pages 59 and 56.)

Traditional Home and Folk Remedies
Drink lemon and honey or cider vinegar to clear the mucus and to strengthen the immune system.

Herbalism

Clean away discharge with a warm infusion of herbs such as chamomile or golden seal, which are antiseptic. (*See page 104.*)

Herbal remedies to boost the immune system include chamomile, echinacea, peppermint, and wild indigo. (*See pages 104 and 111.*)

Herbs to help clear the catarrh include elderflowers, euphrasia, golden rod, and hyssop. (*See page 116.*)

Herbs which are able to reduce catarrh include golden rod, ground ivy, and elderflower. (*See page 116.*)

Aromatherapy

Dilute essential oils of lavender, chamomile, eucalyptus, or rosewood in a light carrier oil. Warm and massage around the ear and neck. (*See pages 133–157.*)

Homeopathy

Kali mur., when there are cracking sounds in the affected ear, accompanied by swollen glands in the neck.

Lycopodium, when there is deafness and a roaring sound is experienced in the affected ear. (*See page 187.*)

Pulsatilla, for a full feeling in the ear, and weepiness. Mercurius, when there is thick, smelly discharge.

Vitamins and Minerals

Chronic infection can be caused by a build-up of catarrh (*see page 305*). Reduce consumption of dairy produce and any other possible allergens, including wheat.

Take cod liver oil and vitamin C to give a boost to the immune system. (*See pages 254 and 238.*)

EARACHE

See Middle Ear Infections, *page 300.*

EAR WAX

Ear wax is a sticky, fatty secretion produced by the glands in the outer ear to protect the eardrum by trapping dust and small objects. Normal soft wax is disposed of naturally by the ear, but hard or dried wax accumulates. An excess of ear wax obstructs the ear canal, and the blockage may be worsened by swimming or bathing since the wax absorbs water.

Symptoms

- a sensation of fullness or aching in the ear
- partial hearing loss caused by inflammation in the ear canal

TREATMENT

Chinese Herbalism

Drop a little warmed almond oil into the ear to soften the wax, making it easier to remove.

Traditional Home and Folk Remedies

A little warmed garlic oil, dropped into the ear, will soften the wax and occasionally dislodge it. (*See page 70.*)

Use an ear candle (available from health stores) to heat and draw out excess wax.

Herbalism

Make a warm infusion of chamomile, elderflowers, or marigold, or put a few drops of the tincture into some warm water. Using a dropper, place the liquid in the ear canal and stop with a cotton ball. Repeat several nights running until the wax has softened and is absorbed by the cotton. (*See pages 104, 116, and 102.*)

Aromatherapy

Put a few drops of warm chamomile oil, blended in a light carrier oil, into the ear canal and block gently with a cotton ball. Repeat until wax has softened.

Homeopathy

Causticum, when there is a build-up of wax with some related loss of hearing. (*See page 174.*)

> **CAUTION**
> Constant prodding or cleaning of the ear can lead to excessive ear wax production.

NASAL PROBLEMS
SINUSITIS

Sinusitis is an inflammation of the sinuses—the air-filled cavities located in the bones around the nose. When this occurs the lining of the sinuses swells, causing a blockage in the channel that drains them. A build-up of mucus discharge results, creating intense pressure and pain. Sinusitis usually develops as a complication of a viral infection such as a cold, but pollution or tobacco can also be triggers. Severe symptoms should be referred to your physician.

Symptoms
- nasal congestion with thick, stretchy mucus
- nosebleeds and sneezing
- loss of sense of smell
- headache with a sensation of pressure in and around the head
- severe pain around the eyes and cheeks (particularly on bending down), sometimes feeling like toothache

More than 50 percent of cases are caused by bacterial infection.

In one U.S. study, 50 percent of sufferers had an immune-system problem.

10 percent of all cases are caused by dental problems.

The proximity of the paranasal sinuses to the brain makes sinus infections potentially dangerous.

Inflammation of the sinuses may develop from an allergy or from bacteria introduced through the nasal channels, causing an infection accompanied by pain and tenderness.

Chronic sinusitis may result from either form or a combination of both.

Maxillary sinusitis can result from a cold or can be caused by swimming in contaminated water.

Rarely, extraction of a molar tooth will break the floor of the maxillary sinus, leaving an opening for bacteria to enter and cause infection.

Frontal and ethmoid sinusitis share symptoms of localized headache, surface tenderness, and, occasionally, swelling of the eyelids.

Sphenoid sinusitis can cause blurred vision because of the proximity of this sinus to the optic nerves.

TREATMENT
Ayurveda
Treatment will involve the elimination of kapha with nasya (inhalation of oils). Herbal treatment may be prescribed, including coriander for sinus problems and related headaches. Detoxification will be appropriate. (*See page 10.*)

Chinese Herbalism
Bi Yan Pian pills are very good for sinusitis, especially with sticky yellow nasal discharge, which is hard to get out.

A herbal prescription of Cang er Zi San, when there is lots of green nasal discharge, headache and pain.

Xin Yi San, when there is lots of clear or white nasal discharge, nasal congestion, and pain.

Peppermint, honeysuckle, tangerine peel, and zanthium fruit may all be useful. (*See pages 52 and 45.*)

Traditional Home and Folk Remedies
Peppermint is antispasmodic and decongestant. Infuse some fresh or dried leaves in a bowl of boiling water, and inhale the steam.

Combine the juice of a fresh peeled and pulped horseradish root with the juice of two or three lemons, and take a half-teaspoon between meals. Use for several months until the mucus in the sinus clears. (*See pages 71 and 74.*)

Herbalism
Elderflower is excellent for catarrh and sinusitis. Drink an infusion as required to reduce symptoms and encourage healing. (*See page 116.*)

Drink an infusion of golden seal every two hours during an acute attack.

Aromatherapy
Try steam inhalations of lavender, eucalyptus, and tea tree, which are anticatarrhal and antibacterial. Lavender in particular will act as an anti-inflammatory and ease any painful symptoms. (*See pages 147, 145, and 148.*)

Homeopathy
Kali bich. is the main remedy, particularly for thick, sticky mucus that accumulates in the throat, and which is difficult to clear. (*See page 185.*)

Try Hep. sulf. if Kali bich. does not help. (*See page 183.*)

Pulsatilla, for sinusitis accompanied by weepiness and pain above the eyes. (*See page 193.*)

Vitamins and Minerals
Many cases are caused by food allergy or intolerance. See a practitioner if you suspect this is the cause.

> **CAUTION**
> Golden seal is not appropriate for people with high blood pressure, or for pregnant women.

CATARRH

Catarrh is the term used to describe the overproduction of thick phlegm by the mucous membranes of the air passages to the lungs, the larynx, the nose, and sinuses. Cells which produce and secrete a watery mucus are present in the mucous membranes, which line the passages, and they are composed of large, thin-walled veins whose blood supply serves to warm incoming air. Inflammation of the membranes as a result of a cold or flu is the usual cause, but other triggers include smoking, inhalation of dust, chronic sinusitis, upper respiratory tract infection, and allergy. A series of colds in close succession may lead to chronic catarrh. Complementary therapists believe that chronic catarrh that is not obviously due to viral or bacterial infection, allergy, chemical irritants, or dry air (all of which irritate or inflame the mucous membranes) is a symptom of general toxicity of the body—catarrh is the body's attempt to rid itself of toxins that are not being adequately dealt with by the liver, or properly excreted by the kidneys, bowels, and skin.

Symptoms
- blocked, possibly painful nose, or excessively runny nose
- cough with phlegm
- earache
- ulcers may develop on the septum (the bone that separates the nostrils)
- possibly nosebleeds

TREATMENT

Ayurveda
Coriander can help to relieve sinus problems and prevent the build-up of catarrh. Brown the seeds and boil them in water with root ginger. Boil until the liquid is reduced and drink (with a little honey) as required. (*See page 24.*)

Chinese Herbalism
Drink ginger or sage tea, and drink onion water with a pinch of cayenne pepper.

Traditional Home and Folk Remedies
Peppercorns will help to clear catarrh. Chew one at a time, followed by a little hot water, and continue until the symptoms have gone. (*See page 83.*)

Eating either raw or cooked onions helps to purge stubborn catarrh. (*See page 70.*)

Try a drop of fresh lemon in each nostril—slightly painful, but enormously powerful! (*See page 74.*)

Mustard powder can be added to a foot bath to help decongest nasal passages and clear catarrh. (*See page 84.*)

Herbalism
Herbs such as golden rod, elderflower, and eyebright are anti-catarrhal and astringent. When catarrh is accompanied by infection, supplement with echinacea and garlic. (*See pages 116, 105, and 98.*)

Poke root is a good tonic and acts to prevent and reduce catarrh.

Aromatherapy
Thyme and eucalyptus oils may be inhaled to ease symptoms, and it is a good idea to keep niaouli by the bed, as it can help you to sleep. (*See pages 133–157.*)

Many oils are decongestant and expectorant, including chamomile, hyssop, mint, niaouli, pine, and clary sage. Rub into the chest and temples in a light carrier oil, or place several drops in a bowl of boiling water and inhale. (*See pages 133–157.*)

Homeopathy
Chronic catarrh should be treated constitutionally, but the following remedies may be helpful:

Arsenicum for thick, yellow discharge which makes the nose and the surrounding area sore. (*See page 167.*)

Pulsatilla, for yellow or green catarrh that is not painful, accompanied by feelings of weepiness. (*See page 193.*)

Nat. mur., for catarrh resembling raw egg white, with a dry nose and the loss of taste and smell. (*See page 190.*)

Calcarea, for yellow and smelly catarrh. (*See page 171.*)

Sulfur, when there are dry scabs inside the nose, causing bleeding, and when the nose is stuffier indoors than outdoors. (*See page 198.*)

Vitamins and Minerals
Increase your intake of vitamin C and zinc, which help to reduce symptoms. (*See pages 238 and 249.*)

If you are prone to chronic catarrh, cut down on intake of dairy produce, which may exacerbate the condition.

It may also be caused by over-consumption of sugar and too many refined carbohydrates.

Ensure that your home is free of dust and avoid smoking.

HAY FEVER

Hay fever (also known as allergic rhinitis) is an allergic reaction to airborne irritants such as grass, tree, or flower pollens. These allergens (and others including dust, animal fur, feathers, spores, plants, and chemicals) trigger a reaction which causes swelling of the nasal membrane and the production of the antibodies which release histamine. It is this chemical substance that is responsible for the characteristic allergic symptoms.

Symptoms
• runny nose, congestion, and sneezing
• red, itchy eyes
• sore throat
• wheezing, which can develop into asthma

TREATMENT
The timing of the symptoms will depend on the type of pollen at fault: tree pollen, grass pollen; and weeds such as nettles, golden rod, and mugwort. In the autumn, spores and mold are likely to cause hay fever.

At least 22 million Americans suffer from hay fever in some form.

Most cases involve some dermatitis (in the form of urticaria or hives), and temporary asthma is common during the hay fever seasons in susceptible people.

German researchers have found that three bananas contain enough magnesium to quell a hay fever attack.

Babies born in the spring, when more pollen is in the air, are more likely to develop hay fever later in life.

Chinese Herbalism
Bi Yan Pian/Nose inflammation pills, for Wind Cold or Wind Heat to the face; sneezing, itchy eyes, facial congestion and sinus pain, acute and chronic rhinitis, and nasal allergies.

A herbal prescription of Yu Ping Feng San/Jade screen helps prevent hay fever, and guards against allergies.

Cang er Zi Tang/ Xanthium powder, for allergic rhinitis with a thickened yellow catarrh or a blocked nose.

Traditional Home and Folk Remedies
A teaspoon of local honey, before and during the season, helps many people. (*See page 87.*)

Eat plenty of fresh garlic to boost the immune system, and to act as an anticatarrhal agent. (*See page 70.*)

Herbalism
Strengthen resistance with a tea of elderflowers and yarrow for some weeks before the pollen season starts.

Soothe itchy eyes with an elderflower, eyebright, or chamomile compress. Eyebright tea or capsules will relieve symptoms.

Aromatherapy
Chamomile in the bath and in massage will help to ease symptoms. (*See page 137.*)

Steam or dry inhalations of lavender and/or eucalyptus can help for sneezing and runny nose. Also use in the bath. (*See pages 147 and 145.*)

Melissa may soothe and calm the allergic reaction.

Homeopathy
Hay fever can be deep-seated and take some time to cure, and treatment should be constitutional. However, there are preventive remedies, including the following:

THE HEALING REMEDIES SOURCEBOOK

Allium, for hay fever where the sufferer has a burning nasal discharge. (*See page 163.*)

Sabadilla, for hay fever with a sore throat.

Arsenicum, when there is a constant need to sneeze.

Euphrasia, when the eyes are itching and red.

Flower Essences

Rescue Remedy or Emergency Essence will help to ease symptoms during an attack, and help to produce a more positive frame of mind. (*See page 229.*)

Vitamins and Minerals

Vitamin C combined with bioflavonoids will act as a natural antihistamine to control symptoms.

Taking extra pantothenic acid may help to relieve hay fever symptoms. (*See page 236.*)

Bee pollen can help prevent allergies when taken for several weeks before the hay fever season. (*See page 256.*)

Royal jelly is also a useful hay fever treatment.

Homeopathy

Aconite, for a sudden nosebleed. (*See page 163.*)

Arnica, for a nosebleed brought on by injury or bruising.

Phosphorus, for a nosebleed brought on by blowing the nose violently. (*See page 192.*)

Rhus tox., for nosebleeds after strenuous exercise.

Lachesis, for nosebleeds occurring in hot weather.

Flower Essences

Rescue Remedy or Emergency Essence will help in cases of emotional distress, and a few drops diluted in water and placed in the nostril may help to encourage the healing process. (*See page 229.*)

> **CAUTION**
> Nosebleeds which do not stop within a couple of hours should be checked by a physician. Do not stem the bleeding too quickly in those suffering from high blood pressure—allow the bleeding to continue for 10 minutes before taking action.

NOSEBLEEDS

Nosebleeds are very common, resulting either from persistent probing, an injury, infection of the mucous membrane, or from drying and crusting. Injury or infection which damages the moist lining of the nose can quite easily rupture tiny local blood vessels and cause bleeding; more often, bleeding occurs for no apparent reason. There is some association between nosebleeds and high alcohol intake.

TREATMENT

Traditional Home and Folk Remedies

Lemon is a natural styptic. Place a drop in the offending nostril, on the end of a cotton bud. (*See page 74.*)

Aromatherapy

A drop of lavender oil, placed in the nostril on a cotton bud, will encourage healing and help to staunch the flow of blood. (*See page 147.*)

DENTAL PROBLEMS

GINGIVITIS

Gingivitis is inflammation of the gums. It may sometimes occur as a result of infection or ill-fitting dentures, but most usually it is caused by an accumulation of plaque and impacted food around and under the gums. Left untreated, gingivitis may lead to loosening of the affected tooth (periodontitis) through damage to the membrane securing it. It is a very common problem, particularly during pregnancy. Gingivitis may also result from systemic disorders such as vitamin C deficiency (scurvy) and endocrine disturbances (diabetes mellitus). Prevention and treatment include good oral hygiene and control or correction of local and systemic factors. The incidence of gingivitis appears to increase with age: at 10 years old, 15 percent of the U.S. population suffer; by the age of 50, more than 50 percent have gingivitis. A blood test can now detect gum disease six months before symptoms set in.

TREATMENT

Traditional Home and Folk Remedies
Peach pit tea is useful for mouth infections. Rinse your mouth with the hot tea three times a day.

Herbalism
Depending on the problem, some herbs, such as myrrh, are highly astringent and antiseptic, and may be useful locally. Other treatments may be used internally to increase the patient's resistance.

Golden seal can make an effective poultice, and will treat any infection.

Comfrey mouthwash will help to heal mouth abrasions, and reduce swelling and bleeding. (*See page 119.*)

Homeopathy
Gingivitis may be treated homeopathically. One of the following specific remedies may be taken every 4 hours for up to three days:

Mercurius, when the gums are spongy and the breath smells bad. (*See page 189.*)

Kreosotum, when the gums are red, inflamed, and swollen, and bleed easily, with the roots of the teeth exposed.

Nat. mur., when gums bleed easily, there are ulcers and a taste of pus in the mouth, accompanied by sensitive teeth. (*See page 190.*)

Phosphorus, for gums which bleed easily when touched, gaps between teeth and gums. (*See page 192.*)

Silicea, for painful, swollen gums, very sensitive to cold, and which bleed easily. (*See page 195.*)

Abscesses generally seem to respond well to Hep. sulf., Belladonna, Silicea, or Mercurius. (*See pages 183, 168, 195, and 189.*)

Vitamins and Minerals
Apart from a visit to a dental hygienist, followed by daily brushing and flossing, a healthy diet will promote healthy gums.

Vitamin C is important for the production of collagen. Most tissues in the body are made from this. (*See page 238.*)

Co-enzyme Q10 supplements have been found beneficial in some cases of gum disease.

Symptoms
- swollen and tender gums which bleed easily after brushing
- halitosis (bad breath) if areas of tissue death occur
- possibly earache from referred pain

TOOTHACHE

Aching or pain in a tooth is generally a result of tooth decay (or "caries"). When the hard enamel of the tooth is damaged, this allows infecting organisms to enter the tooth, which results in inflammation and pain. If a tooth is sensitive to heat, cold, or sweet things, or gives pain lasting for more than a few minutes, nerves in the tooth may be inflamed due to advanced decay. If pain is absent, except when you bite, your tooth or filling may be broken. In either case, it is recommended that you see your dentist within 48 hours. Toothache after a filling is not unusual, on contact with cold air or drinks.

Dental caries is a bacterially caused destruction of the enamel and dentine of the tooth. If untreated, it leads to an infection of the dental pulp and an abscess of the apex of the tooth. The bacteria produce both acid and enzymes to break down the tooth. Sweet foods that stick to the tooth increase the activity of the bacteria. Saliva tends to protect against caries, so decreased saliva flow usually increases caries. Tooth shape and hereditary factors also determine susceptibility to the disease.

TREATMENT

Ayurveda
Crush a clove of garlic and apply to the tooth. (*See page 16.*)

Dip a small cotton ball into cinnamon oil and apply to the affected area. (*See page 23.*)

Chinese Herbalism
Treatment would address Heat in the Stomach, and decayed or damaged teeth.

Gypsum and ginseng might be used to relieve heat.

Herbalism

A herbalist might recommend tinctures of echinacea or myrrh to encourage healing and reduce the risk of infection. (*See page 105.*)

Cayenne can act as a local anesthetic for painful teeth and gums. (*See page 103.*)

Fennel may be applied to the cheek in the form of a poultice, which will reduce inflammation and ease symptoms. (*See page 107.*)

Aromatherapy

Peppermint or clove oils can be applied directly to the area to act as a natural analgesic. (*See page 150.*)

Oil of coriander will reduce inflammation and pain. (*See page 142.*)

Rub a little lavender oil on to the face and jaw to ease pain and distress. (*See page 147.*)

Homeopathy

Chamomilla, when there is unbearable pain, made worse by cold air, or warm food and drinks. (*See page 188.*)

Mercurius, for tender spongy gums which bleed easily, and when there is great thirst and shooting pains.

Apis, when gums feel tight and swollen, and the toothache burns and stings. (*See page 165.*)

Staphisagria, for severe toothache made worse by cold air, food, and pressure, and where the cheeks are red and swollen.

Plantago, for nervy teeth, aggravated by cold air and pressure, but which are better on eating.

Belladonna, for throbbing pain and a dry mouth.

Aconite, when pain comes on quickly. (*See page 163.*)

Arnica, for pain after a filling or an extraction.

Flower Essences

Rescue Remedy or Emergency Essence can be applied to the affected area, and taken internally to reduce pain and encourage healing. (*See page 229.*)

CAUTION

Toothache is an indication of an underlying problem, which should be investigated by a dentist immediately.

TOOTH ABSCESS

In cases of badly neglected decay, infection may gain access to the root canal of the affected tooth or teeth. Inflammation of the tissues around the root causes tissue destruction and the collection of pus, forming an abscess. A tooth abscess may spread sideways under the gum to form what is known as a gumboil, which may open, giving relief from pain. Plaque re-forms within 24–48 hours of brushing, so regular brushing is essential to prevent decay. Some research shows that allergy sufferers—whose immune activity is heightened—have fewer cases of tooth decay. Periodontal disease is the second most common infectious ailment in the U.S.

Symptoms

- intense pain, which may be intermittent, or continuous and throbbing
- increased pain on biting or chewing
- swelling and inflammation of the surrounding gum
- in severe cases there may be fever

TREATMENT

Traditional Home and Folk Remedies

Break the large ridges of a cabbage, heat gently, and apply to the abscessed tooth. (*See page 73.*)

Split a fig and heat it. Apply to the abscessed tooth.

Rinse your mouth with apple cider vinegar to reduce inflammation and infection. (*See page 87.*)

Chew fresh sage leaves or garlic, for antiseptic effect. (*See page 70.*)

Herbalism

Comfrey mouthwash or ointment will help to heal and draw out the infection. (*See page 119.*)

Clove oil will reduce inflammation and ease the pain.

A hot garlic compress, applied to the area, will help to draw out infection and encourage healing. (*See page 98.*)

A tincture of myrrh can be used as an antiseptic and healing mouthwash.

Aromatherapy

Dab on some clove oil, or suck a clove, for its analgesic and antiseptic properties.

Make a gargle containing a few drops of antiseptic oils, such as chamomile, clove, lemongrass, or niaouli. (*See pages 133–157.*)

Homeopathy
Mercurius, where there is copious saliva and the gums are spongy. (*See page 189.*)

Gunpowder, for the discharge of pus from boils on the gums.

Hypericum and Calendula, used in solution as a mouthwash. (*See pages 184 and 172.*)

Belladonna, at the first hint of an abscess.

Hep. sulf., when the abscess is in place. (*See page 183.*)

DENTAL DISCOMFORT FOLLOWING TREATMENT

Discomfort following dental treatment is usually caused by injury (perhaps to a nerve) or bruising around the tooth that has been worked on. This may occur immediately after treatment, or pain may follow initial discomfort after an anesthetic has worn off. There may also be some blood loss. Persistent pain following treatment may signal infection.

TREATMENT
Traditional Home and Folk Remedies
Oil of clove or macerated cloves can be applied to the area to prevent infection, reduce the inflammation and prevent discomfort. (*See page 76.*)

Homeopathy
Arnica should be taken immediately after treatment, every hour for up to 10 doses. (*See page 163.*)

Ruta, for infections after teeth have been removed. (*See page 194.*)

Phosphorus, for bleeding after a tooth has been extracted. Take every 10 minutes for 1 hour. (*See page 192.*)

Hypericum, for pain occurring after treatment. (*See page 184.*)

Ledum, for pain after an injection. (*See page 186.*)

Flower Essences
Rescue Remedy or Emergency Essence will help to reduce the effects of trauma, and encourage the healing process.

GRINDING OF TEETH

Habitual grinding or clenching of the teeth is known as bruxism. It is usually performed unconsciously, but is audible to others. It is common among children and the elderly, and often occurs during sleep. In severe cases the enamel of the teeth may be worn away. There may be some links with anxiety and with alcohol consumption.

TREATMENT
Ayurveda
An Ayurvedic medical practitioner would balance the tri-doshas, and use panchakarma for balancing the vatha. (*See page 10.*)

Chinese Herbalism
A Chinese herbalist might suggest ginseng, Chinese angelica, and white peony root with thorowax root for relaxation. Treatment would be designed to strengthen the Spleen and enliven Liver qi. (*See page 35.*)

Traditional Home and Folk Remedies
Oats contain thiamine and pantothenic acid, which are gentle nerve tonics. (*See page 72.*)

Herbalism
Herbal remedies would be used to calm the nervous system and to relax you. Skullcap and valerian are useful herbs, blended together for best effect. Drink as a tea three times a day while suffering the symptoms. (*See pages 118 and 123.*)

Lady's slipper and limeflowers may ease anxiety and tension that may exacerbate the condition. (*See page 121.*)

Aromatherapy
A relaxing blend of essential oils of lavender, geranium, and bergamot in sweet almond oil or peach kernel oil may be added to the bath to calm nerves and prevent attacks. (*See pages 133–157.*)

Homeopathy

Constitutional treatment will be appropriate if there are emotional causes, but some of the following remedies may be useful:

Arsenicum, for grinding of teeth during sleep, especially between midnight and 2 or 3a.m. (*See page 167.*)

Zinc, when the gums bleed and teeth become loose.

Phytolacca, when there is an overwhelming urge to clench the teeth.

Flower Essences

Remedies would be useful if there is an emotional cause underlying the condition. (*See page 204.*)

Elm, for anxiety accompanying a feeling of being unable to cope. (*See page 226.*)

Red chestnut, for anxiety over the welfare of others.

Aspen, for anxiety for no apparent reason.

FEAR OF DENTAL TREATMENT

Fear of dental treatment (dental phobia) is an extremely common phenomenon—some studies show that nearly 80 percent of the U.S. population suffer some feelings of fear about dental treatment. Full-scale phobia is one of the most common types of phobia in both the U.K. and the U.S. Sufferers develop intense feelings of anxiety and panic from an association between dentists and pain and discomfort, despite the fact that modern dental technology has eliminated much of the pain of treatment. Both adults and children may be affected (children are particularly vulnerable if they sense that their parents are frightened).

Most modern dentists are aware of the nervousness affecting many people, and may offer home visits or sedation, anesthetics, hypnosis, and other forms of relaxation.

Symptoms
- rapid pulse
- profuse sweating
- high blood pressure
- trembling
- nausea

TREATMENT

Ayurveda

Lemon or lime may be suggested for dizziness, and individual treatment would be prescribed according to your specific needs. (*See page 10.*)

Chinese Herbalism

A herbalist may prescribe cooling herbs, and Gui Pi Wan, to help with emotional problems.

Ginseng and Chinese angelica and senega root may also be useful. (*See pages 54, 41, and 56.*)

Herbalism

Valerian tea can help to reduce tension. Drink an infusion as required. (*See page 123.*)

Aromatherapy

The effect of certain smells can help to release tension and induce a feeling of calm. Some of the best oils to try are bergamot, chamomile, clary sage, geranium, jasmine, juniper, lavender, marjoram, melissa, and ylang ylang, which are sedative. They can be used in the bath, in massage with a light carrier oil (such as sweet almond), or in a vaporizer. Carry a bottle of diluted oils with you and apply to the temples or pulse points before dental treatment. (*See pages 133–157.*)

Homeopathy

Aconite, for intense fear. Take before and after treatment. (*See page 163.*)

Gelsemium, for shaking and weak legs and knees, and overall apprehension. (*See page 180.*)

Chamomilla, for a child' who throws a tantrum about seeing the dentist. (*See page 188.*)

Flower Essences

Mimulus, for fear of known things. Make a personal remedy, and take a few drops every time you think of the dentist. Take hourly before going for treatment. (*See page 220.*)

Rescue Remedy or Emergency Essence will help to reduce feelings of fear and panic. Take hourly before treatment, and also during treatment. (*See page 229.*)

MOUTH AND THROAT PROBLEMS
SORE THROAT

A sore throat (or pharyngitis) is an inflammation of the pharynx—the area of the throat between the back of the nose and the beginning of the trachea and vocal cords. It is usually caused by infection, which can be viral or bacterial in origin. A sore throat is a feature of illnesses such as tonsillitis and may also signal the onset of glandular fever, flu, or scarlet fever. If scarlet fever is not treated with antibiotics it may lead to rheumatic flu or kidney failure. Inflammation of the throat can also be caused by heavy smoking or drinking, abuse of gargles or mouthwashes, general vitamin deficiency, or food allergy; it can also be a symptom of blood disorders such as anemia. A sore throat will usually resolve itself in a few days, but infection, accompanied by high fever and malaise, may take up to three weeks. Streptococcal sore throat, or strep throat, is an inflammation of the throat and tonsils caused by bacteria and is the most common type of strep infection. Onset is usually sudden and is accompanied by pain, redness, and swelling in throat tissues, pus on the tonsils, fever, headache, and malaise. If left untreated, strep throat can lead to rheumatic fever.

Symptoms
- hoarseness and thirst
- pain, causing difficulty in swallowing
- possibly a burning sensation
- slight fever
- enlarged and tender lymph nodes in the neck
- possibly earache

TREATMENT
Ayurveda
Dasamoola rasayna, an oral syrup, will treat a sore throat.

Crush a piece of root ginger to extract the juice, and add to a tablespoon of honey and 3 tablespoons of lime. Sip four times a day.

Chinese Herbalism
Yin Qiao Jie du Pian pills, for a sore throat accompanied by flu symptoms, swollen lymph nodes, and headaches.

Sang Ju Gan Mao Pian or Sang Ju Yin Pian, for a sore throat with symptoms of cold.

Liu Wei di Huang Wan, for Kidney Yin-Deficient sore throat. Also for chronic dry sore throat, with hot palms and soles, and night sweats.

Honeysuckle tea may be useful. (*See page 52.*)

Traditional Home and Folk Remedies
Gargle with salt water to ease symptoms and reduce inflammation. (*See page 88.*)

Apply an apple cider vinegar compress to the throat to ease symptoms. (*See page 87.*)

Gargle with honey water, which acts to encourage healing and deal with infection. (*See page 87.*)

White cabbage juice is anti-inflammatory and will draw out infection. (*See page 73.*)

A hot honey and lemon drink will reduce symptoms and encourage healing. (*See pages 87 and 74.*)

Herbalism
Eat fresh garlic whenever possible, to absorb its antibacterial and antiviral properties. (*See page 98.*)

A gargle of red sage will help to soothe a sore throat. (*See page 116.*)

Golden seal powder, added to a cup of hot water, can be infused and drunk as required.

Tincture of calendula can be added to a cup of boiled water for a mouthwash to encourage healing and treat infection. (*See page 102.*)

Burdock or comfrey teas will ease the pain. (*See pages 100 and 119.*)

> **CAUTION**
> Do not take golden seal while pregnant.

Aromatherapy
A steam inhalation of benzoin, lavender, or thyme will ease the discomfort and help to treat the infection. (*See pages 133–157.*)

THE HEALING REMEDIES SOURCEBOOK

Massage a little lavender oil, blended in a light carrier oil, into the neck. (*See page 147.*)

Dab the throat with diluted tea tree oil on a cotton bud—it is analgesic and fights infection, which will help to ease symptoms and treat the cause. (*See page 148.*)

Homeopathy

Belladonna, for sore throat accompanied by a red face and fever. (*See page 168.*)

Gelsemium, when swallowing is painful, with weakness, exhaustion, pain in the neck and ears. (*See page 180.*)

Apis, when the pain is worse on the right side of the body, and improves after cold drinks. (*See page 165.*)

Lachesis, when pain is worse on the left side, there is a feeling of constriction, and pain is worse when swallowing saliva but better when swallowing food. (*See page 200.*)

Aconite, for a sore throat that comes on suddenly, with a burning throat and swollen tonsils. (*See page 163.*)

Vitamins and Minerals

* Increase vitamin C intake. (*See page 238.*)
* Suck a zinc lozenge. (*See page 249.*)

TONSILLITIS

Tonsillitis is an inflammation of the tonsils located at the back of the throat. It is generally due to either viral or bacterial infection (often by the streptococcal bacteria), and causes swelling and redness of the tonsils, possibly with white or yellow spots of pus. The adenoids may also become inflamed and infected. Tonsillitis can occur at any time but is particularly common during childhood. In rare cases complications such as quinsy (an abscess behind the tonsil), kidney inflammation, or rheumatic fever may develop.

Symptoms

* swelling and tenderness of the lymph nodes in the neck
* sore throat with pain on swallowing
* headache, earache, and general weakness and malaise
* fever
* bad breath
* constipation

Tonsillitis is more common in children than in adults.

Tonsillitis usually develops suddenly as a result of a streptococcal infection but may also be caused by a viral infection.

In chronic tonsillitis the tonsils tend to flare up in episodes of acute infection, causing scarring that makes them difficult to treat in subsequent attacks.

TREATMENT

Ayurveda

Apply a cloth with mustard oil to the forehead to ease the pain and reduce fever. (*See page 19.*)

Root ginger can be chewed, and mixed with honey and lemon to make a soothing drink.

Chinese Herbalism

Treatment would be aimed at Fire, Poison, Wind, and Heat. Avoid spicy food and drink honeysuckle tea.

Traditional Home and Folk Remedies

Blackcurrant tea or juice (hot) will treat infection and relieve the sore throat.

Drink plenty of hot honey and lemon or honey and apple cider vinegar to fight infection and boost immunity. (*See pages 87, 74, and 87.*)

Herbalism

A red sage gargle will address infection and reduce symptoms. (*See page 116.*)

Herbs to boost the immune system include echinacea, garlic, myrrh, sage, and wild indigo. (*See pages 105, 98, and 116.*)

Cleavers, marigold, and poke root will help the lymphatic system. (*See page 102.*)

Herbs to reduce fever by inducing sweating are chamomile, elderflowers, yarrow, and limeflowers. (*See pages 104, 116, 97, and, 121.*)

Agrimony, elderflowers, plantain, and raspberry leaves tone the mucous membranes, and clear the catarrh and inflammation. (*See pages 97, 116, 112, and, 114.*)

Herbs to soothe painful tonsils include comfrey, marshmallow, and mullein. (*See pages 119 and 99.*)

Aromatherapy

Thyme oil is a powerful antiseptic and has a local anesthetic effect to reduce the discomfort. Use in a vaporizer, and add to a light carrier oil and massage into the neck.

Lavender and benzoin can be added to a cup of cooled, boiled water and gargled. (*See pages 147 and 156.*)

Tea tree oil, applied neat to the tonsils on the end of a cotton bud, fights infection and discomfort. (*See page 148.*)

Homeopathy

Chronic tonsillitis must be treated constitutionally, but for acute conditions try:

Belladonna, for a sore, tender throat, with shooting pains and a stiff neck. (*See page 168.*)

Hep. sulf., for a feeling that there is a fishbone caught in the throat, and when pain is alleviated by warm drinks, the breath is foul, and there is yellow pus. (*See page 183.*)

Lycopodium, for a throat sore on the right side, and where the tongue is dry and puffy but not coated, the throat is better after cold drinks, and worse between 4 and 8a.m. or p.m. (*See page 187.*)

Mercurius, when the throat is dark red, swollen, and sore, and worse on the right side, and when the breath smells and there are hot sweats. (*See page 189.*)

Phytolacca, for a rough, constricted, hot throat, with red, swollen tonsils and pain extending to the ears. The throat is worse on the right side and with heat.

Vitamins and Minerals

Cod liver oil tablets, along with vitamin C and garlic, will speed up the healing process. (*See pages 254 and 238.*)

LARYNGITIS

Laryngitis is an inflammation of the voice box (the larynx) in which the larynx and vocal cords become swollen and sore, distorting the vocal apparatus. Acute laryngitis is usually a complication of a sore throat, cold, or other upper respiratory tract infection, and should last for only a few days. It can also be an allergic reaction to inhaled pollen. Chronic laryngitis is more persistent and may be caused by long-term irritation from smoking, overuse of the voice, or excessive coughing. It can be an occupational hazard for singers and teachers.

Symptoms
- the throat is inflamed and mucus-coated in acute laryngitis
- the larynx is dry and inflamed in chronic laryngitis
- hoarseness
- difficulty in raising the voice above a whisper
- dry, irritating cough

TREATMENT

Ayurveda
Hollyhock is useful for throat inflammation.

Chinese Herbalism
Treatment would address poisoned Heat in the lungs, and the following herbs may be appropriate: peppermint, honeysuckle flowers, mulberry, lily, and licorice.

Traditional Home and Folk Remedies
Drink a glass of honey and lemon or honey and apple cider vinegar in hot water as required to reduce any inflammation and infection, and encourage healing.

Herbalism
Drink an infusion of red sage, or gargle, to reduce inflammation. (*See page 116.*)

Echinacea both treats and prevents laryngitis—drink an infusion three times daily. (*See page 105.*)

Aromatherapy
Gargle with a drop of geranium, pepper, rosemary, or tea tree oil in a glass of boiled water, as required, to prevent and treat inflammation and infection. (*See pages 133–157.*)

Massage the throat area with a drop of lavender or tea tree oil in a light carrier oil. (*See pages 147 and 148.*)

Try a steam inhalation of sandalwood or thyme to ease inflammation and reduce infection. (*See pages 155 and 156.*)

Homeopathy
Treatment would be constitutional, but some of the following remedies may help:

Aconite, when symptoms come on suddenly, and there is restlessness and anxiety. (*See page 163.*)

Spongia, for a dry, barking cough—particularly useful for croup. (*See page 196.*)

Lachesis, for chronic laryngitis, particularly if you talk a great deal. (*See page 200.*)

Hep. sulf., when symptoms are worse in the morning and after exposure to cold; symptoms are accompanied by a loose cough and a choking feeling. (*See page 183.*)

Apis, where the problem has been caused or exacerbated by allergy, and there is redness and swelling.

Ignatia, when the condition sets in after a trauma of some sort. (*See page 184.*)

Baryta carb., when you lose your voice often, without any obvious cause. (*See page 170.*)

Vitamins and Minerals
- Eat a diet rich in vitamin C to increase resistance to infection. (*See page 238.*)
- Avoid alcohol.

ORAL THRUSH

Oral thrush is a fungal infection which appears as raised creamy spots on the lining of the mouth, lips, and throat. The Candida albicans fungus occurs naturally in the mouth and other moist, warm areas of the body, but if excessive growth is allowed to take place infection can result. This may occur if the bacteria that usually keep it in check are themselves under attack by antibiotics, or if the immune system is compromised for any other reason. Oral thrush is most common in the young and elderly, and in people who wear dentures. Women also appear to be more susceptible than men.

Symptoms
- pain, soreness, and irritation in the affected area
- raised creamy spots in the mouth

TREATMENT
Chinese Herbalism
Gentian and Oriental wormwood may be prescribed to treat fungal infections of the mouth.

Traditional Home and Folk Remedies
Eat fresh live yogurt, and dab on to the affected patches, as required. (*See page 79.*)

Olive oil prevents yeast becoming fungus in the body, and should be drunk or used in cooking, as often as possible. (*See page 81.*)

Rub raw garlic on to the affected areas, and incorporate plenty of raw garlic into your diet. (*See page 70.*)

Lemon will help to soothe discomfort and encourage healing. Drink a cup of hot lemon and honey in water three times daily. (*See pages 74 and 87.*)

Herbalism
Aloe vera mouthwash has an antifungal effect. (*See page 99.*)

Barberry prevents the growth of fungus, and stimulates the immune system. Take three times daily.

Caprylic acid is a good antifungal agent. Take three capsules with each meal.

Chew fresh juniper berries to reduce inflammation and attack the Candida fungus.

Aromatherapy
Add a few drops of myrrh, tea tree, or lavender oil to a cup of boiled water and rinse the mouth several times daily to destroy fungal infection. (*See pages 133–157.*)

Homeopathy
Constitutional treatment to boost immunity will be offered, but the following remedies may also be useful:
- Capsicum, when patches are hot and sore and worse after cold drinks.
- Borax, at first symptoms.
- Arsenicum, for thrush associated with mouth ulcers and which occurs when you are run down. (*See page 167.*)
- Mercurius, when your tongue is hot and trembling, and you have more saliva than usual. (*See page 189.*)

Vitamins and Minerals
Take acidophilus tablets, and eat plenty of ripe bananas to encourage the growth of healthy bacteria in the body, which will reduce the severity of attacks and act to prevent them. (*See page 256.*)

MOUTH ULCERS

Mouth ulcers are white, gray, or yellow open sores with an outer ring of red inflammation, and occur when the mucous membrane or skin surface becomes pitted, resulting from an erosion or disintegration of the tissues. They appear on the inside of the lips, cheeks, or floor of the mouth, and may occur as a result of aggressive tooth brushing, ill-fitting dentures, accidentally biting the side of the mouth, or eating very hot food. They can also be triggered by stress or being run down, and can be a feature of Crohn's disease, ulcerative colitis, and celiac disease, or food allergy. Women may be particularly prone to mouth ulcers around menstruation. In children, contact with the herpes simplex virus that causes cold sores may manifest itself as mouth ulcers. Mouth ulcers are common, affecting one in five U.S. adults.

Symptoms
- pain and stinging in affected area, particularly when eating acidic or spicy foods
- dry mouth

TREATMENT
Ayurveda
Rub the tongue with a piece of ginger, and chew fresh root ginger to treat fungal infections of the mouth.

Aloe vera is useful for mouth ulcers associated with the herpes virus. (*See page 17.*)

Herbalism
Tincture of myrrh can be added to a cup of boiled water and used as a mouth rinse to destroy infection or infestation. Use the tincture neat and apply to sores in the mouth with a cotton bud.

Rub a little aloe vera gel into the affected area.

Aromatherapy
Mix a drop of geranium and lavender oil in a cup of boiled water and gargle as required. (*See pages 151 and 147.*)

Homeopathy
Arsenicum, when ulcers are on the edges of the tongue, with burning pains. (*See page 167.*)

Mercurius, for ulcers that erupt on the palate or tongue, and which are yellow and spongy. (*See page 189.*)

Kali bich., for ulcers that feel thick and firm, and sting.

Vitamins and Minerals
Take supplements of vitamins A, E, and B2. (Vitamin E oil can be applied directly to the ulcers.)

BAD BREATH

Bad breath (or halitosis) is often caused by accumulated food debris as a result of poor dental hygiene, smoking, and alcohol consumption. It may be accompanied by dribbling during sleep and a yellowish, thickly coated tongue. Bad breath can also be a symptom of many disorders including gingivitis, tonsillitis, sinusitis, oral thrush, diabetes, acute bronchitis, liver failure, cancer of the mouth, throat, larynx, lungs, or esophagus, chronic gastritis, underproduction of saliva, and constipation.

TREATMENT
Ayurveda
Chew fresh coriander or cardamom seeds after meals—they will act as a digestive and discourage bad breath.

Chinese Herbalism
Treatment would be aimed at stomach damp heat, using golden thread, peppermint tea, giant hyssop, and radish seeds. (*See page 47.*)

Traditional Home and Folk Remedies
Drink a combination of fresh carrot, celery, watercress, and cucumber juice with some paprika.

Herbalism
Chew fresh rosemary leaves, or make a mouthwash with a pinch of cloves, cinnamon, anise seed, and rosemary. Steep in a cup of sherry for a week, and then strain. Use daily as required. (*See page 114.*)

Chew fresh watercress, which is rich in chlorophyll and vitamin C.

Chew walnut bark and rub it on the gums, then gargle with lemon water.

Chew fresh parsley, mint, or tarragon. (*See page 111.*)

Aromatherapy

Add a drop of myrrh essential oil to a cup of cool, boiled water, and rinse the mouth daily. (*See page 142.*)

Thyme or fennel oil will be equally effective.

Homeopathy

Nux vomica, for breath that smells sour, particularly after meals or drinking alcohol. (*See page 198.*)

Petroselinium, for breath that smells of onions.

Nitric acid for bad breath with loose teeth and mouth ulcers.

Pulsatilla for bad breath after eating fatty foods, and which is accompanied by a dry mouth and no thirst. (*See page 193.*)

Mercurius, for breath that smells, with copious saliva and a yellow, furry tongue. (*See page 189.*)

Vitamins and Minerals

Store your toothbrush in grapefruit seed extract to destroy bacteria which may be encouraging bad breath.

COLD SORES

See under Skin and Hair, *page 279.*

LUNG AND RESPIRATORY DISORDERS

ASTHMA

Asthma is a condition in which the muscles of the bronchi (the air tubes of the lung) contract in spasm, obstructing the flow of air and making breathing out, in particular, very difficult. Asthma is becoming increasingly common, especially among children, and may be triggered by a number of factors, including allergens (such as house dust or pets), pollution, infection, emotional trauma, or physical exertion. Asthma is divided into two categories: intrinsic, for which there is no identifiable cause for attacks, and extrinsic, which is caused by something, usually inhaled, that triggers an attack.

In many asthma patients, inflammation of the lining of the airways leads to increased sensitivity to a variety of environmental triggers that can cause narrowing of the airways, resulting in obstruction of airflow and breathing difficulty. In some patients, the mucous glands in the airways produce excessive thick mucus, further obstructing airflow.

An asthma attack may be brief or last for several days. Typically, an attack begins within minutes after exposure to a triggering agent. Some patients have only occasional or "seasonal" symptoms, while others have daily symptoms.

Symptoms
- difficulty in breathing
- an increase in pulse rate
- wheezing, especially on breathing out
- a persistent dry cough
- a sensation of tightness around the chest

The prevalence of asthma is only about 1 or 2 percent worldwide, but in the U.S. asthma affects about 6 percent of children.

In the U.S. asthma affects 1 in 20 adults, affecting over 7 million adults and 3 million children, or roughly 4 percent of the population.

Children under 16 and adults over 65 are most commonly affected.

The incidence of hospitalization for children suffering from asthma and asthma-related illness has increased by 500 percent over the last 30 years.

The incidence of asthma in the U.K. population has increased 30 times over the last 30 years.

Asthma is on the increase in the Western world, and although orthodox medicine can control all the worst symptoms, there is no sign of a cure being found.

Drinking caffeine is said to open the airways and reduce symptoms by one-third in asthma sufferers.

- Ipecac., for wheezy children who cough until they vomit up a little mucus. (*See page 175.*)
- Arsenicum, for waking between midnight and 2a.m., accompanied by difficult breathing. (*See page 167.*)
- Bryonia, for asthma at the end of a cold, with a hard, dry cough. (*See page 170.*)
- Nat. sulf., for asthma in damp weather, with a loose cough and yellowish mucus. (*See page 191.*)
- Lachesis, for asthma that starts in spring or autumn, or at menopause. (*See page 200.*)

TREATMENT

Ayurveda
Ginger and stramonium may be used to treat asthma.

Chinese Herbalism
The cause of the illness is considered to be Phlegm produced by weakness of the Spleen and Kidneys. Almond and ephedra may be prescribed to open the Lungs.

Herbalism
Any of the herbs suggested for stress (*see page 266*) will help you to relax, which should decrease the incidence of attacks.

Elecampane can be infused to treat asthma. Drink daily if you are prone to attacks.

During a mild attack, grindelia, hyssop, wild cherry bark, and motherwort will help. (*See page 110.*)

Turmeric has a bronchodilatory effect, and it can be sipped sprinkled in a cup of warm water.

Aromatherapy
A steam inhalation of chamomile, eucalyptus, or lavender essential oils can be taken during an attack and immediately afterwards to ease panic and to help open the airways. (*See pages 133–157.*)

Pine oil in the bath or a vaporizer will reduce the incidence of attacks. (*See page 152.*)

Bergamot, clary sage, neroli, chamomile, and rose are antispasmodic, as well as being relaxant, and they will be particularly useful for attacks brought on by stress.

Homeopathy
Chronic asthma must be treated constitutionally, but the following remedies can be used for mild attacks, while waiting for medical attention:

Flower Essences
Take Rescue Remedy when you feel symptoms coming on. This will ease symptoms and prevent a full-blown attack. (*See page 229.*)

Vitamins and Minerals
Increase your intake of vitamin B6, which is said to reduce the frequency and severity of attacks. (*See page 237.*)

COUGHS

Coughs are necessary to expel foreign bodies and mucus from the trachea and airways of the lungs. Coughing is a symptom rather than an illness, and can indicate sinusitis, croup, bronchitis, pneumonia, flu, viruses, the early stages of measles, asthma, whooping cough, or an excess of catarrh from the nose or sinuses, due to irritation or infection.

A dry cough may be caused by mucus from infections or colds, chemicals in the atmosphere, a foreign object or nervousness which constricts the throat. A loose, wetter cough is caused by inflammation of the bronchial tubes produced by an infection or allergy. A constant nighttime cough, or one which recurs with each cold and is hard to get rid of, may indicate asthma.

Various terms describe the type of cough:
An acute cough starts suddenly, and is usually resolved within a day or two.

A chronic cough persists, sometimes for many weeks.

A productive cough brings up lots of catarrh or mucus.

A nonproductive cough brings up very little or no mucus, and usually sounds harsh and hard.

TREATMENT

Ayurveda

Brown 4 tablespoons of coriander seeds in a frying pan, then boil with 4 cups of water, with 4 slices of root ginger. Reduce to 2 cups of liquid, strain, and drink.

Other herbs to consider are sunflower, henbane, and stramonium.

Traditional Home and Folk Remedies

A tincture of garlic (place several garlic cloves in brandy and leave for 2 or 3 weeks, then strain) or garlic syrup (tincture, or fresh garlic mixed with a little honey) will help the body to fight infection. It also works to cleanse the blood. (*See page 70.*)

Ginseng in hot herbal tea warms the body and eases symptoms.

Honey and lemon will ease coughs and encourage healing. (*See pages 87 and 74.*)

Mustard powder, mixed with a little water, can be made into a poultice and applied to the chest area. (*See page 84.*)

Apply a warm roasted onion poultice to the chest, or drink a warm onion broth to cleanse and reduce congestion.

Herbalism

Peppermint tea can be drunk to soothe. (*See page 111.*)

Add lightly macerated licorice root sticks to your herbal drink to ease. (*See page 108.*)

Aniseed, marshmallow, and wild cherry bark are useful for unproductive, irritating coughs. (*See page 99.*)

Use golden seal, plantain, and thyme if infection is present. (*See pages 112 and 122.*)

Aromatherapy

Inhale the steam from a few drops of eucalyptus oil in boiling water, as it is expectorant and decongestant.

Pine oil, in a vaporizer, will ease coughing and act to restore the lungs. (*See page 152.*)

Massage frankincense or sandalwood into the chest and back. (*See pages 135 and 155.*)

Essential oil of myrrh reduces mucus and phlegm.

Homeopathy

Pulsatilla, for a loose, wet, rattling cough, which is worse in the morning and when in bed at night.

Ant. tart, is especially useful for elderly people who suffer from persistent rattling cough, and are full of loose mucus but cannot seem to bring it up. (*See page 164.*)

Rumex, for a very tickly cough, when cold air irritates the nose and throat.

Bryonia, for a dry cough where the chest feels sore from coughing. (*See page 170.*)

Phosphorous, for a tickling cough in delicate people with weak chests. (*See page 192.*)

Drosera, for a violent tickly cough with retching and pain in the ribs. (*See page 178.*)

Chamomilla, for a dry, irritating cough with wheezing, and which is worse at night and makes you feel irritable. (*See page 188.*)

> **CAUTION**
> If a cough lasts for more than 10 days, or is accompanied by fever, difficult breathing, blue lips, drowsiness or difficulty speaking, contact your physician.

FLU

Also known as influenza, flu is a viral disease of the upper respiratory tract, spread by the contaminated droplets (via coughing and sneezing) of other sufferers. The three main types of flu are caused by three different viruses—A, B, and C. Type C, once caught, confers immunity. Types A and B, however, are constantly mutating so that our bodies cannot build up resistance against them. Incubation of the virus is generally one or two days, during which time it is highly infectious, and therefore notoriously impossible to contain.

TREATMENT

When new strains of influenza virus arise, they spread rapidly around the world, infecting millions of people and causing many deaths.

Flu victims 50 years old or older, children, and immune-deficient people are at risk of developing pneumonia and other secondary infections.

Over the age of 65, pneumonia and flu are the fifth leading cause of death.

The disease is produced by any one of three types of Orthomyxovirus virus (A, B, and C), of which there are many strains.

Vaccines have been developed that have been found to be 70–90 percent effective for at least six months against either A or B types, and a genetically engineered live-virus vaccine is under development.

Vaccination is considered especially important for older people, patients with cardiac or respiratory diseases, and pregnant women.

The incidence of infection is highest among school-age children, partly because of their lack of previous exposure to various strains.

Approximately every ten years, influenza pandemics have been caused by new strains of type-A virus.

Epidemics, or regional outbreaks, have appeared every 2 to 3 years for influenza A, and every 4 to 5 years for influenza B.

Symptoms
- high fever, possibly accompanied by shivering
- sore throat, and possibly a dry, unproductive cough
- runny nose and sneezing
- breathlessness and general weakness
- headache, stiff and aching joints, and muscular pain
- nausea and loss of appetite

TREATMENT

Ayurveda
Heat mustard oil and apply as a compress to the head to reduce fever. (*See page 19.*)

Crush root ginger, add to a little honey and lime, and drink as required.

Bitter orange, sunflower, and coriander may be useful in treating flu. (*See page 24.*)

Traditional Home and Folk Remedies
Some warmed apple juice (preferably fresh) can ease the fever.

Barley water is a traditional remedy for high fever—particularly one caused by infection and inflammation.

Ginseng powder can be added to herbal teas to restore.

Drink hot lemon and honey in a cup of warm water to ease inflammation and fever. (*See pages 87 and 74.*)

Gargle with lemon juice to kill germs and help to stop the spread of the virus. (*See page 74.*)

Herbalism
Drink an infusion of boneset to relieve aches and pains and clear congestion.

Fenugreek with lemon and honey will help to bring down fever and soothe aching limbs.

Ginseng is a great all-round restorer and will help to bring down body temperature to normal. (*See page 112.*)

Use wormwood, sage, and licorice to prevent flu. (*See pages 116 and 108.*)

Aromatherapy
Gargle with tea tree oil to prevent the spread of infection.

Use a eucalyptus or peppermint inhalation to unblock sinuses and the chest. (*See pages 145 and 150.*)

Massage tea tree and geranium oil into the chest and head to reduce symptoms and fight infection.

Oils which act to bring down fever include bergamot, chamomile, melissa, and tea tree. (*See pages 133–157.*)

Homeopathy
Gelsemium, for occasions when muscular weakness, aching, and heaviness predominate. (*See page 180.*)

Rhus tox., for flu that starts after getting wet, where there is a lot of aching in joints rather than muscles. Accompanied by restlessness and an inability to get comfortable. (*See page 194.*)

Bryonia, for a bad headache and dry cough, with a desire to lie quite still. (*See page 170.*)

Eupatorium perfoliatum, for intense aching in the back and limbs, together with shivery chills.

Arsenicum, when you feel debilitated, often with loss of fluids, and with accompanying watery diarrhea and sometimes vomiting. (*See page 167.*)

Baptisia, for gastric flu, when you feel "wiped out," and your body feels bruised, or scattered around the bed; also with sudden bouts of diarrhea or vomiting. (*See page 169.*)

Vitamins and Minerals

Eat plenty of foods rich in vitamin C, bioflavonoids and zinc, which will encourage healing, help to fight infection, and boost the action of the immune system. (*See pages 238, 256, and 249.*)

Royal jelly acts as a tonic and an antiviral agent. (*See page 260.*)

Freshly made apple juice is a good home remedy, providing vitamin C to help to combat injection. Using a juice extractor enables this to be made quickly and easily.

The apple juice can be poured into a pan and gently warmed, but it must not be boiled or overheated or the vitamin content will be severely reduced.

EMPHYSEMA

Emphysema is a progressive disease in which the tiny air sacs in the lungs (alveoli) break down, reducing the area available for gas exchange. This means that insufficient oxygen reaches the vital organs, and too much carbon dioxide enters the bloodstream. Emphysema is particularly common among heavy smokers and sufferers of asthma and chronic bronchitis. Industrial pollutants may also be a cause, as well as hereditary factors.

The exact cause of pulmonary emphysema is unknown. Cigarette smoking is closely associated with the disease, and in some cases a genetic link is suspected, in that a significant number of people with emphysema lack a gene that controls the liver's production of a protein called alpha-1 antitrypsin, or AAT. Emphysema rarely occurs before the age of 40, and women appear to be less prone, although with the increase in the numbers of women smoking this may change.

Symptoms

- breathlessness, especially on exertion
- a cough producing sputum
- chest may become barrel-shaped as the disease progresses
- a blue tinge to the skin (cyanosis)
- respiratory failure may eventually occur

TREATMENT

Ayurveda

Boil 2 or 3 cloves of garlic in 2 cups of water until tender. Crush into the water and drink to relieve chest pain.

Stramonium may be useful.

Herbalism

Peppermint tea will soothe inflammation and help to open lungs. (*See page 111.*)

Slippery elm bark soothes the chest and lungs, and can be added to any herbal tea. (*See page 123.*)

Aromatherapy

Massage oils of cedarwood, peppermint, or eucalyptus into the chest daily, to open lungs and reduce coughing. (*See pages 135–157.*)

Make an inhalation of eucalyptus, and use as required to expel phlegm. (*See page 145.*)

Homeopathy

Emphysema cannot be cured, but the symptoms can be alleviated and the condition arrested by constitutional treatment.

See coughs (*page 318*), bronchitis (*page 322*), and asthma (*page 317*) for remedies that fit specific symptoms.

PLEURISY

Pleurisy (or pleuritis) is an infection, viral or bacterial in origin, caused by an inflammation of the pleura— the sac-like membrane surrounding the lungs. The two layers of the inflamed pleura rub together to cause the characteristic creaking noise in the chest that makes diagnosis so easy. A surplus of pleural fluid may also be produced by the inflammation, causing a pleural effusion which can be detected on physical examination. In a very few cases, pleurisy may be an indication of more serious diseases such as lung cancer or pulmonary embolism, while chronic pleurisy may be a symptom of tuberculosis. Before the advent of antibiotics, pleurisy was a life-threatening condition and one of the most common causes of death, particularly in children. Today, the condition is usually easily diagnosed and treated in the early stages.

> **CAUTION**
> If you do not feel better after a day (taking doses every hour), see your physician.

Symptoms
- stabbing pain, usually at a particular point in inhalation or on coughing

TREATMENT

Traditional Home and Folk Remedies
Apple cider vinegar compresses will reduce inflammation and encourage healing. (*See page 87.*)

Herbalism
Comfrey root or leaf tea compresses can be applied to the chest to ease inflammation. (*See page 119.*)

Wrap a bruised wet plantain leaf across the chest to soothe symptoms. (*See page 112.*)

Combine a handful of sage leaves and corn silk to strengthen the kidneys and expel water from the system. (*See page 116.*)

Aromatherapy
The following anti-inflammatory oils can be used in gentle massage of the chest and back, or in the bath or an inhaler to encourage healing: bergamot, calendula, chamomile, myrrh. (*See pages 133–157.*)

Lavender can be sniffed during an attack to calm you and help fight infection. (*See page 147.*)

Homeopathy
During an acute attack, the following remedies may be useful:
- Aconite, for a sudden sharp pain, usually after exposure to cold wind. (*See page 163.*)
- Cantharis, for breathlessness and burning pains with mild fever and a dry cough. (*See page 173.*)
- Belladonna, for sudden pain and a hot flushed face accompanied by thirst. (*See page 168.*)
- Hep. sulf., for slower recovery, with fluid on the lungs.
- Bryonia, for pain that is made worse by movement, and which is accompanied by thirst and general irritability.
- Sulfur, for sharp, cutting pains that are made worse by movement. (*See page 198.*)

BRONCHITIS

Bronchitis is an inflammation of the lining of the bronchi (the air tubes of the lungs). Acute bronchitis, in which mucus infected with bacteria is expelled from the lungs, often follows a viral illness such as a cold or flu. Smoking and a damp, dusty, or foggy atmosphere can lead to chronic bronchitis resulting from long-term irritation of the air passages.

Symptoms
- a cough, dry at first but with gradually increasing sputum
- possibly chest pain
- shortness of breath and wheezing
- in cases of chronic bronchitis symptoms may begin in winter, but then persist throughout the year

Smokers are 50 times more susceptible to bronchitis.

Male sufferers outnumber female sufferers by ten to one.

Ayurvedic breathing exercises and yoga generally assist breathing and shortness of breath.

Acute bronchitis is usually caused by infection by one of the many viruses that cause the common cold or influenza, and is frequently associated with measles.

Acute chemical bronchitis may be caused by the inhalation of irritating fumes, such as smoke, chlorine, ammonia, and ozone.

Chronic bronchitis results from prolonged irritation of the bronchial membrane, causing coughing and the excessive secretion of mucus for extended periods. By far the most common cause of chronic bronchitis is cigarette smoking, but air pollution, industrial fumes, and dust are also recognized lung irritants.

TREATMENT

Ayurveda
Heat mustard oil and apply as a compress to the head to reduce fever. (*See page 19.*)

Crush root ginger, add to a little honey and lime, and drink as required.

Hollyhock may be appropriate, as well as bitter orange and stramonium.

> **CAUTION**
> If your temperature rises above 102 degrees, of if you cough blood, call your physician.

Chinese Herbalism
The source is believed to be external Wind, Cold, or Heat in cases of acute bronchitis, and internal Deficient Spleen or Lung, or internal Mucus for chronic bronchitis.

Acute conditions will respond to fritillary bulb, plantain seed, and balloon flower root. (*See pages 50 and 56.*)

Chronic conditions would respond to honeysuckle flowers, mulberry leaves, gardenia fruit. (*See page 52.*)

Traditional Home and Folk Remedies
Honey and lemon work to fight infection and ease coughs. (*See pages 87 and 74.*)

Combine mustard seed powder and water to make a poultice to decongest the chest. (*See page 84.*)

Onions will soothe inflamed membranes and induce perspiration. (*See page 70.*)

Herbalism
Anise diluted in a small amount of water soothes a hacking cough.

Wild cherry bark extract added to any herbal drink relieves coughing.

Coltsfoot can be added to licorice and honey to alleviate coughs.

Rub garlic oil into the chest to fight infection and encourage healing. (*See page 98.*)

Drink ginseng in hot water, as it will help to eliminate infection and ease coughing fits. (*See page 112.*)

Peppermint tea will soothe the cough and help to bring out the infection. (*See page 111.*)

Aromatherapy
Oils to help clear the congestion include eucalyptus and thyme, which can be inhaled as required.

Ginger oil can be diluted and rubbed into the chest for chronic bronchitis, to dispel mucus. (*See page 157.*)

Juniper, myrrh, and rosemary will help to prevent mucus, and act to detoxify the body. (*See pages 133–157.*)

Homeopathy
The following remedies can be offered for acute bronchitis; chronic bronchitis must be treated constitutionally:
- Pulsatilla, for symptoms that are worse in stuffy rooms, and for a cough which is dry at night and loose in the morning. (*See page 193.*)
- Ipecac., for nausea, vomiting, and suffocation feelings.
- Bryonia, for a dry, stabbing cough accompanied by a headache and great thirst. (*See page 170.*)
- Phosphorus, for a tight, tickly cough, when you are pale, anxious, and thirsty for cold water. (*See page 192.*)
- Aconite, for sudden onset bronchitis, with a dry cough and chills. (*See page 163.*)

Vitamins and Minerals
Increase your intake of vitamins B, C, and A, and zinc. (*See pages 234–238 and 249.*)

TRACHEITIS

Tracheitis is an acute inflammation of the lining of the trachea (windpipe). It is usually viral in origin but can sometimes be bacterial. It is often associated with an infection elsewhere in the upper respiratory tract, such as bronchitis or influenza. Tracheitis is the most common cause of painful attacks of croup in young children. In cases where the bronchi of the lungs become infected (laryngotra-cheobronchitis), the walls of the airway swell, which can lead to asphyxia in small children.

TREATMENT
Ayurveda
Hollyhock may be useful for throat irritation.

Herbalism
Comfrey root or leaf tea compresses on the throat and neck will help ease inflammation. Wrap a bruised, wet plantain leaf across the throat to soothe symptoms.

Aromatherapy
Anti-inflammatory oils can be used in gentle massage of the chest, neck, and head, or in the bath or an inhaler to encourage healing. Try bergamot, calendula, chamomile, and myrrh. (*See pages 133–157.*)

Homeopathy
Rumex, for a raw feeling in the throat, a tickly cough, and where the throat is sore to the touch.

Stannum, when there is sweet yellow phlegm and pain after coughing.

Bryonia, when pain is made worse by talking, smoke, and warm rooms. (*See page 170.*)

Phosphorus, for a hacking cough, thirst for cold drinks, and a raw feeling. (*See page 192.*)

Kali bich., for sticky phlegm that is difficult to expel.

Vitamins and Minerals
Take extra vitamin C and zinc to boost the immune system. (*See pages 238 and 249.*)

HYPERVENTILATION

Hyperventilation is the term used to describe the act of breathing more quickly and deeply than normal, and which causes excessive loss of carbon dioxide from the blood. This can lead to alkalosis (an increase in blood alkalinity). It can occur at high altitudes, as a result of heavy exercise, during panic attacks, or as a response to poisoning (as in an aspirin overdose). Hyperventilation associated with uncontrolled diabetes or with kidney failure represents the body's efforts to eliminate excess carbon dioxide in dealing with acidosis. Chronic hyperventilation is association with a combination of fatigue and over-arousal (lack of sleep, plus stress, for instance); it may also stem from organic problems in the brain, or in the lungs themselves. Acute attacks are usually a reaction to emotional or physical trauma.

Symptoms
- a feeling of not getting enough air
- the muscles of the forearms and calves may go into spasm

TREATMENT

Ayurveda
An Ayurvedic medical practitioner would balance the tri-doshas, and use panchakarma for balancing the vátha.

Chinese Herbalism
A Chinese herbalist might suggest ginseng, Chinese angelica, and white peony root with thorowax root for relaxation. Treatment would be designed to strengthen the Spleen and enliven Liver. (*See page 35.*)

Traditional Home and Folk Remedies
Oats contain thiamine and pantothenic acid, which act as gentle nerve tonics. (*See page 72.*)

Herbalism
Herbal remedies would be used to calm the nervous system and to relax you. Skullcap and valerian are useful herbs, blended together for best effect. Drink this as a tea three times daily while suffering symptoms.

Lady's slipper and limeflowers may also work to ease factors which may be causing the condition.

Aromatherapy
A relaxing blend of essential oils of lavender, geranium, and bergamot in sweet almond oil or peach kernel oil may be used in the bath at times of great stress and anxiety.

Homeopathy
Take Aconite every 5 minutes for up to six doses in an acute attack. (*See page 163.*)

Constitutional treatment will be necessary for chronic conditions.

Flower Essences
Rescue Remedy or Emergency Essence will help to calm you in an attack. (*See page 229.*)

Elm, for an attack linked to anxiety accompanying a feeling of being unable to cope. (*See page 226.*)

Aspen, for an attack caused by anxiety for no reason.

Vitamins and Minerals

Increase your intake of B vitamins, which work on the nervous system. (*See pages 235–238.*)

Avoid caffeine in any form.

HICCUPS

A hiccup is a common irritation of the diaphragmatic nerves which causes involuntary inhalation of air. A lowering of the diaphragm and the sudden closure of the vocal cords result in the characteristic hiccup sound. Hiccups may be brought on by indigestion and drinking carbonated drinks, and can also occur during pregnancy and as a result of alcoholism. Most attacks last only a few minutes, usually with a brief interval in between attacks. Frequent, prolonged attacks of hiccups, which are extremely rare, may lead to severe exhaustion.

> **CAUTION**
> While hiccups are usually quite innocuous, they may be a feature of more serious disorders such as pleurisy, hiatus hernia, and pneumonia.

Symptoms
- prolonged episodes of hiccups may be accompanied by chest pain
- if persistent, hiccups can eventually be exhausting

TREATMENT

Chinese Herbalism
The cause is thought to be Heat, Cold, or Food Stagnation. Berilla stems, rhubarb, and ginger will be used to treat hiccups.

Traditional Home and Folk Remedies
Squirt some lemon juice to the back of your throat, or suck a piece of fresh lemon. (*See page 74.*)

Give babies a sip of water with honey.

Homoepathy
Take one of the following remedies every 15 minutes for up to 6 doses:
- Nux vomica, for hiccups after eating, and accompanied by belching. (*See page 198.*)
- Arsenicum, for hiccups which are worse after cold drinks and accompanied by a chilly feeling. (*See page 167.*)
- Ignatia, when hiccups come on after emotional upset, eating, drinking, or smoking. (*See page 184.*)
- Mag. phos., for a sore chest and retching. (*See page 188.*)
- Cicuta, for violent, noisy hiccups.

COMMON COLD

The common cold is an infection of the upper respiratory tract which may be caused by any one of up to 200 strains of virus. These are spread either by inhaling droplets coughed or sneezed by others, or, more probably, by direct hand-to-hand contact with sufferers. When infection occurs, the walls of the respiratory tract swell and produce excess mucus, giving rise to the typical cold symptoms of stuffy or runny nose, throat discomfort, malaise, and occasional coughing. Colds can produce fevers of up to 102°F (39°C) in infants and children, but such fevers in adults indicate that the infection is probably influenza. The incubation period is from 1–3 days, after which symptoms occur, and most colds run their course in 3–10 days. Infants and elderly people are susceptible to complications such as sinusitis, ear inflammations, and pneumonia.

In conventional medicine, colds are treated with rest and fluids, in addition to antihistamines, decongestants, and cough medicines, as needed. Aspirin is recommended only when symptoms are severe, because it increases viral shedding and makes the sufferer more contagious. Vaccines are of little use in prevention because so many kinds of viruses are involved. Research suggests that interferon (a protein produced by animal cells when they are invaded by viruses, which is released into the bloodstream or intercellular fluid to induce healthy cells to manufacture an enzyme that counters the infection) could prevent the spread of colds and may prove useful to people at high risk of complications.

Symptoms
- sneezing and runny nose
- mild fever
- headache
- coughing and a burning or sore throat
- catarrh

TREATMENT

Ayurveda
Brown 4 tablespoons of coriander seeds in a frying pan, then boil with 4 cups of water, with 4 slices of root ginger. Reduce to 2 cups of liquid, strain, and drink. (*See page 24.*)
   Sunflower may be useful. (*See page 27.*)

Chinese Herbalism
Plantain seed, peppermint, mulberry, honeysuckle, and skullcap may be prescribed to address weakness of the Lung, Cold, and Wind. (*See pages 52 and 61.*)

Traditional Home and Folk Remedies
Barley water with lemon and honey will encourage healing and shorten the duration of a cold. (*See page 74.*)
   Cinnamon is an excellent warming herb, and can be added to food and drinks, or as an oil to a vaporizer, to treat and prevent colds and flu.
   Fresh garlic, eaten daily, will discourage the onset of a cold. Garlic will also work to reduce fever.
   Honey, eaten fresh or added to herbal teas, will encourage healing and prevent secondary infections occurring. (*See page 87.*)
   Steep lemons in hot water, and a little honey; drink regularly in the cold season, or during a cold, to restore yourself and prevent infection. This will also treat coughs. (*See pages 74 and 87.*)
   A mustard poultice on the chest or mustard added to a foot bath will act as a decongestant. (*See page 84.*)

Herbalism
Ginger promotes perspiration and helps soothe the throat. (*See page 126.*)
   The herb echinacea will encourage immune response, and acts as a natural antibiotic. (*See page 105.*)
   Peppermint helps to reduce the symptoms of a cold. (*See page 111.*)

Ginseng powder, added to any warming herbal tea, will boost the immune system and help the body to fight the infection. (*See page 112*)

Aromatherapy
Tea tree and lemon oils help to fight infection. Massage, in a light carrier oil, into the chest and head, or place in the bath or a burner. (*See pages 148 and 140.*)
   Lavender oil in the bath will help you sleep, to aid recovery—particularly good if there is a cough. (*See page 147.*)
   Eucalyptus oil can kill bacteria and soothe inflamed mucous membranes. (*See page 145.*)

Homeopathy
Aconite, in the first stage of a cold. (*See page 163.*)
   Belladonna, for colds with a high temperature and great thirst. (*See page 168.*)
   Mercurius, for colds that begin with a sore throat, with swollen glands. (*See page 189.*)
   Gelsemium, for flu-like symptoms, weakness, and achiness. (*See page 180.*)
   Allium, for streaming nose and eyes where the discharge makes the nose red raw. (*See page 163.*)
   Pulsatilla, for runny nose with thick, yellow or green mucus. (*See page 193.*)
   Nat. mur., for colds with a crop of cold sores; sneezing and watery eyes. (*See page 190.*)
   Dulcamara, when the nose is stuffed up with catarrh in rainy or windy weather. (*See page 197.*)
   Bryonia, if you feel like a bear with a sore head. (*See page 170.*)

Vitamins and Minerals
Citrus fruit is rich in vitamin C, which will help the body to fight infection. (*See page 238.*)
   Zinc is known to reduce the duration of a cold; suck a zinc lozenge at the first signs. (*See page 249.*)
   Royal jelly acts as a tonic and an antiviral agent.
   Both ginger and coriander are useful in treating colds. To make a decoction, brown 4 tablespoons of coriander seeds. Once the seeds are browned, add 4 cups of water and bring to the boil. Add 4 slices of root ginger and reduce the liquid to 2 cups and strain. Drink to reduce a fever.

HEART, BLOOD, AND CIRCULATORY DISORDERS

HIGH BLOOD PRESSURE

Blood pressure is the force with which the blood presses against the arterial walls as it circulates. In a person with high blood pressure, or hypertension, this force is greater than normal and causes the arterial walls to narrow and thicken, putting extra strain on the heart. Blood pressure fluctuates even in healthy individuals. It tends to increase with physical activity, excitement, fear, or emotional stress, but such elevations are usually transient. Most physicians will not make the diagnosis of hypertension unless the pressure is high on at least three separate occasions. Obesity, alcohol and sugar intake, and hereditary and ethnic factors all contribute, as will diabetes, kidney disease, and pregnancy. It is usually only when the secondary complications—damage to the arteries, brain, eyes, or elsewhere in the body—have developed that symptoms occur, by which time the condition is serious.

Symptoms
- mild hypertension has no symptoms
- severe hypertension: headaches, shortness of breath, visual disturbances, giddiness
- In the U.S. at least 50 million people have hypertension
- Hypertension is usually described as being a systolic pressure greater than 139, or a diastolic pressure greater than 89, or both. The World Health Organization defines it as being consistently above 160mm. Hg. systolic, and 95mm. Hg. diastolic
- In the U.K. high blood pressure is extremely common, affecting 10–20 percent of the adult population
- High blood pressure is more frequent and more severe in African Americans than in the white U.S. population, and in both races in the south-eastern United States than in the rest of the nation
- It is uncommon in children and adolescents
- In young adulthood and early middle age, high blood pressure occurs more frequently in men than in women; thereafter the reverse is true
- Hypertension occurs worldwide and is most prevalent in Japan and northern China
- In societies that consume little or no salt the incidence of hypertension is extremely low

> **CAUTION**
> Routine blood pressure checks should be undertaken by everyone as a matter of course. Sustained high blood pressure can cause severe damage to the heart, kidneys, and eyes, and should not be ignored. Do not take herbal remedies while taking conventional medicine without consulting your physician.

TREATMENT

Ayurveda
The Ayurvedic products Dashamoola and Sarpaganda are used for treating high blood pressure.

Chinese Herbalism
Internal Wind is believed to be the cause, and treatment will calm Liver Yang and Blood Wind. The herbs used might include chrysanthemum flowers, peony root, astragalus. (*See pages 53 and 42.*)

Traditional Home and Folk Remedies
Eat plenty of fresh raw garlic, which acts as a tonic to the circulatory system and maintains its health. (*See page 98.*)

Herbalism
Hawthorn berries, infused, are a good heart tonic.
Cramp bark can be used to encourage the arteries to dilate. (*See page 125.*)
Limeflowers and yarrow are also useful in the treatment of high blood pressure. (*See pages 121 and 97.*)

Aromatherapy
Lavender will soothe and relax. (*See page 147.*)
Regular massage with oils of lavender, marjoram, and ylang ylang can have a beneficial effect.

Homeopathy
Constitutional treatment is appropriate.

Vitamins and Minerals

Increase your intake of dietary fiber, and of potassium, calcium, and magnesium, which have a balancing effect on the circulation and encourage the action of the heart. (*See pages 258, 245, and 241.*)

LOW BLOOD PRESSURE

Low blood pressure, or hypotension, is an abrupt fall in blood pressure due possibly to the heart's failure to maintain it or to severe loss of fluid from the circulation. It is perhaps most commonly noticed on standing up suddenly from a sitting or prone position, but can also result from severe hemorrhage, burns, gastroenteritis, or dehydration.

Blood pressure is conventionally written as two numbers, systolic pressure over diastolic pressure. Systolic pressure is the maximum blood pressure that occurs during the contraction of the heart; diastolic pressure is the lowest pressure measured during the interbeat period. The medically acceptable upper limit for blood pressure in an adult has been lowered in recent years and is now considered to be 140/90mm. Hg.

Symptoms

- fainting (due to the blood volume circulating being insufficient to supply the brain and lungs): older people in particular and those taking drugs against hypertension may experience fainting episodes, accompanied by paleness, a weak pulse, and dilated pupils

Chinese Herbalism

Treatment would be aimed at Deficient qi in the Blood and Heart. Ginseng and Chinese angelica might be used.

Herbalism

Broom is useful for treating low blood pressure, as it tones the arteries.

Ginger, hawthorn tops, and rosemary will also be useful as they are stimulating and work to encourage circulation. (*See pages 126, 104, and 114.*)

Aromatherapy

Regular massage with oils of black pepper, lemon, sage, or rosemary, which stimulate and warm, will be useful.

Homeopathy

Treatment would be constitutional, but the following remedies may help if you feel a tendency to faint:

- Veratrum, for fainting caused by anger.
- Coffea, for fainting brought on by excitement.
- Ignatia, for fainting caused by an emotional shock or trauma. (*See page 184.*)
- Aconite, for fainting caused by fright, and characterized by tension and pale, clammy skin. (*See page 163.*)
- Cocculus, when caused by lack of sleep.
- Gelsemium, when you feel weak and shaky.

CAUTION

Low blood pressure is not formally regarded as a disease in the U.K. in the way that hypertension, or high blood pressure, is. Genuine hypotension can, however, be fatal, and must be given urgent medical attention.

ENLARGED SPLEEN

The spleen is located on the left side of the body below the ribs and is responsible for removing dead blood cells from the blood. It varies in size and weight according to the amount of blood it contains in storage and its immune functions. In adult humans the spleen functions both as an immunologically active organ and as a filter for white and red blood cells. All of the blood in the human body passes through the spleen approximately every 90 minutes. Slight enlargement of the spleen is normal during and after digestion, and the size of the spleen in adults usually ranges from 3½–8oz. (100–250g.). Abnormal enlargement, or splenomegaly, may occur in the course of a number of diseases, including: malaria, typhoid, hemolytic anemia, leukemia, Hodgkin's disease, glandular fever, septicemia, and syphilis. An enlarged spleen becomes firmer and can easily be felt on physical examination.

Symptoms

Symptoms will vary according to the cause of enlargement,
but the general area of the spleen will be very tender.

TREATMENT

Herbalism

Any of the herbs that help the immune action will be
useful, including the following:

- Licorice can enhance recovery, stimulating white
  blood cell and antibody formation and efficiency.
- Garlic helps to prevent infections of all kinds, including
  those which have become resistant to a dose of antibiotics.
- Echinacea is widely used to treat chronic and acute
  infections, cleansing the blood and lymphatic system,
  and stimulating production of white blood cells and
  antibodies. (*See page 105.*)
- Ginseng can boost immunity and encourage the body to
  deal efficiently with stress, as well as stimulating white
  blood cell production and aiding recovery after illness.

Homeopathy

Treatment would be constitutional, but the following
may help, depending on the cause:

- Quercus, for an enlarged spleen associated with
  cirrhosis of the liver, and swollen ankles.
- Nat. mur., for a swollen spleen with constipation, salt
  cravings, and oversensitive reactions. (*See page 190.*)

ANEMIA

Anemia is a deficiency of hemoglobin—the chemical
that carries oxygen—in the red cells of the blood.
The most common cause of anemia is iron deficiency
resulting from excessive blood loss (through trauma,

surgery, childbirth, or heavy menstrual bleeding), poor
diet, or failure to absorb iron from food. Other causes of
anemia include: excessive destruction of red blood cells
(hemolytic anemia); vitamin B12 deficiency (pernicious
anemia); and the inherited disorders of sickle cell anemia
and thalassemia. Of all sufferers, 20 percent are women,
and 50 percent are children.

The most common type of anemia is iron deficiency
anemia, most often resulting from chronic blood loss;
also from lack of iron in the diet, impaired absorption of
iron from the intestine, or an increased need for iron, as
occurs during pregnancy.

Iron is an essential component of the hemoglobin,
which carries oxygen to the tissues in chemical
combination with its iron atoms.

Pernicious anemia is a chronic inherited disease of
middle-aged and older people in which the stomach fails
to produce a factor needed for the absorption of vitamin
B12, which is essential for mature red blood cells.

Aplastic anemia is the result of the failure of bone
marrow cells to manufacture mature red cells. It is
usually caused by toxic chemicals (for example, benzene)
or by radiation.

Symptoms

- weakness and fatigue
- breathlessness on minimal exertion
- pale skin and lips
- headaches, dizziness, and possibly fainting in severe cases
- in pernicious anemia there may be: nosebleeds, a sore
  tongue, "pins and needles" in the hands and feet

TREATMENT

Ayurveda

There are a number of Ayurvedic products available,
including Kalyanaka ghritha (oral ghee), Kishor (oral
pills) and Avipathi choorna (oral powder), which would
complement a treatment program.

Chinese Herbalism

The cause would be attributed to a Spleen not transforming qi, and Gui Pi Wan (return spleen tablets) would be useful.

Traditional Home and Folk Remedies

Nettle tea is rich in iron; drink daily.

Beet and carrot juice may be drunk to treat the condition. (*See page 76.*)

Herbalism

Chinese angelica root may be helpful. Take as tincture, decoction, or tea. (*See page 100.*)

Alfalfa, dandelion root, nettles, watercress, and yellow dock are rich in iron. (*See pages 121, 124, and 115.*)

Aromatherapy

Lavender essential oil is helpful where the anemia is associated with palpitations and dizzy spells. (*See page 147.*)

Massage with Roman chamomile essential oil. (*See page 137.*)

Homeopathy

Ferr. phos. helps assimilation of iron from food. (*See page 179.*)

Nat. mur., for anemia with constipation, headache, and a tendency to cold sores. (*See page 190.*)

Calc. phos., for anemia during a growth spurt, and irritability. (*See page 171.*)

Picric acid, for anemia with mental overload.

Vitamins and Minerals

Iron-rich foods include oats, egg yolks, pumpkin seeds, and watercress. (*See page 243.*)

Calcium, copper, vitamin C, and B vitamins must be present for the body to assimilate iron; ensure you have a sufficient intake in your diet. (*See pages 241–242 and 235–238.*)

Vegetarians should take extra vitamin B12. (*See page 238.*)

Avoid drinking tea at mealtimes as this makes iron absorption less efficient.

ANGINA

Angina (known medically as angina pectoris) is chest pain caused by a narrowing of the arteries, with the result that the blood supply to the heart muscle is not enough to meet its demands for oxygen and nutrients. The pain most commonly occurs after physical exertion, a heavy meal, cold weather, or various other circumstances requiring the heart to work harder. Groups likely to be susceptible to angina include smokers, diabetics, and the overweight.

Cardiovascular diseases such as angina have been a major health problem in the U.S. for years and comprise the leading cause of death.

Nearly 1 million people die each year of cardiovascular disease. An estimated 50 million Americans have cardiovascular disease and are unaware of it.

The death rate from cardiovascular diseases has declined since the mid-1970s, due to modification of risk factors for disease, and improvements in diagnosis and treatment.

At first, angina may only be evident during periods of exercise or emotional stress, resolving when the activity ceases. Later, it may occur even at rest.

Symptoms

- severe pain in the chest, often spreading up to the neck and down the left arm
- a feeling of tightness in the chest
- there may also be pain between the shoulder blades

TREATMENT

Chinese Herbalism

Treatment would be aimed at stagnant qi in the Blood and Heart. Herbs used may include safflower, cinnamon twigs, red sage root, peony root, and macrosten onion bulb. (*See pages 44 and 53.*)

Herbalism

Hawthorn berries, made into an infusion, are a good tonic for the heart. (*See page 104.*)

Motherwort is useful for the treatment of angina. Sip a motherwort decoction three times daily. (*See page 110.*)

Balm and limeflowers are tonics for the heart and the circulatory system, and regular infusions will help ensure their healthy functioning. (*See page 121.*)

Homeopathy

Treatment would be constitutional, but the following remedies may help in mild attacks:

Cactus, for a constricted chest and trouble breathing.

Lilium, for a bursting feeling in the heart, with palpitations and some pain in the right arm.

Naja, for an irregular pulse, accompanied by anxiety and fearfulness.

Glonoinum, for a fluttering heart, a sensation of blood rushing, difficulty breathing, and faintness, which are made worse by heat. (*See page 181.*)

Vitamins and Minerals

Increase your intake of dietary fiber and oily fish (such as sardines, herring, salmon, and mackerel).

Raw garlic aids the functioning of the circulatory system, and helps treat the condition.

CAUTION

Prolonged or more severe cases of angina can be a precursor to a heart attack and should receive urgent medical attention.

PALPITATIONS

The average heart beats about 72 times a minute and pumps about 3,600 gallons (13,6401.) of blood a day. During exercise, the pumping action automatically increases three- or fourfold, in response to the tissues' demand for increased oxygen. Palpitation refers to a fast or irregular heartbeat. Palpitations are quite common and usually harmless, often brought on by physical exertion or fright. Frequent or prolonged palpitations, however, may be an indication of heart disease, particularly if accompanied by dizziness, fainting, or chest pain. The sensation of a "missed" beat is due to a premature ectopic beat followed by a compensatory gap before the next beat. This can be induced by excitement, anxiety, or stimulants such as caffeine and nicotine.

Symptoms

- pounding in the chest following exercise
- uncomfortable awareness of a rapid heart rate when anxious

TREATMENT

Chinese Herbalism
Treatment would be aimed at addressing a Heart Blood deficiency, and may include the use of asparagus root and wild jujube seed. (*See page 62.*)

Herbalism
Motherwort, drunk as an infusion, may help if palpitations are linked to anxiety or stress. (*See page 110.*)

Broom, limeflowers, mistletoe, and valerian are useful herbs for treating palpitations. (*See pages 121 and 123.*)

Aromatherapy
If your palpitations are linked to emotional causes, calming oils such as ylang ylang, marjoram, lavender, and mandarin will help. Place a few drops in the bath, or use in regular massage. Carry a bottle with you, and sniff in times of distress. (*See pages 133–157.*)

Peppermint, aniseed, lavender, melissa, rosemary, and neroli essential oils can be used separately or combined in a good massage oil to treat palpitations. (*See pages 133–157.*)

Homeopathy
Nux vomica, when palpitations are brought on by overindulgence. (*See page 198.*)

Nat. mur., for strong palpitations and chest constriction, made worse by heat. (*See page 190.*)

Cactus, for violent palpitations which are worse before menstruation, with dizziness, shortness of breath, and flatulence.

Pulsatilla, when palpitations are brought on by heat or rich fatty foods. (*See page 193.*)

Lachesis, for fainting, a constricted feeling, and anxiety.

Flower Essences
Rescue Remedy or Emergency Essence will help to calm panic and anxiety associated with the onset of palpitations. (*See page 229.*)

GANGRENE

Gangrene is the decay and eventual death of tissue as a result of inadequate blood supply. This may be caused by injury, burns, frostbite, or by disorders such as atherosclerosis, embolism, thrombosis, and diabetes. Excessive smoking can also lead to gangrene.

Symptoms
- if the affected area is not infected, it will typically be dry, and brown or black in color
- if bacteria have entered the affected tissue, festering occurs, leading to "wet" gangrene
- infection of the affected area by one of the clostridia family of gas-producing soil bacteria leads to "gas" gangrene. This is characterized by swelling of the tissues, particularly the muscles, which spreads rapidly to healthy tissues causing discoloration, and severe illness
- antibiotics can sometimes prevent gangrene from spreading

TREATMENT

Homeopathy
The following symptoms can be used on an emergency basis, for up to 10 doses:

Echinacea, when the wound turns septic and also smells foul.

Euphorbia, for wet gangrene in a chronic ulcer.

Lachesis, for pain which is worse after sleeping, and when the affected area is blue or purple. (*See page 200.*)

Arsenicum, when the skin is ulcerated, cold makes the pain worse, and you feel restless. (*See page 167.*)

Vitamins and Minerals
Vitamin E taken orally and applied to the wound or gangrenous area will promote healing. (*See page 239.*)

> **CAUTION**
> Treatment is urgent, and you should be seen by your physician.

ATHEROSCLEROSIS

Atherosclerosis is a degenerative disease of the arteries in which a fatty patch (atheroma) consisting mainly of cholesterol builds up on the wall of an artery. This eventually hardens and partially blocks the artery, causing the formation of a blood clot behind it. It is a progressive condition, generally worsening with age, and is most dangerous when the arteries supplying blood to the heart and brain are affected. Contributing factors to the development of atherosclerosis include smoking, high blood pressure, high blood cholesterol, heredity, and diabetes.

Atherosclerosis can lead to:
- heart attack and angina, where the coronary arteries (supplying the heart) are affected
- stroke, where the carotid arteries (supplying the brain) are affected
- severe pain in the legs on walking when the femoral arteries (supplying the legs) are affected
- severe anemia

TREATMENT

Traditional Home and Folk Remedies
Increase your intake of olive oil, which breaks down cholesterol and fatty deposits in the blood. (*See page 81.*)

Drink barley water daily to ensure that your heart is healthy. (*See page 78.*)

Garlic, onions, and yogurt all have a beneficial effect on the heart. (*See pages 70 and 79.*)

Herbalism
Lavender oil helps to regulate the heart and may prevent heart attack. Use the herb in the bath, or the oil in a vaporizer or gentle massage.

Rosemary—fresh, dried, or as an oil—can be used to stimulate the circulatory system. (*See page 114.*)

Hawthorn berries and tops, and limeflowers are both useful herbs for arterial diseases. (*See pages 104 and 121.*)

Aromatherapy
Regular massage with juniper and lemon can help to break down fatty deposits in the body. (*See pages 146 and 140.*)

Homeopathy

Baryta carb., if you suffer from high blood pressure and palpitations. (*See page 170.*)

Phosphorus, for treating fainting spells, salt cravings, and nervousness. (*See page 192.*)

Glonoinum, for tight congested headache and pounding arteries. (*See page 181.*)

Vanadium, for fainting, dizziness, liver problems, feeling that the heart is being compressed.

Vitamins and Minerals

Increase your intake of dietary fiber, and reduce your intake of salt and sugar.

Increase your intake of foods with bioflavonoids, to improve artery health. (*See page 256.*)

ANEURYSM

An aneurysm is a swelling or bulge in the wall of an artery that can vary in shape, size, and cause. A potentially fatal complication is rupture of the vessel, resulting in massive hemorrhage. It may occur in the main artery, the aorta, as a result of weakness in the muscular wall, possibly through atherosclerosis, syphilis, or a congenital defect. It can eventually rupture, causing fatal internal bleeding. It can also develop in the left ventricle of the heart (ventricular aneurysm) following a heart attack, and can lead to heart failure or an embolism. Aneurysms can also occur in the blood vessels of the brain. These are often congenital.

Symptoms
- severe headaches
- painful spine from the pressure of the swelling in the aorta, which can also cause: a cough, voice loss, and difficulty in swallowing
- in a dissecting aneurysm the wall of the affected artery splits, forcing blood between the layers

There are many different types of aneurysms:
- Arterial aneurysms may be due to atherosclerosis, trauma, infectious injury, or a congenital defect. They occur most often in elderly people.
- Aortic aneurysms usually occur in the abdominal portion of the aorta, generally below the arteries leading to the kidney.
- A relatively common type of aneurysm—giant aneurysms—cause a hemorrhage in the brain.
- Defects in eye arteries may result in multiple aneurysms of the retina.
- Dissecting aneurysms, also called aortic dissection, begin suddenly as a tear in the inner vessel lining followed by entry of blood.
- A ventricular aneurysm may occur following a heart attack. Scar tissue forms over the dead heart cells and creates a patch over the weakened area, which may then bulge when the heart contracts.

Aromatherapy

Oils like chamomile and cypress will bring about the contraction of the capillaries. Use in the bath or in a vaporizer. (*See pages 137 and 143.*)

Homeopathy

For a burst aneurysm, ring for emergency help and take Aconite every 5 minutes until help arrives. (*See page 163.*)

Constitutional treatment is appropriate for a developing aneurysm, but the following treatments will help until you receive treatment:

Baryta carb., for raised blood pressure, palpitations, possible atherosclerosis, and pallor. (*See page 170.*)

Lycopodium, for aneurysm of the aorta, where symptoms worsen between 4 and 8p.m. (*See page 187.*)

Kali iod., for bone pain, which is worse at night and when in warmth.

Vitamins and Minerals

Eat plenty of garlic and brewer's yeast, which will encourage the healthy functioning of the circulatory system. (*See page 257.*)

Increase your intake of oily fish.

Vitamins C and E will encourage the healthy functioning of the circulatory system. (*See pages 238 and 239.*)

VARICOSE VEINS

Varicose veins are swollen and twisted veins, most commonly found in the legs but also in the rectum (where they are known as hemorrhoids), the scrotum, and the esophagus. The swelling is caused by a weakness in the valves of the veins, which leads to increased pressure on the vein walls. This can be the result of deep vein thrombosis, obesity, pregnancy, prolonged sitting or standing, constipation, prolapse, or it may be hereditary.

Symptoms
- extremely sore, swollen, and tender veins
- swelling of the legs
- bruising and discoloration
- burning sensation
- aching calves
- irritated and flaky skin
- ulcers
- in severe cases, a vein may rupture and bleed

TREATMENT

Chinese Herbalism
The source of the problem is bad circulation, stagnant qi, and stagnant Blood, and the following herbs would be used: angelica, cinnamon twigs, and astragalus; honey might be used externally. (*See pages 41, 42, and 44.*)

Traditional Home and Folk Remedies
Raw beetroot should be eaten daily, for its healing and strengthening action.

A mustard poultice may help to encourage circulation in the area. (*See page 84.*)

Herbalism
Calendula oil, or marigold tea as a compress can be applied. (*See page 102.*)

Herbs to repair and tone the veins include hawthorn berries, horse chestnut, prickly ash and yarrow—all of which can be infused and drunk. (*See pages 104 and 97.*)

Aromatherapy
Rosemary oil, blended with a light carrier oil, can be massaged into the legs. (*See page 154.*)

Essential oils of juniper and lavender can be diluted and massaged into the surrounding area, or used in the bath. (*See pages 146 and 147.*)

Homeopathy
Hamamelis, for bruised, sore veins, and piles. (*See page 182.*)

Carb. veg., for mottled and marbled skin. (*See page 173.*)

Pulsatilla, especially during pregnancy, and if warmth makes symptoms worse. (*See page 193.*)

Ferr. phos., for pale legs that redden easily, but are better on walking. (*See page 179.*)

Vitamins and Minerals
Increase your intake of vitamins E and C, and bio-flavonoids, which improve blood vessel health. (*See pages 239, 238, and 256.*)

Increase your intake of dietary fiber, which will prevent constipation.

Rutin helps to keep the vein walls in good shape.

RAYNAUD'S DISEASE

Raynaud's disease is a disorder in which the arteries of the fingers and (less often) the toes go into spasm on exposure to cold. Raynaud's disease is more common in women than men, and its onset usually occurs in young adulthood. It affects mainly young women, has no known cause, and is rarely serious. Raynaud's phenomenon, however, caused by disease or occupational hazard, is more problematic: inflammation of the arteries of the fingers and toes occurs, sometimes leading to the formation of a blood clot.

Symptoms
- tingling sensation, burning, and numbness in fingers or toes
- affected areas turn white, then blue, then red
- painful ulcers or even tissue death (gangrene) can occur in cases where the disease persists for years

TREATMENT

Ayurveda
Massage hands and feet with a mixture of warm mustard and sesame seed oils. (*See page 19.*)

Chinese Herbalism

Cinnamon twigs and Chinese angelica may be useful. (*See pages 44 and 41.*)

Herbalism

Cayenne pepper can be added to any herbal tea to stimulate the circulation and warm the body. (*See page 103.*)

Fresh ginger can be chewed, and the juices swallowed, to improve circulation and act as a tonic to the heart.

Aromatherapy

Rubefacient oils such as black pepper, lemon, and rosemary can be massaged into the affected area to increase circulation and warmth. (*See pages 133–157.*)

Homeopathy

Constitutional treatment is advised, but the following may help:
- Carb. veg., for icy, mottled-looking skin. (*See page 173.*)
- Lachesis, for blue or purple skin, worse after sleep.
- Pulsatilla, for symptoms that are made worse by heat or hanging the limb. (*See page 193.*)
- Arsenicum, for swelling, burning and itching made worse by exposure to cold. (*See page 167.*)
- Cactus, for icy cold, swollen hands and feet.
- Secale, for burning sensation in fingers or toes.

Vitamins and Minerals

Increase your intake of iron, and ensure that you take plenty of foods rich in vitamin C alongside, which helps the absorption of iron. (*See pages 243 and 238.*)

BRUISING

Bruising (or ecchymosis) results from the release of blood from the capillaries into the tissues under the skin. The characteristic bluish-black mark on the skin lightens in color and eventually fades as the blood is absorbed by the tissues and carried away. Bruising usually occurs as a result of an injury, but can occasionally be spontaneous and an indication of an allergic reaction, or more serious diseases such as leukemia and hemophilia.

> **CAUTION**
> A case of bruising without any obvious cause requires medical investigation as it may be an outward symptom of a more serious condition.

Symptoms
- pain on pressure
- in severe cases, pain on attempting to move the affected area

TREATMENT

Traditional Home and Folk Remedies

Macerated and heated cabbage leaves can be applied to the affected area. (*See page 73.*)

A mustard poultice or black pepper oil draws the blood away from the bruise. (*See pages 84 and 83.*)

A vinegar compress can be used for all bruises or swelling. Avoid the eye area. (*See page 87.*)

Witch hazel tincture can be used to relieve swellings and bruises. Apply to a cool compress. (*See page 78.*)

Use roasted onions in a poultice to help heal bruising.

Herbalism

Bathe the area in witch hazel, which disperses the blood and encourages healing. (*See page 109.*)

Homeopathy

Arnica, where there is bruising due to trauma or injury.

Hamamelis, for bruising with broken skin, or due to poor circulation. (*See page 182.*)

Ruta. grav., for bruising that feels as if it is in the bone.

Hypericum, when bruising involves nerve endings, such as fingers and toes. (*See page 184.*)

Homeopathic remedy and tincture of Calendula will ease symptoms. (*See page 172.*)

Flower Essences

Rescue Remedy can be applied to the bruised area, to encourage healing and prevent the negative effects of trauma.

Crushed agrimony roots and leaves can be used as a compress for bruises or taken internally. (*See page 210.*)

Comfrey is exceptional for healing, and can be applied as a compress or poultice on the bruise.

Daisy is also known as bruisewort; bruise the leaves and flowers and add them to wheat germ oil.

Vitamins and Minerals

Increase your intake of vitamin C and bioflavonoids, to help the health of the capillaries. (*See pages 238 and 256.*)

Zinc strengthens the integrity of the capillaries.

DISORDERS OF THE DIGESTIVE SYSTEM

NAUSEA AND VOMITING

Nausea (a feeling of sickness) and vomiting are symptoms of various disorders, which include gastroenteritis, inner ear infection, migraine, excessive food or alcohol intake, hiatus hernia, pancreatitis, indigestion, food poisoning, gallstones, or liver disease. They may also be caused by hormonal changes in pregnancy and menstruation, travel, or by certain smells and sights. Nausea may be accompanied by a feeling of faintness and dizziness. Vomiting is usually preceded by nausea, and may be accompanied by sweating, excessive salivation, and a slowing of the heart rate. A constant feeling of nausea with no vomiting, but with a headache and abdominal pain, is most likely to be stress- or anxiety-related.

> **CAUTION**
> If nausea or vomiting are accompanied by severe pain lasting for more than one hour, or if vomit is blood-stained, seek urgent medical advice.

TREATMENT

Chinese Herbalism

Treatment would be aimed at ascending Stomach qi, and useful herbs may include root ginger, Ren Dan, Shen Chu Cha, Xiang Sha Yang Wei Pian, or Bu Zhong Yi Qi Wan.

Er Chen Wan pills, a classical formula to dissolve Phlegm, resolve Spleen Damp and harmonize the center (digestive organs), as well as symptoms brought on by food retention in the Stomach.

Herbalism

Drinking ginger tea or chewing a piece of crystallized ginger warms the stomach and allays cold nausea. This can be used for relief of sickness in pregnancy or during travel. (*See page 126.*)

Persistent nausea may indicate liver trouble: seek advice. Take decoction or coffee made of dandelion root. (*See page 121.*)

Homeopathy

Sepia, when you feel nauseous at the thought or smell of food, but feel better for eating. (*See page 196.*)

Nux vomica, when nausea is made better by vomiting, and may be caused by overindulgence. (*See page 198.*)

Lactic acid, when there is profuse salivation and a history of anemia.

Tabacum, for nausea and vomiting relieved by uncovering the abdomen.

Arsenicum, when nausea and vomiting are accompanied by diarrhea, and symptoms are worse between midnight and 2a.m. (*See page 167.*)

Phosphorus, for cravings for cold water, which is then vomited, with blood in the vomit and burning pains in the stomach. (*See page 192.*)

Pulsatilla, for vomiting after rich, fatty food, with some tearfulness. (*See page 193.*)

Arnica, when vomiting follows a head injury.

Aconite, when vomiting and severe pain last for more than one hour, and are not relieved by vomiting.

Flower Essences

Rescue Remedy or Emergency Essence will be useful for prolonged or distressing vomiting; it will help to reduce panic and calm the mind and body. (*See page 229.*)

Vitamins and Minerals

Take vitamin B6 for morning sickness (consult your doctor first) and for travel sickness. It is appropriate for children if given in half-doses. (*See page 237.*)

THE HEALING REMEDIES SOURCEBOOK

JAUNDICE

Jaundice refers to a yellowing of the whites of the eyes and of the skin caused by bilirubin—a natural coloring substance. Under normal circumstances, bilirubin is released by red blood cells and passed to the intestine in bile, via the liver. If the liver is diseased, however, or if there is bile duct blockage, it accumulates in the blood, causing the characteristic yellow staining of tissue. Newborn infants frequently develop mild jaundice, which lasts several days until a normal excess of red blood cells is destroyed. This condition is not normally considered to be serious. But erythroblastosis fetalis, a serious form of jaundice in infants, generally is due to a Rh factor incompatibility. Adolescents and young adults who have a viral inflammation of the liver often develop jaundice; jaundice in middle-aged adults is commonly due to gallstones. In older adults jaundice may signal cancer of the liver or the bile ducts. It is often the first symptom of liver damage in heavy drinkers.

> **CAUTION**
> Jaundice is not a disease in itself, but is an indication of an underlying disorder such as hepatitis, gallstones, hemolytic anemia, cirrhosis of the liver, pancreatitis, or pancreatic cancer. The cause of jaundice should always be investigated immediately.

Symptoms
- yellowing of the skin and the whites of the eyes
- darkened urine
- pale-colored stools

TREATMENT
Chinese Herbalism
Treatment would be aimed at Dampness in the Gall Bladder and Liver, and useful herbs may include gardenia fruit, oriental wormwood, and the bark of the cork tree.

Herbalism
Any of the following herbs can be used to tonify the liver: golden seal, verbena, barberry, blue flag, dandelion, and wild yam. (*See pages 125 and 121.*)

Aromatherapy
Oils that strengthen the liver include chamomile, cypress, lemon, peppermint, rosemary, and thyme. Use one or a blend of these oils in massage, or in a vaporizer in your room. (*See pages 133–157.*)

Homeopathy
Constitutional treatment would accord with the cause of the jaundice.

Crotalus is appropriate for jaundice caused by hemolytic anemia.

Vitamins and Minerals
- Drink fresh carrot and lemon juice daily.
- Avoid alcohol and caffeine.
- Eat plenty of fresh fruit and vegetables, as well as whole grains and cereals.

HIATUS HERNIA

A hiatus hernia occurs when part of the stomach slides up through the esophageal opening in the diaphragm into the chest. As a result of this the stomach's contents regurgitate into the esophagus, which may cause damage and inflammation (esophagitis). The underlying cause of hiatus hernia is unknown, but this common condition tends to occur more often in obese people (and especially in women in later middle age), and in those who smoke. In some cases it is present at birth.

Symptoms
- severe heartburn (a burning pain behind the breastbone) that worsens on bending, straining, and lying down
- if esophagitis occurs there may be associated symptoms of acid in the mouth, difficulty in swallowing, and ulceration

TREATMENT
Chinese Herbalism
Treatment would be individual, but there are a number of herbs which will restore the balance. (*See pages 39–62.*)

Homeopathy

Constitutional treatment would be suggested, but the remedies for indigestion will be appropriate. (*See page 340.*)

Calc. fluor., a tissue salt, will help elasticity.

APPENDICITIS

The appendix is 1–8in. (2–20cm.) long, about as thick as a pencil, and hollow. It consists mostly of lymphoid tissue, like the tonsils and adenoids, and is easily invaded by micro-organisms. One out of every 15 people develops appendicitis, the inflammation of an infected appendix. This is a medical emergency that usually requires the surgical removal of the appendix.

> **CAUTION**
> Perforation of the appendix can lead to peritonitis—
> a serious, potentially fatal inflammation of the
> membrane lining the abdominal cavity.

Symptoms
- pain and tenderness beginning in the center of the abdomen, moving to the right and down toward the groin
- possibly nausea and vomiting
- fever

TREATMENT
Herbalism

Treatment is aimed at preventing the condition in people who have a "grumbling" appendix, with inflammation and recurring abdominal pain. The following herbs will help to resolve inflammation and irritation: agrimony, chamomile, echinacea, licorice, and wild yam. These can be combined or taken separately, up to 3 times a day. (*See pages 97, 104, 105, and 108.*)

Homeopathy

Urgent medical treatment will be required, but the following remedies can be offered, every 15 minutes, while waiting for help:

- Lachesis, for cutting, tearing pains, a distended abdomen and irritability. (*See page 200.*)
- Bryonia, for intense pain over the appendix area.
- Belladonna, for pain that is made worse by movement, accompanied by a red, flushed face. (*See page 168.*)

After an operation, the following remedies help:
- Arnica, to prevent bruising and encourage healing.

Flower Essences

Rescue Remedy or Emergency Essence can be given while waiting for help, to calm and reduce anxiety. (*See page 229.*)

Vitamins and Minerals

Eat plenty of fresh fruits and vegetables, and avoid getting constipated.

Never use laxative preparations, which will aggravate the condition.

GASTROENTERITIS

Gastroenteritis is an acute inflammation of the stomach and intestine, causing violent upset. It may be due to bowel organisms such as salmonella or other bacterial toxins or viruses that may contaminate food or water; food intolerance; or excessive alcohol intake. The symptoms and their severity will vary according to the cause. It can also be a side-effect of certain drugs. Gastroenteritis is most serious in the elderly and in babies because of the danger of dehydration through vomiting and diarrhea.

> **CAUTION**
> If symptoms persist for more than 48 hours, or are
> accompanied by severe pain, call for emergency help.

Symptoms
- fever
- abdominal pain
- nausea and vomiting
- diarrhea
- in severe cases there may be shock and collapse

THE HEALING REMEDIES SOURCEBOOK

TREATMENT

Traditional Home and Folk Remedies

Very ripe bananas will ease nausea, act as a gentle constipant, and help to restore the healthy bacteria in the intestines.

Live yogurt, taken by the teaspoon throughout the day, can help to restore bacteria to the stomach and digestive tracts. (*See page 79.*)

Honey is a natural antibiotic and anti-inflammatory. Mix a few teaspoonfuls in a cup of warm water and sip. Freeze into ice cubes if you find hot drinks difficult to manage. (*See page 87.*)

Herbalism

Make an infusion of comfrey root and meadowsweet to treat the infection and relieve the associated symptoms. (*See pages 119 and 106.*)

Arrowroot or slippery elm tea can be sipped during the worst symptoms to soothe the digestive tract, and afterwards to help restore bowel health. (*See page 123.*)

Aromatherapy

Massage chamomile and geranium essential oils into the abdomen to bring relief from pain and discomfort. (*See pages 137 and 151.*)

Homeopathy

The following remedies can be taken hourly, as required:

- Arsenicum, for burning abdominal pains, accompanied by great thirst. (*See page 167.*)
- Pulsatilla, for symptoms which are worse at night, and tearfulness. (*See page 193.*)
- Baptisia, if a salmonella infection is suspected—stools dark, bloody, and smelly, nearly liquid. (*See page 169.*)
- Mercurius for diarrhea, where there is blood and mucus in the stools. (*See page 189.*)
- Phosphorus, for a burning sensation when stools are passed, with vomiting and cravings for cold water, which is then vomited. (*See page 192.*)
- Sulfur for burning diarrhea which is at its worst around 5a.m., with a red, itchy anus. (*See page 198.*)

Vitamins and Minerals

Take acidophilus to restore the healthy flora in the intestines, which will help to fight infection. (*See page 256.*)

2 million people in the U.S. suffer from food poisoning each year.

The most common type of food poisoning, accounting for nearly 70 percent of cases, is due to Salmonella typhimurium, a bacterium commonly found in meat, eggs, and milk.

The Staphylococcus bacteria, another type of food poisoning, multiply rapidly at room temperature and are usually transmitted by careless food handling; workers may sneeze or cough on food, or may have infected pimples or wounds on the hands or face and transmit the bacteria to the food.

If food contaminated by the bacterium Clostridium botulinum is improperly canned or bottled the bacteria are able to produce a toxin, which produces the disease botulism. The mortality rate can be as high as 65 percent.

Diarrhea and vomiting may result from infection by the protozoan Entamoeba histolytica, acquired by eating uncooked vegetables or drinking contaminated water (amoebic dysentery).

Certain rare strains of the bacteria Escherichia coli can cause food poisoning in young children, the elderly, and people with impaired immune systems. E. coli, normally found in the intestines and fecal matter of humans and animals, can survive in meat if the meat is not cooked past 155°F.

STOMACH ULCERS

Peptic ulcers occur most commonly in the duodenum, near the junction with the stomach, and in the stomach wall. They usually occur singly as round or oval wounds. The erosions are usually shallow, but can penetrate the entire wall, leading to hemorrhage and possibly death. When gastric juices (consisting of hydrochloric acid, mucus, and a digestive enzyme called pepsin) act upon the walls of the digestive tract, a peptic ulcer results. Peptic ulcers tend to become chronic.

The peptic ulcer develops when there is imbalance between the normal "aggressive" factors, the acid-peptic secretions, and the normal "resistance" factors, such as mucus and rapid cellular replacement. Physical and mental stress are thought to be triggers, as are hereditary factors, smoking, excessive alcohol intake, and non-steroidal anti-inflammatory drugs (NSAIDs). Gastric (stomach) ulcers affect both men and women, usually over the age of 40, while duodenal ulcers are more common in men. Ulcers in the lower esophagus are relatively rare and are usually associated with hiatus hernia (*see page 337*) and esophagitis. Peptic ulcers affect approximately 10 percent of the U.S. population. Duodenal ulcers are two to three times more common than gastric ulcers, and people with blood group O are more likely to get them.

Symptoms

- gastric ulcers: a gnawing, burning pain, which is worse during or after eating, nausea, and vomiting
- duodenal ulcers: intermittent upper abdominal pain characteristically relieved by eating; pain usually begins around mid-morning and sufferers are often woken up by it at night
- peptic ulcers:, may bleed, causing blood in vomit and dark, blackish stools, occasionally a peptic ulcer perforates, causing severe pain and shock

TREATMENT

Ayurveda
Suitable herbs which might be suggested include bitter orange, coriander, and kalanchoe. (*See page 24.*)

Chinese Herbalism
Treatment would be aimed at unblocking stagnant Stomach qi, excess Heat, and a weak Spleen. Suitable herbs may include dandelion, ginseng, and corydalis tuber. (*See page 54.*)

Herbalism
Licorice has a soothing effect on the stomach and the mucous membranes, and a decoction can be drunk three or four times each day to ease symptoms. (*See page 108.*)

A decoction of marshmallow root is healing. (*See page 99.*)

Comfrey or slippery elm may also be of help. (*See pages 119 and 123.*)

Aromatherapy
Oils of chamomile, frankincense, geranium, and marjoram can be diluted and massaged into the abdomen. (*See pages 133–157.*)

Homeopathy
Treatment would be constitutional, but the following remedies may be appropriate:
- Nux vomica, for pain which is worse after eating. (*See page 198.*)
- Anacardium, when pain is relieved by eating. (*See page 164.*)
- Kali bich., for pain in a small, distinct position in the stomach area. (*See page 185.*)
- Phosphorus, for burning pains and vomiting which are better for cold drinks. (*See page 192.*)
- Bryonia, for a feeling of a stone in the stomach and sensitivity to touch. (*See page 170.*)

INDIGESTION

Indigestion (or dyspepsia) is a general term which usually refers to abdominal discomfort, nausea, heartburn (burning sensation or pain behind the breastbone), hiccups, and flatulence. Indigestion refers to discomfort in the upper abdomen—gastric distress—often brought on by eating too much, by eating too quickly, or by eating very rich, spicy, or fatty foods. Nervous indigestion is a common effect of stress. Indigestion is also commonly caused by excessive smoking, excessive alcohol or caffeine consumption, pregnancy, or anxiety. It can also be a feature of several diseases, including esophagitis (inflammation of the lining of the esophagus), gastroenteritis (*see page 338*), peptic ulcer (*see page 339*), and gallstones (*see page 342*).

Symptoms
- abdominal discomfort
- nausea
- heartburn (burning sensation or pain behind the breastbone)
- hiccups
- flatulence

TREATMENT

Ayurveda

Crush fresh root ginger to extract the juice. Mix with the juice of a lime and a lemon, add a pinch of salt, and drink.

Chinese Herbalism

Treatment would address a weakness of the Spleen and Stomach. Rice and wheat sprouts would be used.

Herbalism

Try an infusion of peppermint or fennel tea after meals or when feeling full and windy. (*See pages 111 and 107.*)

Improve the general tone of the digestive tract with bitter aperient herbs such as dandelion, gentian, and wormwood, taken 20 minutes before food. (*See page 120.*)

A cold stomach can be warmed by eating three cardamom pods, or a pinch of ginger or cayenne.

Fresh dill, added to boiling water and steeped, will reduce flatulence and gas pains.

Traditional Home and Folk Remedies

Eat a slice of fresh pineapple after meals to ease symptoms.

Clove tea and cinnamon tea are both digestive and will soothe away the symptoms. (*See page 76.*)

Fennel, eaten raw or cooked, or the bruised seeds infused and drunk, acts as a digestive.

Peppermint leaves can be infused and drunk to relieve indigestion, and to soothe any gas pains. Peppermint oil can be rubbed into the abdomen for instant relief.

Drink a little warmed vinegar and honey in a cup of hot water to ease digestive complaints. (*See page 87.*)

Homeopathy

Chronic indigestion should be treated constitutionally, but the following remedies may be useful during an attack:

- Carb. veg., after rich foods, with gas and belching.
- Nux vomica, after spicy food, and overindulgence in cigarettes and alcohol. (*See page 198.*)
- Arsenicum, when there is burning pain, particularly between midnight and 2a.m. (*See page 167.*)
- Pulsatilla, for an attack brought on by rich food, and accompanied by a bad taste in the mouth, nausea, and weepiness. (*See page 193.*)

- China, for windy stomach, and a bloated and sluggish feeling, and where stools have the appearance of chopped egg. (*See page 175.*)
- Lycopodium, for a bloated stomach with heartburn, and a full feeling even when hungry, especially where food causes instant discomfort. (*See page 187.*)
- Graphites, for burning pains which are relieved by food or milk, but followed by ingestion. (*See page 181.*)
- Bryonia, for a heaviness in the stomach, which is worse after food, with heartburn, nausea, and faintness; and which is made worse by movement but improved by lying down. (*See page 170.*)

TRAVEL SICKNESS

Travel or motion sickness is a sensitivity to the constant passive movement of the body while in a car, boat, airplane, train, or bus. Some people may even experience it in lifts. Why only some people experience travel sickness is unclear. The syndrome appears to arise from sensory mismatch, when the information coming to the brain from various sensory inputs does not add up, as when the eyes report a steady horizon, but the balancing (vestibular) system reports a rocking motion. Travel sickness appears to be more common in women, and children under the age of two. Elderly people do not seem to be so troubled by the problem. Severe travel sickness can cause a complete lack of coordination.

Symptoms

- progressive nausea
- vomiting
- pallor, faintness, and dizziness
- abdominal discomfort
- headache
- sweaty palms and face
- increased salivation

TREATMENT

Ayurveda

Ginger, chewed fresh, may help symptoms.

Oral syrup of Vilwadi lehya will be useful.

Chinese Herbalism
Sipping a warm drink with grated root ginger may be helpful.

Herbalism
Chew fresh angelica leaves, and hang them in the car while traveling. (*See page 100.*)

Chew fresh or crystallized ginger to ease nausea. (*See page 126.*)

Fennel or chamomile tea will ease the symptoms. (*See pages 107 and 104.*)

Fresh peppermint leaves can be chewed, or drink an infusion to soothe and settle the stomach. (*See page 111.*)

Homeopathy
Take the following remedies hourly when symptoms begin:
- Nux vomica, for a feeling of chilliness, which is improved by vomiting. (*See page 198.*)
- Arnica, when you are overtired and irritable. (*See page 167.*)
- Cocculus, for nausea with a metallic taste in the mouth.
- Sepia, when nausea is made worse by the smell of food and improved by eating. (*See page 196.*)
- Tabacum, for nausea with giddiness, and pale, cold sweat, with a band around the head.

GALLSTONES

Gallstones are hard stone-like masses occurring in the gall bladder or in the bile duct. They are usually about the size of a pebble, and most are composed of cholesterol, calcium, or both. Abnormal composition of bile (too much cholesterol, for example), blockage of bile outflow, infection, or hereditary factors may all cause gallstones. Risk factors include obesity, advancing age, a high-fat diet, and food intolerance. Far more women than men are affected by gallstones. Gallstones occur in about 10 percent of the U.S. population, particularly in women. There may be from one to ten or more stones, ranging in size, about 1–25mm. across. Gallstones are rare in childhood, but become progressively more common with age. Autopsies show that 20 percent of all women have gallstones when they die. The use of oral contraceptives may cause gallstones to form earlier than they would have otherwise.

Symptoms
- acute upper abdominal pain
- possibly high fever
- inflammation of the gall bladder (cholecystitis)
- there may be some jaundice if the stones cause bile duct obstruction
- severe pain if a stone passes from the bile duct into the duodenum (biliary colic)

TREATMENT
Ayurveda
Kalonchoe can be used to treat gallstones.

Chinese Herbalism
Herbs such as lysimachia, pyrrosia leaf, and rhubarb may break up and dissolve small stones. (*See page 60.*)

Herbalism
The following herbs will dissolve the gallstones, but it will take several months. Blend infusions of balmony, dandelion leaves, stone root, and fringetree bark. Take two or three times a day. (*See page 121.*)

Aromatherapy
Massage lavender and rosemary oils over the gall bladder area to relieve the pain. (*See pages 147 and 154.*)

Homeopathy
Treatment would always be constitutional, but the following remedies may help until you are able to seek advice:
- Berberis, for relief of normal symptoms.
- China, if Berberis is not effective. (*See page 175.*)

Vitamins and Minerals
Reduce your intake of all fats, except olive oil, which has been proved to break up gallstones.

Increase your intake of dietary fiber, and ensure that you drink plenty of water.

HEPATITIS

Hepatitis is a disorder involving inflammation of the liver. Hepatitis A, once called infectious hepatitis, is the most common cause of acute hepatitis and is usually transmitted by food and water contaminated by human waste. Hepatitis B is spread mainly by blood or blood products, but can be transmitted from mother to fetus, and by intimate contact, including sexual intercourse. It often causes an initial episode of liver disease and occasionally leads to chronic hepatitis. Hepatitis C is the most common form of viral hepatitis. Type C is transmitted in blood and blood products (which are now screened for the virus), and it may be present in the body for many years before it damages the liver. Hepatitis C is a leading cause of chronic hepatitis and is considered a serious public health threat.

Hepatitis C accounts for 10–40 percent of all hepatitis, and 90–95 percent get the disease from blood transfusions.

Another strain of hepatitis C is uncommon in Europe and the U.S., but common in Mexico, Africa, and Asia, and usually contracted from contaminated water.

According to recent research, 25 percent of people in the U.S. who receive blood transfusions will develop hepatitis.

Of those contracting chronic hepatitis, most are women under the age of 45.

Chronic hepatitis leads to cirrhosis and liver damage.

Acute hepatitis may arise secondary to various infections that involve the liver.

Symptoms
- loss of appetite
- dark urine
- fatigue
- sometimes fever
- the liver may become enlarged
- jaundice may occur, giving the skin a yellow tinge
- hepatitis may be acute or chronic: the acute form can subside after about two months or, rarely, can result in liver failure

TREATMENT

Chinese Herbalism
Hepatitis A would require treatment for excess liver and gall bladder Damp Heat. Suitable herbal remedies include gardenia fruit and oriental wormwood.

Hepatitis B would require treatment for deficient qi and a weakened liver. Suitable herbs include peony root, mulberry, ginseng, licorice, and astragalus. (*See pages 53, 54, 50, and 42.*)

Herbalism
Liver tonics may be taken daily to encourage healing and rejuvenation. Any of the following herbs can be used: golden seal, verbena, barberry, blue flag, dandelion, and wild yam. (*See pages 125, 121, and 105.*)

Traditional Home and Folk Remedies
Drink barley or rice water as an overall tonic. (*See pages 78 and 82.*)

Aromatherapy
Oils which act as tonics to the liver include juniper, grapefruit, chamomile, and cypress. Massage them, in a little carrier oil, into the abdominal area, or add a few drops to your bath. (*See pages 133–157.*)

Homeopathy
Chronic hepatitis, which is rare, will be treated constitutionally. Cases of acute hepatitis may respond to the following:
- Bryonia, for symptoms that come on after exposure to cold, with sharp pain in the liver area. (*See page 170.*)
- Mercurius, for a yellow tongue and bad breath, with jaundice and sensitivity to cold and heat. (*See page 189.*)
- Hydrastis, for swollen, tender liver, and catarrh.
- Lachesis, when the liver feels tender and swollen, and the abdomen is distended and painful. (*See page 200.*)

Vitamins and Minerals
Plenty of fluids are necessary to cleanse the system.

Extra vitamin C will help overcome the infection. (*See page 238.*)

CIRRHOSIS OF THE LIVER

The liver is the second-largest organ in the human body, after the skin. It is a spongy, reddish-brown gland that lies just below the diaphragm in the abdominal cavity, and it serves to metabolize carbohydrates and store them as glycogen; metabolize lipids (fats, including cholesterol and certain vitamins) and proteins; manufacture a digestive fluid, bile; filter impurities and toxic material from the blood; produce blood-clotting factors, and destroy old, worn-out red blood cells.

The liver is able to regenerate itself after being injured or diseased; but if a disease progresses beyond the tissues capacity to regenerate new cells, the body's entire metabolism is severely affected. Severely impaired livers are sometimes replaced, and in the early 1990s the one-year survival rate was 76 percent.

Cirrhosis of the liver is the replacement of normal tissue by nonfunctioning fibrous tissue, causing scarring (or fibrosis). Cirrhosis occurs as the last stage in a range of liver disorders which have been so damaging as to cause a breakdown in the livers regeneration process. Normal liver function is prevented and any remaining healthy liver cells are cut off from the blood supply they need. Cirrhosis may be caused by hepatitis B, poisoning, and long-term alcohol abuse.

Symptoms
- appetite and weight loss
- continuous indigestion
- nausea and vomiting with general malaise
- loss of muscle power
- itching of the skin
- bad breath
- bleeding varicose veins (caused by the blood's attempt to use an alternative route from the liver back to the heart)
- vomiting blood

TREATMENT
Herbalism
Good liver tonics include barberry, dandelion root, golden seal, vervain, wild yam, and yellow dock. Make an infusion of one or more and sip two or three times daily. (*See pages 121, 125, 105, and 115.*)

Aromatherapy
Oils which work as a tonic to the liver and improve its function include chamomile, cypress, grapefruit, juniper, lemon, and orange. Mix a few drops in a warm carrier oil and massage into the abdomen, or add a few drops to your bath (*see pages 133–157*).

Homeopathy
Constitutional treatment with an experienced homeopath will be necessary, but the following remedies will help until you have arranged treatment.

Arsenicum, when there is fluid retention, and the patient feels chilly, restless, and worse between midnight and 2a.m. (*See page 167.*)

Phosphorus, when there is jaundice, a craving for cold water (which makes symptoms worse), and a tendency to bleed easily. (*See page 172.*)

China, when the liver is swollen and painful, and you feel chilly and full of wind. (*See page 175.*)

PANCREATITIS

A long, thin organ, the pancreas has both digestive and endocrine functions, and for this reason contains two completely different types of cells. It measures about 5-6in. (12–15 cm.) in length and is situated within the curve of the duodenum.

Pancreatitis is an inflammation of the pancreas which can be either acute or chronic. Acute pancreatitis may be caused by interference (often from gallstones) with the outflow of digestive juices from the pancreas, as a result of which the pancreas begins to digest itself. Heavy drinking is another cause, and is almost always responsible for cases of chronic pancreatitis. Chronic pancreatitis is more common in men than in women and is most commonly due to heavy drinking. The dominant feature of chronic pancreatitis is upper abdominal and back pain. Diagnosis of pancreatitis can be difficult since it closely resembles peptic ulcer and acute appendicitis. Pancreatic cancer is the fourth leading cause of cancer death in the U.S.

Symptoms

- acute pancreatitis: severe central abdominal pain, spreading to the back and shoulder, then the whole abdomen
- nausea, vomiting, and shock
- chronic pancreatitis: constant pain, often in the back
- weight loss
- if bile duct obstruction occurs there will be jaundice

TREATMENT

Herbalism

Soothing herbs include licorice and yellow dock, drunk as an infusion in an attack. (*See pages 108 and 115.*)

Treatment would be individual, according to the cause of the illness.

Homeopathy

For acute pancreatitis, ring for emergency medical attention, and give Aconite, every 10 minutes, until help arrives.

For chronic pancreatitis, constitutional treatment is necessary, but the following remedies may help in an attack:

- Phosphorus, when there is jaundice and a craving for cold drinks that are then vomited up. (*See page 172.*)
- Iris, for watery stools, a burning sensation in the bowels, and cutting pains in the abdomen.
- Mercurius, for stabbing pains in the abdomen, a chilly feeling, jaundice, and offensive sweat. (*See page 189.*)
- Arsenicum, for burning pains which are worse between midnight and 2a.m., feeling chilled and restless.

CROHN'S DISEASE

For sufferers of Crohn's disease, segments of the bowel become inflamed, ulcerated, and greatly thickened, while the sections in between remain normal. Any part of the bowel may be affected, but usually it is the last part of the small intestine, the terminal ileum, that is involved. It is a chronic disease whose cause is unknown, although there may be a genetic factor. Complications of Crohn's disease include arthritis, red swellings on the skin, mouth ulcers, eye inflammation, gallstones, urinary infections, and kidney stones. Crohn's most often affects young adults and people over sixty.

Crohn's disease commonly occurs between the ages of 20 and 40 and is four times more common in Caucasians and Jews than any other ethnic group.

Crohn's may be hereditary, affecting multiple family members.

Crohn's mainly affects the small intestine, but can occur anywhere along the digestive tract. Bowel obstruction and various other complications which arise may require surgical intervention.

Symptoms

- spasms of lower abdominal pain
- diarrhea
- appetite and weight loss
- anemia
- rectal bleeding in older sufferers

TREATMENT

Ayurveda

Henbane can be used for bowel spasms and colic. It has sedative and antispasmodic actions.

Coriander can help with diarrhea and the pain of Crohn's disease. It is an anti-inflammatory. (*See page 24.*)

Hollyhock is often used to treat bowel irritation.

Herbalism

An infusion of peppermint can help protect the gut lining from irritation, and help to soothe the griping of the condition. The bitters stimulate and cleanse the bowels, and have an antiseptic and antibacterial action.

Hops have an antispasmodic action which reduces tension in the body, relieving colic and spasm in the gut. The bitters in hops also enhance the action of the digestive system.

Aromatherapy

Lavender oil will help you to relax and to reduce the effects of stress. Add it to your bath water, or use in an overall body massage for best effect. (*See page 147.*)

Roman chamomile oil, rubbed into the abdomen, may help to soothe pain. (*See page 137.*)

Homeopathy

Treatment would be constitutional, but some of the following remedies may be appropriate:

- Colocynthis, for diarrhea accompanied by griping pains, and also copious, thin, frothy stools.
- Pulsatilla, for symptoms made worse by onions, rich food, and cold drinks, with diarrhea worse at night. (*See page 193.*)

Vitamins and Minerals

You may need to take extra vitamin A, B, and D, and zinc supplement daily. (*See pages 234–239 and 249.*)

You may be allergic to some foods, such as dairy produce or wheat—see a nutritional therapist for advice.

Avoid sugar and other refined carbohydrates.

Place chopped peppermint leaves in a pot and pour boiling water over the herb. Cover with a lid. Allow the peppermint to infuse for approximately 4 minutes before pouring.

CONSTIPATION

Constipation refers to unduly infrequent or irregular bowel movements, with difficulty, discomfort, and sometimes pain on passing dry, hard feces. It is usually harmless but may be an indication of an underlying disorder, especially in adults over the age of 40. Constipation may result from: insufficient fiber in the diet, immobility, hemorrhoids (*see page 350*), an anal fissure (*see page 349*), iron tablets, hypothyroidism (*see page 380*), or hormonal changes, such as those in pregnancy. Dietary causes include inadequate fluid intake; a lack of vitamin B1, B5, B6, potassium, magnesium, and zinc; too much animal protein, too many dairy products, too much vinegar, pepper, salt, spices, and aluminum. If the diet is not at fault, the cause may be eating meals too fast, not taking enough exercise, tension, anxiety, depression, taking antibiotics, abusing laxatives, or abuse of certain over-the-counter drugs, such as cough mixtures.

Symptoms
- pain during bowel movements

- weight loss
- sufferers may experience headaches, furred tongue, loss of appetite, nausea, fatigue, and depression, all arising largely from anxiety about constipation

TREATMENT

Chinese Herbalism

Constipation is believed to be caused either by Heat, stagnation of qi, Deficiency (of qi, yang, Blood, or yin), or interior Cold. Some suitable pills include:

- Ma Ren Wan, for Heat (dry stools, thirst, dark urine).
- Run Chang Wan, for chronic constipation of any kind, especially in old age or after childbirth.
- Mu Xiang Shun Qi Wan, for qi stagnation.

Herbalism

Laxative herbs, which can be drunk as herbal infusions up to three times daily, include licorice, marshmallow root, rhubarb root, buckthorn, and senna leaves.

Aromatherapy

Massage a few drops of marjoram, rosemary, or fennel oil, diluted in grapeseed oil, into the abdomen, to relieve constipation. (*See pages 133–157.*)

Homeopathy

Constipation is regarded as a constitutional problem, but the following remedies can help with occasional symptoms:

- Lycopodium, when there is flatulence but no need to open bowels for long periods of time; then stools are hard, and passed with pain. (*See page 187.*)
- Nux vomica, for constipation that alternates with diarrhea. (*See page 198.*)
- Sepia, when the belly feels full. (*See page 196.*)
- Opium, when there is no desire to pass stool.
- Silicea, when there is a burning sensation after a bowel movement. (*See page 196.*)
- Causticum, for a stitch-like pain accompanying a bowel movement. (*See page 174.*)
- Bryonia, for large, hard, dry stools, with congestion in the abdomen causing distension, and a burning feeling in the rectum. (*See page 170.*)
- Alumina, when there is no desire to open bowels until the rectum is full; the stool may be covered in mucus.

Vitamins and Minerals

Increase your intake of dietary fiber, which will help to bulk out stools.

Acidophilus will encourage the health of the intestines and make bowel movements more normal. (*See page 256.*)

Chronic constipation may respond to an increased intake of B-complex vitamins, particularly if it follows a course of antibiotics. Vitamin B1 is most effective. (*See page 235.*)

DIARRHEA

Diarrhea occurs when normal reabsorption of water from the stools has not taken place, so that stools are characteristically loose and runny. The two basic mechanisms involved in diarrhea, which may operate independently or together, are excessive accumulation of fluid in the intestinal tract and excessive propulsive action in the intestines. Excessive fluid in the intestines can result from conditions that decrease the absorption of water from the colon, or from conditions that cause water to be secreted into the intestines, as in cholera and other infections. The body secretes excess water in order to "flush" disease and toxins. Excessive propulsive action may be caused by nervous and chemical factors or by partial obstruction of the intestine. Diarrhea is a feature of many conditions, including dysentery, food poisoning, cholera, typhoid, gastroenteritis, and parasitic infestation. It can also be brought on by stress or anxiety, and in babies it may be caused by lactose intolerance. Chronic diarrhea may be caused by Crohn's disease (*see page 345*), ulcerative colitis, or cancer of the colon.

> **CAUTION**
> Consult a physician regarding episodes of diarrhea lasting more than 48 hours, particularly if there is fever and/or vomiting.

Symptoms

Depending on the cause, associated symptoms may include:
- abdominal cramps
- vomiting
- wind

TREATMENT

Ayurveda
Cassia pods, henbane, and coriander can be used to treat diarrhea. (*See pages 20 and 24.*)

Chinese Herbalism
The full condition is caused by Cold Damp or Damp Heat; the empty condition is due to a Spleen, Stomach, or Kidney yang deficiency. (*See page 33.*)

Skullcap root may be suitable for acute diarrhea, as well as golden thread, kapok flowers, and dandelion root.

For chronic diarrhea, a treatment of psoralea fruit, codonopsis root, and astragalus may be given.

Huo Xiang Zheng Qi Wan/Agastache upright qi powder, for gastric flu. (*See page 40.*)

Mu Xiang Shun Qi Wan and Shen Ling Bai Zhu Wan, 2 pills taken together for alternating diarrhea and constipation (Liver qi stagnation with Spleen qi deficiency). The latter can be taken for chronic loose stools with poor appetite, tiredness, etc. (*See page 43.*)

Liu Jun Zi Pian, or Six Gentlemen Tablet, for loose stools, diarrhea, indigestion resulting from Spleen qi deficiency.

Xiang Sha Liu jun Zi Wan, for loose stools, diarrhea, and indigestion, accompanied by nausea.

Traditional Home and Folk Remedies
Carrot juice or soup is very helpful, especially for infants. (*See page 76.*)

Herbalism
For acute diarrhea take a gentle laxative such as dock to clear away the cause of the irritant.

A few drops of myrrh tincture in water will clear many infections.

For chronic and nervous diarrhea use chamomile or marigold mixed with a soothing, astringent herb such as raspberry leaf. (*See pages 104, 102, and 114.*)

Homeopathy

Chronic diarrhea should be treated constitutionally, but acute attacks may be treated with one of the following remedies:

- Aconite, for diarrhea that comes on suddenly, where the patient has a distended abdomen. (*See page 163.*)
- Pulsatilla, for diarrhea which is worse at night and made worse by rich foods. (*See page 193.*)
- Colocynthis, for diarrhea accompanied by griping pains, with yellowish, thin, and copious stools.
- Arg. nit., for diarrhea caused by anxiety, characterized by episodes of belching and cravings for sweet and salty food. (*See page 166.*)
- China, for stools accompanied by wind, and made worse by fruit. (*See page 175.*)
- Phosphoric acid, when stools contain undigested food and you feel better after passing them.

Vitamins and Minerals

Increase your intake of potassium, which is easily lost in diarrhea and vomiting. (*See page 245.*)

Increase your intake of vitamins B1 and B3, which will address the digestive system. (*See pages 235 and 236.*)

Drink plenty of water, to flush the system.

Take a multivitamin and mineral supplement with food when you are able to eat properly again, to replace lost nutrients.

Take plenty of fresh acidophilus for at least a month after an attack, to ensure the health of the bowels. (*See page 256.*)

IRRITABLE BOWEL SYNDROME (IBS)

Irritable bowel syndrome (or spastic colon) is a very common disorder with recurrent abdominal pain, intermittent diarrhea alternating with constipation. This may be caused by a disturbance in the muscle movement in the large intestine, triggered by anxiety, stress, or food intolerance. IBS affects far more women than men.

- 10–20 percent of the population suffers or has suffered from IBS.

- Up to 50 percent of all health cases dealt with by gastroenterologists are caused by IBS.
- The vast majority of sufferers are women, and the young to middle-aged are particularly vulnerable.

Symptoms

- cramp-like abdominal pain, usually after eating, relieved by going to the toilet
- swelling of the abdomen
- excessive wind and abdominal rumblings
- headache and back pain
- general malaise
- a sensation of fullness halfway through a meal
- undue awareness of bowel action
- anxiety

TREATMENT

Ayurveda

Coriander and hollyhock are suitable herbs to treat IBS.

Chinese Herbalism

Treatment would address weakness of the Kidneys and Spleen, excess Damp in the intestines, and stagnation of Liver qi. Some suitable herbs might include rhubarb, dandelion, magnolia, and angelica. (*See pages 60 and 41.*)

Herbalism

Slippery elm has a soothing action along the length of the gut. (*See page 123.*)

Try calming herbal teas such as chamomile, peppermint, and balm, all of which have an antispasmodic action. (*See pages 104 and 111.*)

Chew fresh ginger to help relieve spasms. (*See page 126.*)

Aromatherapy

Massage the abdomen with lavender or chamomile oils, which have antispasmodic qualities.

Detoxifying oils include juniper, garlic, fennel, and rose; add to your bath water or use in massage.

Homeopathy

Treatment must be constitutional, but the following remedies may provide some relief:

Arg. nit., when there is flatulence, constipation alternating with diarrhea, and mucus in the stools.

Cantharis, for burning pain in the abdomen, great thirst, nausea, and accompanying cystitis. (*See page 173.*)

Colocynthis, for griping pains brought on by anger.

Colchicum, for water stools, and tearing pains and nausea made worse when food is smelt.

Flower Essences

Consider whether or not your condition is stress-related (*see* Stress, *page 266*) and choose a remedy that fits your emotional symptoms. (*See page 209.*)

Rescue Remedy is useful during attacks, to calm.

Mimulus will help if you are frightened by the thought of eating or of experiencing another attack.

Vitamins and Minerals

Vitamin A is necessary to keep the intestinal tract healthy.

Take acidophilus to encourage the growth of healthy bacteria. (*See page 256.*)

A deficiency of zinc and vitamin B6 is indicated in many cases; ensure that your intake is adequate.

Dietary fiber helps to detoxify.

ANAL FISSURE

An anal fissure is a tear in the lower anal canal, close to the anal sphincter, and is often associated with internal hemorrhoids. The condition is fairly rare, but is most common in middle age, although it affects some children. When the stool is passed, the split is irritated, causing the sphincter muscles to go into painful spasm. Constipation is the root cause in most cases. Usually it heals quickly without complications but occasionally it may be chronic, spreading to the sphincter muscle and ending in infection. In some cases an anal fissure may be linked with other gut diseases.

Symptoms

- pain during bowel movements
- minor bleeding
- irritation and discomfort

TREATMENT

Ayurveda

The following preparations may be helpful if the fissure is caused by constipation: Abhayarishta (an oral tonic), Gin (oral pills), or Sukumara ghrita (oral ghee).

Traditional Home and Folk Remedies

Dab a little olive oil on to the fissure to encourage healing and relieve pain. (*See page 81.*)

Fresh lemon juice, applied to the fissure, will prevent infection and dull the pain. (*See page 74.*)

Herbalism

Dandelion coffee is a mild laxative, and can be drunk, as required, on a daily basis. (*See page 121.*)

Take a drink made of a cup of psyllium or flax seeds in a cup of water before bedtime to moisten stools and encourage regular bowel movements.

Butternut, cascara, licorice, and yellow dock, decocted and mixed with a little honey, can help to stimulate bile, which will help produce normal bowel movements. (*See pages 108 and 115.*)

Slippery elm and cinnamon will lubricate. (*See page 123.*)

Comfrey root can help to heal the sore and inflamed tissues. (*See page 119.*)

Aromatherapy

Apply a few drops of neat lavender or tea tree oil to the fissure to encourage healing and prevent infection. It may sting. (*See pages 147 and 148.*)

Homeopathy

Constitutional treatment would be appropriate, particularly if you are prone to fissures, but the following remedies, taken four times daily, may help:

- Nitric acid, for sharp pains during the passing of stools, also afterwards; constipation, irritability.
- Ratanhia, for relieving a burning sensation in the rectum which worsens after a bowel movement (loose or constipated).
- Aesculus, for sore, burning pain in the fissure, and an aching lower back, with stools large and hard.

Vitamins and Minerals

Acidophilus encourages the health of the bowels, and so should be taken daily as required. (*See page 256.*)

Eat plenty of foods that are high in dietary fibers, including whole grains, fresh, raw vegetables and fruits, and dried fruits.

PILES (HEMORRHOIDS)

Piles are swollen (or varicose) veins in the lining of the anus. The varicosity may be just above the anal canal, causing "internal" hemorrhoids, or at the lower end of the canal, causing "external" hemorrhoids. The latter may even protrude outside the anus ("prolapsed" hemorrhoids). Piles are caused by increased pressure on the veins of the anus, most commonly as a result of chronic constipation with straining, pregnancy, and childbirth. There may, however, be a congenital predisposition. Piles affect 50–75 percent of the U.S. population, and become more common with age.

Symptoms
- pain and bleeding during bowel movements
- soreness and itching around the anus
- possibly a mucus discharge from prolapsed hemorrhoids

TREATMENT

Ayurveda
There are several Ayurvedic preparations available from health food stores, including Abhayarishta, which is an oral tonic, and Dadimadi ghritha (oral ghee).

Traditional Home and Folk Remedies
Red potato can be cut into a slim cigar shape and inserted into the anus to relieve symptoms. (*See page 84.*)

Sit on a cold bowl of water, or use a cold bidet, several times daily to reduce inflammation and swelling.

Herbalism
Make a small witch hazel compress, and keep it on the affected area for as long as possible to reduce inflammation and encourage healing. (*See page 78.*)

Pilewort ointment is useful, and should be applied two or three times daily.

Bayberry and yellow dock are both astringent herbs, and can be added to cocoa butter, which can then be shaped into a suppository and placed in the anus. (*See page 115.*)

Internally, a course of dandelion root, horse chestnut, stone root, or yarrow can be helpful.

Externally, horse chestnut can be applied.

Clear congestion in the area with a good diet and teas of bitter herbs such as dock or. dandelion root. (*See page 121.*)

Aromatherapy
Apply a local compress of astringent essential oils of cypress, frankincense, lavender, or myrrh. (*See pages 123–157.*)

Add a little rosemary oil to a warm bath to improve the circulation. (*See page 154.*)

Homeopathy
Ratanhia, for pain that feels like splinters on the anus when passing a stool.

Hamamelis, for a bruised, sore, and congested feeling.

Sulfur, for hot, burning, and itching piles. (*See page 198.*)

Sepia, for the sensation of having a ball in the rectum, along with a tendency to prolapse. (*See page 196.*)

WIND

Wind (or flatulence) refers to the expulsion from the body of an excessive amount of air or gas, via the anus (breaking wind) or the mouth (belching or burping). Gas discharged via the anus is called flatus and comprises a number of gases, including hydrogen sulfide, which is responsible for the characteristic unpleasant smell. Wind can be caused by excessive swallowing of air (aerophagy), which may be a response to stress, or a consequence of eating too quickly. It is also a feature of disorders such as indigestion and irritable bowel syndrome. Certain foods such as pulses and beans produce more flatus than others. Gas is formed in the large intestine as a result of the action of bacteria on carbohydrates and amino acids in digested food; the gas consists of hydrogen, carbon dioxide, and methane. Gas formed in the intestine is passed only through the anus.

Symptoms
- besides its characteristic sounds, flatulence can also often cause abdominal discomfort

> **CAUTION**
> Excessive flatulence accompanied by weight loss, severe abdominal pain, or bleeding during bowel movements requires medical attention.

TREATMENT

Ayurveda
Ayurvedic preparations available include Digesic, which is an oral tablet, as well as Gasex and Ramabana.

Henbane may also be useful.

Chinese Herbalism
Treatment would be aimed at stagnant Stomach energy, and suitable herbs include magnolia bark, and orange or lemon peel.

Traditional Home and Folk Remedies
Charcoal is excellent for reducing gas in the stomach and intestines.

Celery seeds can reduce flatulence. (*See page 71.*)

Herbalism
Fresh dill, added to boiling water and steeped, will reduce flatulence and gas pains.

Try making an infusion of sweet flag, drinking half a cup before meals.

Homeopathy
The following remedies can be taken in every 30 minutes, for up to 6 doses:
- Lycopodium, when gas feels stuck, is painful, and is made worse by onions, garlic, and fried foods. (*See page 187.*)
- Arsenicum, for a burning discomfort. (*See page 167.*)
- Arg. nit., for the feeling that the stomach is full of gas. (*See page 166.*)

DISORDERS OF THE URINARY SYSTEM
KIDNEY STONES

Kidney stones (calculi) may occur .anywhere in the kidneys or ureters and are the result of the crystallization of various substances in the urine, often when the body is dehydrated, causing the urine to be more concentrated. Dehydration alone, however, will not cause the formation of stones, and there is usually some other factor involved, such as kidney disease, infection, a bodily disturbance, or certain drugs. Most stones are combinations of calcium, magnesium, phosphorus, and oxalate. Collections of small kidney stones are known as "gravel," while much larger ones are called "staghorn" calculi.

The most common types of stones contain various combinations of calcium, magnesium, phosphorus, or oxalate. Up to 80 percent of stones are formed mainly of calcium.

Kidney stones affect approximately 1 in 1,000 Americans—an estimated 10 percent of U.S. men and 3 percent of U.S. women.

Most common in the south-eastern U.S., known as the "stone belt."

Less common types are due to inherited disorders characterized by excretion of abnormal amounts of cystine or xanthine.

Recurrence of most stones can be prevented by therapy based on analysis of the stones, the urine, and the blood.

Kidney stones range in size from less than 2/10in. (5mm.) to over 1in. (2.5cm.) in diameter.

They tend to run in families, and four out of every five patients with kidney stones are male, usually between the ages of 20 and 30.

Differences in dietary and fluid intake may put certain people at higher risk for kidney stones.

Symptoms
- if a stone is lodged in the ureter it may cause agonizing pain—ureteric colic—through muscle contractions; the pain may spread to the lower abdomen and the groin

- often there is blood in the urine
- if stones cause blockage of the urinary tract, this can cause serious damage to kidney function

TREATMENT

Chinese Herbalism
Herbs which may help with correcting Kidney deficiency include ginseng, water plantain, poria, cinnamon twigs, and ephedra. (See pages 44 and 54.)

Traditional Home and Folk Remedies
Include 2 tablespoons of extra virgin olive oil in your diet each day. (See page 81.)

Fresh lemon juice, drunk in a little hot water every morning, will help to flush the kidneys and break down kidney stones. (See page 74.)

Herbalism
Herbs that can be used to dissolve the stones include celery seed, gravel root, parsley, and stone root. Sip a decoction three times daily.

During an acute attack, try infusions of corn silk, coughgrass, or yarrow. (See page 97.)

Aromatherapy
Oils used to treat kidney stones include fennel, geranium, juniper, and lemon. These can be added to a light carrier oil and massaged into the bladder area, or used in the bath.

Homeopathy
Treatment would be constitutional, but the following remedies may be useful for up to 10 doses:
- Tabacum, for pains shooting to the urethra, causing nausea and cold sweat.
- Nux vomica, for right-sided pain, causing nausea and vomiting, an urgent need to empty the bowels, accompanied by weak urine flow and irritability.
- Berberis, for stitching pain in the lower ribs and hips when urinating, which worsens if moving about.
- Lycopodium, for pain in the right side which stops at the bladder, and which is worse between 4 and 8p.m.

Vitamins and Minerals
Drink plenty of water (about 12 cups [3l.] a day) to flush the kidneys.

Avoid long-term use of vitamin C, calcium, or vitamin D supplements. (See pages 238, 241, and 239.)

Extra magnesium and vitamin B6 will help.

BLADDER STONES

Most bladder stones (calculi) are made up of crystals of calcium oxalate or uric acid. They are caused by the precipitation from solution of substances present in the urine. The stones may cause obstruction to urinary output, resulting in infection, although often they remain unrecognized. They occur with greater frequency in developing countries, and may be a result of a diet low or deficient in phosphate and protein. Bladder stones mainly affect men. Gout sufferers may experience bladder stones, and any disease which causes a high level of calcium in the blood and urine, such as hyperparathyroidism, may contribute to the formation of stones.

Symptoms
- difficulty in passing urine
- stress incontinence
- if infection develops there may also be: burning pain on passing urine, small amounts of urine, cloudy in appearance and with an unpleasant smell, fever, a dull ache in the lower abdomen

TREATMENT

Chinese Herbalism
Herbs which may help include ginseng, water plantain, poria, cinnamon twigs, and ephedra.

Traditional Home and Folk Remedies
Fresh lemon juice, drunk in a little hot water every morning, will help to flush the bladder and break down bladder stones. (See page 74.)

Barley or rice water will help to encourage the flow of urine and act as a tonic to the urinary system.

Herbalism

Herbs that can be used to dissolve the stones include celery seed, gravel root, parsley, and stone root. Sip a decoction three times daily.

During an acute attack, try infusions of corn silk, coughgrass, or yarrow. (*See page 97.*)

Aromatherapy

A number of essential oils work on the urinary tract, including tea tree, sandalwood, juniper, and eucalyptus. They should be applied in repeated hot compresses over the bladder area. (*See pages 133–157.*)

Homeopathy

Treatment would be constitutional, but the following remedies may be useful for up to 10 doses:

- Lycopodium, for red sediment in the urine and a frequent urge to urinate, particularly at night. (*See page 187.*)
- Sarsaparilla, for slimy, sandy urine, with severe pain around the urethra when the flow stops.
- Uva ursi, when stones stop the flow of urine, which contains blood and mucus.

Vitamins and Minerals

Drink plenty of water (about 12 cups [3l.] a day) to flush the bladder.

Extra vitamin C acts as a natural diuretic and will help to flush the urinary system. (*See page 238.*)

CYSTITIS

Cystitis is inflammation of the urinary bladder and/or urethra (the tube through which urine passes from the bladder out of the body). Inflammation usually occurs as a result of infection, bruising, or irritation. In the case of infection the bacteria involved are most often Escherichia coli, which will have traveled from the anus, via the urethra, to the bladder. Irritation and bruising can be caused by barrier contraceptives and sexual intercourse. Other causes of cystitis include chemical irritants (soap, bubble bath, bath oils), poor hygiene, insufficient drinking, food irritants, fruit juices, pregnancy, and menopause. Cystitis is far more common in women than in men.

More frequent in women because of the close proximity of the urethra and the vagina to the anus.

- 50–80 percent of the bacteria in our bodies are resistant to allopathic (conventional) treatment.
- Prevalent in women during childbearing years, especially during pregnancy.
- Drugs such as methenamine mandelate, nitrofurantoin, and cyclophosphamide may also cause cystitis.

Symptoms

- burning pain on passing water
- frequent and urgent need to pass water, although little if any is passed
- dragging pain in lower abdomen and lower back
- nausea and possibly vomiting
- possibly unpleasant smelling urine, that may contain blood

TREATMENT

Ayurveda

Hollyhock is a diuretic, and can treat cystitis.

Boil 4 tablespoons of coriander seeds in 4 cups of water until the liquid is reduced to 2 cups. Strain and drink with a little honey. (*See page 24.*)

Chinese Herbalism

Plantain seeds would be used to address Damp Heat.

Traditional Home and Folk Remedies

Eat live yogurt; use as a douche to ease symptoms and prevent recurrence. (*See page 79.*)

Cranberry juice discourages bacteria from sticking to the walls of the bladder. (*See page 85.*)

Garlic tincture added to food or warm drinks eases cystitis. (*See page 70.*)

Drink barley water and lemon juice daily. (*See pages 78 and 74.*)

Herbalism

Herbs used to treat cystitis include urinary antiseptics and diuretics. Drink infusions of buchu, corn silk, coughgrass, uva ursi, and yarrow. (*See pages 101 and 97.*)

Aromatherapy
Add antiseptic bergamot, lavender, and sandalwood to the bath. (*See pages 133–157.*)

Homeopathy
Chronic cystitis should be treated constitutionally, but take the following in an attack:
- Cantharis, for burning urine.
- Staphisagria, for cystitis after intercourse.
- Mercurius, for violent pain with blood in the urine. (*See page 189.*)
- Apis, for stinging pain that is better for cold water. (*See page 165.*)
- Sarsaparilla, for burning after urinating.

Vitamins and Minerals
Drink plenty of water to flush the urinary system.

Take 1g. of vitamin C daily, which acts as a natural diuretic and boosts the immune system. (*See page 238.*)

URETHRITIS

Urethritis is an inflammation of the urethra (the tube through which urine passes out of the body). In women it is usually caused by a bladder infection, while in men it may be a symptom of other diseases, including gonorrhea and Reiter's syndrome. It may also result from damage to the urethra, from a catheter for example. Nonspecific urethritis (NSU) is a milder form thought to be caused in most cases by chlamydia, although the cause may not be established. NSU may be caused by a large number of different types of micro-organisms, including bacteria and yeasts. Other possible causes include exposure to irritant chemicals, such as antiseptics and some spermicidal preparations. Urethritis may be followed by scarring and the formation of a urethral stricture (narrowing of a section of the urethra), which can make the passing of urine difficult.

Symptoms
- burning sensation and sometimes severe pain on passing urine
- blood in urine and possibly a pus-filled yellow discharge

- in NSU the symptoms are milder and the discharge in men is usually clear
- in women there may be no symptoms, with occasionally increased discharge

TREATMENT
Ayurveda
Hollyhock is diuretic, and can be used to treat urethritis.

Boil 4 tablespoons of coriander seeds in 4 cups or water until the liquid is reduced to 2 cups. Strain and drink with a little honey. (*See page 24.*)

Traditional Home and Folk Remedies
Eat live yogurt, and use as a douche to ease the symptoms of infection and inflammation, and prevent recurrence of the urethritis. (*See page 79.*)

Cranberry juice, drunk daily, discourages bacteria from sticking to the urinary tract. It treats and prevents urethritis. (*See page 85.*)

Garlic tincture, added to food or warm drinks, will ease inflammation and fight infection. (*See page 70.*)

Drink barley water, several cups a day, with some lemon juice. (*See pages 78 and 74.*)

Herbalism
Herbs used to treat urethritis include urinary antiseptics and diuretics. You may drink infusions of any of the following herbs, alone or in combination: buchu, corn silk, coughgrass, uva ursi, and yarrow.

Buchu will help to clear infection. Take as a tea, three times daily.

Aromatherapy
Bergamot, lavender, and sandalwood are soothing and antiseptic. Add them to the bath water every evening.

Homeopathy
For NSU, antibiotics should be taken, as prescribed, but the following may be helpful if it is not NSU:
- Cantharis, when the urine burns and is violently painful.
- Staphisagria, for cystitis after intercourse.
- Mercurius, for violent pain with blood in the urine.

- Apis, for stinging pain that is better for cold water. (*See page 165.*)
- Sarsaparilla, for burning pain which comes on after urinating.

Vitamins and Minerals
Drink plenty of water (12 cups [3l.] daily) to flush the urinary system.

Take 1g. of vitamin C daily, which acts as a natural diuretic and boosts the immune system. (*See page 238.*)

Vitamin C builds healthy mucous membranes. (*See page 238.*)

Take acidophilus after a course of antibiotics. (*See page 256.*)

INCONTINENCE

Incontinence is the inability to retain feces in the rectum, or an uncontrollable involuntary passing of urine. Incontinence, or involuntary urination, is extremely common. The most common form is stress incontinence, in which a small quantity of urine is "leaked" when there is increased pressure in the abdomen, as in laughing, sneezing, or coughing. Stress incontinence is often experienced after childbirth, as a result of injury or strain to the pelvic floor muscles, whose function it is to support the bladder and keep the urethra closed. Other causes include senile dementia, prostate enlargement, damage to nerve control as a result of stroke, multiple sclerosis, or local cancer, and bladder stones.

Fecal incontinence (lack of normal control over passing feces) may occur in diarrhea, or if the controlling muscles have been damaged by disease or childbirth. Another cause is fecal impaction, which is often caused by long-standing constipation. (*See* Constipation on *page 346* and Diarrhea on *page 347* for treatment of fecal incontinence.)

TREATMENT
Chinese Herbalism
Treatment would address Kidney Yang Deficiency with internal Cold, and the best herb to use is golden lock, taken as a tea.

If the condition accompanies prolapse, treatment will be given for Deficient qi, using central qi pills. This will help with the control of fecal and urinary incontinence.

Herbalism
The seeds of the ginkgo biloba plant act as a tonic to the kidneys and bladder, and have been used for incontinence and excessive urination. (*See page 108.*)

Horsetail has toning and astringent properties, which make it useful both for incontinence and frequent urination. (*See page 106.*)

Homeopathy
Treatment would be based on the cause of the incontinence, but some of the following might be useful:

Causticum, for incontinence made worse by coughing or laughing.

Ferr. phos., for an inability to control the bladder, with pain and a frequent urge to urinate. (*See page 179.*)

Nux vomica, for irritability and involuntary dribbles of urine. (*See page 198.*)

Pulsatilla for stress incontinence which is made worse by sitting down. (*See page 193.*)

Sepia, for incontinence related to weak pelvic floor muscles, accompanied by the feeling that the abdomen is falling out of the vagina. (*See page 196.*)

Flower Essences
A number of the remedies will help with negative emotions and distress. Some to try are:
- Walnut, if incontinence is the result of change, such as pregnancy, a new baby, or menopause. (*See page 218.*)
- Sweet Chestnut, if you suffer from despair.
- Agrimony, if you hide behind a cheerful face.
- Crab Apple if you feel unclean.

Vitamins and Minerals
Increase your intake of dietary fiber, which will prevent constipation and straining, a common cause of incontinence.

Drink plenty of water to ensure regular use of the bladder muscles.

DISORDERS OF THE REPRODUCTIVE SYSTEM: FEMALE

BREAST PROBLEMS

The female breast consists mainly of a round mass of glandular tissue comprising about 15–20 lobes, each having a duct leading to an opening on the nipple; the duct system and glandular tissue develop fully with pregnancy. The amount of fat sheathing the glandular tissue determines the size of the breast. Connective tissues, or stroma, form the foundation or framework of the breast. The layer of ligaments directly beneath the breast sends strands into the breast itself, providing the firm consistency of the organ. The deep layer of connective tissue sends strands in the opposite direction into the covering of the chest muscles.

Breast cancer is an important medical problem, with women of age 35 or older at increasing risk of developing some form of the disease. Physicians urge that women conduct monthly self-examinations of their breasts to detect potentially cancerous lumps, because the disease is more easily curable when found at an early stage. Another screening method is the X-ray process called mammography. Medical groups agree that women of 50 and older should have a yearly mammograph test. Some groups also advise an initial test for women between 35 and 40, and a test every one or two years for women between 40 and 50.

Some typical breast problems are:
- Tenderness, associated with pregnancy and PMS.
- Abscesses, which start as a bacterial infection in the breast tissue, producing swelling, redness, pain, and possibly fever. They usually occur in women who are breast-feeding. (*See also* Breastfeeding Problems, *page 357.*)
- Cysts, non-cancerous fluid-filled capsules in the ducts of the breast, appearing in groups or singly, occur mainly between the ages of 30 and 50, and in many women they cause one or more breasts to become lumpy and tender in the week or so before a menstrual period starts.

- Duct ectasia, blockage and inflammation of the milk ducts, is one of the most common causes of breast pain, particularly in women aged 40 to 50. It produces hot, red areas on the breast, a lump, and sometimes a watery discharge.
- Duct papillomas are benign, wart-like tumors in the ducts which, if not removed, may turn malignant. Their cause is uncertain, but may be hormonal.
- Fat necrosis, when fatty material released from the fat cells as a result of a blow to the breast forms into a hard lump of scar tissue, causing dimpling on the skin.
- Fibroadenoma, a benign breast tumor which is usually round, firm, and rubbery, causing no pain, can be moved around beneath the skin using the fingertips. These lumps are very common and most women will have one at some stage.

> **CAUTION**
> Pregnant women should not take celery seed without a physician's approval.

TREATMENT

Ayurveda
Barberry can be applied externally for its antibiotic and antifungal action. It also shrinks tumors (benign and cancerous), when it is taken internally. (*See page 18.*)

Calamus oil will stimulate lymphatic drainage, and can be used for treating most breast problems. (*See page 15.*)

Celery seed is diuretic, and can be useful when breast problems are related to swellings. (*See page 18.*)

Chinese Herbalism
A poultice made from powdered dried rhubarb root can be applied to the breast to ease pain and swelling.

Madder root and dandelion may also be useful.

Traditional Home and Folk Remedies
Apply a bruised white cabbage leaf to the breast when there is infection, to heal and draw out the pus. (*See page 73.*)

Apply continuous compresses of strong peach tea to the affected area for infection.

Bruised parsley leaf poultices can be used for hard and lumpy breasts.

Herbalism

The herbs that are most useful for preventing and treating breast problems are those that encourage the action of the lymphatic system: cleavers, golden seal, marigold, marshmallow, nettles, and yellow dock.

Consider taking the herb agnus castus for breast problems related to hormones (particularly premenstrually, and during menopause).

Aromatherapy

Geranium oil can be used in the bath for relief of tenderness and edema, or massage it, blended into a little carrier oil, into the affected area. (*See page 151.*)

Juniper, rosemary, lavender, and fennel oils will help to regulate hormone imbalance and relieve the symptoms of breast diseases. (*See pages 133–157.*)

Homeopathy

For pain associated with PMS, try:
- Carb. an., for breast enlargement with shooting pains.
- Conium, for swelling, pain, and tenderness.
- Nat. mur., when the breasts are retaining water.

Cysts should be dealt with constitutionally, but the following remedies may be useful in the short term:
- Pulsatilla, for sudden, inexplicable pains. (*See page 193.*)
- Conium, when the affected area is hard and painful.
- Phytolacca, for breasts that are more tender premenstrually, and when you are stressed.

For an abscess, try:
- Bryonia, for the early stages, with hardened breasts and pain. (*See page 170.*)
- Belladonna, for the early stages when there are red streaks. (*See page 168.*)
- Hep. sulf., for localized pain with irritability.
- Silicea, for cracked, oozing nipples and feelings of exhaustion. (*See page 195.*)

For lumps, the following may be useful:
- Graphites, for hard, swollen, thickened breasts with blistered and sore nipples. (*See page 181.*)
- Belladonna, when the breasts are red, throbbing, and heavy. (*See page 168.*)

- Mercurius, for when the breasts are painful and full of milk at the time of menstruation. (*See page 189.*)

Vitamins and Minerals

Cut down on salty food to prevent water retention.

Supplements of evening primrose oil and vitamin B6 may be useful. (*See pages 254 and 237.*)

Cut down on caffeine, which can encourage the formation of cysts and lumps in the breast.

Breast pain and lumps may be alleviated by increasing your daily intake of vitamin A. (*See page 234.*)

Women with low levels of selenium may have a greater risk of suffering fibrocystic breast disease.

Apply vitamin E cream to heal cracked nipples.

BREAST-FEEDING PROBLEMS

After the birth of a child a mother's breast begins to produce milk, a natural process designed to provide complete nourishment for a baby for several months after its birth. Before milk is produced the mother's breast produces colostrum, a deep-yellow liquid containing high levels of protein and antibodies. A newborn baby who feeds on colostrum in the first few days of life is better able to resist the bacteria and viruses that cause illness. The mother's milk, which begins to flow a few days after childbirth when the mother's hormones change, is a blue-white color with a very thin consistency. If the mother is well nourished the milk provides the baby with the proper balance of nutrition. The fat contained in human milk, compared with cow's milk, is more digestible for infants and allows for greater absorption of fat-soluble vitamins into the bloodstream from the baby's intestine. Calcium and other important nutrients in human milk are also better utilized by infants. Antigens in cow's milk can cause allergic reactions in a newborn child, whereas such reactions to human milk are rare. Human milk also promotes growth, largely due to the presence of certain hormones and growth factors.

Breast-fed babies have a very low risk of developing meningitis or severe blood infections, and have a 500–600 percent lower risk of getting childhood lymphoma. Breast-fed babies also suffer 50 percent fewer middle ear infections.

Typical breast-feeding problems are:

- Aching breasts, usually caused by engorgement either through increased blood pressure or overproduction of milk. Symptoms include fever, with hard, lumpy, and painful breasts.
- Blocked duct, a small red lump on the breast or a white lump on the nipple caused by rushed feeds, or by not emptying the breast properly.
- Cracked nipples, possibly caused by poor feeding position or by using damp breast pads.
- Mastitis, inflammation of the breast, usually caused either by a blocked duct or by infection. Symptoms include fever, redness and pain in the affected breast.
- Slow let-down reflex, that is to say a delay in the breast's milk-releasing response.
- Sore nipples, tenderness caused by prolonged suckling.
- Vaginal dryness caused by the suppression of estrogen production during lactation.

TREATMENT

Ayurveda
Cumin can increase milk production. (*See page 25.*)
Fenugreek seeds will increase milk production.

Chinese Herbalism
Dandelion, peony bark, Chinese gentian, and madder root can be used for relieving mastitis. (*See page 53.*)

Traditional Home and Folk Remedies
Bruise parsley leaves, and apply them to hardened or knotty breasts during breast feeding.

Feed your baby a little diluted dill tea to prevent wind, which may be causing his or her breastfeeding problems.

Herbalism
Calendula cream will soothe and encourage the healing of sore and cracked nipples, and is safe for the baby to swallow.

Caraway, aniseed, dill, and fennel promote the flow of breast milk, and can be taken in the form of teas or infusions.

Compresses of marshmallow and slippery elm can often help with engorgement. (*See pages 99 and 123.*)

Red sage will dry up breast milk almost instantly, if necessary. (*See page 116.*)

Dilute tinctures of St. John's wort and marigold in boiled water and dab on to cracked nipples after each feed.
Take echinacea for any infection. (*See page 105.*)

Aromatherapy
Lavender oil, in a bath or in a vaporizer, can encourage the letdown reflex. Better still, try massaging your baby with 1 drop in a light carrier oil before a feed, to relax you both. Caraway and verbena oils can be massaged into the breasts to stimulate the production of milk. (*See pages 133–157.*)

Calendula and chamomile oils are anti-inflammatory, and can be applied to the breasts to ease inflammation and pain. Wash off before feeding. (*See pages 135 and 137.*)

Peppermint oil, in cold compresses, can reduce the flow of milk when there is engorgement. (*See page 150.*)

Homeopathy
Chamomilla, Pulsatilla, Sulfur, and Graphites for sore and cracked nipples. (*See pages 188, 193, 198 and 181.*)

Pulsatilla and Calcarea, for hard, engorged breasts.
Agnus will help with loss of breast milk.
Calcarea, for poor-quality milk, when the mother is prone to chills.

Aconite, for sudden, excessive milk production, or, equally, sudden loss of milk caused by shock.

Bryonia, for hard and swollen breasts. (*See page 170.*)
China, for exhaustion from breast-feeding.
Ignatia, for loss of milk due to grief or trauma.

Flower Essences
Apply Rescue Remedy or Emergency Essence cream to the nipples when they are sore or cracked, to soothe and encourage healing. (*See page 229.*)

Take either essence internally for distress caused by pain.
Olive is useful for overwhelming fatigue. (*See page 220.*)
Walnut is useful for helping with change—in this case, the birth of your baby. (*See page 218.*)

Vitamins and Minerals
Breast-feeding mothers need plenty of protein, vitamins, and iron.

Drink plenty of fluids while breast-feeding.
Apply vitamin E oil to sore and cracked nipples to help them heal. (*See page 239.*)

THE HEALING REMEDIES SOURCEBOOK

MENSTRUAL PROBLEMS

The most common menstrual problems are dysmenorrhea (painful menstruation), menorrhagia (heavy menstrual bleeding), and amenorrhea (no menstrual bleeding). In primary dysmenorrhea there is either an increased level of or increased sensitivity to prostaglandin, the hormone-like substance that produces uterine contractions. Secondary dysmenorrhea (unusual menstrual cramps) begins at least three years after menstruation begins and may be caused by endometriosis, fibroids, a pelvic infection, stress, or a thyroid disorder. The symptoms for both include sharp pain or a dull ache in the lower abdomen and lower back, headaches, sweating, diarrhea. In severe cases there may be vomiting and fainting. Menorrhagia is best described as bleeding that is so heavy that it interferes with normal life. It may be caused by fibroids, polyps, pelvic infection, endometriosis, hypothyroidism, blood-clotting disorders, stress, or use of an IUD or injectable contraceptive. Primary amenorrhea refers to menstruation not starting by the age of 18. This is usually due to low body weight or heredity. Secondary amenorrhea occurs when menstruation stops for more than six months due to pregnancy, weight loss, starting oral contraceptives, severe shock, stress, anemia, thyroid disorder, or a fibroid.

TREATMENT

Ayurveda
Aloe vera can induce menstruation. (*See page 17.*)

Basil can be used to promote menstruation.

Caraway relaxes uterine tissue and is beneficial for menstrual cramps. (*See page 19.*)

Cardamom will help digestive problems associated with menstruation. (*See page 26.*)

Cedar stimulates the menstrual cycle, and celery seeds can treat irregular menstruation.

Chinese Herbalism
Excessive flow is considered to be caused by Heat in the Blood; scanty flow, late menstruation, and painful menstruation are due to Cold in the Blood.

Warming herbs, such as ginger, ginseng, and cinnamon, may be used. (*See pages 54 and 44.*)

Cornelian Asiatic cherry can be used in the treatment of heavy menstrual bleeding. (*See page 46.*)

Traditional Home and Folk Remedies
Dried carrot powder taken daily may help to regulate the menstrual cycle. (*See page 76.*)

Cayenne pepper regulates bleeding. Add a few grains to any herbal tea.

Cinnamon bark will help to control menstrual flow.

Diluted lemon juice cleanses the system and helps to control bleeding. (*See page 74.*)

Beets help to regulate menstrual problems.

Strawberry leaves, taken over a long period, can help to regulate menstrual flow and ease pain.

Herbalism
Cramp bark is helpful for menstrual cramps.

Lady's mantle is an astringent and is useful for heavy menstrual bleeding. Take three times daily, as required. (*See page 98.*)

Yarrow will help to regulate menstruation. (*See page 97.*)

Raspberry leaves can help to control an excessive flow of blood. (*See page 114.*)

Thyme tea, drunk each morning and evening, can control excessive flow. (*See page 122.*)

Angelica root can help to promote menstruation which is delayed. (*See page 100.*)

Catnip tea, drunk each evening and morning during menstruation, will help to ease pain.

Peppermint tea will ease any bloating and pain during menstruation. (*See page 111.*)

Aromatherapy
Antispasmodic oils, such as clary sage, cypress, and lavender, will help to ease cramps. (*See pages 133–157.*)

Clary sage and fennel oils, massaged into the lower back, can help to regulate hormone balance, and, through that, the menstrual cycle. (*See pages 133–157.*)

Heavy menstrual bleeding can be treated with geranium, rose, or cypress essential oils. Add to the bath water or use in a local massage. (*See pages 133–157.*)

Homeopathy

China, for spasmodic bleeding with dark clots and cramps. (*See page 175.*)

Belladonna, for pain, bright red blood, and nagging headache. (*See page 168.*)

Ipecac., for heavy bleeding and bright red blood with nausea. (*See page 175.*)

Sepia, for a bearing-down type pain. (*See page 196.*)

Aconite, for menstruation that stops after an emotional shock. (*See page 163.*)

Ignatia, for menstruation that stops after grief, trauma, or loss. (*See page 184.*)

Colocynthis, for cramping pain which is improved by pressure.

Sabina, for pain and dark red blood with clots.

Chamomilla, for pains that resemble labor pains. (*See page 188.*)

Vitamins and Minerals

Vitamin B6, taken twice daily, can help prevent menstrual cramps. (*See page 237.*)

Iron and zinc will help in cases of heavy menstrual bleeding. (*See pages 243 and 249.*)

Take vitamin A and B6 for heavy bleeding.

Bioflavonoids can help to balance hormone levels and regulate the menstrual cycle. (*See page 256.*)

Deficiencies of zinc and vitamin B6 can result from absence of menstruation. (*See pages 249 and 237.*)

PREMENSTRUAL SYNDROME (PMS)

Premenstrual syndrome is the term used to describe a huge range of symptoms, at least some of which are experienced by most women (especially those over 30) every month between ovulation and menstruation. The symptoms may be physical, emotional, or behavioral in character and are thought to be caused either by hormonal imbalance (possibly due to recent childbirth or a gynecological disorder) or by marginal (sub-clinical) nutritional deficiencies which can affect the fine hormone balance in the body. Interestingly, women who regularly consume caffeine are more likely to suffer from severe PMS, and there is sometimes a connection with a thyroid condition.

Symptoms

- physical, breast enlargement and tenderness, bloated abdomen, headaches/migraines, pelvic discomfort, fluid retention and weight gain, constipation or diarrhea, greasy hair and skin, tiredness
- emotional irritability and confusion, anxiety, disturbed sleep, depression and, in severe cases, suicidal thoughts
- behavioral clumsiness and lack of coordination, poor concentration, violent or aggressive outbursts

TREATMENT

Ayurveda

Calamus root stimulates the adrenals, which will help PMS associated with stress.

Caraway is useful for digestive problems associated with PMS, and is a natural diuretic. (*See page 19.*)

Myrrh is used for treating many conditions relating to menstruation. (*See page 23.*)

Angelica is specific for PMS. (*See page 17.*)

Chinese Herbalism

PMS is believed to be caused by an imbalance of Spleen, Kidneys, and Liver, and can be treated with angelica, peony, hoelen, and skullcap. (*See pages 41, 53, and 61.*)

Traditional Home and Folk Remedies

Swelling can be prevented by eating plenty of fresh, crunchy apples in the week prior to menstruation.

Celery is also a good diuretic, and acts on the kidneys to encourage their action. (*See page 71.*)

Eat fresh grapes to prevent bloating.

Barley water, which is rich in B vitamins, can be drunk freely throughout your menstrual cycle to ease symptoms.

To ease irritability and other emotional symptoms, eat plenty of oats. (*See page 72.*)

Herbalism

Try an infusion (herbs steeped in boiling water) of agnus castus or false unicorn, which have a balancing effect on the hormones.

Herbs which help to reduce some of the symptoms of stress and anxiety include oats, vervain, and passiflora.

Water retention can be eased with couchgrass or dandelion teas, drunk two or three times each day during the premenstrual phase. (*See page 120.*)

Rosemary, oats, cinnamon, and lemon balm will help to lift the spirits. (*See pages 114 and 102.*)

Skullcap, wood betony, and vervain are good for addressing tension, anxiety, and depression.

Cornsilk and burdock are useful for symptoms associated with bloating. (*See page 100.*)

Cleavers and poke root will help with monthly breast tenderness.

Take valerian for extreme tension. (*See page 123.*)

Chamomile, cinnamon, and peppermint will help with nausea and vomiting. (*See pages 104 and 111.*)

Yellow dock and wormwood will balance the blood sugar levels. (*See page 115.*)

Aromatherapy
Try essential oils of geranium and rosemary in your bath to relieve symptoms, including water retention and irritability. (*See pages 151 and 154.*)

Clary sage and rose may help with depression. (*See pages 154 and 155.*)

A light massage (whole body, or over the abdominal area) with lavender oil or clary sage will balance hormones and ease symptoms. (*See pages 147 and 155.*)

Homeopathy
Treatment will be constitutional, but useful remedies include:
- Lachesis, for symptoms which are worse first thing in the morning; also good for painful breasts. (*See page 200.*)
- Nux vomica., for irritability and chilliness, constipation, frequent urination, and various food cravings. (*See page 198.*)
- Sepia, for irritability, weepiness, emotional flatness, feeling turned off by sex, and cravings for sweet or salty foods. (*See page 196.*)
- Kali carb., for tension, exhaustion, feeling overweight, and where the symptoms become worse around 3a.m.
- Pulsatilla, for suddenly bursting into tears, nausea, depression, irregular menstruation, and painful breasts. (*See page 193.*)

- Lycopodium, for bad temper, depression, and a craving for sweet things. (*See page 187.*)
- Sulfur, when the main symptom is a craving for sweets.

Flower Essences
Mustard, for depression.
Scleranthus, for mood swings.
Olive, for fatigue.
Crab Apple, for feeling repulsive and unliked.

Vitamins and Minerals
Evening primrose oil, with the following supplements: vitamins C, E, and B6, magnesium, zinc, iron, and chromium. These should be taken continuously for one month, and subsequently during the fortnight preceding menstruation.

INFERTILITY

The term infertility, or failure to reproduce, is generally applied when failure to conceive follows regular, unprotected sex over an 18-month period. Infertility indicates a fault in the reproductive system and is very often treatable.

TREATMENT
Ayurveda
Cloves can tone the uterus, and garlic has a rejuvenating effect on the reproductive system. (*See page 26.*)

Saffron is aphrodisiac, and can help when infertility is associated with sexual problems. (*See page 24.*)

Chinese Herbalism
Infertility is believed to be caused by Damp Heat and imbalance of yin and yang. Golden lock tea may be useful, but treatment is always individually prescribed, so see a practitioner.

Traditional Home and Folk Remedies
Oats are calming, and can help with the effects of stress, as well as toning the body. Eat as often as possible.

Herbalism

Agnus castus is an excellent hormone regulator and will help if your menstruation is irregular, or you are not ovulating for hormonal reasons. It may also be useful if you are prone to early miscarriage.

False unicorn root helps to regulate the ovaries and strengthen the endometrium.

Balm, passiflora, and skullcap will help to reduce the effects of stress, which may be causing the condition.

Aromatherapy

Rose oil is said to increase sperm count and quality, as well as acting as a mild aphrodisiac. Add a few drops to your partner's bath, or perhaps engage in a little gentle massage, with 2 or 3 drops of rose essential oil in a mild carrier oil such as sweet almond oil. (See page 154.)

A few drops of geranium and melissa can be used neat in the bath, or diluted in a gentle carrier oil and massaged over the abdomen on a regular basis. (See pages 151 and 149.)

Tea tree and lavender oils are anti-infective and anti-inflammatory, and can be useful in abdominal massage, for treating any pelvic infection or inflammation which may be preventing the woman conceiving. (See pages 148 and 147.)

If infertility is causing the patient great anxiety, one of the relaxing oils, such as lavender, marjoram, or chamomile, can be used in the bath, or try it in a vaporizer.

When repeated attempts to get pregnant have failed and you need a little encouragement to continue with love-making, ylang ylang is a lovely, relaxing oil that acts as an aphrodisiac. Use as a massage oil or in the bath.

Homeopathy

Treatment would be constitutional, but the following remedies may be helpful:
- Conium, when breasts are tender, with areas of hard swelling, and sexual desire is suppressed.
- Saline, for previous miscarriages before 12 weeks.
- Sepia for irregular menstruation, and a feeling of chilliness, weeping, and irritability. (See page 196.)

Flower Essences

White Chestnut may be useful if you are extremely upset or tormented by the problem. (See page 209.)

For despondency, try Gorse. (See page 226.)

Vitamins and Minerals

Cutting out alcohol, smoking, and drugs may be suggested for the period before conception.

Eating plenty of whole foods rich in vitamins and minerals will not only ensure that sperm and egg are healthy, but that the woman's body is a welcoming home for the growing embryo. Good nutrition increases the chances of conception and gives the baby every chance of being healthy.

Vitamin E and B6 may be supplemented, as low intake is often linked to a low sperm count. Vitamin E may regulate the production of cervical mucus in women. (See pages 239 and 237.)

Increase intake of EFAs (essential fatty acids): in oily fish, fish liver oils, seeds, nuts, pulses, beans, evening primrose oil, unrefined vegetable oils), to stimulate sex hormone production.

Zinc deficiency has been linked to infertility.

Causes of infertility include:
- Age. Fertility declines in women over the age of 35.
- Cervical mucus may be too thick and sticky, or contain hostile antibodies.
- Endometriosis, when pieces of the womb lining migrate to the Fallopian tubes or the ovaries, causing tube blockage or clogging of the area.
- Fibroids, benign growths of muscle.
- Narrowed or scarred cervix, which may have resulted from surgery in the cervical area.
- Ovulation problems due to congenital abnormality, damage to the ovaries, or hormonal problems.
- Pelvic infections. Scar tissue from infections can cause blockage of the Fallopian tubes.
- Polycystic ovaries, repeated or multiple ovarian cysts.
- Smoking, which can cause constriction of blood vessels supplying the reproductive organs, which then inhibits their action.
- Stress. There are possible links between stress and infertility.
- Womb problems such as adenomyosis, where scar tissue forms on the womb wall, an abnormal womb shape, and polyps.
- Approximately 10–15 percent of couples, or one in every seven marriages, in the United States is affected by infertility.

- In approximately 40 percent of cases, infertility is due to a female factor, 40 percent of cases are due to a male factor (*see page 374*), and in the remaining instances no cause can be found despite thorough evaluation.
- In as many as 35 percent of couples, multiple conditions causing infertility can be identified.
- In female infertility, ovulatory dysfunction, including lack of ovulation and poor progesterone production, is responsible for approximately 15 percent of infertility cases.
- Fallopian tube obstruction and pelvic adhesions, which may result from pelvic inflammatory disease, endometriosis, and postnatal infections, account for 30 percent of infertility cases.
- Cervical factors, which may impede the passage of sperm into the uterus, are responsible for approximately 5 percent of infertility cases.
- Uterine factors, including polyps, adhesions, leiomyomata (fibroid tumors), and congenital anomalies, may interfere with implantation of the embryo. Approximately 5 percent of infertility cases are caused by these abnormalities.

MISCARRIAGE

Spontaneous abortion, or miscarriage, occurs when the embryo fails to develop, when there is complete or incomplete expulsion of the embryo or fetus, and placenta, or when the fetus dies prior to 20 weeks. If fetal death occurs at 20 weeks or more after the last period, it is termed a late fetal death or a stillbirth.

Up to three-fourths of conceptions abort spontaneously. Most occur before the woman's pregnancy can be confirmed, prior to six weeks after her last period. These constitute about one-fifth of confirmed pregnancies and about one-tenth of all pregnancy hospitalizations in the United States.

In many cases the womb sheds an embryo because it is not developing normally. Often, however, there is no explanation for miscarriage at all, although the following may be at greater risk: women over 40, pregnancies resulting from fertility treatment, twin or multiple pregnancies, and pregnancies where the placenta is faulty.

Symptoms

- of a threatened miscarriage: bleeding, clots or a dark discharge from the vagina, mucus in the vaginal blood, abdominal pain, possibly cramp-like pain similar to menstrual cramps, back pain
- of inevitable miscarriage: opening of the cervix and continuous bleeding (inevitable abortion), emptying of the uterus, after which the cervix closes and bleeding stops (complete abortion), partial emptying of the uterus, after which the cervix remains open and bleeding continues (incomplete abortion)

TREATMENT

Ayurveda
Herbs to tone the uterus and improve circulation may be useful, but treatment must be undertaken by a registered practitioner.

Chinese Herbalism
Dodder seeds are used to prevent miscarriages. (*See page 48.*)

Herbalism
Herbs for threatened miscarriage include false unicorn root decoction, which should be sipped every few minutes.

Cramp bark can help to relax the uterus and prevent miscarriage. (*See page 125.*)

Black haw can be used to avert miscarriage and ensure relaxation.

Tonic herbs to prevent miscarriage include red raspberry leaves mixed with a little vervain. (*See pages 114 and 125.*)

Following miscarriage, you can use raspberry leaves to aid the healing of the uterus, and antiseptic herbs such as thyme or echinacea to help prevent infection.

Rosemary and wild oats will help to support the nervous system following the trauma of miscarriage. (*See pages 114 and 102.*)

Aromatherapy
Lavender is relaxing, and can be used daily in the bath to calm—particularly if you are concerned about miscarriage. Use only in a vaporizer if you have a history of miscarriage. It will be useful following a miscarriage to help your body get back to normal. (*See page 147.*)

Rose has an affinity with the reproductive system, and can be used in a vaporizer (not applied) to help prevent miscarriage. (*See page 154.*)

Homeopathy
Arnica, where there is risk of miscarriage following an accident or injury. (*See page 167.*)

Take Hypericum, following amniocentesis, to prevent miscarriage. (*See page 184.*)

Ipecac., for threatened miscarriage, when the blood is bright red with abdominal cramps. (*See page 175.*)

Sabina, if the blood is dark and clotting, usually at the end of the first trimester.

Flower Essences
Rock Rose, for helplessness and terror. (*See page 216.*)

Mimulus, for gnawing fear of miscarriage.

Star of Bethlehem, for shock. (*See page 220.*)

Gentian, for despondency following a very early miscarriage. (*See page 215.*)

Walnut, to help you adjust to the new situation.

CAUTION

Sudden, severe abdominal pain between the fifth and tenth weeks of pregnancy may indicate an ectopic pregnancy (one that develops in the fallopian tube). This is a life-threatening condition requiring urgent medical attention.

PREGNANCY PROBLEMS

Women may experience problems during pregnancy, often as a result of hormonal changes. Some of the most common problems women experience are:

ANEMIA (*see page 329*)

BACKACHE, due either to postural changes made to accommodate the extra weight, or to the position in which the baby is lying

BLEEDING GUMS, caused by hormonal changes which lead to a thickening and softening of the gums

CONSTIPATION, when normal bowel action is slowed down by an increase of progesterone

CRAMPS, which occur mainly in the feet, calves, and thighs due to inefficient circulation (as a result of increased progesterone), and possibly calcium deficiency

FAINTING, caused by a shortage of blood to the brain due to lowered blood pressure and an increased demand for blood to the womb

FLATULENCE, since digesting food is moved more slowly, which allows wind to build up

FLUID RETENTION, when an upset in the balance of salt and potassium in the cells causes swelling in the hands, legs, and feet

HEARTBURN, a burning sensation in the upper chest, and possibly a sour taste in the mouth, which are caused by acidic juices rising back up the esophagus

INSOMNIA, caused by general inevitable bodily discomfort towards the end of pregnancy

MORNING SICKNESS, nausea and/or vomiting usually in the first three months of pregnancy, but not necessarily confined to the morning

PELVIC PAIN, pain in the groin or inside of the thighs when walking, caused by pressure on the pelvic nerves

PILES (*see page 350*)

STRETCH MARKS, fine red lines (which eventually turn silver) appearing on the breasts, abdomen, and thighs, and caused by stretching of the skin

VARICOSE VEINS

TIREDNESS, characterized by a desire to sleep a lot in the first three months

INCREASED VAGINAL DISCHARGE, probably thickish and white

TREATMENT
Ayurveda
Aloe vera con be applied externally to prevent stretch marks. (*See page 17.*)

Ginger, for recurrent nausea in pregnancy.

Eating caraway seeds deals with constipation and digestive problems. (*See page 19.*)

Cardamom suppresses vomiting when eaten with a banana. (*See page 26.*)

Cayenne, used externally, can ease muscle pain.

Clove tones muscles and expectant mothers are recommended to eat them in the last month of pregnancy to strengthen the uterus. (*See page 26.*)

Licorice, for constipation, and digestive problems.

Long pepper, for muscle soreness, digestive problems, and constipation. (*See page 30.*)

Mustard can help with muscle and joint pain, and acts as a laxative. (*See page 19.*)

Chinese Herbalism

Teasel root, ginseng, and acanthopanax root, for persistent back pain. (*See page 54.*)

Peony root and astragalus, for high blood pressure. (*See pages 53 and 42.*)

Ginseng, licorice, and tangerine peel, for an acid stomach. (*See pages 54, 50, and 45.*)

Gui Pi Wan, for anemia.

Astragalus, for overwhelming exhaustion.

Wild jujube and fleeceflower stem, for insomnia. (*See page 57*)

Dittany bark, for itching.

Ginger, for morning sickness.

Water plantain, poria, cinnamon twigs, and ephedra, for edema.

Gentian and oriental wormwood, for thrush.

Traditional Home and Folk Remedies

Eating yogurt will cool the pain of heartburn.

Use a witch hazel compress on varicose veins—either in the legs or the vulva. (*See page 78.*)

For relief of varicose veins in the legs or vulva, apply neat lemon juice. (*See page 74.*)

Garlic helps the circulation, and can prevent cramping, varicose veins, and piles.(*See page 70.*)

Apply a witch hazel compress to piles to reduce inflammation and encourage healing. (*See page 78.*)

Drink a glass of honey and apple cider vinegar in warm water before bed to help you sleep peacefully.

Celery juice can help you sleep when taken before bedtime. (*See page 71.*)

Chamomile, fennel, and thyme have antifungal properties, and can be used as a compress and pressed against the vagina to ease and treat thrush.

Herbalism

Dandelion tea is a mild diuretic, and so will help with edema. (*See page 121.*)

Chamomile or peppermint tea will ease heartburn. (*See pages 104 and 111.*)

Dandelion leaves, nettles, chives, sorrel, and coriander leaves are rich in iron, which will prevent anemia.

Chamomile, fennel, burdock, and ginger are gentle laxatives, safe for preventing constipation. (*See pages 104, 107, 100, and 126.*)

Lavender, vervain, and lemon balm will soothe the nerves and relax muscles. (*See page 125.*)

Nettles, meadowsweet, and celery seeds are rich in calcium, which can help to prevent cramping.

Lemon balm and chamomile tea can help prevent nausea, as can ginger and fennel. Take as infusions as required. (*See pages 104, 126, and 107.*)

Slippery elm helps to soothe the digestive tract, and can help morning sickness and weak digestion. (*See page 123.*)

Hops can be used for treating severe vomiting.

False unicorn root and agnus castus can balance the hormones, which will prevent many symptoms.

Calendula, marjoram, and comfrey are astringent and can be applied to the legs or vulva as required.

Peppermint and cleavers can be drunk as an infusion to improve circulation and treat varicose veins.

Chamomile, catnip, and vervain can help with insomnia, when taken before bedtime or during the night.

Chamomile, dandelion root, nettle, and licorice can be taken three times daily for piles.

Calendula flowers can be infused, added to coconut oil, and rubbed into the skin to prevent stretch marks.

Aromatherapy

Lavender oil can be rubbed into the temples for headaches, and into the back for muscle pains. (*See page 147.*)

Geranium, fennel, marjoram, and ylang ylang can be added to the bath to prevent constipation.

Roman chamomile and marjoram are excellent in a full-body massage to ease the muscular pains of pregnancy. (*See pages 137 and 151.*)

Thyme, cypress, lavender, and lemon oils can be added to the bath water to strengthen the veins and increase circulation. (*See pages 133–157.*)

Essential oil of geranium can be added to the bath for piles. (*See page 151.*)

A gentle massage with lavender, chamomile, or lemon balm can relax and help you sleep. (*See pages 133–157.*)

Add a few drops of tea tree or cinnamon oil to a cup of cool water and apply to the vaginal area on a clean cloth to treat thrush. (*See pages 148 and 137.*)

A light massage of lavender and neroli, in a carrier oil, can prevent stretch marks. (*See pages 147 and 139.*)

Massage lavender, geranium, or ginger oils into the lower back to ease pain and reduce tension. (*See pages 133–157.*)

Homeopathy

Nat. mur., for help with water retention. (*See page 190.*)

For anemia (*see page 329*), try Kali carb., when the back feels weak and tired, and there are unpleasant dragging pains.

Belladonna, when there is a hard tense feeling in the lower abdomen. (*See page 168.*)

Nux vomica., for nausea that is worse in the morning, and when the vomit contains mucus. (*See page 198.*)

Ipecac., for nonstop nausea and vomiting.

Pulsatilla, for nausea which comes on in the evening.

Ferr. phos., for nausea a few hours after eating.

Nat. mur., for nausea with an aversion to bread and fat, with a craving for salt and great thirst. (*See page 190.*)

Capsicum, for heartburn with a burning sensation behind the breastbone.

Phosphorus, for heartburn with a craving for cold drinks that are then vomited. (*See page 192.*)

Sulfur, for heartburn that is worse around 11 a.m.

Flower Essences

Olive is useful for dealing with general exhaustion.

Crab Apple may help with relief of nausea.

Rescue Remedy or Emergency Essence may be useful for vomiting. (*See page 229.*)

Vitamins and Minerals

Ensure you get plenty of iron, to prevent and treat anemia. Take vitamin C together with iron, in order to aid iron absorption. (*See pages 238 and 243.*)

Folic acid is necessary during pregnancy for the healthy development of the fetus. (*See page 237.*)

Dietary fiber will help to prevent constipation.

Eat plenty of foods rich in calcium to prevent cramp.

Supplements of vitamin B6, zinc, and magnesium may help with nausea. (*See pages 237, 243, and 245.*)

Vitamins C and E, and bioflavonoids, zinc, and brewer's yeast will help to heal damaged blood vessels which are the cause of varicose veins. (*See pages 238, 239, 256, 243, and 257.*)

Take acidophilus for thrush. (*See page 256.*)

Ensure you have plenty of vitamins E, C, zinc, silicon, and pantothenic acid, which can help to prevent stretch marks. (*See pages 238, 239, 243, and 248.*)

Vitamin E oil can be applied neat to areas that are likely to become stretched, including the perineum.

LABOR PAINS

Labor pains are caused by womb contractions. In the first stage of labor the contractions slowly dilate the cervix until it is wide enough to allow the baby's head to pass through. During the second stage, more powerful and more frequent contractions push the baby into the lower part of the birth canal and into the world. In the third stage, continued contractions help to expel the placenta. The pain itself varies at different stages. At first it may be no more than a dull discomfort eased by moving around. Later it may be likened to severe menstrual cramps which reach a peak then die out as the contraction ends. Pain may be felt in the lower abdomen, lower back, and the legs. The pain experienced appears to be different between women, and is related to their "pain threshold." Most women describe severe, in many cases almost unbearable, pain.

TREATMENT

Ayurveda
Basil is heating and can help to induce labor.

Chinese Herbalism
Chinese angelica and peony root, for abdominal pains experienced during and after childbirth.

Jing Jie may be useful as a painkiller, and will help to prevent hemorrhaging.

THE HEALING REMEDIES SOURCEBOOK

Herbalism

Blue cohosh can be taken throughout labor to tone the uterus and help keep contractions strong.

Raspberry leaf, black cohosh, and motherwort can help during the second stage of labor. (*See page 114.*)

Angelica root and raspberry leaf can help with the delivery of the placenta. (*See pages 100 and 114.*)

Chamomile tea can be sipped to soothe and calm.

Ginger may be used to speed up a slow labor.

Aromatherapy

Clary sage, jasmine, and rose can be massaged into the lower back to relax the mother between contractions. (*See pages 133–157.*)

Melissa oils can help to relieve the pain of childbirth, and should be used throughout the labor. (*See page 149.*)

Rub lavender oil into the lower back, or add it to the water of a birthing pool to ease pain. (*See page 147.*)

Homeopathy

Coffea, for violent, unbearable pain when the mother cries out and is understandably nervous between contractions.

Belladonna, for violent contractions, with delirium and staring eyes. (*See page 168.*)

Nux vomica., when the pains are accompanied by a need to pass water or a stool, and the mother is irritable.

Secale can speed a slow labor, when the uterus seems unable to contract any longer.

Carb. veg. is useful when the mother becomes exhausted during labor. (*See page 173.*)

Caulophyllum for weak, irregular contractions.

Gelsemium, if the mother is anxious and trembles, and contractions are not productive. (*See page 180.*)

Flower Essences

Rescue Remedy can be sipped for anxiety and tension.

Olive, for overwhelming fatigue. (*See page 220.*)

For overstraining, use Vervain. (*See page 226.*)

Sweet Chestnut is good for utter despair, and for the feeling that the baby will never be born. (*See page 212.*)

Impatiens, when things do not seem to be happening fast enough. (*See page 218.*)

POST-DELIVERY PROBLEMS

Almost all women suffer from problems of some kind following the trauma of childbirth, whether physical or emotional. These may include:

ABDOMINAL SORENESS, usually resulting from a Cesarean section, from which it can take up to 12 weeks to recover

ANEMIA caused by blood loss during delivery (*see page 329*)

BACKACHE, which may very well relate to back strain during the birth process

BREAST-FEEDING PROBLEMS (*see page 357*)

EXHAUSTION as a result of the birth, coupled with sheer lack of sleep due to the needs of a crying baby

HAIR LOSS caused by normal hormonal changes after the birth

HEADACHE, which may be severe and last up to 48 hours after the delivery, for those who have an epidural injection

PILES (*see page 350*)

POSTNATAL DEPRESSION (*see page 368*)

PROLAPSE (*see page 371*)

SORENESS in the genital area, caused by stitches from a tear or episiotomy, which may last for some days

TREATMENT

Ayurveda

Aloe vera will encourage healing, and soothe spasm and inflammation. (*See page 17.*)

Vetovert is excellent for exhaustion and depression.

Turmeric can be used for bruising.

Saffron is a good overall herb for postnatal problems.

Chinese Herbalism

San Qi will relive swelling, stop hemorrhaging, and disperse bruising. (*See page 54.*)

Tian Ma (castrodia rhizome) will help relieve headaches which come on after childbirth. (*See page 49.*)

Ginseng will help to restore, boost energy levels, prevent infection, and encourage healing. (*See page 54.*)

Herbalism

Good pain-relieving herbs include pulsatilla, black cohosh, lavender, and wild yam. (*See page 105.*)

St. John's wort and calendula will help healing.

An infusion of calendula can be used to assist in healing the perineum. (*See page 102.*)

Witch hazel can be applied to the perineum to encourage healing and soothe pain. (*See page 109.*)

A comfrey compress can be applied to the perineum to speed healing. (*See page 119.*)

Golden seal will help with bleeding, as will beth root and false unicorn root.

Golden seal and myrrh are excellent for dispelling uterine infections.

Cramp bark will help with uterine infections, pain, and cramping. (*See page 125.*)

Black haw is useful for any afterpains suffered.

Beth root and horsetail can be added to the bath for incontinence and weak pelvic floor muscles. (*See page 106.*)

Nettles, chickweed, and coriander will act as tonics for fatigue. (*See page 124.*)

Aromatherapy

Geranium, rose, and clary sage act as uterine tonics and help the pelvic tissues to regain their elasticity after the birth.

Lavender is useful for relief of afterpains. (*See page 147.*)

Chamomile, massaged into the abdomen, helps relieve pain and cramps. (*See page 137.*)

Jasmine has a tonic action on the womb. (*See page 147.*)

Apply lavender and chamomile, diluted in a little apricot kernel oil, to the affected area for sore stitches. (*See pages 147 and 137.*)

Homeopathy

Coffea, for sharp afterpains and exhaustion. (*See page 177.*)

Nux vomica., for afterpains associated with an urgent need to pass water. (*See page 198.*)

Pulsatilla, for pains if part of the placenta is retained.

China, for exhaustion following loss of blood.

Carb. veg., for exhaustion with sweating. (*See page 173.*)

Sepia, for exhaustion with bearing-down pains.

Belladonna, for troublesome incontinence. (*See page 168.*)

Pulsatilla, for piles. (*See page 193.*)

Ferr. phos., for bleeding (the blood is bright red, clots easily), accompanied by a burning face. (*See page 179.*)

Secale, for a post-partum hemorrhage.

Pulsatilla, for continuing labor pains and dark red blood.

Arnica, to encourage healing and prevent bruising.

Hypericum or Arnica tincture, diluted in water, to cleanse the perineum and any stitches. (*See pages 184 and 167.*)

Ledum, where stitching has been necessary.

Vitamins and Minerals

Ensure that you are getting plenty of iron, which can help with fatigue. (*See page 243.*)

Vitamin B and chromium stabilize energy levels.

Vitamin E will encourage healing, and can be applied to stitches. (*See page 239.*)

POSTNATAL ILLNESS (PNI)

The term postnatal illness covers the varying degrees of anxiety, fearfulness, and depression experienced by women after the birth of a baby. Its cause is thought to be the massive drop in pregnancy hormones, aggravated by general exhaustion and discomfort in the days following delivery. Mild "baby blues" usually begin three to four days after delivery, and last only a few days. Some women experience symptoms for several weeks. Many women suffer from baby blues, but in a few women the symptoms, initially a natural response to a new situation, last for much longer than a few weeks and seriously undermine their ability to cope. Postnatal depression (PND) generally starts within weeks of the birth and may last for a year or more. In extreme cases there may be postnatal psychosis, characterized by virtual breakdown. Postnatal depression is most common in women with other stresses—marriage or relationship problems, anxiety about coping with a new baby, financial problems—as well as hormonal imbalances, blood sugar problems, and previous episodes of postnatal depression.

Symptoms

- baby blues: irritability, tearfulness and vulnerability, mild depression and anxiety, fears about responsibility

- postnatal depression: constant feeling of sadness, unable to cope, feelings of guilt and inadequacy, loss of sex drive, excessive worrying
- postnatal psychosis: hyperactive, manic and euphoric, depressive, with panic attacks and insomnia, almost schizophrenic behavior, hallucinations

TREATMENT

Ayurveda
Camphor clears the mind and helps the nervous system. (*See page 22.*)

Cumin may be useful. (*See page 25.*)

Licorice strengthens the nerves. (*See page 27.*)

Individual treatment will be necessary to lift the spirits and to address any hormonal problems.

Chinese Herbalism
Angelica, peony root, licorice, and thorowax root may be useful. (*See pages 41, 53, and 50.*)

Ginseng will help to restore and to strengthen the whole person. (*See page 54.*)

Chinese senega can reduce insomnia and bouts of depression.

Dodder seed may help to restore hormone imbalances to normal. (*See page 48.*)

Herbalism
Agnus castus can help to restore the hormone balance in the body.

St. John's wort and oats are nervine, and will help to reduce stress symptoms and anxiety. (*See page 110.*)

Rosemary or lemon balm teas or tinctures will help the nervous system and lift depression. (*See page 114.*)

False unicorn root balances the hormones and can be added to any herbal preparation.

Aromatherapy
Clary sage has a balancing effect on hormones, and so can help to treat and prevent post-natal illness.

Jasmine and bergamot are overall tonics and relaxants, and can be used daily, either in the bath or in massage, to ease symptoms. (*See pages 147 and 140.*)

Ylang ylang and neroli are specific to PND, and can be used in a long, enjoyable, warm bath in order to ease symptoms. (*See pages 136 and 139.*)

Homeopathy
Treatment would be constitutional, but the following remedies may help:

Pulsatilla, for curtailing episodes of weepiness.

Nat. mur., for coping with feelings of irritation, guilt, and withdrawal. (*See page 190.*)

Sepia, for allaying exhaustion, lack of interest, and irritability. (*See page 196.*)

Flower Essences
Rescue remedy or Emergency Essence will help after the trauma of the birth. (*See page 229.*)

Gorse is good for feelings of hopelessness. (*See page 226.*)

Mustard, when you feel as if you are under a dark cloud for no apparent reason. (*See page 224.*)

Olive will help to address exhaustion. (*See page 220.*)

Walnut will help you to deal with change.

Sweet Chestnut is for fits of utter despair.

Vitamins and Minerals
Some experts believe that nutritional deficiencies are at the root of the problem; ensure you eat plenty of foods rich in vitamins C and B, calcium, iron, magnesium, and also potassium. (*See pages 235–238, 241, 243, and 245.*)

Tyrosine and tryptophan, amino acids, can help to ease postnatal depression. (*See page 230.*)

MENOPAUSE SYMPTOMS

Menopause is the cessation of menstruation and a woman's reproductive capacity. It usually occurs around the age of 50, but may happen prematurely, or artificially after removal of the ovaries. Most symptoms that occur during menopause result directly from the estrogen deficiency produced by the failing ovaries. Interestingly, Japanese women suffer far fewer symptoms of menopause because they eat more plant estrogens like tofu, soya, and miso.

Symptoms

- back pain
- dry, thinning hair
- very heavy periods (flooding)
- very light periods
- hot flashes, mostly affecting the face and neck, and varying in frequency and duration
- incontinence, one of the most common menopausal symptoms; through wear and tear, childbearing, and lack of estrogen
- osteoporosis
- psychological problems such as irritability, anxiety, insomnia, and poor memory
- increased hair growth on the face, stomach, or chest, due either to an increase in the male hormone, androgen, or the drop in estrogen production
- vaginal looseness, a feeling of slackness, or of something protruding into the vaginal passage— possibly a prolapsed uterus, or a section of the urethra, bladder, or rectum dropping downward as a result of lost muscle tone
- about 20–25 percent of menopausal women experience pain during intercourse, called dyspareunia. Mostly, this is due to thinning of the vaginal wall and a lack of lubrication, both caused by estrogen deficiency

TREATMENT

Ayurveda

Calamus root can be good for memory problems and mental stress. (*See page 15.*)

Celery seeds and cedar are balancing, and may help with menstrual problems. (*See page 21.*)

Cinnamon is especially powerful during menopause, and is particularly useful for low libido and edema.

Coriander is cooling, and acts as a diuretic and diaphoretic. It is also thought to be aphrodisiac.

Aloe vera cools and cleanses the liver when taken internally, helping with any "hot" symptoms of menopause, including flashes, sweats, and swelling. (*See page 17.*)

Chinese Herbalism

Shan Zhu Yu can be used or flooding, with ginseng for heavy sweating and hot flashes. (*See page 46.*)

Chinese senega may be useful for irritability, insomnia, and depression.

Angelica, peony root, and thorowax root are the ideal herbs to treat the symptoms of menopause, which is believed to be a weakness of the Kidneys, deficient Blood, and an imbalance between Kidney and Liver. (*See page 35.*)

Herbalism

Valerian will help with anxiety and tension, and combined with skullcap relaxes the nervous system. (*See pages 123 and 118.*)

Ginseng will help with anxiety and irritability, and increases mental alertness. It will also boost vitality and prevent feelings of fatigue. (*See page 112.*)

Herbal laxatives include butternut, blue flag, and senna.

Shepherd's purse, lady's mantle, yarrow, golden seal, beth root, and periwinkle help with heavy bleeding.

Dandelion cleanses the liver and helps the body to detoxify, which can reduce the risk of breast growths and other cell changes. (*See page 121.*)

Milk thistle can be used to treat lumpy and painful breasts. (*See page 118.*)

Agnus castus can be used for breast tenderness and any problems of menopause, as it works to normalize the levels of female hormones.

Black cohosh can restore female hormonal balance and help to prevent night sweats and hot flashes. Other herbs to consider are licorice, alfalfa, and Dong Quai. (*See page 108.*)

American ginseng can increase libido, as can agnus castus and black cohosh. (*See pages 112 and 126.*)

Ginkgo biloba can help with memory and concentration problems. (*See page 108.*)

Cramp bark is antispasmodic and will help with painful menstruation. (*See page 125.*)

Burdock root helps with dry and scaly skin, and licorice or chamomile, applied directly to the skin, will soothe and soften. (*See pages 100, 108, and 104.*)

Valerian can help improve the quality of sleep and treat insomnia. (*See page 123.*)

Passiflora will help you to sleep.

Motherwort can restore thickness and elasticity to the walls of the vagina, and dong quai can help with dryness. (*See page 110.*)

Dandelion is a natural diuretic and will help with any swelling associated with water retention.

Aromatherapy

Clary sage will lift your mood and help to deal with fluctuating hormones. (*See page 155.*)

Chamomile, diluted in a little carrier oil, is adaptogenic, and will balance hormone levels causing night sweats, hot flashes, and other symptoms. (*See page 137.*)

Essential oils of damian, and geranium or ylang ylang are aphrodisiacs for low libido. (*See page 136.*)

Fennel can be massaged into the abdomen for water retention and symptoms of hormonal imbalance.

Homeopathy

Sepia is enormously useful, and can treat hot flashes, headaches, irritability, and heavy menstrual bleeding.

Conium, for loss of libido.

Graphites, for weight gain, hot flashes, and scanty menstrual bleeding. (*See page 181.*)

Lachesis, for flooding, irritability, memory loss and concentration problems, hot flashes, and headaches.

Pulsatilla, for depression, weepiness, and changeable moods. (*See page 193.*)

Sanguinara, for tender breasts and flooding.

Flower Essences

Mustard, for depression with no identifiable cause.

Olive, for fatigue. (*See page 220.*)

Mimulus, for fear of aging and death. (*See page 220.*)

Walnut, for life changes. (*See page 218.*)

Vitamins and Minerals

Take magnesium and vitamin B-complex for anxiety and irritability. (*See pages 245 and 235–238*)

Vitamin E, linseed oil, acidophilus, and vitamin B-complex will help with tender and lumpy breasts. (*See pages 239, 256, and 235–238.*)

For constipation, try extra vitamin C. (*See page 238.*)

Coenzyme Q10 will help lack of energy and fatigue; check that you are not anemic.

Quercetin can help with migraine and headaches associated with menopause, as can vitamin C and E.

Vitamin C can help regulate heavy bleeding (flooding) when combined with bioflavonoids. (*See page 238.*)

Vitamin A, zinc, iron, and vitamin B-complex can also help with heavy menstrual bleeding.

Selenium may help to reduce hot flashes and night sweats, as will vitamin C, which is a more effective preventive than HRT. (*See pages 247 and 238.*)

Zinc, vitamin C, vitamin E, and magnesium will help with painful menstruation.

Linseed oil, evening primrose, vitamin B-complex, and zinc can be taken for skin problems.

Magnesium is helpful for insomnia and sleep problems. (*See page 245.*)

A vitamin E capsule can be placed inside the vagina for vaginal dryness. (*See page 239.*)

PROLAPSE

Prolapse occurs when the uterus and/or vagina slip downward due to a weakening or stretching of the structures that would normally keep them in place. It occurs when ligaments and muscles which hold the uterus and vagina in place become weak or slack with age, or as a result of childbirth, allowing the uterus to bulge into the vagina and press on the bladder or rectum. If prolapse is complete a large part of the vagina or uterus may actually protrude through the vaginal opening, causing soreness or ulceration, and encouraging infection. The risk of a prolapse may be heightened by a chronic cough, chronic constipation, or obesity. Neither prolapse is serious at first, but may become so if neglected. Surgery to tighten pelvic floor muscles may be necessary if exercises do not improve the muscle tone. A ring pessary, fitted behind the pubic bone, may be necessary in an elderly woman. Sixty-five percent of all women who prolapse do so before the age of 55. Women who have had several children, or a difficult labor, seem to be more prone to prolapse.

Symptoms
- a sensation of something dropping down
- dragging feeling in lower abdomen
- backache
- fatigue
- in addition to the above, prolapse of the vagina may involve: frequent urge to pass water, stress incontinence, possibly urine infections

TREATMENT

Chinese Herbalism
Treatment would be aimed at Deficient qi, and Central qi pills would be useful.

Herbalism
Motherwort, Lady's mantle, and life root can help to restore the tone of the uterus and vagina.

Use astringent herbs such as horsetail, shepherd's purse, false unicorn, and bayberry. These can be taken as teas, tisanes, decoctions, pills, etc. They can also be used as a poultice and applied to the abdomen. Barberry stimulates the uterus to contract: do not use in pregnancy.

For a prolapse after menopause, try sage, calendula, ginseng, and wild yam: all estrogenic.

Chickweed ointment or douche can soothe and heal soreness of the vagina or cervix.

Pessaries with glycerin and golden seal can be helpful.

Aromatherapy
Massage the lower abdomen and back with diluted oils of rosemary and lemon to improve the circulation and tighten tissues. (*See pages 154 and 140.*)

Homeopathy
Sepia, for a pressing feeling that something is coming out.

Aloe, for long-standing prolapse with a feeling of fullness and sometimes morning diarrhea.

Vitamins and Minerals
Uterus glandular tissues give support to your uterus.

Vitamin E increases the elasticity of the tissues, and helps them respond to stress more effectively.

OVARIAN CYSTS

A cyst is an abnormal sac or cavity that contains liquid or semi-solid material enclosed by a membrane. Ovarian cysts most commonly occur in women between the ages of 35 and 55. Usually they are benign, but they can sometimes cause problems because of their size. Ovarian cysts may be caused by slight ovulation disorders, or by swelling of the lining of the ovary through fluid collection. The most common ovarian cyst is a follicular cyst that contains watery fluid. Pseudomucinous cysts contain a thick mucous fluid and can lead to complications if they rupture or become infected.

Symptoms
- pain, once the cyst has grown large enough to cause problems
- abdominal discomfort
- possibly an increase in the size of the abdomen
- breathlessness
- may lead to varicose veins (*see page 334*) or piles (*see page 350*)
- repeated or multiple cysts may affect fertility

TREATMENT

Chinese Herbalism
Dodder seeds can balance the reproductive system.

San qi, for general relief of pain. (*See page 54.*)

Tree peony may be useful. (*See page 53.*)

Herbalism
False unicorn root or blue cohosh can help to restore the function of the reproductive system.

Kelp can be added to ensure normal thyroid function.

Take dandelion root to help the liver metabolize estrogen.

Agnus castus acts to restore estrogen levels.

Aromatherapy
Basil, marjoram, and lavender can be massaged into the abdomen to ease pain and restore balance.

Clary sage will help to balance hormones.

Homeopathy
Treatment should be constitutional, but the following remedies may be useful.

Colocynthis, is for small round cysts which cause boring pain which is improved by pressure.

Apis, for stinging pains, particularly in the right ovary.

Lachesis, for local pain which is worse in the morning, and occurs mainly in the left ovary. (*See page 200.*)

Ledum, for driving pain through the ovary and womb.

Flower Essences

Take Rescue Remedy or Emergency Essence to restore a sense of calm during pain and discomfort.

Vitamins and Minerals

Increase your intake of iodine, since thyroid problems may be at the root of the cysts. (*See page 244.*)

Vitamin E is helpful for preventing and treating cysts.

The B-complex vitamins will help to re-establish hormone balance and the metabolism of estrogen by the liver.

PELVIC INFLAMMATORY DISEASE (PID)

Pelvic inflammatory disease (PID) is an umbrella term for infections and inflammations that have penetrated the reproductive system, i.e. the ovaries (ovaritis), Fallopian tubes (salpingitis), and the uterus (endometritis). Left untreated, these infections can develop and recur for years. Possible causes of PID are gonorrhoea and chlamydia cystitis (*see page 353*), various viruses, or the natural flora of the vagina. Triggers include anything that allows a lurking infection to travel, such as childbirth, abortion, surgery on the reproductive system or in the pelvic area, or an IUD (intrauterine device, which prevents pregnancy).

Symptoms
- acute: fever with shaking, painful intercourse, unusual vaginal discharge, vaginal bleeding after sex or in mid-menstrual cycle, severe lower abdominal pain, back pain
- chronic: weight loss, backache and lower abdominal pain, nausea, diarrhea, tiredness, pain on urination, reduced fertility (caused by scarring which blocks the Fallopian tubes)

TREATMENT

Ayurveda

Aloe vera relieves inflammation, soothes muscle spasms, and purifies the blood. (*See page 17.*)

Angelica has antibacterial properties and can help with pain. (*See page 17.*)

Gotu kola may be useful if the infection is linked to STDs.

Chinese Herbalism

Peony root can be used for abdominal pain. (*See page 53.*)
Cinnamon treats pain and other symptoms. (*See page 44.*)
Pseudoginseng root (San Qi) may be useful. (*See page 54.*)

Traditional Home and Folk Remedies

Peel a clove of garlic, wrap it in gauze, and tie a piece of string to one end. Place in the vagina and change daily.

Herbalism

Fresh garlic, taken as often as possible throughout the day, can act to fight infection and boost the immune system.

Echinacea will help to boost immunity as well as addressing the infection. (*See page 105.*)

Thyme and parsley will help to fight infection.

Blue cohosh has an affinity with the reproductive system. Take daily.

False unicorn root and myrrh combine well.

Aromatherapy

Add lavender, rosemary, or geranium oils to the bath water to relax and help to fight infection. (*See pages 133–157.*)

Homeopathy

Treatment should be constitutional, but the following may help:

Mercurius, for chills and sweat that is unpleasant, and where the condition is improved by rest. (*See page 189.*)

Apis, for stinging, burning pains, mainly on the right side.

Aconite, for sudden onset, with mild fever and anxiety.

Belladonna, for sudden onset, with red face and burning.

Colocynthis, is for cramping pains relieved by pressure.

Vitamins and Minerals

Include vitamin C, E, and zinc in your diet to boost the immune system. (*See pages 238, 239, and 249.*)

Acidophilus encourages the growth of healthy bacteria, and is especially useful if you have taken a course of antibiotics. (*See page 256.*)

THRUSH

Thrush is a variant of oral thrush (*see page 315*) and, in addition to the mouth, can live in the vagina, bowel, and skin. Aggravating factors include high sugar intake, tight clothing, poor personal hygiene, and scented bath oils. Women suffer more frequently from thrush than men.

PAINFUL INTERCOURSE

Many women experience pain or discomfort during sexual intercourse (called dyspareunia) at different points in their lives, and it may be attributed to a number of causes:

ENDOMETRIOSIS, when cells from the womb's lining migrate outside the womb, usually to the Fallopian tubes or the ovaries. Because they are still under the influence of the menstrual cycle's hormones they grow and bleed each month, resulting in blood-filled cysts and scarring.

FIBROIDS, which are noncancerous growths in or on the walls of the uterus.

PELVIC INFLAMMATORY DISEASE (PID), an umbrella term for infections and inflammations that have penetrated deep into the reproductive system.

SEXUALLY TRANSMITTED DISEASES (STDs).

THRUSH (*see above*).

CHILDBIRTH. The labor and delivery process can cause soreness and discomfort for some weeks, particularly if the woman has had an episiotomy.

MENOPAUSE (*see page 369*).

TREATMENT

See treatment for Thrush *on page 315*, Menopause *on page 370*, Pregnancy Problems *on page 364*, and PID *on page 368*.

Aromatherapy

Lavender and marjoram are relaxing, and can help you to get over the emotional trauma of painful sex. Try a full-body massage with your partner before intercourse.

Homeopathy

Treatment would be constitutional, and would depend on the cause of the pain.

Calcarea iod., for treating small fibroids with a yellow discharge.

Aurum mur., for a swollen uterus and painful contractions of the vagina associated with fibroids.

Aconite, for sharp pain that comes on suddenly.

Sepia or Belladonna, when the problem is associated with prolapse. (*See pages 196 and 168.*)

Flower Essences

Mimulus, for fear of pain during sex. (*See page 220.*)

Rescue Remedy or Emergency Essence, taken before making love, to calm and reduce feelings of panic and anxiety. (*See page 229.*)

Vitamins and Minerals

Take plenty of vitamin A and E, which will help restore the health of the reproductive system.

Acidophilus will help to maintain the balance of healthy flora in the body. (*See page 256.*)

Vitamin E capsules can be placed in the vagina to ease pain and dry ness. (*See page 239.*)

DISORDERS OF THE REPRODUCTIVE SYSTEM: MALE

INFERTILITY

The term infertility is generally applied when failure to conceive follows an 18-month period of regular, unprotected sexual intercourse. It is usually a sign that something in the body is not working properly. The most common cause of infertility in men is a low sperm count (possibly due to environmental pollution). Poor sperm quality, inadequate mobility of sperm, no sperm at all, or an abnormality in the penis may also be responsible. In some cases the problem may be hormonal. Risk factors include smoking, excessive alcohol consumption, raised temperature around the testes (caused by tight trousers, or by varicose veins on the scrotum), certain prescription drugs, stress, or infection with mumps. A diet lacking in vitamins and minerals can also cause a man to be less fertile. One research study discovered that organic farmers had twice the sperm count of other men!

Infertility in humans is defined as the failure to conceive after a year to 18 months of unprotected sexual intercourse.

Approximately 10–15 percent of couples, or one in every seven marriages in the United States, is affected by the problem of infertility.

In approximately 40 percent of cases, the cause of infertility is due to a female factor (*see page 361*); 40 percent of cases are due to a male factor; and in the remaining instances no cause can be found despite thorough evaluation.

In as many as 35 percent of couples, multiple conditions causing infertility can be identified.

TREATMENT

Ayurveda
Saffron is used for the treatment of infertility. (*See page 24.*)

Sandalwood can help with impotence and acts as an aphrodisiac. (*See page 31.*)

Clove, ginger, cardamom, cinnamon, vetiver, and coriander are aphrodisiac, which may help.

Chinese Herbalism
Infertility is believed to be caused by Damp Heat, and an imbalance of yin and yang; treatment will be according to the nature of your infertility. The following combinations may be useful: Yi Zhi Ren, He Shou Wu, Gou Qi Zi, Du Zhong, and Wu Wei Zi, for problems associated with sperm. (*See pages 40, 57, and 52.*)

Herbalism
Remedies such as damiana and saw palmetto have hormonal effects, stimulating the male reproductive system while also acting as useful nerve restoratives. (*See pages 122 and 117.*)

Aromatherapy
Rose oil is said to increase sperm count and quality, as well as acting as a mild aphrodisiac. Add a few drops to your partner's bath, or perhaps engage in a little gentle massage, with 2 or 3 drops of rose essential oil in a mild carrier oil such as sweet almond oil. (*See page 154.*)

If infertility is causing anxiety, any of the relaxing essential oils, such as lavender, marjoram, or chamomile, can be vaporized or used in a bath. (*See pages 133–157.*)

When repeated attempts to get pregnant have failed and you need a little encouragement to continue with love-making, ylang ylang is a lovely, relaxing oil that will act as an aphrodisiac. (*See page 136.*)

Homeopathy
Treatment would be constitutional, but the following remedies may be helpful:

Conium, for inability to sustain an erection.

Lycopodium, for an increased desire for sex, but where intercourse is spoiled by anticipation of failure.

Flower Essences
White Chestnut, for worrying thoughts. (*See page 209.*)

Pine, for guilty feelings. (*See page 221.*)

Olive, for exhaustion and overwhelming fatigue.

Vitamins and Minerals
There is a possibility that a zinc deficiency might cause problems with male fertility. Studies in the U.S. have shown that zinc is essential for sperm formation, and men who have zinc deficiencies may produce zero or reduced sperm counts. Zinc is also linked to a man's sex drive.

Cutting out alcohol, smoking, and drugs may be suggested for both partners for the period before conception.

Vitamins E and B6 may be supplemented, as a deficiency is often linked to a low sperm count.

An increased intake of EFAs (essential fatty acids, found in oily fish, fish liver oils, seeds, nuts, pulses, beans, evening primrose oil, and unrefined vegetable oils) stimulates sex hormone production.

PROSTATE PROBLEMS

The prostate is a small sex gland which surrounds the urethra (urine tube) under the bladder. Its function is to produce the fluid which transports and nourishes sperm as it is ejaculated. Common prostate problems include:

BENIGN PROSTATIC HYPERPLASIA (BPH), a slow, noncancerous enlargement of the prostate, progressively constricts the urethra, causing obstruction in the flow of urine. Incomplete emptying of the bladder as a result causes a frequent urge to urinate at night as well as during the day.

PROSTATITIS, inflammation of the prostate gland, is common in younger men and may be chronic or acute. Symptoms include a frequent urge to urinate, burning pain, and difficulty in urinating, lower back pain, painful ejaculation, and inflamed testes.

PROSTATE CANCER, the second most common form of cancer in men. The prostate is enlarged, as in BPH, but is felt to be hard on examination. As well as an urge to urinate more frequently, there may be blood in the urine and pain on urinating. If the cancer is advanced there may also be bone pain and weight loss.

CANCER of the prostate occurs in 1 of 8 American men. Prostate cancer is more common after the age of 55; approximately 80 percent of all cases occur in men over 65; by the age of 80, 80 percent of all men have the cancer to some degree. Cancer of the prostate also becomes increasingly common in men over the age of 60; its development is stimulated by male hormones and retarded—to a variable extent—by female hormones. A male baby has a 13 percent chance of contracting prostate cancer, and a 3 percent chance of dying from it. For early detection of prostate cancer, the ACS (American Cancer Society) recommends that men over age 40 should have an annual digital rectal examination. After age 50, men should have an annual prostate-specific antigen blood test.

BENIGN PROSTATIC HYPERTROPHY occurs in half of all men over the age of 50, and in three-quarters over the age of 70—a total of about 10 million men.

TREATMENT

Ayurveda
Gotu kola is cooling, rejuvenating, and diuretic. (*See page 22.*)

Cedar and celery seed are natural diuretics and will encourage urination. (*See pages 21 and 18.*)

Cinnamon is diuretic and analgesic, which will help ease the discomfort. (*See page 23.*)

Coriander is diuretic and aphrodisiac, which will help address the low libido that is associated with this condition.

Chinese Herbalism
Prostate problems are believed to be caused by excess dampness and stagnant qi. The herbs cinnamon bark, cork tree bark, and water plantain will be useful treatments.

Panax ginseng is recommended for an enlarged prostate.

Traditional Home and Folk Remedies
Watercress leaves are tonic and should be eaten as often as possible to help alleviate the problem. (*See page 81.*)

Sesame seeds have a beneficial effect in maintaining and enhancing sexual vigor.

Pumpkin seeds are a male sexual tonic, and are used in the treatment of prostate problems.

Herbalism
Saw palmetto is able to reduce inflammation of the prostate.

Couchgrass and horsetail can be given to help encourage urination, and can be drunk freely throughout the day as a natural diuretic.

Aromatherapy
Clary sage and geranium, which have estrogen-like oils, can be used in whole-body massage or in the bath to treat the condition. (*See pages 155 and 151.*)

Bergamot, chamomile, and myrrh are anti-inflammatory, and will ease symptoms, particularly of prostatitis.

Benzoin, sandalwood, frankincense, and cedarwood are all diuretic, and can be used both in the bath and for a full-body massage. (*See pages 133–157.*)

Homeopathy
Constitutional treatment would be required, but in the meantime the following remedies can be taken four times daily for 3 to 4 weeks:

Arg. nit., for impotence because erection is lost on penetration, and for pain on intercourse and low libido.

Sabal, for difficult or painful urination, and spasms of pain. Also for enlarged prostate, and if intercourse is painful.

Pulsatilla, for thick yellow discharge from the penis and an urgent desire to urinate. (*See page 193.*)

Thuja, for burning at the neck of the bladder and a frequent need to urinate. (*See page 200.*)

Baryta carb., for a frequent urge to urinate, a slow stream of urine, and premature ejaculation. (*See page 170.*)

Iodum, for loss of potency, with shrunken testicles and hard prostate gland.

Vitamins and Minerals

Lecithin, calcium, and magnesium may help treat prostate disorders. (*See pages 255, 241, and 245.*)

An increased intake of zinc can help to prevent and treat prostatitis. (*See page 249.*)

Evening primrose has been successfully used for prostate problems. (*See page 254.*)

Cold-pressed linseed oil can help if the condition is mild but recurrent.

Flower pollen is widely used to treat problems of the prostate gland. (*See page 256.*)

ERECTION PROBLEMS

Failure to achieve an erection that is firm enough, or sustained for long enough, to allow normal sexual intercourse is generally known as impotence. Its cause may be physical (organic), psychological, or a combination of both. Organic impotence may be due to an imperfect blood supply to the penis, an age-related loss of male sex hormones, diabetes, medicinal drugs, or various neurological conditions. Psychological factors such as lack of desire, depression, or fear of failure may be responsible for impotence, and alcohol, while enhancing sexual desire, can actually impede performance.

It is now believed that up to 85 percent of cases have a physical cause.

The Association for Male Sexual Dysfunction recognizes over 200 drugs that may cause it, including alcohol, antihistamines, antidepressants, narcotics, diuretics, sedatives, and nicotine.

Primary impotence is the case in which the male has never maintained an erection of long enough duration to engage in sexual intercourse.

Secondary impotence is when a previously potent male loses the ability to maintain an erection during intercourse.

Fear of failure and performance anxiety are frequently underlying negative psychological sources of impotence.

TREATMENT

Ayurveda

Sandalwood is good for impotence, and accompanying anxiety and nervousness. (*See page 31.*)

Cinnamon tones the muscles and is noted for treating impotence. (*See page 23.*)

Ginger is warming and can help improve matters.

Saffron is used for impotence and anxiety.

Clove, ginger, cardamom, cinnamon, vetiver, and coriander are aphrodisiac, which may help.

Chinese Herbalism

Ginseng can improve vitality and help to reduce feelings of anxiety. (*See page 54.*)

Impotence is believed to be caused by a weakness of the Kidneys and Liver, with Liver qi stagnation, and cibot root may be useful.

Chinese angelica, white peony root, and thorowax will help feelings of anxiety. (*See pages 41 and 53.*)

Traditional Home and Folk Remedies

Watercress leaves are tonic and should be eaten as often as possible to help alleviate the problem. (*See page 81.*)

Sesame seeds have a beneficial effect in maintaining and enhancing sexual vigor.

Pumpkin seeds are a male sexual tonic.

Avocado pear is excellent if you suffer from sexual problems. (*See page 82.*)

Herbalism

Peppermint leaves stimulate and warm the body, and will help to reduce feelings of anxiety. (*See page 111.*)

Anise is a powerful tonic: drink small amounts to treat impotence.

Remedies like damiana and saw palmetto have dual hormonal effects, stimulating and toning the male reproductive system, and restoring nerves. (*See pages 122 and 117.*)

Aromatherapy

Essential oils of clary sage, sandalwood, and ylang ylang are natural aphrodisiacs and will help you to relax. Try a full-body massage, or a few drops in the bath. (*See pages 133–157.*)

Homeopathy

Lycopodium, when you feel surges of desire, but anticipate failure. (*See page 187.*)

Agnus, for an erection that is not firm enough for successful penetration.

Conium, for an erection which does not last.

Caladium, for erections which occur during sleep, but disappear on waking, and a lack of erection even when sexually excited.

Flower Essences

Larch, for lack of sexual confidence and feelings of inadequacy. (*See page 218.*)

Gentian, for a sense of failure. (*See page 215.*)

Sweet Chestnut, for despair and hopelessness.

Crab Apple, for feeling unclean on any level.

Vitamins and Minerals

Avoid alcohol, drugs, and caffeine, which constrict the blood vessels and inhibit the blood flow needed to achieve an erection.

Molybdenum can prevent impotence and sexual difficulties. (*See page 246.*)

Zinc is required for the healthy functioning of the reproductive organs, and should be included in a varied, healthy diet. (*See page 249.*)

L-tryptophan may help to prevent feelings of anxiety from causing sexual difficulties. (*See page 253.*)

EJACULATION PROBLEMS

For men, orgasm is usually accompanied by ejaculation. A single ejaculate contains about 300 million sperm in a fluid medium called semen. Ejaculation is a two-phased process. In the emission phase seminal fluid accumulates in the bulb of the prostate. In the expulsion phase the neck of the urinary bladder closes to ensure that no urine will mix with the semen, and the muscles at the base of the penis and of the penile urethra contract to force the semen out of the urethral opening. Some men experience a "retrograde," or dry, ejaculation as a result of genetics, illness, medication, surgery, or damage to the valves of the urethra that control the flow of semen.

In most cases ejaculation problems are psycho-sexual in origin, and not due to any physical abnormality, so that a man may experience sexual failure with one partner, but function quite normally with another. There are two main problems: premature ejaculation and absence of ejaculation. Premature ejaculation is very common indeed and refers to the occurrence of the male orgasm at the time of penetration, or very soon after. In extreme cases it may even take place before physical contact is made. Premature ejaculation is usually a feature of early sexual experience, or a sign of performance anxiety. The absence of ejaculation is very rare but can occur as a result of overindulgence, inadequate stimulation of the penis, or age-related loss of penile sensitivity.

TREATMENT

Ayurveda

An Ayurvedic medical practitioner would balance the tri-doshas, and use panchakarma for balancing the vátha.

Sandalwood may help to relieve anxiety, and has an anesthetic effect on the area which can reduce premature ejaculation. (*See page 31.*)

Saffron may be helpful. (*See page 24.*)

Chinese Herbalism

Treatment may address a weakness of the Kidneys and Liver, and deal with Liver qi stagnation. Cibot root may work well.

Problems causing or associated with anxiety may be treated with ginseng, Chinese angelica, white peony root, and thorowax root. (*See pages 41 and 53.*)

Traditional Home and Folk Remedies

Oats contain thiamine and pantothenic acid, which act as gentle tonics for the nerves and will relax and calm you. Take regularly. (*See page 72.*)

Herbalism

Herbal remedies would be used to calm the nervous system and to relax.

Skullcap and valerian are useful herbs, and should be blended together for best effect. Drink this as a tea three times daily to calm. (*See pages 118 and 123.*)

Lady's slipper and lime blossom may also work to ease anxiety and tension associated with the condition.

Remedies like damiana and saw palmetto have hormonal effects, stimulating and toning the male reproductive system and restoring nerves. (*See pages 122 and 117.*)

Aromatherapy

A relaxing blend of essential oils of lavender, geranium, and bergamot in sweet almond oil or peach kernel oil may be used in the bath at times of great stress and anxiety.

Homeopathy

Constitutional treatment will be necessary, but the following remedies may be of some use:

Lycopodium, for an increased sexual desire; lack of self-confidence and expectation of failure with premature ejaculation. (*See page 187.*)

Nux vomica., for impatience, craving excitement, short temper, and use of stimulating drugs. (*See page 198.*)

Graphites, for loss of sex drive, premature or non-existent ejaculation. (*See page 181.*)

Nitric acid, for irritability, self-criticism, and extreme sensitivity.

Ignatia, for problems caused by grief or disappointment.

Mercurius, when thrush or urethritis causes the problem. (*See page 189.*)

(*See also* Prostate Problems, *page 316*).

Flower Essences

Try Elm for anxiety accompanying a feeling of being unable to cope. (*See page 226.*)

Larch may help with lack of self-confidence.

Gentian may be useful for a sense of failure. (*See page 215.*)

Rescue Remedy or Emergency Essence, taken before intercourse, can help to calm and relax you. (*See page 219.*)

Vitamins and Minerals

Increase your intake of B vitamins, which work on the nervous system, and avoid caffeine or other stimulants in any form. (*See pages 234–238.*)

PRIAPISM

Priapism is the name given to prolonged and painful erection in the absence of sexual interest. It is caused by failure of the blood to return from the penis to the circulation after a period of sexual activity. This may be because of a disturbance in the nervous system's control of blood flow, due to a disease of the spinal cord or brain. It may also be caused by clotting due to leukemia or sickle-cell anemia, inflammation of the prostate, bladder stones, or urethritis.

> **CAUTION**
> A long-sustained erection can be dangerous as there is a risk of thrombosis, which may cause permanent loss of erectile function.

TREATMENT

Ayurveda

Angelica can improve circulation. (*See page 17.*)

Black pepper increases blood circulation and feeds the nervous system. (*See page 30.*)

Calamus oil massage will improve circulation in the area. (*See page 15.*)

Cayenne pepper is analgesic and warming. (*See page 20.*)

Chinese Herbalism

Gui Zhi may be useful when the yang qi has failed to move fluids through channels. (*See page 44.*)

Dang Gui will reduce pain and invigorates blood circulation. (*See page 41.*)

Herbalism

Herbs which encourage circulation include:
- Broom, which tones the arteries.
- Ginger, hawthorn tops, and rosemary, which are stimulating and work to encourage circulation.
- Lavender and vervain, which are calming, and can be sipped during an attack to ease symptoms. (*See page 125.*) (*See also* the sections on Prostate Problems, *page 376;* Urethritis, *page 354;* and Bladder Stones; *page 352.*)

Aromatherapy

Local massage with rosemary or peppermint is stimulating and will help normalize the blood flow in the area.

Massage the area with diluted juniper, marjoram, myrrh, or tea tree, which will act as a tonic.

Bergamot is anti-inflammatory, and may be used in local massage or in the bath to ease inflammatory conditions causing priapism. (*See page 140.*)

Homeopathy

Treatment would be constitutional, but during an attack the following remedies may help:

Carb. veg., for sluggish circulation, and possibly piles and varicose veins. (*See page 173.*)

Kali brom., for the treatment of impotence.

Cantharis, for a painful erection.

Vitamins and Minerals

Vitamin E is suggested. (*See page 239.*)

Vitamin C, which affects the health of the circulatory system, may be useful. (*See page 238.*)

DISORDERS OF THE ENDOCRINE SYSTEM

THYROID PROBLEMS

The thyroid gland, found in the neck, is responsible for controlling the general level of activity of the body. An overactive gland (hyperthyroidism) causes a racing heart, increased digestion, and enormous physical energy. Untreated, this condition can lead to heart failure and extreme weight loss, among other things. An underactive gland (hypothyroidism) leads to apathy, overwhelming fatigue, heart problems, menstrual problems, and weight gain. Thyroid problems are very common and, fortunately, they can be diagnosed long before they become serious, and various remedies can then be applied. Occasionally thyroid disease forms part of a wider disease process, including diabetes and rheumatoid arthritis. Other causes of thyroid disease include iodine deficiency, which may exist from birth and features in mental retardation, enlargement of the thyroid gland (goiter), inflammation, and, rarely, cancer.

Disorders of the thyroid include:

Iodine deficiency. Iodine is an essential element in the thyroid hormone. Deficiency of iodine is rare, but can cause cretinism—physical and mental retardation featuring poor feeding, constipation, a characteristic cry, and a large tongue.

Hypothyroidism, underaction of the thyroid. Features slowing of physical and mental processes, sensitivity to cold, obesity, no sweating, loss of hair, a puffy face, coronary artery disease. Untreated, hypothyroidism may lead to coma.

Hyperthyroidism, overaction of the thyroid. Features weight loss, increased appetite, palpitations, anxiety, irritability, dislike of heat, sweating, and infrequent menstruation. Untreated it may lead to heart failure.

In the U.K. researchers discovered that one in ten people suffering from Parkinson's disease also suffered from hyperthyroidism.

Over 5 million people in the U.S. suffer from thyroid problems; 90 percent of them are women.

Goiter. Various conditions can cause goiter, an enlargement of the thyroid gland

If goiter is caused by a low dietary intake of iodine, it is termed endemic (colloid) goiter.

Overproduction of hormones in the thyroid gland, which may follow emotional or physical stress, results in toxic diffuse goiter (Grave's disease) or toxic nodular goiter (Plummer's disease), both of which are characterized by nervousness, sweating, weight loss, and hyperactivity.

Cancer. Thyroid cancer is quite rare and is usually found as a single firm lump in the neck. It may spread to the lymph nodes in the neck and can involve the vocal cords, causing hoarseness or loss of the voice.

TREATMENT

Ayurveda
An Ayurvedic medical practitioner may suggest panchakarma Method for detoxification. (*See page 11.*)

Hyperthyroidism is believed to be caused by Heat in the Liver, and marine plants and seaweed are prescribed.

Chinese Herbalism
Bugleweed is excellent, and should be drunk three times daily for hyperthyroidism.

Bladderwrack helps to regulate the function of the thyroid gland. Take three times daily, in any form.

Aromatherapy
Geranium oil balances hormone production, and will help to ensure that the thyroid gland is working effectively. Use the oil in the bath, or in an overall massage for best effect. (*See page 151.*)

Homeopathy
Treatment will be constitutional and aimed at controlling acute symptoms. Long-term control of the condition should be undertaken by a physician. However, specific remedies which may help control symptoms are:

Hyperthyroidism:
Iodum, when the sufferer feels hot, cannot stop activity, is obsessive, and probably dark-haired and brown-eyed.

Nat. mur., for symptoms accompanied by constipation, palpitations, and earthy-colored complexion.

Belladonna, when symptoms include a flushed face and staring eyes. (*See page 168.*)

Lycopus, when the heart is pounding and racing.

Hypothyroidism:
Arsenicum can be taken for up to five days, twice daily, while constitutional treatment is being sought.

Vitamins and Minerals
Nutritional deficiencies (for example, zinc, Vitamin A, selenium, and iron) and a toxic overload are thought to be the main factors involved in the onset of hypothyroidism. Ensure that you eat a good healthy diet, with plenty of fresh organic vegetables, seafood, and onions.

Garlic and onions are both particularly valuable if the patient's thyroid gland is underactive.

Supplement your diet with natural thyroid hormones created from iodine, and the amino acid tyrosine for hypothyroidism. (*See pages 244 and 230.*)

Garlic is a rich source of iodine, which can help regulate thyroid function. (*See page 244.*)

GOITER

Goiter is an enlargement of the thyroid gland, visible as a swelling on the neck, and is fairly common. In order for the thyroid to produce hormones it requires iodine in the diet for their synthesis. If there is insufficient iodine in the diet the gland increases its activity and swells, resulting in a goiter. The nontoxic enlargement of the thyroid due to insufficient iodine is common and easily remedied by eating more fish and iodized salt, thereby increasing iodine intake. Conditions of which goiter is a feature are:

GRAVE'S DISEASE, where the thyroid is overactive and enlargement is accompanied by excessive hormone production.

HASHIMOTO'S THYROIDITIS, where the thyroid is underactive due to antibodies to thyroid hormone. Causes an ache in the neck and difficulty in swallowing.

SUB-ACUTE THYROIDITIS, probably a viral infection which causes inflammation and pain.

DYSHORMONOGENESIS, a genetic enzyme deficiency which interferes with normal hormone synthesis.

TUMORS of the thyroid gland, which may be benign or malignant.

Symptoms

- swelling at the front of the neck, which may vary from a small lump to a very large mass
- difficulty in swallowing or breathing in severe cases
- hyperthyroidism (overactive thyroid): weight loss, increased appetite, warm, dry skin, tremor, insomnia, bulging eyes
- hypothyroidism (underactive thyroid): tiredness, muscle weakness, weight gain, flaky skin, hair loss, deepening voice

TREATMENT

Herbalism
Bladderwrack, brown seaweed, can help goiter caused by an underactive thyroid. (*See page 107.*)

Bugleweed is used to treat an overactive thyroid.

Aromatherapy
Clary sage has a balancing effect on hormones, and since it is now believed that an underactive thyroid may be linked to an excess of female hormones, this may be a useful oil. (*See page 155.*)

Homeopathy
The following remedies, taken twice daily for up to 2 weeks, should improve the condition:

- Iodum, for someone who is always in a hurry and feeling hot.
- Spongia, for a long-standing condition, where there is a hard lump. (*See page 196.*)
- Calcarea, for a pale, chilly, overweight person.
- Fluoric acid, for elderly sufferers who are young-thinking, vigorous, and with varicose veins.

Vitamins and Minerals
Increase your intake of salt, fish, seafish, and kelp to ensure adequate iodine. (*See page 244.*)

DIABETES

The most common form of diabetes is diabetes mellitus. It is caused by a lack of, or insufficient, insulin (the hormone produced by the pancreas), as a result of which the body is unable to process glucose. This causes a high level of glucose in the blood, and low absorption of the vital energy-producing glucose by the tissues. In Type I (insulin-dependency) diabetes the sufferer produces little or no insulin and requires lifelong monitoring. Blood sugar levels can swing wildly between hypoglycemia (featuring strange feelings, abnormal behavior, and a risk of coma) and hyperglycemia (causing overproduction of ketones, and coma). Type I usually first appears in those who are under the age of 35, particularly adolescents, and develops rapidly. Type II, maturity-onset diabetes, is thought to be caused by the body's cells' lack of response to insulin. It usually affects people aged 40 and over, and there is an association with obesity and pregnancy. The onset of Type II is gradual and may go unnoticed for some time.

Diabetes affects over 10 million people in the United States and causes about 300,000 deaths each year.

An estimated 5 million adults have undetected Type II diabetes, and another 20 million have a glucose intolerance that could lead to diabetes.

Complications due to diabetes are the third most frequent cause of death in the U.S.

Damage to the retina from diabetes is the main cause of blindness in the U.S.

Its prevalence increases with age, from about 0.2 percent in persons under 17 years of age to about 20 percent in persons aged 65 years and over, and is greater in females.

Prevalence is inversely related to family income and varies markedly among ethnic groups, with occurrence about two times higher in non-Caucasians than in Caucasians.

Symptoms

- excessive thirst
- excessive urination
- weight loss
- fatigue, weakness, and apathy

- hunger
- bad breath
- complications include: nerve damage (causing damage to the eye muscles and double vision as a result); damage to blood vessels affecting the eyes (sometimes causing blindness), kidneys, circulation in the legs; organic impotence; arterial disease and gangrene

TREATMENT

Ayurveda

An Ayurvedic practitioner would recommend oral preparations from herbs that act upon the levels of glucose in the blood. There have been good results from treatment, with some cases being resolved within as little as 2 months.

For non-insulin-dependent diabetes, boil and cut one karella into small pieces and eat with the seeds every morning and evening.

Chinese Herbalism

Lilyturf root, grassy privet, lotus seed, and Chinese yam are suggested.

Treatment aimed at nourishing the Spleen, Kidneys, and Stomach would use Chinese yam, lotus seed, and mulberry.

Herbalism

Onions and garlic lower blood sugar levels. Ensure that you have plenty in your diet; take garlic oil supplements if not. (*See page 98.*)

Fenugreek seed works to control blood sugar levels. Drink daily.

Alfalfa is recommended for diabetics, and it should be taken daily.

Homeopathy

Constitutional treatment will be balancing and can be taken alongside conventional medication. In some cases the condition has been completely cured through homeopathy, but it must be undertaken by a registered practitioner.

Vitamins and Minerals

Brewer's yeast contains chromium, which helps to normalize blood sugar levels and metabolism. Take 2–3 tablespoons daily. (*See page 257.*)

ADDISON'S DISEASE

Addison's disease is a disorder of the adrenal glands which leads to insufficient output of cortisol and aldosterone—the steroid hormones which help the body to react to stress and control water balance, respectively. The disease is caused by an inflammation followed by atrophy of the outer layer (cortex) of the adrenal gland. This in turn is caused by abnormal action of the immune system in which it behaves towards the gland tissue as though it were foreign. Addison's is therefore known as an auto-immune disease. Addison's disease is usually due to damage by an auto-immune reaction, tuberculosis, or fungal infections. Addison's disease is rare, and generally has a slow onset and chronic course, with symptoms developing gradually over months or years. Acute episodes, called Addisonian crises, can be brought on by infection, injury, or other stresses, and they occur because the adrenal glands cannot increase their production of steroid hormones which normally help the body to deal with stress. The condition was invariably fatal before hormone treatment became available in the 1950s.

Symptoms
- weakness
- fatigue
- low blood pressure
- excessive urination
- dehydration
- skin discoloration, as the pituitary gland attempts to compensate for insufficient adrenal output by overproducing another hormone which stimulates the pigment cells

TREATMENT

Herbalism

Treatment to stimulate the endocrine system; herbs to boost the immune system may also be appropriate. Treatment would be individual.

Aromatherapy

Oils which strengthen the adrenal system include: rosemary, ginger, and lemongrass. (See pages 133–157.)

Homeopathy

Treatment would be constitutional; however, the following treatments may help. If you don't feel any better after a week or so, see your doctor.

Silicea, when your feet are sweaty and smelly, cold weather makes the symptoms worse, and you feel really exhausted. (See page 195.)

Nat. mur., for when you have constipation, dry lips, a craving for salt, and symptoms which are made worse by sun. (See page 190.)

Arg. nit., for apprehension, salt and sweet cravings, and tremors. (See page 166.)

HYPOGLYCEMIA

Hypoglycemia is a condition in which there is an abnormally low level of glucose in the blood. It is extremely dangerous because the brain is dependent on a constant supply of glucose. The most common cause of hypoglycemia is a relative insulin overdose by diabetics (i.e. the actual amount of insulin taken may be correct, but the intake of carbohydrate or the amount of exertion may have used up the supply too quickly). Excessive exercise and insufficient carbohydrate may, in fact, lead to hypoglycemia in non-diabetics.

The condition occurs in association with a number of diseases, most notably insulin overdose in diabetics.

Repeated severe attacks can cause permanent brain damage.

There are two main types of hypoglycemia: organic and functional.

Any endocrine malfunction in the pancreas and adrenal glands, as well as the pituitary, thyroid, or sex glands, may result in organic hypoglycemia. Alcoholism, which impairs the liver's ability to produce glucose, can also lead to organic hypoglycemia, as can other disorders of the liver and tumors of the liver or pancreas.

Functional hypoglycemia is a temporary condition of markedly lowered blood sugar, most commonly occurring 2–3 hours after a meal high in carbohydrates.

50 percent of sufferers over the age of 50 have a thyroid problem.

Symptoms
- headache and faintness
- rapid pulse and palpitations
- profuse sweating
- mental confusion and loss of memory
- irrational and disorderly behavior
- slurred speech
- numbness, temporary paralysis
- fits and, eventually, potentially fatal coma

TREATMENT

Ayurveda

Plants which act on blood sugar levels will be prescribed, as well as detoxification treatment to ensure that the system is working efficiently. (See page 10.)

Traditional Home and Folk Remedies

Onions and garlic will help to regulate blood sugar levels. Eat raw or cooked, as often as possible. (See page 70.)

Chinese Herbalism

Chinese yam and lotus seed will help to normalize blood sugar levels.

Homeopathy

Homeopathic treatment would be constitutional, but well worth it, because in many cases the condition can be cured completely.

Flower Essences

Take Rescue Remedy if you feel an attack coming on. It will calm you and help to reduce the severity. (*See page 229.*)

Vitamins and Minerals

Take extra Vitamin C and B-complex tablets, chromium (to regulate blood sugar levels), magnesium, potassium, zinc, and manganese.

OBESITY

Obesity is the excessive storage of energy in the form of fat, and applies to a bodyweight that is more than 20 percent over the recommended maximum for a person's height. The main cause of obesity is excessive calorie intake, but other factors include a low basal metabolic rate, genetic factors, emotional problems, metabolic disorders such as thyroid problems, taking steroids, or insulin. Obesity can aggravate or trigger other conditions such as heart attack, gallstones, arthritis, hiatus hernia, varicose veins, kidney disorders, and fertility problems. In particular, the chances of suffering from high blood pressure, stroke, and maturity-onset diabetes are greatly increased by obesity. Obese women are more likely to be at risk from cancer of the ovaries, womb, and breast; obese men are at risk from cancer of the colon, rectum, and prostate. The strain on the joints of the back, knees, and hips from extra weight can also cause problems.

Affects approximately 20–30 percent of the U.S. population.

Fat should account for up to 25 percent of body weight in a healthy woman, and 17 percent in a healthy man.

Individuals who weigh more than 20 percent above their supposed "ideal bodyweight" according to the standard height and weight tables of the Metropolitan Life Insurance Company may be judged as obese.

At least one-third of Americans are 20 percent or more overweight.

25–50 percent of adult Americans are currently on a diet; $30 billion is spent on diet aids annually.

One in every four U.S. teenagers carries enough weight to put them at risk of later health problems.

Obesity may be classified according to the age of onset, family history, degree of obesity, and adipose tissue cell size and distribution.

Obesity significantly increases the risk of premature death, heart attack, diabetes mellitus, hypertension, atherosclerosis, gall bladder disease, osteoarthritis, and certain cancers.

Obese individuals with an apple shape (fat in the upper body or abdomen) are at greater risk of medical diseases than those with a pear shape (fat confined to the lower body or hips).

THE BODY MASS INDEX

The Body Mass Index (BMI) is reached by dividing your weight in pounds, multiplied by 703, by your height in inches squared. So, if you weigh 176 lbs. and are 6 ft., 6in. tall, your BMI is 176 times 703, divided by 6,084 – which is 20.3.

If you have a BMI of 27 or more, you double the risk of high blood pressure, heart disease, and gallstones, and are 14 times more likely to contract diabetes.

If it is over 30, you have 4 times the risk of heart disease, high blood pressure, and gallstones, and are 30–50 times more likely to contract diabetes. You are also 4 times more likely to get degenerative arthritis.

$$BMI = \frac{(weight\ (lbs) \times 703)}{height\ (inches)^2}$$

IDEAL BMI	20–25
OVERWEIGHT	BMI 25–30
OBESE	BMI 30+
UNDERWEIGHT	BMI 20 or less

TREATMENT

Ayurveda

Treatment would be aimed at addressing an addiction to food, accompanied by marma puncture and a diet modified to your dosha type. (*See page 10.*)

A complete detoxification will encourage weight loss naturally.

Chinese Herbalism

Increase your intake of foods that are bitter, pungent, astringent, and hot, which will encourage your body to eliminate waste more efficiently. Cut down on salty, sweet, and sour foods.

Traditional Home and Folk Remedies

Drink a glass of freshly squeezed grapefruit juice every morning to cleanse, help break down fats, and suppress appetite.

Herbalism

Bladderwrack may help to encourage the metabolism.

Nettles are good diuretics and generally help the metabolism. Try drinking nettle tea before meals.

Homeopathy

Constitutional treatment is most appropriate, but some of the following remedies might be useful:

Graphites, if you suffer from constipation and skin problems, and feel cold. (*See page 181.*)

Kali carb., if you are clogged with catarrh, have a backache, and feel cold.

Ferr. phos., if you are oversensitive and get flushed easily.

Capsicum, if you are lazy, have a red face, and suffer from burning sensations in the digestive tract.

Calcarea, if you suffer from indigestion, and crave hot food and eggs.

Vitamins and Minerals

Bee pollen stimulates the metabolism and helps to curb appetite. Take up to 1 teaspoon daily. (*See page 256.*)

Brewer's yeast will help to reduce various cravings for food and drink. (*See page 257.*)

Chromium supplements will help to ensure that your blood sugar levels are stable, and regulate appetite.

Phenylalanine, taken on an empty stomach before bed, encourages weight loss. (*See page 252.*)

GOUT

Gout is an acute disease of the joints. It is caused by the deposition of chalky crystals around the joints, tendons, and other body tissues when there is an abnormally high level of uric acid in the body. Severe inflammation and tissue damage result, and possibly structural damage to the kidneys and stone formation. Primary gout appears to involve a hereditary factor.

Symptoms

The first sign of gout is usually excruciating pain and inflammation of the innermost joint of the big toe (or, less frequently, the ankle, knee joint, wrist, or elbow). An attack can last for days or weeks and then subsides, but usually there are recurrences, until eventually gout is a constant presence.

TREATMENT

Chinese Herbalism

Painful joints are said to be caused by Wind Cold, and some of the most useful herbs to relieve Cold and Damp include cinnamon, aconite root, angelica root, and wild ginger. (*See page 44.*)

Traditional Home and Folk Remedies

Raw apple and cucumber juice will help to reduce the severity and incidence of attacks. (*See pages 80 and 75.*)

Herbalism

Drink plenty of water and cleansing infusions such as celery seed tea.

Bring down the acute inflammation with a compress made of crushed cabbage leaf.

Nettle tea is helpful in preventing attacks. (*See page 124.*)

Aromatherapy

Rub a few drops of lavender and frankincense, mixed in a little grapeseed oil, into the affected joints.

Pine, rosemary, or juniper oils, which increase circulation, can be added to the bath or added to a foot bath to ease the condition. Rub them neat into the affected joints.

Homeopathy

Homeopathic treatment would be constitutional, but in an attack one of the following remedies may be appropriate:
- Pulsatilla, for fleeting pains. (*See page 193.*)
- Lycopodium, for symptoms that are worse between 4–8p.m. (*See page 187.*)
- Urtica, for joints that feel hot and itchy. (*See page 201.*)
- Arnica, for painful joints which feel bruised.
- Ledum, for joints that are cold and swollen, and are improved by moving around. (*See page 186.*)

Vitamins and Minerals

A good diet is the key. Eat plenty of fresh, green vegetables and avoid high-protein foods such as red meat and seafood.

Eat food containing plenty of vitamin C (or take supplements of 1g daily). (*See page 238.*)

Avoid alcohol, which increases uric acid.

Charcoal tablets may help to reduce the levels of uric acid in the body. (*See page 257.*)

DISORDERS OF THE IMMUNE SYSTEM
GLANDULAR FEVER

Glandular fever, or infectious mononucleosis as it is also known, is caused by the Epstein-Barr virus (a herpes virus). The virus multiplies in the white blood cells, eventually harming the immune system's efficiency. Glandular fever is usually transmitted via saliva, hence its nickname of the "kissing disease." While symptoms may last for only six weeks, recovery is slow and fatigue and low energy levels may linger for months. The disease occurs most commonly in adults 15–30 years old, but one attack confers immunity.

Symptoms
- flu-like symptoms, including fever, sore throat, headache
- fatigue and lethargy
- swollen lymph glands in the neck, armpits, and groin
- a rash of small, slightly raised red spots
- chest pain, with breathing difficulty and a cough
- enlarged spleen and possibly damaged liver and jaundice

TREATMENT
Chinese Herbalism

Tonic herbs such as astragalus, ganoderma, and ginseng will help your overall constitution.

Salvia, millettia, and peony will improve the Blood, and give the circulation a boost. (*See page 53.*)

Chinese angelica can restore energy and stimulate white blood cells and antibody formation. (*See page 41.*)

Traditional Home and Folk Remedies

Apply apple cider vinegar to the neck glands daily. Drink it in a cup of warm water to encourage healing.

Ginseng acts to balance the glands. Chew the fresh or dried root, or add the powder to hot herbal teas. It will prevent fatigue and stimulate you.

Herbalism

Herbs to promote healing include cleavers, echinacea, and nettles, all of which stimulate immune activity as well as fighting infection. (*See pages 105 and 124.*)

Balm, oats, and skullcap, if depression accompanies the fever. (*See pages 102 and 118.*)

Infusions of yarrow and elderflower will help to control fever and also induce sweating.

Aromatherapy

Essential oils can be used in the bath, or in massage, which also has therapeutic benefits. Oils to consider are eucalyptus, lavender, rosemary, and tea tree, which will encourage immune activity and fight the virus.

Homeopathy

Constitutional treatment is recommended, but the following remedies may be useful, taken up to six times daily, for two days.

Belladonna, for sudden high fever, with a reddish face and agitation. (*See page 168.*)

Mercurius, for tender glands and smelly sweat.

Calcarea, for chilliness, sweating, a sour taste in the mouth, and fatigue.

Cistus, for a chilly feeling, with painful neck and glands, exacerbated by cold air and mental exertion.

Baryta carb., for swollen glands. This is particularly useful for children. (*See page 170.*)

Flower Essences

Flower essences are often used by practitioners to help you cope with the physical and emotional effects of glandular fever.

Olive will help if you feel exhausted on all levels.

Mustard controls feelings of depression that have no identifiable cause. (*See page 224.*)

Gorse will help with feelings of hopelessness.

Vitamins and Minerals

Take extra vitamin C, B-complex, and zinc.

Evening primrose oil will help to encourage healing.

Royal jelly will help fight feelings of fatigue and depression, and stimulate the immune system.

Eat plenty of foods containing antioxidants.

ALLERGIES

An allergy is the immune system's abnormal response to contact with a specific substance. The system overreacts when faced with foreign substances or organisms—allergens—and deals with them as if they were harmful, as it would with invading bacteria, for example. The result is an allergic reaction, also known as a histamine reaction (histamine being the substance produced in response to attack). Common allergens include certain foods, grass pollens, spores, fabrics, drugs, household chemicals, and stress. Some of the most common allergic responses are urticaria (*see page 282*), dermatitis (*see page 279*), asthma (*see page 317*), and hay fever/rhinitis (*see page 306*). An estimated 35 million people in the United States suffer from various allergies, some of which are mistaken for the common cold.

Symptoms

- sneezing and runny nose; excess catarrh
- wheezing
- urticaria
- anaphylactic shock (sometimes fatal), causing breathing difficulty, edema, constriction of air tubes, and heart failure

TREATMENT

Ayurveda

Cleansing and detoxification will be followed by a varied diet of organic foods.

Herbal preparations to boost immunity may be appropriate, including Chebulic myrobalan (Harithaki), which helps in cases of eczema; bitter orange for asthma and other respiratory allergies; and stramonium.

Chinese Herbalism

Bi Van Pian/Nose inflammation pills, for Wind Cold or Wind Heat to the face, indicated by sneezing, itchy eyes, facial congestion and sinus pain, acute and chronic rhinitis, and nasal allergies. Herbal prescriptions will be offered.

Yu Ping Feng San/Jade screen helps prevent hay fever and guards against allergies.

Cang Er Zi Tang/xanthium powder, for allergic rhinitis, with thick yellow catarrh, or blocked nose.

Traditional Home and Folk Remedies

Eat the local honey if you suffer from hay fever.

Honey and apple cider can be drunk in a glass of warm water to restore and prevent allergies.

Drink nettle tea to increase resistance.

Apply nettle tea to skin, or use Urtica urens cream or homeopathic remedy for urticaria.

Herbalism

Echinacea acts as a natural antibiotic while building the immune system. Take three times daily, as an infusion, or a few drops of tincture in a glass of warm water, during attacks or when you are run down. (*See page 105.*)

Other useful herbs include chamomile, elderflower, red clover, and yarrow. (*See pages 104, 116, and 97.*)

Add a small amount of ginseng powder to herbal drinks to overcome the tendency to allergic attacks, such as hay fever. (*See page 112.*)

Eat the local honey in a cup of warm water with 2 tablespoons of apple cider vinegar to reduce the reaction to allergens. This is particularly useful during the hay fever season.

Herbs to boost immunity include garlic, angelica, borage, and wild yam. (*See pages 98, 100, and 105.*)

Strengthen the weakened area with tonic teas, 2 cups taken over a period of time: the sinuses with elderflower tea; the stomach with chamomile, linden, and a warming digestive like cardamom; the skin with chamomile washes and rosemary in the bath.

Aromatherapy
Place a few drops of Roman chamomile in a vaporizer or on a light bulb to treat an allergic reaction, including asthma.

Melissa, in the bath or a vaporizer, soothes and reduces a reaction's severity. (*See page 149.*)

Lavender essential oil, in a light carrier oil, can be massaged into the chest or other affected area to reduce spasm and generally boost immunity. (*See page 147.*)

Homeopathy
Homeopathic treatment has proved to be very successful in the treatment of allergies. Remedies will be prescribed according to your individual case, so it is best to see a registered practitioner to ensure that prescription is exact.

Urtica, for urticaria. (*See page 201.*)

Pulsatilla or Arg. nit., for relief of conjunctivitis.

Apis, for bee stings. (*See page 165.*)

Anaphylactic shock is a medical emergency, and you must summon emergency medical care immediately. The following remedies can be given until help arrives:

Aconite, when the patient is frightened and restless.

Veratrum, when the skin is cold and mottled, and the victim is in a cold sweat.

Arnica, for shock brought on by injury. (*See page 167.*)

Flower Essences
If suffering a sudden allergic reaction, take Rescue Remedy or Emergency Essence. (*See page 229.*)

Vitamins and Minerals
Take steps to boost immunity, by increasing intake of magnesium (seafood, beans, and nuts), B vitamins (yeast extract, meat, or yeast), zinc (eggs, nuts, and seeds), vitamin A (fish and yellow and green vegetables), iron (liver, sesame seeds, and dried fruit), and vitamin C (fresh fruit and vegetables).

A diet high in protein will help to build up immunity, while roughage from fruit, vegetables, nuts, seeds, and pulses will keep the digestive tract working and encourage the growth of beneficial bacteria in the gut (called flora), which helps the body to resist infection.

Acidophilus, taken daily, will also work to encourage bowel health. (*See page 256.*)

Evening primrose oil and blackcurrant seed oil are rich sources of essential fatty acids, which can prevent allergies in susceptible people. (*See page 254.*)

Pollen supplements are useful for preventing allergies, in particular hay fever. (*See page 256.*)

HODGKIN'S DISEASE

Hodgkin's disease (or Hodgkin's lymphoma) is a cancer that attacks the lymphatic tissue and the lymph nodes in particular. As the tissue becomes more and more damaged, relatively minor infections may become life-threatening. Late in the disease's development the bone marrow may also be affected. The cause of Hodgkin's is unknown, although it is thought that cancer-causing viruses are involved. In the United States, about 30 people out of every million have this ailment; it is more common in males between the ages of 20 and 40, although both sexes can suffer from the condition. Untreated, Hodgkin's disease is invariably fatal.

Symptoms
- painless enlargement of lymph nodes, which acquire a rubbery feel
- liver and spleen enlargement
- anemia and fever
- appetite and weight loss
- night sweats
- possible secondary effects caused by pressure on other structures from enlarged nodes, neurological damage, obstruction to veins, difficulty in swallowing and breathing, jaundice

TREATMENT

Aromatherapy

Extra treatments to try are fennel, garlic, juniper, and rose, which can be used in the bath or in a vaporizer to detoxify the body. (*See pages 133–157.*)

Tea tree and lavender essential oils strengthen the body's defenses. (*See pages 148 and 147.*)

Oils which strengthen the action of the adrenals include geranium and rosemary, along with peppermint and thyme. (*See pages 133–157.*)

Vitamins and Minerals

Eat as much fresh fruit and vegetables as you can, paying particular attention to those containing antioxidants.

Reduce your intake of animal fats and avoid processed foods.

A deficiency of vitamin C has been found in conjunction with certain tumors. Ensure you get plenty in your diet.

Vitamin A can protect against cancer in smokers to some degree. (*See page 234.*)

Digestive enzymes may be offered to halt activities of trophoblastic cancer cells.

Vitamin E is said to prevent a number of cancers. Ensure that you get plenty in your diet or take supplements.

DISORDERS OF THE MUSCULOSKELETAL SYSTEM

OSTEOPOROSIS

In osteoporosis (meaning porous bones) the bones lose their density, becoming fragile and brittle. This is caused by alterations, with age, of the amounts of the various growth and sex hormones which control chemical changes in the bones, leading to progressive calcium and protein loss. Osteoporosis affects far more women than men, and may be triggered or accelerated by a sedentary lifestyle, loss of activity, a low-calcium diet, smoking, heavy alcohol consumption, hereditary factors, or prolonged lack of estrogen. An overactive thyroid gland, chronic liver disease, and prolonged use of corticosteroids all predispose a person to osteoporosis.

Bone mass reaches a peak in women between the ages of 30 and 45; between the ages of 55 and 70, a woman will have lost 30–40 percent of her bone mass.

Most common in Caucasian women after menopause.

Affects more women than heart disease, stroke, diabetes, breast cancer, and arthritis.

50 percent of women between the ages of 45 and 75 suffer from some osteoporosis; 30 percent of these suffer from serious bone deterioration.

Costs approximately $3.8 billion in treatment in the U.S. each year.

Aggravated by a variety of factors, including smoking, excessive alcohol consumption, and a sedentary lifestyle.

A "dowager's hump" is an abnormal curvature of the spine in the upper back. Typically affecting older women, the curvature is a result of collapse of the spinal column, caused by osteoporosis.

Symptoms

- loss of height from shrinkage of the spinal bones
- sudden breakage of a bone in the spine, with severe pain and disfigurement
- reduced ribcage movement, causing shortness of breath and pain
- wrist, forearm, neck, or hip fractures resulting from minor stumbles or falls

TREATMENT

Chinese Herbalism

The condition is believed to be caused by Kidney Deficiency, and can be treated with cibot rhizome, drynaria tuber, and eucommia bark. (*See page 49.*)

Cinnamon twigs will help to reduce pain. (*See page 44.*)

Herbalism

Drink a cup of comfrey leaf and bay leaf tea three times daily.

Many herbs, such as hops or sage, contain estrogen-like substances which can protect the bones against loss.

If you are in pain, use analgesic herbs such as white willow, meadowsweet, or wild yam. (*See pages 115, 106, and 105.*)

Herbs that contain calcium include nettles, parsley, dandelion leaves, kelp, and horsetail, which can be drunk as often as possible. (*See pages 124, 120, and 106.*)

Take estrogenic herbs, which discourage the loss of calcium from the bones, including calendula, ginseng, false unicorn root, sage, hops, blue cohosh, wild yam, and licorice.

Herbs which encourage the digestion and absorption of minerals from food include yellow dock root, rosemary, wormwood, and yarrow. (*See pages 115, 114, and 97*)

Homeopathy

Constitutional treatment will be necessary, but the following remedies may be useful to deal with bone pain:

Ruta grav., for pain at the nape of the neck and lumbar.

Aurum, for pains that are worse at night, mainly in the skull, nose, or palate. (*See page 169.*)

Calcarea phos., for limbs that feel achy, numb, and chilly.

Fluoric ac., for stabbing pain.

Vitamins and Minerals

Recent evidence suggests that an increased intake of magnesium may help prevent the worst effects of osteoporosis. Magnesium sources include nuts, and brewer's yeast.

Calcium can also be very helpful. Recommended doses are between 1,000mg and 1,500mg a day. (*See page 241.*)

Vitamin D helps the body absorb calcium.

Increase your intake of foods containing boron, which reduces the body's excretion of calcium and magnesium, and increases the production of estrogen.

Fluoride may be useful for preventing and treating the condition because it stimulates new bone formation.

RHEUMATISM

Rheumatism is a very general term applied to aches, pains, and stiffness in bones and muscles, occurring as a result of viral infection, food allergy, emotional stress, or an underlying joint disease. The following may all come under the umbrella term rheumatism:

FIBROSITIS (*see page 398*)
HYPERTHYROIDISM (*see page 381*)

MYOSITIS, in which inflammation of muscles causes pain and weakness. It may develop from a bacterial or viral infection

POLYMYALGIA RHEUMATICA, featuring pain and stiffness in the shoulders, neck, back, and arms, possibly due to a blood disorder

VITAMIN D DEFICIENCY, which causes bone pain and muscle weakness

PALINDROMIC RHEUMATISM is a disease that causes frequent and irregular attacks of joint pain, especially in the fingers, but leaves no permanent damage to the joints.

PSYCHOGENIC RHEUMATISM is common in women between the ages of 40 and 70, although men also contract this disease. Symptoms include complaints of pain in various parts of the musculoskeletal system that cannot be substantiated medically.

One of the most common forms of rheumatism is rheumatoid arthritis, affecting 1–3 percent of the population. Rheumatoid arthritis usually occurs between ages 35 and 40, but can occur at any age. It characteristically follows a course of spontaneous remissions and exacerbations, and in about 10–20 percent of patients remission is permanent.

TREATMENT

Ayurveda

Ginger, coriander, and aloe vera (when there are hot pains) can be used to treat rheumatism. (*See pages 32, 24 and 17.*)

Angelica is a good tonic and is warming for stiffness and discomfort. (*See page 17.*)

Barberry, taken as a tea or applied as a compress, can be used to treat rheumatic ailments. (*See page 18.*)

Basil relieves arthritis and rheumatism. (*See page 29.*)

Rub calamus oil into the affected joints to improve circulation and drainage.

Camphor is indicated for arthritis, rheumatism, and many other musculoskeletal problems. (*See page 22.*)

Chinese Herbalism

The condition is thought to be caused by qi stagnation, excess Wind, Damp, and Heat. Chinese herbalists use achyranthus root and cork tree bark. (*See page 55.*)

Traditional Home and Folk Remedies

Chew a tiny quantity of horseradish leaves, which is said to prevent attacks. (*See page 71.*)

Herbalism

Useful herbs, which may be taken internally or applied as a compress to the affected part of the body, include bogbean, feverfew, meadowsweet, and white willow.

Use a little cayenne pepper oil to warm the area and reduce pain and stiffness. (*See page 103.*)

A poultice of slippery elm may be of benefit.

An infusion of celery seed may help reduce the level of acid in the blood, which is a contributory factor in rheumatism.

Aromatherapy

Bergamot and myrrh reduce inflammation. Use in the bath, or massage the local area. (*See pages 140 and 142.*)

There are many oils which can reduce swelling and inflammation and encourage the healing process. Try massage with pine, lemon, or juniper, in a suitable carrier oil. (*See pages 133–157.*)

Massage with oil of black pepper or eucalyptus can stimulate the circulation and relieve stiffness.

Lavender oil calms pain and helps to relieve stiffness.

Homeopathy

Aconite, for sharp pains which tend to come on suddenly.

Bryonia, for pains that are worse in dry cold weather and on movement. (*See page 170.*)

Pulsatilla, for pains that move from joint to joint, and muscle to muscle. (*See page 193.*)

Rhus tax., for stiffness that is worse in the morning or after rest. (*See page 194.*)

Mercurius, for pain that is worse at night and for heat.

Calcarea hypophos., for sharp pains in the wrists and hands.

Causticum, for pains in the jaw and neck, with spasm.

Flower Essences

Rub a little Rescue Remedy into the affected area.

Vitamins and Minerals

Many cases of rheumatism respond to a dietary change, and it is suggested that the following foods are eaten as often as possible to reduce muscular and joint inflammation: cabbage, celery, turnip, lemon, dandelion, and oily fish.

Drink plenty of water, which will flush the system and act as a detoxicant.

Eliminate members of the "nightshade" family of plants from your diet, as these can cause joint problems. These include potatoes, peppers, eggplant (aubergine), and paprika.

Evening primrose oil is a rich source of gamma-linolenic acid, which is necessary for the production of prostaglandins, which may have an anti-inflammatory effect.

FRACTURES

A fracture is a break or crack in a bone. It may occur as a result of excessive force through injury (particularly in sports), an accident such as a car crash, or disease. A simple fracture is one where the soft tissue overlying the broken bone is still intact; a compound fracture is one where the skin is damaged so that the fractured bone is exposed and therefore vulnerable to infection. Fractures caused by disease (such as osteoporosis, or a tumor or cyst) are known as pathological fractures. In such cases there is a weakening of bones that predisposes them to break more easily. An estimated 200,000 hip fractures occur in people over the age of 65 each year. The tendency to fracture increases with age.

CAUTION

If you suspect a fracture, see your physician immediately.

Symptoms

- swelling, pain, and tenderness
- inability to move the affected part
- possibly a protruding bone, deformity, and discoloration

TREATMENT

Ayurveda

Aloe vera will help to encourage the healing of broken bones, and can be applied externally as a gel, or taken internally.

Chinese Herbalism

Die da wan (bodily injury pills) and Imperial ted da wine resolve bruising, and promote healing in damaged tissue. They can be taken after you have received medical attention.

Herbalism

A comfrey poultice can be applied to the affected area to encourage healing. (*See page 119.*)

Use an infusion of comfrey, horsetail, and mouse ear and apply locally (when the plaster cast has been removed) to help heal the broken bones. (*See pages 119 and 106.*)

Comfrey root can be taken internally (in small amounts) to set the bone and encourage healing. (*See page 119.*)

Aromatherapy

Elemi oil can help to encourage the circulation after a plaster cast has been removed.

Lavender in a vaporizer will help to relax and calm. (*See page 147.*)

Thyme, rosemary, and marjoram can be diluted and massaged into the area, or applied as a compress, to soothe pain and promote healing. (*See pages 133–157.*)

Homeopathy

Arnica, every 10 minutes after the injury, then every 8 or 10 hours thereafter, as necessary. (*See page 167.*)

Symphytum ("knitbone") can be used for up to 3 weeks to promote healing. Do not take this unless you are sure the bone is aligned, for the healing is profound.

Flower Essences

Rescue Remedy or Emergency Essence can be given at the time of the injury, and taken as required to calm and to treat any shock. (*See page 229.*)

Vitamins and Minerals

Increase your calcium, magnesium, and phosphorus intake. (*See pages 241, 245, and 247.*)

Increase your intake of vitamin A. Foods such as carrots are a good source. (*See page 234.*)

SPRAINS AND STRAINS

A sprain is the result of an overstretching or tearing of the ligaments which bind the joints together, caused by a sudden pull. Severe sprains may lead to dislocation of the affected joint (particularly common in the case of the shoulder), and repeated injury of this nature can cause a loss of the ligaments' elasticity. The most commonly strained or sprained joint is the ankle, which is usually sprained as a result of going over on the outside of the foot so that the complete weight of the body is placed on the ankle. The back, fingers, knees, and wrists are also commonly sprained.

Symptoms
- swelling in the affected area
- pain in the affected joint, sometimes severe

TREATMENT

Chinese Herbalism

San Qi is useful after injury, for swelling and pain. (*See page 54.*)

Die Da Wan will help with injuries to the soft tissues, inflammation, and bruising.

Traditional Home and Folk Remedies

Cider vinegar can be used as a compress in order to relieve pain and swelling. (*See page 87.*)

Apply a poultice of raw onions to the sprain.

Raise the affected limb and apply a cold compress as soon as possible. Strains should be bandaged with an elastic bandage to provide support, but take care not to bind too tightly and cut off circulation. Keep the limb elevated until the swelling goes down and some normal movement is possible.

Herbalism

Burdock can be taken internally in the form of a tea, or applied as a poultice to the affected area. (*See page 100.*)

Ginger can be added to bath water or a foot bath, or applied as a compress to encourage healing. (*See page 126.*)

Chamomile can be taken internally to calm and reduce pain. (*See page 104.*)

Aromatherapy

Use a little lavender oil in a foot bath, or on a cold compress applied to the area. Avoid massaging the area, which will increase inflammation. (*See page 147.*)

A compress with essential oils of sweet marjoram and rosemary can be used to heal and to reduce inflammation.

Homeopathy

Arnica should be taken internally until the injury has healed.

Ruta grav. can be taken the day after the injury occurs.

A cold compress with Arnica tincture should be applied hourly for the first 8 hours to reduce swelling.

Flower Essences

Rescue Remedy can be taken internally to calm. A few drops on a cold compress, applied to the injury, can help to reduce pain. When the swelling has gone down, a little Rescue Remedy cream can be massaged into the joint.

Vitamins and Minerals

The following nutrients help to encourage healing in the body: vitamin C and E, beta carotene, zinc, and selenium.

NECK PROBLEMS

Constant movement of the neck, along with its position and the number of structures within it, makes it particularly vulnerable to problems, which include:

CERVICAL OSTEOARTHRITIS—the cartilage of the vertebrae of the neck wear away, most commonly in middle age, causing pain, stiffness, and sometimes tenderness to touch.

CERVICAL RIB—this is an abnormal floating rib or pair of ribs attached to the lowest vertebra of the neck, which can cause compression of various nerves and arteries.

CERVICAL SPONDYLOSIS—neurological damage is caused in the neck region as a result of compression of the spinal cord or nerve roots by an outgrowth of bone. Sufferers develop a walking disorder (spastic gait) and weakness in the arm muscles. Cervical spondylosis can begin from the age of 25 onward.

LOCKED NECK—overstrain of ligaments or muscle spasms caused by an awkward or sudden movement, often occurring during sleep.

NECK RIGIDITY—stiffness and pain caused by neck muscle spasms. A classic symptom of meningitis.

NECK SWELLING—swelling of any of the structures in the neck may be caused by tumors, allergy, bleeding, or inflammation. It can be extremely dangerous, seriously interfering with breathing. It may also affect swallowing.

TORTICOLLIS (WRY NECK)—an abnormality in the head's position caused by permanent twisting of the neck, due possibly to muscle damage sustained at birth, a whiplash injury, a visual problem, or shortening of the skin of the neck through scarring.

WHIPLASH INJURY—a sudden force (such as a car collision) causes a violent bending of the neck in one direction, followed by reflex muscle contraction which throws the neck in the opposite direction. The ligaments connecting the vertebrae are stretched or torn, causing prolonged pain and disability.

> ### CAUTION
> A stiff neck accompanied by headache, nausea, vomiting, and abnormal sleepiness may indicate meningitis, and immediate medical attention is required.

TREATMENT

Ayurveda

Barberry can be taken internally for pain. (*See page 18.*)

Mustard oil relieves muscular pains and stiffness.

Turmeric and St. John's wort are also excellent for relieving stiffness, pain, and inflammation.

Chinese Herbalism

The cause of stiffness and "freezing" may be caused by weak yang qi, external Cold and Damp. Useful treatments include cinnamon twigs and turmeric. (*See page 44.*)

Traditional Home and Folk Remedies

Drink celery juice to ease nerve pain. (*See page 71.*)

Apply fresh horseradish to the affected area (do not leave on for long, or it will numb and burn).

Apply bruised juniper berries to muscular swellings. Local heat will help to relax tense muscles.

Herbalism

St. John's wort has sedative, painkilling properties. It can be drunk as an infusion or applied to the affected area in an oil.

Valerian can reduce tension and help you to sleep.

The following herbs reduce inflammation and relieve pain: Jamaican dogwood, St. John's wort, vervain, and white willow. (*See pages 110, 125, and 115.*)

Aromatherapy

A drop of juniper, mustard, or pepper oils, diluted in some carrier oil, can be massaged into the affected area. Wrap warmly afterward. (*See pages 133–157.*)

Wintergreen oil is good for muscular pains: massage into the affected area.

Rosemary is stimulating and analgesic, and can be massaged into the area to relieve pain and stiffness.

Take hot baths with lavender, juniper, pine, or nutmeg to warm, reduce pain, and encourage the healing process.

Homeopathy

Cimicifuga, for a stiff neck.

Causticum, for dull pain at the nape of the neck, together with stiffness between the shoulders.

Bryonia, for pain made worse by the slightest touch.

Dulcamara, for pain at the top of the nape of the neck, as if from lying in an awkward position.

Lacnanthes, for pain down the right side of the neck, and in the upper arm and elbow.

Flower Essences

Rub Rescue Remedy cream into the affected area.

Star of Bethlehem can be taken internally after an injury to reduce the effects of shock and trauma. (*See page 220.*)

BACK PROBLEMS

Aches or pains in the back are due to mechanical disorders, which may cause or arise from damage to ligaments, muscles, vertebral joints, or disks. These may occur as a result of poor posture, lack of exercise, obesity, unaccustomed lifting or maneuvers, pregnancy, stress, or depression. A slipped disk is one of the most common causes of back pain, and this in turn may cause sciatica. Types of back pain vary according to the underlying cause.

A slipped disk does not, in fact, slip, but it herniates when the outer layer of the disk degenerates and the soft interior material extrudes into the spinal column, causing pain and sciatica.

Most back pain is caused by a muscle strain. Injuries are the second most common cause of pain.

Nearly 80 percent of all adults suffer from back pain at some time.

The U.S. National Center for Health Statistics reports that back pain is the sixth most common reason for visits to the emergency room, and accounts for 13 million visits to general physicians' offices eacn year.

In the U.K., the Back Pain Association estimates that every year over 3 million Britons consult a family physician because of back trouble.

In the U.S., around 60 million working days are lost each year through back pain, and that figure is rising.

Symptoms
- muscle spasms
- lower back pain, ranging from mild to excruciating
- stiffness
- referred pain or pins and needles in other areas

TREATMENT

To make a cramp bark decoction, add the bark to a pan of water. Use 1 teaspoonful of bark per cup of water.

Cover the pan, bring the mixture to the boil, and simmer for about to to 15 minutes.

Pour the decoction through a strainer and store it in a dark glass bottle if you are not using it immediately.

Ayurveda

Aloe vera can be taken for inflammation, and applied externally for pain and inflammation. (*See page 17.*)

Massage the painful area with mustard oil to reduce pain and aching. (*See page 19.*)

Use cayenne externally for soreness and stiffness.

Chinese Herbalism

Teasel root, ginseng, and acanthopanax can be used to relieve pain.

Jing Jie can be used to stop swelling and to kill pain.

Pseudoginseng root can be used to relieve swellings and for general relief of pain. (*See page 54.*)

Traditional Home and Folk Remedies

It may be helpful to chew a small quantity of horseradish leaves every day to ease pain. (*See page 71.*)

A mustard poultice, applied to the area, will ease pain and reduce any congestion in the area.

Herbalism

Massage cramp bark cream into the back. Or take cramp bark decoction, tincture, or capsules. (*See page 125.*)

Rub macerated comfrey or St. John's wort to relieve pain.

The following herbs reduce inflammation and relieve pain: Jamaican dogwood, St. John's wort, vervain, and white willow. (*See pages 110, 125, and 115.*)

Aromatherapy

Relaxing in a warm bath to which lavender oil has been added can be very soothing. (*See page 147.*)

Pain due to fatigue or tension can be treated with a massage of ginger, juniper, marjoram, or rosemary; the same oils can be added to the bath. (*See pages 133–157.*)

Massage with ginger or black pepper can be used when there is acute pain. (*See pages 157 and 153.*)

Marjoram can help to treat the muscular problem in the longer term, as well as reducing pain. (*See page 151.*)

Bergamot and myrrh are anti-inflammatory, useful for massage or in the bath. (*See pages 140 and 142.*)

Homeopathy

Treatment would be constitutional, but the following remedies may be useful:

Calc. fluor., for backache that is worse when starting to move but eases if you continue to move.

Arnica, for bruising and pain resulting from an injury.

Ruta grav. helps relieve pain at the nape of the neck and in the lumbar region. (*See page 194.*)

Aconite, for sharp pain made worse by exposure to cold or dry weather. (*See page 163.*)

Rhus tox., when the lower back feels stiff and bruised, especially after resting and in damp weather. (*See page 194.*)

Sulfur, for violent sharp pain on stooping. (*See page 198.*)

Bryonia, for pain that comes on in cold dry weather and is made worse by movement. (*See page 170.*)

LUMBAGO

Lumbago is the term used to describe any persistent or recurrent lower back pain. It is muscular in origin and usually concerns the large group of muscles surrounding the spine. Lumbago may vary in severity from a dull ache to severe pain; often it is experienced as a sudden excruciating pain on bending, on standing up from sitting, on twisting around, or on lifting heavy objects. It is generally brought on or exacerbated by cold, damp weather conditions, muscle strain, poor posture, obesity, and pregnancy. Lumbago is one of the most commonly reported complaints, and it generally becomes more frequent with age.

TREATMENT

Ayurveda

Saffron is anodyne and has antispasmodic properties.

Chinese Herbalism

Apart from physical injury, the cause may be excess internal Cold. Treatment would include tincture of achyranthes root and acanthopanax bark.

Herbalism

Rub a little oil made from comfrey or St. John's wort into the affected area, to relieve the pain. (*See pages 119 and 110.*)

The following herbs reduce inflammation and relieve pain: Jamaican dogwood, St. John's wort, vervain, and white willow. (*See pages 110, 125, and 115.*)

Aromatherapy

Add a little mustard, rosemary, and thyme oils to the bath to relieve pain. Hot baths are most effective. (*See pages 133–157.*)

Juniper, oregano, pine, and rosemary poultices ease inflammation and pain. (*See pages 133–157.*)

Homeopathy

Aconite can be taken when the pain comes on suddenly and is made worse by cold dry weather. (*See page 163.*)

Arnica, for pain that comes on after injury. (*See page 167.*)

Rhus tox., for a painful lower back that feels bruised and stiff, and that improves with movement. (*See page 194.*)

Sulfur, for violent sharp pain on stooping. (*See page 198.*)

Bryonia, for pain that comes on in cold dry weather and is made worse by movement. (*See page 170.*)

Ant. tart., for pain with nausea and vomiting.

Flower Essences

Agrimony is useful for those who make light of the pain and do not let it show in front of others. (*See page 210.*)

Hornbeam, for weariness at the prospect of doing daily tasks that cause pain. (*See page 212.*)

SCIATICA

Sciatica is the name given to the aching or pain along the route of the sciatic nerve. This is the largest nerve in the body, running from the spinal cord, through the buttock and the back of each leg. Sciatica is usually caused by pressure on the roots of the sciatic nerve, most commonly from a prolapsed disk (*see page 395*), but other possible causes include pregnancy and childbirth, heavy lifting, stress, or a tumor. The type of pain varies from mild to more severe and "shooting" in nature. There may also be associated symptoms. Sciatica and other back pains may be eased by lying on the floor for 15 minutes. Prop the head up on a small pile of paperback books and keep the knees bent. Repeat daily.

> **CAUTION**
> See your physician if you have prolonged sciatica.

Symptoms

- a burning sensation and muscle weakness
- numbness or pins and needles in the leg, foot, or toes
- muscle spasms in buttock or leg
- diminished reflexes in knees and ankles

TREATMENT

Ayurveda

Saffron is used for neuralgia and is warming.

Mustard oil can be rubbed into the affected area to warm it. (*See page 19.*)

Chinese Herbalism

Sciatica is believed to be caused by Heat stagnation in the Liver. Gou Teng may be useful, and San Qi can help with the general relief of pain. A practitioner will select herbs specific to your symptoms and the cause of the condition.

Traditional Home and Folk Remedies

Take a warm bath to which nettles have been added to help relieve the pain.

Celery juice or tea can alleviate some forms of sciatica.

Rub fresh lemon over the affected area—it works!

Herbalism

Apply bruised juniper berries to the affected area for pain relief.

Coltsfoot leaf or tincture can be used in a soothing compress (hot) and applied on the affected area.

Elderberry wine is a traditional remedy for sciatica.

For pain relief, try cajeput cream or ointment rubbed on the affected area.

Aromatherapy

Lavender oil is antispasmodic and anti-inflammatory. Use in the bath or in local massage. (*See page 147.*)

Chamomile compresses or massage will reduce the irritation and lessen the pain. (*See page 137.*)

Mix a few drops of juniper, mustard, or pepper essential oil in a little carrier oil and rub into the affected area. Cover with warm clothing. (*See pages 133–157.*)

Oregano and thyme can be added to the bath to relieve the symptoms. (*See page 151.*)

Homeopathy

Colocynthis, is for shooting pains down the right leg to the foot, causing numbness.

Rhus tox., for tearing pain which is better for heat and movement. (*See page 194.*)

Arsenicum, for sciatic pain in an elderly person.

Lycopodium, for pain in the right leg, and which is worse between 4 and 8p.m. (*See page 187.*)

Carbon sulf., for pain in the left leg, which is worse for heat and cold.

Gelsemium, for burning pains worse at night.

FIBROSITIS

Fibrositis (or fibromyalgia) is a chronic stress- or occupation-induced condition in which a series of muscular spasms causes intermittent aches and pain, usually in the back and trunk. It seems to be triggered by cold weather conditions or emotional upset. Fibrositis is most common in middle-aged and elderly people, and may occur more often in anxious people, and in those who spend time sitting in a cramped position. Tender areas (there are nine specific spots) are felt on the affected muscles. Pain and stiffness may be felt in the neck, shoulders, chest, buttocks, knees, and back. In some cases the attacks are accompanied by exhaustion and disturbed sleep. Fibrositis is not considered to be a medical term, and some doctors refuse to recognize the condition because investigation usually fails to reveal any detectable reason for the symptoms.

Symptoms
- aches and pain in muscles or tendons
- tenderness in particular spots on the affected muscles

TREATMENT

Ayurveda
Barberry, taken as a tea or as a compress, treats fibrositis.

Basil can provide pain relief. (*See page 29.*)

Rub calamus oil into the affected joints to improve circulation and drainage.

Camphor can be rubbed into the affected area to warm and encourage healing. (*See page 22.*)

Chinese Herbalism
Gan Caeo is good for spasm in the legs.

Bai Shao helps spasm in the feet and hands.

Ginseng will be useful as an overall tonic.

Traditional Home and Folk Remedies
Apply compresses of apple cider vinegar to the affected area; use several cups of vinegar in bath water.

Make a honey and vinegar drink, with 1 tablespoon of each in a cup of hot water, and drink.

Herbalism
A decoction of cramp bark taken 4 or 5 times a day should bring relief. Cramp bark can also be taken as a tincture or in capsule form. The ointment is useful for massaging into the affected area. (*See page 125.*)

Make a fresh peppermint poultice and apply to the area of spasm. (*See page 111.*)

Aromatherapy
Essential oil of lavender relieves pain and reduces inflammation. Use in the bath or in a gentle massage of the affected area. (*See page 147.*)

Chamomile, lavender, and rosemary are anti-inflammatory and pain-relieving, and are good for local massage or using in compresses. (*See pages 133–157.*)

Black pepper, eucalyptus, marjoram, and benzoin will improve the circulation and reduce stiffness.

Homeopathy
Aconite, for pain that starts suddenly and worsens with movement. (*See page 163.*)

Arnica, for muscles that feel bruised and are made worse by movement. (*See page 167.*)

Bryonia, for fibrositis in the back, neck, and limbs, which worsens with movement. (*See page 170.*)

Chamomilla, for pain, stiffness, and bad temper.

Ledum, for a cold feeling in the muscles, with pain and stiffness alleviated by cold. (*See page 186.*)

Nux vomica., for pain and stiffness which are worse in damp weather and improved by pressure. (*See page 198.*)

Rhus tox., for muscles stiff from overuse, which are better for movement. (*See page 194.*)

Causticum, for tearing pains in the muscles, with stiffness, and which are made worse by cold.

Flower Essences
Rub a little Rescue Remedy cream into the affected area to encourage healing and provide pain relief. (*See page 229.*)

Take Rescue Remedy or Emergency Essence during an attack to calm and restore. (*See page 229.*)

Vitamins and Minerals
Royal jelly may help to relieve symptoms. (*See page 260.*)

Take extra calcium, magnesium, and vitamin C to encourage the health of the muscles and joints.

ARTHRITIS

Athritis is an inflammation of the tissues of one or more joints, usually with pain, swelling, and redness. The two most common forms of arthritis are osteoarthritis and rheumatoid arthritis. Other disease processes and infections which cause arthritis include gout, psoriasis, tuberculosis, rubella, and gonorrhea.

Osteoarthritis is a degenerative disorder in which the cartilage between the joints wears away. The body attempts to repair this damage by producing bony outgrowths at the margins of affected joints, but these, in fact, cause pain and stiffness. It is usually age-related and affects the hips, knees, spine, and shoulders in particular. Obesity is an aggravating factor.

Rheumatoid arthritis is a chronic, progressive disorder. It most commonly arises between the ages of 30 and 40, affecting women more often than men. Its exact causes are not clear, but it is thought that there may be immunological (perhaps triggered by infection) and genetic factors at work. The synovial membrane lining the joint becomes inflamed, spreading over and eroding the cartilage, causing the characteristic pain and stiffness. Anemia, joint infections and pericarditis are all complications of rheumatoid arthritis.

Over 50 million Americans suffer from arthritis.

Rheumatoid arthritis affects 1–3 percent of the American population (about 2.1 million people).

The usual age of onset for arthritis is between 30 and 40, but the disease may start at any age and may even strike children (juvenile rheumatoid arthritis or Still's disease).

Juvenile rheumatoid arthritis affects 71,000 young Americans each year, 6 times as many girls as boys, and figures are increasing.

Women are affected by rheumatoid arthritis three times as often as men, and about 16 percent of the female population over 65 have the disease.

Osteoarthritis rarely attacks before the age of 40, but most people over the age of 60 suffer from it.

Symptoms
- osteoarthritis: intermittent pain in affected joints, gradually becoming more frequent, progressive movement limitation, audible creaking in affected joints, swelling and redness
- rheumatoid arthritis: morning stiffness, taking up to an hour for the joints to loosen; weakness and inflammation of the ligaments, tendons, and muscles; eventually there may be deformity of joints (typically the fingers/hands), causing pain and debility; eye inflammation; bursitis; general feelings of being unwell include lethargy, appetite and weight loss, muscle pain

TREATMENT
Ayurveda
Ginger, coriander, and aloe vera can be used to treat arthritis.

Angelica is a good tonic and is warming. (*See page 17.*)

Barberry, taken as a tea or applied as a compress, can be used to treat arthritis. (*See page 18.*)

Basil can provide relief from the pain of arthritis and rheumatism. (*See page 29.*)

Rub calamus oil into the affected joints to improve circulation and drainage. (*See page 15.*)

Camphor is indicated for the treatment of arthritis and rheumatism, and many other musculoskeletal problems.

Chinese Herbalism
The source of the problem is considered to be Wind Damp. Painful joints are caused by Wind Cold. Arthritis with hot, swollen, but not painful, joints is considered to be caused by Wind Heat.

Treatment would include cinnamon twigs to release qi; aconite root, angelica root, and wild ginger to relieve Cold and Damp. (*See pages 44 and 41.*)

Gentian and cork bark tree can be used for Wind Heat. (*See page 55.*)

Pupleuri root, licorice, and Chinese skullcap are recommended for their powerful anti-inflammatory effects.

Osteoarthritis is thought to be a weakness in the Kidneys, and Blood stagnation. Use cinnamon twigs, tinospora stem, angelica, and ledebouriella root. (*See pages 44 and 41.*)

Traditional Home and Folk Remedies
Eating nettles or drinking nettle tea is an old remedy for arthritis. The "stings" in stinging nettles contain histamine, which is anti-inflammatory.

Vinegar and honey is another old remedy.

Apple cider baths or ginger root baths can help to reduce symptoms and encourage healing. (*See page 80.*)

Apples are good detoxifiers. Eat them daily to improve symptoms and cure the condition. (*See page 80.*)

Herbalism
Apply a poultice of slippery elm and cayenne to the affected joints. (*See pages 123 and 103.*)

Herbs that work to heal arthritis include feverfew, meadowsweet, celery seed, and white willow. They can be taken internally, or used externally, as required.

Bladderwrack capsules, tablets, or powder used regularly may prevent the progress of the disease. (*See page 107.*)

For aching joints, try a liniment made with tincture of comfrey and a few drops of black pepper essential oil.

Dandelion root and horsetail tea or tincture is recommended for degenerative arthritis.

For inflamed hand joints, take a decoction or tincture of Devil's claw. (*See page 109.*)

Siberian ginseng is beneficial for rheumatoid arthritis.

Aromatherapy
Use juniper oil in the bath or in a massage oil blend. It is stimulating and anti-rheumatic. (*See page 146.*)

Massage petitgrain into the limbs for osteoarthritis.

Lemon and cypress oils are detoxifying, and can be used in the bath and in massage to help the body eliminate poisons. (*See pages 140 and 143.*)

Chamomile, lavender, and rosemary are anti-inflammatory and pain-relieving; use in local massage or compresses.

Black pepper, eucalyptus, marjoram, and benzoin will improve the circulation in the area and reduce stiffness.

Homeopathy
Bryonia is useful for arthritis where stitching pains occur in swollen pale or red joints. (*See page 170.*)

Colchicum, when it is worse in warm weather, with inflamed joints, irritability, and sensitivity to touch.

Rhododendron, when it is worse in stormy weather.

Rhus tox., when the arthritis symptoms include pain and stiffness, and are made worse after rest and in cold damp weather, as well as improving with movement. (*See page 194.*)

Pulsatilla, when pain moves from one joint to another.

Apis, for hot, stinging pain. (*See page 165.*)

Vitamins and Minerals
There is some evidence to show that the antioxidants—Vitamins A, C, and E, plus selenium—may have beneficial effects on arthritis. (*See pages 234, 238, 239, and 247.*)

Magnesium is required to form the synovial fluid which surrounds the joints, and an adequate intake will ensure health. (*See page 245.*)

Cod liver oil and evening primrose oil capsules are reported to help rheumatoid arthritis. (*See page 254.*)

Copper may help relieve the symptoms of rheumatoid arthritis, and many sufferers use copper bracelets.

CAUTION

Bladderwrack should be avoided by anyone suffering from an overactive thyroid. Devil's claw should not be used during pregnancy; it is best avoided if you suffer from stomach acidity or ulcers. Do not use Siberian ginseng during pregnancy unless advised to do so by a qualified herbalist.

CRAMP

Cramp is a painful muscular spasm which occurs most frequently in the feet and legs, but can also affect the abdomen, arms, and hands (writer's cramp). Excess salt loss through sweating is the most common cause, and pregnancy, prolonged sitting or standing, strenuous or unaccustomed exercise, or lying in an unusual position may all be triggers. The muscle contraction is usually short-lived, lasting minutes only, but in some cases it may be prolonged, and repeated. Many old people suffer from night cramps. Some research indicates that a vitamin E deficiency may be partly to blame, and there may also be an imbalance of magnesium and calcium in the body.

> **CAUTION**
> Seek medical advice if cramp in the chest occurs during or after exercise, as this may be angina.

Symptoms

- twitching, followed by severe pain and a sensation of contortion in the affected muscle

TREATMENT

Ayurveda

Yarrow is antispasmodic and can help to prevent and treat cramp. (*See page 15.*)

Aloe vera, taken internally and applied externally, can soothe muscular spasm. (*See page 17.*)

Basil, caraway, celery seed, garlic, and myrrh all help.

Chinese Herbalism

Gan Cao is good for spasm and cramps in the abdomen and legs. (*See page 50.*)

Bai Shao helps cramps in the feet and hands.

Traditional Home and Folk Remedies

Apply compresses of apple cider vinegar to the affected area, and use several cups of vinegar in the bath. (*See page 87.*)

A pinch of salt and a sip of lemon juice before bed may prevent night cramps. (*See page 74.*)

Make a honey and vinegar drink, with 1 tablespoon of each in a cup of hot water, and drink. This works by distributing calcium throughout the bloodstream, which can reduce chronic cramp. (*See page 87.*)

Herbalism

A decoction of cramp bark taken four or five times a day should bring relief. Cramp bark can also be taken as a tincture or in capsule form. The ointment is useful for massaging into the affected area. (*See page 125.*)

Make a fresh peppermint poultice and apply directly to the area affected by the spasm. (*See page 111.*)

Olbas oil is effective for sports-induced muscle cramps and spasm.

Aromatherapy

Lavender is antispasmodic and can be usefully employed for cramp as a massage oil. (*See page 147.*)

Rub the affected area with geranium essential oil.

Use melissa and chamomile oils for abdominal cramps, diluted in a light carrier oil. (*See pages 149 and 137.*)

Homeopathy

Take Mag. phos. (6c) every five minutes when cramp occurs. It is especially useful for writer's cramp and cramp that occurs after excessive exercise. (*See page 188.*)

For menstrual cramp, take Mag. phos. every 30 minutes.

Cuprum metallicum, for the spasm and subsequent pain.

Arnica, for cramps caused by muscle fatigue following prolonged exercise. (*See page 167.*)

Flower Essences

Rub a little Rescue Remedy cream into the affected area to encourage healing and provide pain relief. (*See page 229.*)

Take Rescue Remedy or Emergency Essence during an attack to calm and restore. (*See page 229.*)

Vitamins and Minerals

Increase your intake of calcium if you are susceptible to cramp. (*See page 241.*)

Vitamin D is essential for the absorption of calcium.

Vitamin E supplements have been proved to help prevent night cramps. (*See page 239.*)

Increase your intake of salt and magnesium.

Calcium tablets taken with vitamin C are said to prevent night cramps. (*See page 241.*)

RESTLESS LEGS

Restless legs is the term used to describe a condition associated with insomnia in which the legs ache and are constantly moved around in order to achieve comfort.

It is thought to be due either to problems in the nervous system, or to hereditary factors. It is more common in older people and smokers, and it may be triggered by cold, damp weather conditions or overexertion of muscles. There is also an association with diabetes, vitamin B and iron deficiency, excess caffeine intake, and withdrawal from drugs.

Symptoms
- tickling sensation under the skin
- burning or prickling sensation
- aching, twitching, and jerking
- restlessness relieved by movement

TREATMENT

Ayurveda
Warming herbs such as mustard (seeds and oil) and turmeric may be recommended. (*See pages 19 and 25.*)

Black pepper stimulates circulation and nervous system.

Camphor stimulates the nervous system and body tissues.

Cumin is useful for nervous conditions and is generally warming. (*See page 25.*)

Chinese Herbalism
Restlessness is thought to be caused by yin or Blood Deficiency, and possible treatments are lotus seed sprouts and felskrone root tea.

Herbalism
A chamomile infusion or compress can help dispel the condition. (*See page 104.*)

Valerian root works on the nervous system and can help to calm. (*See page 123.*)

Bruised cloves can be added to any tea to relieve nervous conditions.

Aromatherapy
Benzoin, bergamot, and frankincense have a calming action on the nervous system and can be used in the bath, in a vaporizer, or in local massage to ease. (*See pages 133–157.*)

If you have trouble sleeping, try using a few drops of chamomile, lavender, marjoram, and ylang ylang, which are hypnotic. (*See pages 133–157.*)

Homeopathy
Arsenicum, for general restlessness and feelings of chilliness.

Sepia, for twitching which is worse during the day, and better for exercising. (*See page 196.*)

Belladonna, for legs that jerk into spasm, and for feeling hot, with cold extremities. (*See page 168.*)

Ignatia, when the problem comes on after grief or a broken love affair. (*See page 184.*)

Flower Essences
Rescue Remedy cream can be rubbed into the muscles of the legs, as required, to calm. (*See page 229.*)

Vitamins and Minerals
Vitamin E will help to control the condition.

Iron or vitamin B deficiency may be at the root of the condition, so ensure that you include plenty in your diet.

Cut use of stimulants, such as caffeine and alcohol.

Keep the affected muscles warm, and take hot baths.

Zinc, for trembling, twitching feet, and restless legs.

BURSITIS

Bursitis is inflammation of a bursa (a small fluid-filled sac). Bursas act in a protective capacity, reducing friction around joints. The membrane lining a bursa may increase fluid production in response to infection, injury, prolonged pressure, or rheumatic disease, causing the bursa to swell. This may occur in any of the large joints of the body, such as the ankle or shoulder, and is commonly associated with bunions at the joint between the big toe and the foot. The build-up of calcium deposits on tendons associated with a joint is a frequent precipitating cause. The calcium deposits trigger an inflammatory reaction that can spread to a nearby bursa and even rupture it. Constant kneeling is a trigger for bursitis, causing a condition known as "housemaid's knee."

Symptoms
- restricted movement in the affected joint, caused by swelling
- pain and tenderness in the affected area

TREATMENT

Ayurveda

Ginger, coriander, and aloe vera can be used to treat bursitis. (*See pages 24 and 17.*)

Angelica is a good tonic and is warming. (*See page 17.*)

Barberry, taken as a tea or applied as a compress, can be used to treat pain and inflammation. (*See page 18.*)

Rub calamus oil into the affected joints to improve circulation and drainage. (*See page 15.*)

Chinese Herbalism

Pupleuri root, licorice, and Chinese skullcap are recommended for their powerful anti-inflammatory effects.

Cinnamon twigs, tinospora stem, angelica, and ledebouriella root may also be helpful.

Traditional Home and Folk Remedies

Eating nettles, or drinking nettle tea, is a traditional remedy for pain and inflammation. The "stings" in stinging nettles contain histamine, which is anti-inflammatory.

Apple cider foot baths or ginger root baths can help to reduce symptoms and encourage healing. (*See page 80.*)

Hot or cold compresses on the area will help to disperse swelling.

Herbalism

Apply a poultice of slippery elm and cayenne to the affected joints. (*See pages 123 and 103.*)

Herbs that work to heal bursitis include feverfew, meadowsweet, celery seed, and white willow. They can be taken internally, or used externally, as required.

For relief of aches and pains, try a liniment made with tincture of comfrey and a few drops of black pepper essential oil. (*See page 119.*)

For improving inflamed joints, take a decoction or tincture of Devil's claw. (*See page 109.*)

Siberian ginseng is a beneficial herb. (*See page 112.*)

Aromatherapy

Use juniper oil in the bath or as part of a massage oil blend. It has stimulating and anti-rheumatic qualities.

Chamomile, lavender, and rosemary are anti-inflammatory and relieve pain. Use on a compress or for local massage. (*See pages 133–157.*)

Black pepper, eucalyptus, marjoram, and benzoin will improve the circulation in the area and reduce stiffness.

Homeopathy

Belladonna, for pain which is made worse by the slightest movement, with red hot joints that are swollen and throbbing. (*See page 168.*)

Kali iod., for pains that are worse at night.

Rhus tox., for tearing pains with stiff, swollen joints, and which are made worse by heat and cold.

Pulsatilla, for dragging pain and tightness over the bursa, with chilliness. (*See page 193.*)

Apis, for burning, stinging pain made worse by heat.

Sticta, for shooting pains.

Bryonia, for pain made worse by movement or heat.

Flower Essences

Rub a little Rescue Remedy cream into the affected area to encourage healing and provide pain relief.

Take Rescue Remedy or Emergency Essence during an attack to calm and restore. (*See page 229.*)

TENDINITIS

Tendinitis is an inflammation and thickening of the tendons, usually caused by an injury or overuse of the muscles. There is some association with bursitis (*see page 402*), and indeed the diagnosis is often difficult to make. Bursitis is characterized by a dull pain, whereas the pain of tendinitis is sharp.

Symptoms

- sharp pain and limited movement in the affected area
- swelling
- pins and needles and numbness

TREATMENT

Ayurveda

Turmeric is anti-inflammatory and can be used externally, or taken internally, three times daily, between meals.

Traditional Home and Folk Remedies
Apply a vinegar compress to reduce areas of inflammation.

Wrap a bruised wet plantain leaf around the affected area to reduce swelling and stiffness, and to encourage healing.

Herbalism
Apply a poultice of slippery elm and cayenne to the affected joints. (*See pages 123 and 103.*)

Herbs that work to heal arthritis include feverfew, meadowsweet, celery seed, and white willow. They can be taken internally or used externally, as required.

For aching joints, try a liniment of tincture of comfrey and a few drops of black pepper essential oil. (*See page 119.*)

For inflamed joints in the hand, take a devil's claw decoction or tincture. (*See page 109.*)

Aromatherapy
Chamomile, lavender, and rosemary are anti-inflammatory and pain-relieving. Use in local massage or compresses.

Black pepper, eucalyptus, marjoram, and benzoin improve the circulation in the area and reduce stiffness. Use as cold or warm compresses. (*See pages 133–157.*)

Homeopathy
Ruta grav., for tearing pains and lameness.

Rhus tox., for tearing pains made worse by rest, damp, and movement. (*See page 195.*)

Vitamins and Minerals
The following nutrients in the diet help encourage healing of the soft tissues: vitamin C, beta carotene, zinc, selenium, vitamin E. (*See pages 238, 249, 247, and 239.*)

Bromelain, a digestive enzyme, is an anti-inflammatory agent.

BUNION

A bunion (or hallux valgus) is an inflammation of the soft tissue at the base of the big toe due either to ill-fitting shoes or an inherited weakness. Women are more prone to bunions than men, and there is also an association with flat feet. A bunion pushes the big toe outward at the base and in towards the other toes at the top. In some cases a bunion is so large it may distort the sufferer's shoe. Bunions are known as bursitis (*see page 402*).

Ensure that shoes fit properly and are designed to suit the foot, not the fashion. High-heeled shoes and shoes with narrow toes are especially bad for the feet. Go barefoot as often as is practical, walking on a variety of surfaces to exercise the small bones in the feet. Practice picking up small objects, such as marbles, with the toes.

Symptoms
- pain and discomfort in the affected foot
- the bunion is aggravated by continuous and prolonged pressure

TREATMENT
Ayurveda
Cedarwood can be used as a rub for sore joints and pain. (*See page 21.*)

Camphor can be used externally to ease the pain caused by bunions. (*See page 22.*)

St. John's wort can be taken internally and also used externally in the treatment of bunions. (*See page 28.*)

Mustard, used in a foot bath, will reduce pain and inflammation, and encourage healing. (*See page 19.*)

Chinese Herbalism
Ginger is a useful anti-inflammatory agent.

Other herbs to try, for external use, include: San Qi, for general relief of pain and swelling, and Jing Jie for inflammation, stiffness, and pain. (*See page 54.*)

Herbalism
Treatment to ease inflammation and swelling includes compresses of marshmallow, linseed, comfrey, and slippery elm. (*See pages 99, 119, and 123.*)

Chamomile infusions, taken internally, will help.

Aromatherapy
For inflamed bunions, add a drop of melissa or chamomile essential oil to the massage oil and rub ingently.

Lavender or marjoram oil will relieve pain. (*See pages 147 and 151.*)

THE HEALING REMEDIES SOURCEBOOK

Homeopathy

Antimonium is the most effective remedy. (*See page 164.*)

Apis, for burning, stinging pain made worse by heat.

Sticta, for shooting pains.

Kali iod., for pain which is much worse at night.

Ruta grav., when the bunion feels bruised and painful.

Rhus tox., when the skin is itchy, red, swollen, and burning and the joints are stiff, but pain decreases with moving around. (*See page 195.*)

COMMON CHILDHOOD AILMENTS

SLEEP PROBLEMS

All babies and children need different amounts of sleep, and most of them experience some difficulty sleeping at some point. Common causes of sleep problems in babies are diaper rash, teething, colic, illness, being too hot or cold, or simply being wakeful. Older children may be worried about something at school, or a stressful event in the family home. Illness usually disrupts sleep patterns in some way. Some children experience night terrors, which may cause the child to waken suddenly, screaming.

> ### CAUTION
> If you are concerned about the cause of your child's sleep problems, see your physician.

TREATMENT

Traditional Home and Folk Remedies

A little brewer's yeast, mixed with honey and warm milk, makes a soothing bedtime drink for children from the age of four upward. (*See page 87.*)

Herbalism

Vervain is a gentle sedative, and can help children fall asleep—particularly if they are fighting against it.

Limeflowers will be useful for calming nervous, sensitive children. (*See page 121.*)

Motherwort can be useful for calming a frightened child or baby. (*See page 110.*)

A crying baby may be soothed with an infusion of chamomile, offered an hour or so before bedtime or upon waking. (*See page 104.*)

A strong infusion of chamomile, hops, lavender, or limeflower can be added to a warm bath to soothe and calm a baby or child. (*See pages 104 and 121.*)

Tincture of catmint, added to a little honey, can be given to a distressed child as and when required.

Aromatherapy

A few drops of chamomile, geranium, rose, or lavender can be added to the bath water. (*See pages 133–157.*)

Lavender oil, on a handkerchief tied near the cot or bed, will help your baby or child to sleep. (*See page 147.*)

Lavender or chamomile can be used in a vaporizer in your child's room. (*See pages 147 and 137.*)

A gentle massage before bedtime, with a little lavender or chamomile blended with a light carrier oil, may ease any tension or distress. (*See pages 147 and 137.*)

Homeopathy

Ant. tart, for night terrors.

For constant crying, use Colocynthis or Bryonia.

Phosphorus, for thirst, and alternating anger and affection. (*See page 192.*)

Pulsatilla, for a weepy and clingy child. (*See page 193.*)

Chamomilla, if sleep is being disturbed by teething.

Nux vomica, for irritability, and after a busy, stressful day.

Flower Essences

White Chestnut will be helpful for children with overactive minds. (*See page 209.*)

A distressed child or baby can be given Rescue Remedy, which will calm him or her. (*See page 229.*)

Rock Rose, for night terrors. (*See page 216.*)

Aspen, for anxiety for no identifiable cause.

Walnut will be useful for change—a new baby, school, or house. (*See page 218.*)

A few drops of Mimulus will soothe a child who is afraid of the dark. (*See page 220.*)

Vitamins and Minerals

Avoid cold-energy foods such as bananas and cucumbers, which can cause colic and digestive problems.

A warm glass of goat's milk will encourage sleep without causing any digestive disturbance.

Older children may suck a zinc lozenge before bedtime to help them to go to sleep. (*See page 249.*)

There is mounting evidence that the overprocessing of foods—including artificial colorings, flavorings, preservatives, and other additives—may be a factor, coupled with the depletion of various vitamins and minerals from the processed foods.

Allergy-like intolerance of certain foods, especially milk, wheat, and corn, produces ADHD in some children.

Pollutants such as lead, mercury, cadmium, insecticides, and herbicides may also be causative.

HYPERACTIVITY

Hyperactivity is a behavioral disorder which appears to be becoming more common. A hyperactive child has an excessively high energy level, being restless, inattentive, and easily frustrated. There are often prolonged and regular tantrums, and fidgeting. Intelligence is common among hyperactive children, but there is such a short attention span that they often do not do well at school. Psychiatrists have labeled the problem attention-deficit hyperactivity disorder, or ADHD. (Some children display attention-deficit disorder, or ADD, without hyperactivity.) ADHD appears in children before the age of four, but its signs are often missed until the child attends school.

There is a widespread belief that food additives, such as preservatives, are at the root of the problem, but this has not been conclusively proved. Others believe that minor brain damage may be the cause of hyperactivity.

Symptoms
- restlessness
- inattentiveness
- tantrums
- fidgeting

Up to 3 percent of all children manifest significant symptoms of ADHD, with boys greatly outnumbering girls.

A low frustration threshold predisposes such children to uncontrollable tantrums.

There are many causes of ADHD, only some of which are known. In addition to genetic influences, various factors affecting the pregnant mother have been implicated, including the use of prescription or illicit drugs and the use of alcohol and nicotine.

TREATMENT

Herbalism

Black root and fringe tree may be useful herbs if poor digestion is causing hyperactivity.

Herbs to support a stressed nervous system include vervain and skullcap. (*See pages 125 and 118.*)

Oats act as a tonic to the nervous system. (*See page 102.*)

Chamomile, limeflowers, and skullcap, for tense and anxious children. (*See pages 104, 121, and 118.*)

Borage and licorice will work to address an overworked adrenal gland. (*See page 108.*)

Aromatherapy

Massage may calm hyperactivity in children. If the child can be persuaded to lie quietly for a few minutes, both mother and child may benefit from the feeling of peace and calm created during the massage. Use a little lavender or Roman chamomile oil to calm.

Neroli, rose, and sandalwood essential oils have a calming action on the nervous system.

Add a few drops of Roman chamomile to the bath water to soothe and encourage sleep.

Homeopathy

Constitutional treatment is recommended, but China may be appropriate if food allergies are at the root. (*See page 175.*)

Chamomilla will calm an overexcited, demanding child.

Flower Essences

Vervain, for an overenthusiastic child. (*See page 226.*)

Impatiens, for a child who is talkative, quick thinking, and impatient. (*See page 218.*)

Cherry Plum, for loss of control. (*See page 221.*)

Vitamins and Minerals

Include plenty of vitamin B-complex, vitamin C, zinc, and essential fatty acids in the diet, which help behavioral problems. (*See pages 235–238, and 249.*)

It will probably be necessary to take a good multi-vitamin and mineral tablet each day.

BEDWETTING

Bedwetting is not considered to be a problem until your child is at least five years old. Many children, boys in particular, are slow in getting the message that they should get up to use the toilet at night, but that is no reflection on the state of their health—mental or otherwise. If a child sleeps heavily it may take longer for night dryness, but many children manage it by two or three years of age. Bedwetting in children who have already established a pattern of dry nights is usually caused by stress of some sort, like moving house, changing schools, or family fighting. Children who have never been dry at night may suffer from immature nerves and muscles controlling bladder function. Other medical causes include diabetes, urinary infection, nutritional deficiencies, and food allergies.

TREATMENT

Herbalism

Offer St. John's wort and horsetail teas throughout the day, sweetened with honey, to soothe an irritable bladder and encourage control of the bladder. (*See page 28.*)

If the bedwetting stems from an emotional upset or disturbance, vervain and lemon balm relax and soothe.

Aromatherapy

Massage oil of chamomile into the lower back and tummy while settling your child down to sleep. (*See page 137.*)

Homeopathy

Equisetum, when the wetting occurs during dreams.

Belladonna, when it occurs early in the night.

Kreosotum, when wetting occurs during dreams early in the night and during deep sleep.

Causticum, for wetting in first sleep, and when the problem is worse in clear weather or when your child has a cough. (*See page 174.*)

Plantago, when all else fails.

Flower Essences

Try Wild Rose if your child drifts through life.

Walnut will help if the bedwetting is brought on by change, such as a new house, school, or baby.

Chestnut Bud, if the child does not seem to learn from the experience. (*See page 210.*)

Star of Bethlehem, if bedwetting is related to a trauma or shock. (*See page 220.*)

Mimulus, when the problem is linked to fear.

CRADLE CAP

Cradle cap (seborrheic eczema) is common during the first three months of life and is characterized by a thick encrusted layer of skin on the baby's scalp. Nearly 90 percent of all babies will suffer from cradle cap at some point during the first few months. There will be yellow scales, which form in patches, especially on the top of the head. In severe cases, cradle cap can last for up to three years. Like dandruff, cradle cap is a condition in which the seborrheic glands are overactive, and it is often associated with seborrheic dermatitis, a skin condition in which there are red, scaly areas on the forehead and eyebrows, among other places.

> **CAUTION**
> Try not to loosen crusts that have not pulled away on their own—bleeding and infection may result.

TREATMENT

Traditional Home and Folk Remedies

Massage olive oil into the scalp each evening, and then gently shampoo away in the morning. (*See page 81.*)

Mash an avocado, apply to the scalp, and then gently rinse. Rub the skin of the avocado across the head to moisten and heal. (*See page 82.*)

Overwashing will make the condition much worse. Gently brush away loosened crusts with a soft brush.

Herbalism
Rinse the scalp after washing with an infusion of meadowsweet, which acts as an anti-inflammatory and will reduce any itching. (*See page 106.*)

Burdock may also be used to rinse the scalp after washing your baby's hair. (*See page 100.*)

Butternut can be taken internally (1 drop, three times daily, mixed in water) to encourage healing.

Aromatherapy
Massage a few drops of lavender or lemon oil, mixed in a light carrier oil, into the scalp before bedtime. Rinse gently each morning. (*See pages 147 and 140.*)

Homeopathy
Massage the scalp with Calendula ointment. (*See page 172.*)

Lycopodium, taken internally, is useful if the skin is dry but uninfected. (*See page 187.*)

Flower Essences
Rock Rose is useful if the itching causes distress. Rescue Remedy cream may be massaged into the scalp to reduce symptoms. (*See page 229.*)

Add 2 drops of Rescue Remedy to the rinse water, and use after a shampoo. (*See page 229.*)

IMPETIGO

(*See under* Skin and Hair, *page 289*).

STICKY EYE

Sticky eye is a mild infection of the eyes which causes a yellowish discharge and crusting. It is most common in the first week of life, and is usually the result of a foreign object entering the eye during birth, or from the blood or amniotic fluid. This condition is not serious and usually rights itself without treatment. In an older child, sticky eyes are usually a sign of conjunctivitis, which is a condition in which the conjunctiva of the eye becomes infected (*see page 296*). It may indicate a blocked tear duct.

> **CAUTION**
> Always use very weak herbal infusions for babies and toddlers—one-fifth of the dose for adults. Children should have half doses between the ages of 6 and 12.

TREATMENT
Traditional Home and Folk Remedies
Apply cold bread to closed eyes to reduce the inflammation and soothe itching. (*See page 86.*)

Boil fennel seeds to make an eyewash for conjunctivitis and sore and inflamed eyes.

Honey water can be used to cleanse the eye; it acts to destroy any infection, soothe, and encourage healing. (*See page 87.*)

Herbalism
Infusions of the following herbs can be taken internally to ease the condition: echinacea (which boosts the immune system and acts as a natural antibiotic), eyebright, and golden seal. (*See page 105.*)

Infusions of chamomile, elderflower, eyebright, and golden seal can be applied externally. Some of these herbs can also be bought as a tincture and then used to make a soothing eyewash. (*See pages 104 and 116.*)

Soak a chamomile tea bag and hold to the eyelids to soothe. Use it to gently clean the eyes (a new bag for each eye). (*See page 104.*)

Distilled rosewater or witch hazel can help. (*See page 109.*)

Homeopathy
Euphrasia, for burning, itching eyes. (*See page 179.*)

1 or 2 drops of Euphrasia tincture can also be used to bathe the eyes. (*See page 179.*)

Pulsatilla can be used when there is mucus collecting in the corner of the eyes. (*See page 193.*)

Hep. sulf. will be useful to draw out infection. (*See page 183.*)

EARACHES AND MIDDLE EAR INFECTIONS

Earaches may be caused by inflammation of the lymph nodes in the neck, or by another illness like mumps. There may be an ear infection in the inner, middle, or outer parts of the ear. Occasionally a boil can crop up in the outer ear, which can be very painful. The most common ear infections in children are middle ear infections. These are usually caused by the transmission of infection from the nose or throat by the Eustachian tube. Because this tube is short and small in babies and young children, it is easily blocked, and infection does not have far to travel to the middle ear itself. Ear infections can cause a great deal of pain, and the pressure may burst the eardrum, causing a discharge. Earache is also occasionally a sign of dental problems.

CAUTION
Untreated ear infections may scar the eardrum and cause permanent hearing damage. Infection can also spread from the ear to other parts of the head, which may be life-threatening.

Symptoms
- pain
- possibly a discharge
- possibly fever and a sore throat
- malaise

As many as 95 percent of all children will have at least one ear infection by the age of six.

If untreated, ear infections may become chronic.

Chronic infections may also be associated with allergies, tuberculosis, measles, and other diseases.

Up to 30 percent of children under the age of six suffer from chronic ear infections.

Young children, who have shorter and straighter Eustachian tubes than adults, are especially prone to middle ear infections.

The tendency to ear infections is now believed to be inherited.

Researchers have also linked recurrent middle ear infections in young children to food allergies.

TREATMENT

Traditional Home and Folk Remedies
Witch hazel can be added to a teaspoon of oil of St. John's wort and dropped into the ear. This will take away the pain and inflammation. (*See page 78.*)

Crush fresh garlic and mix with a little honey to encourage the body to fight off the infection. (*See pages 78 and 87.*)

Drink honey and lemon, or a little cider vinegar, in some warm water to help rid the body of catarrh and strengthen immunity. (*See pages 87, 74, and 87.*)

Blackcurrant tea will help to boost the immune system and to reduce catarrh.

Herbalism
Passiflora will help if there is panic.

Echinacea can be taken to boost the immune system and clear the pus. (*See page 105.*)

Apply a hot compress or poultice to the neck and ears using mullein or St. John's wort, which are anti-inflammatory.

Give chamomile tea to drink, to soothe pain and distress.

For an acute attack, use black root and hops to lower fever and reduce the inflammation present.

A few drops of tincture of myrrh or golden seal can be added to a light oil, warmed, and dropped into the ear canal.

Soak a cotton ball with a few drops of warmed garlic oil and press gently into the ear canal. (*See page 98.*)

Aromatherapy
A few drops of neat lavender oil can be placed in the ear on a cotton ball, or gently eased in with a Q-tip. (*See page 147.*)

Gently massage the neck and head around the ear with oil of mullein or lavender in a light carrier oil. (*See page 147*)

Tea tree or lavender oil can be used in a vaporizer for their antiseptic properties. (*See pages 148 and 147.*)

Use a few drops of lavender oil on a handkerchief by the bed to help your child to stay calm and to sleep.

Homeopathy
Hep. sulf. is useful for acute attacks, with an earache accompanying a sore throat; and where the child feels chilly.

Aconite can be used in the early stages, particularly when the symptoms set in suddenly. (*See page 163.*)

Belladonna, when the affected ear is red and hot, and the child is feverish and perhaps delirious. (*See page 168.*)

Chamomille when the child is inconsolable and the pain is made worse if the child is in a draft. (*See page 188.*)

Flower Essences

Rub a little Rescue Remedy into the painful parts just below the ears to stop panicking and reduce inflammation.

Rescue Remedy or Rock Rose will ease panic.

Olive can be used during recuperation. (*See page 220.*)

Vitamins and Minerals

Make sure your child's diet is rich in foods containing vitamin C and zinc, which boost the immune system and help to treat infection.

GLUE EAR

Glue ear is a chronic condition affecting a large number of children. It is characterized by a thick, often smelly, mucus which builds up in the middle ear, due to Eustachian tube obstruction. It impairs hearing, and causes the eardrum to perforate, allowing the mucus to be discharged. Glue ear is common in children who have frequent colds or other infections, which block the Eustachian tube (*see* Earaches and Middle Ear Infections on *page 300* and Outer Ear Infections on *page 301*). There is some indication that overuse of antibiotics may encourage the condition, and many children have excess or chronic catarrh (*see page 305*) which may be linked to food allergies or intolerance. Usually both ears are affected, and it is often accompanied by enlarged adenoids and frequently occurs with viral upper respiratory infections, such as the common cold. The first and often the only sign of glue ear is some degree of deafness.

CAUTION

Severe inattention among children under two years old could well be due to partial deafness caused by glue ear. It is essential that this is investigated in order to avoid long-term speech, comprehension, and intellectual impairment.

TREATMENT

Chinese Herbalism

Herbs to reduce inflammation and Mucus (Phlegm) would be Sheng di Huang or Chinese senega root/Polygala.

Traditional Home and Folk Remedies

Drink lemon and honey or cider vinegar to clear the mucus and to strengthen the immune system.

Garlic is excellent at shifting catarrh and cleansing the blood. Offer as garlic perles, or chop fresh garlic and serve with a teaspoon of honey. (*See page 70.*)

Blackcurrant tea is excellent for catarrh and will encourage healing of the ear.

Herbalism

Chamomile and echinacea are antiseptic, and can be taken internally or added to a foot or hand bath to reduce subsequent infection and to relieve unpleasant symptoms.

Clean away discharge with a warm infusion of antiseptic herbs, such as chamomile or golden seal.

Herbal remedies to boost the immune system include chamomile, echinacea, peppermint, and wild indigo.

Herbs to help clear the catarrh include elderflower, euphrasia, golden rod, and hyssop. (*See page 116.*)

Herbs which work to reduce catarrh include golden rod, ground ivy, and elderflower. (*See page 116.*)

Aromatherapy

Dilute essential oils of lavender, chamomile, eucalyptus, or rosewood in a light carrier oil, warm, and massage around the ear and neck. (*See pages 133–157.*)

Massage the ear area with a few drops of essential oil of lavender blended in a light carrier oil. (*See page 147.*)

A steam inhalation of eucalyptus, chamomile, or lavender can help to reduce catarrh and ease accompanying symptoms.

Apply a hot compress to the nose, ears, and throat made using diluted essential oils of lavender, rosewood, or chamomile. (*See pages 133–157.*)

Homeopathy

Kali mur., when there are cracking sounds in the affected ear, accompanied by swollen glands in the neck.

Lycopodium, when there is deafness and a roaring sound in the affected ear. (*See page 187.*)

Pulsatilla, for a full feeling in the ear, and a feeling of weepiness. (*See page 193.*)

Mercurius, when there is thick, smelly discharge.

Vitamins and Minerals
Chronic infection can be caused by a build-up of catarrh (*see page 305*). Reduce consumption of dairy produce and any other possible allergens, including wheat.

Take cod liver oil and vitamin C to boost the immune system. (*See pages 254 and 238.*)

COLDS

Small children are more susceptible than adults to the viruses causing colds and flu because their immune systems are immature. Do not be surprised if your child seems to contract every cold he or she comes into contact with. (*See* Common Cold *page 325.*)

COUGHS

(*See* Coughs, *page 318.*)

CROUP

Croup is an acute inflammation and narrowing of the air passages, especially the larynx, in young children. The disorder is caused by various viruses, particularly the para-influenza virus, or by bacteria. The primary symptoms are coughing, hoarseness, and noisy, difficult breathing, which can sometimes be alleviated with steam inhalations. The characteristic cough of croup is a definite loud bark or whistle, caused by inflammation of the vocal cords. Infectious croup occurs mainly in the winter, when the larynx (voice box) or trachea (windpipe) become inflamed and swollen after what seems to be simply a cold. Other causes include allergy or the inhalation of a foreign body. Because the larynx swells and blocks the passage of air, breathing can be very difficult, which can panic a child.

> **CAUTION**
> If your child turns blue, call a physician immediately.

TREATMENT
Traditional Home and Folk Remedies
Offer a hot honey and lemon drink to ease the symptoms. Honey has strong antibacterial properties and will be useful if the cause of the croup is bacterial infection.

A little cider vinegar mixed with a mug of warm water can be sipped to ease symptoms. (*See page 87.*)

Blackcurrant tea is helpful and restorative.

Put your child in a bathroom with the door shut and the hot taps running, or fill a bowl with boiling water and gently place your child's head over it, covered by a towel. Steam will open the airways and reduce symptoms. Raise the upper end of the cot or bed so that breathing is easier.

Herbalism
Lobelia and black cohosh will reduce spasm, soften the phlegm, and clear the lungs.

Wild cherry syrup can reduce spasm and help deal with phlegm.

Try infusing lavender flowers or chamomile in a bowl of hot water, then ask your child to lean over it, to help breathing. (*See page 104.*)

Infuse some chamomile, catmint, or wild cherry, and give your child small sips before bedtime and during an attack. (*See page 104.*)

Mix catmint, horehound, and wild cherry together with a little honey or licorice and give by the teaspoonful as necessary.

A foot bath with some thyme or eucalyptus oil added should help. (*See page 122.*)

Aromatherapy
Essential oils of eucalyptus, lavender, pine, chamomile, thyme, and cinnamon can be added, together or individually, to a vaporizer or a foot bath. (*See pages 133–157.*)

A few drops of eucalyptus or lavender can be placed on a handkerchief by the child's cot or bed to ease breathing and encourage the child to relax.

Rub a few drops of lavender oil mixed with petroleum jelly into your child's chest and upper back. (*See page 147.*)

Homeopathy
Spongia is the traditional treatment for croup, and can be taken every 20 minutes during an attack. (*See page 196.*)

Aconite can be taken alongside Spongia. (*See page 163.*)

Phosphorus may be useful when there is a thirst for cold drinks (which may be vomited up). (*See page 192.*)

Drosera, for a deep hoarse-sounding cough, with gasping and retching. (*See page 178.*)

Flower Essences
Rescue Remedy will help to calm the child, which will make breathing easier. (*See page 229.*)

Rock Rose will help if your child is frightened.

Olive can be taken to combat exhaustion after an attack.

THRUSH

Thrush is very common in those with immature or compromised immune systems (*see* Thrush on *page 374*). In children, it is most common in the mouth and diaper area, where it appears as an itchy red rash with a white top.

TREATMENT

See Thrush (*page 374*) for treatment. Remember that children's dosage should be lower. Where treatments require the sufferer to drink a dosage, instead rinse the baby's mouth or dab drops onto the affected area. For aromatherapy treatment, try a vaporizer in the child's room. Diluted Rescue Remedy cream can also be dabbed onto the affected area.

TEETHING PROBLEMS

Your baby's first teeth will probably appear at about six months of age, and there may be problems with teeth coming through until the age of two or three. Most babies experience some discomfort, which can range from quite mild, which may make them clingy and fractious, to severe, accompanied by dribbling, loosened stools, and sleeping problems. A classic symptom is a red patch on one cheek.

> **CAUTION**
> Vomiting is not a symptom of teething. See your physician if your baby seems unwell.

TREATMENT
Traditional Home and Folk Remedies
Rub a little honey into the gums for relief. Make sure it is pasteurized. (*See page 87.*)

Give your baby a cold licorice root to gnaw on.

Cold raw carrots are useful teethers, but watch your baby carefully to make sure he or she doesn't bite off a piece and choke on it. (*See page 76.*)

Herbalism
Syrup made from the marshmallow root will soothe inflamed gums. Add a few teaspoons to your baby's normal meals.

Offer infusions of chamomile or fennel to calm and to soothe. (*See pages 104 and 107.*)

Aromatherapy
Put a few drops of lavender oil on the bedsheets to help your baby to sleep. Essential oils of chamomile and lavender can be added to the bath water to calm a distressed baby.

Rub the gums with a little chamomile oil mixed with a teaspoon of honey. Clove oil also acts as a local anesthetic, and a minute amount can be diluted and rubbed into the gums.

Homeopathy
Chamomilla is the standard remedy for teething, and can be taken up to 6 times daily. (*See page 188.*)

Calc. phos. may also be useful. (*See page 171.*)

Flower Essences
Rub a little diluted Rescue Remedy directly into the gums, or apply to pulse points if your baby is crying inconsolably. A few drops at nighttime will keep your baby calm, enabling him or her to sleep.

Walnut will help the child through the transition.

COLIC

Colic is characterized by apparently unending frantic crying, usually at around the same time of day or night. The legs are drawn up to the abdomen, and the baby appears to be in severe pain. Excessive crying causes the baby to swallow air, which can exacerbate the problem and lead to abdominal bloating. The cause is unknown, but colic may be caused by contractions of the colon, an allergy to something in the formula (if bottle-fed), or the mother's diet (if breast-fed), or simply excessive air which is gulped in through repeated bouts of crying. The most common form of colic is three-month colic, typically coming on in the evening and lasting anything from a few minutes to several hours. Burping or laying the baby over the knee or shoulder usually has little effect.

> **CAUTION**
> Vomiting or diarrhea are not symptoms of colic and treatment must be sought immediately.

TREATMENT

Traditional Home and Folk Remedies
Caraway water can be diluted and given to even a very young baby in a sterilized bottle. Offer a few sips before a feed.

Herbalism
Because colic is exacerbated by tension, relaxing herbs are often suggested—used in the bath, or infused, cooled slightly and taken by bottle. Chamomile, lemon balm, and limeflowers are the most effective.

A warm bath with an infusion of dill, fennel, marshmallow, or lemon balm will soothe a colicky baby.

Aromatherapy
Rub a little very dilute fennel oil into the abdomen before feeds to prevent colic. (*See page 107.*)

A gentle massage of the abdominal area with one or a blend of essential oils of chamomile, dill, lavender, or rose will help to ease symptoms and calm a distressed baby.

If your baby is wakened by discomfort, place a handkerchief with a few drops of lavender oil by the bed.

Try a few drops of lavender or chamomile oil in a warm bath, just before evening feeds. (*See pages 147 and 137.*)

Homeopathy
Chamomilla is useful for babies who seem better when they are held. (*See page 188.*)

Pulsatilla is used for babies who are better in the fresh air and when they are rocked. (*See page 193.*)

Cuprum met. is used when the tummy rumbles, and the child curls fingers and toes in discomfort. (*See page 178.*)

Flower Essences
Rock Rose is excellent for extreme fright. (*See page 229.*)

Rescue Remedy can be used to calm and should therefore help to reduce any spasm. (*See page 229.*)

Vitamins and Minerals
If you are breastfeeding, avoid dairy produce for a few days to see if this helps.

Other foods which should be avoided are spicy, citrus, or gassy foods (beans, onions, cabbage, etc.), and sugar.

VOMITING AND DIARRHEA

There are many causes of vomiting and diarrhea in children, including infections such as gastroenteritis, eating rich or fatty foods (or, indeed, overeating), emotional upsets, and food poisoning. These conditions are not usually serious, unless they recur. Gastroenteritis is usually present if there is fever of 100°F (38°C), vomiting, lack of enthusiasm for feeds, and torpor. Occasionally diarrhea is due to too early reintroduction of milk after an attack of gastroenteritis. Remember that babies and children can dehydrate quickly, and you must ensure that they drink plenty of liquids.

> **CAUTION**
> Babies and children can very easily become dehydrated by vomiting or diarrhea, and it is important that you seek medical treatment urgently. See your physician if there is blood in the vomit or feces.

TREATMENT

Traditional Home and Folk Remedies

Milk and honey are excellent for treating an attack of food poisoning. (*See page 87.*)

Mustard is a natural emetic and can be taken internally, mixed with a few teaspoons of warm water.

Garlic is excellent to fight infection, boost immunities, and cleanse the blood. It is also a natural antibiotic, so is excellent in cases of bacterial infection. (*See page 70.*)

Drink fresh lemon juice, warmed and mixed with a little honey, to cleanse the gut. (*See pages 74 and 87.*)

Drink blackcurrant juice, as a gut astringent.

Raw apple which has gone brown is useful for settling an upset stomach. Offer in small quantities.

Herbalism

Chamomile or melissa tea will help to settle and calm an excited child. (*See page 104.*)

Meadowsweet or marshmallow syrup can help with vomiting. (*See pages 106 and 99.*)

Gentian and barberry can be added to water and sipped frequently.

Chamomile and vervain can be taken internally to soothe a child whose illness is exacerbated or caused by emotional upset, or who is distressed by the vomiting.

Try ginger, crushed or decocted, to ease nausea.

Chamomile, echinacea, peppermint, and thyme can be drunk as infusions or added to a foot bath when infection causes the illness. (*See pages 104, 105, 111, and 122.*)

Aromatherapy

Massage the tummy and chest with a few drops of lavender or chamomile essential oil in a light carrier oil. (*See pages 147 and 137.*)

Use essential oil of thyme or tea tree in a vaporizer for their antiseptic properties. (*See pages 156 and 148.*)

A few drops of lavender essential oil in the bath or by the bedside will calm. (*See page 147.*)

Homeopathy

Nux vomica may help if the child vomits after eating too much, or too quickly. (*See page 198.*)

China, for diarrhea with wind, particularly when the child is very irritable. (*See page 175.*)

Colocynthis, if diarrhea is copious, thin, and yellow, accompanied by episodic pain. (*See page 176.*)

Arsenicum, when there is burning and the child is restless, anxious, and cold. (*See page 167.*)

Veratrum alb., when there is vomiting and diarrhea with cold sweats.

Pulsatilla, after a rich, fatty meal, when there is no thirst.

Flower Essences

Rescue Remedy will relieve the distress caused by vomiting and diarrhea. (*See page 229.*)

Olive flower essence is useful for recuperation.

If the vomiting is caused by emotional problems select a remedy that will help with those problems.

Vitamins and Minerals

Following an attack of vomiting or diarrhea, offer lots of live yogurt and very ripe bananas to restore the proper bacterial balance of the gut.

An acidophilus tablet can be taken for the same purpose. These are available in vanilla flavor. (*See page 256.*)

DIAPER RASH

Diaper rash is caused by contact with urine or feces, which cause the skin to produce less protective oil and therefore provide a less effective barrier to further irritation. It can also be caused by irritating chemicals in feces, not thoroughly rinsing soap or detergent out of diapers, and the chemicals contained in disposable diapers. The baby's buttocks, thighs, and genitals become sore, red, spotty, and weepy in areas touched by diapers. In boys, the foreskin may become inflamed, making urination painful. The rash may become secondarily infected with the Candida fungus if the baby has been given antibiotics or if breast milk has antibiotics in it, or if the mother has oral or genital thrush.

> **CAUTION**
> Any diaper rash which does not heal within a week or so should be seen by a physician.

TREATMENT

Traditional Home and Folk Remedies

Rub the skin of an avocado on the rash to encourage healing.

Wash the bottom with a little diluted cider vinegar and allow it to dry before putting on the diaper.

Live yogurt can be spread on the diaper area to soothe, and to prevent thrush from occurring in the folds of the skin.

Egg white can be painted on the sore bottom and allowed to dry before putting on a diaper. This will encourage the skin to heal and prevent further irritation.

Avoid using soap or other detergents on the diaper area. Rinse carefully with clean water at each diaper change. Frequent diaper changes are suggested, and using a disposable diaper liner may help to reduce irritation. Allow your baby to go for as long as possible with a bare bottom, to allow it to dry and heal. Give plenty to drink.

Herbalism

Buchu will reduce the acidity of the urine.

Marigold ointment can be rubbed on to the diaper area to soothe and to reduce inflammation. (*See page 102.*)

Wash the diaper area with infusions of marigold, rosemary, or elderflower. (*See pages 102, 114, and 116.*)

Powdered golden seal can be applied to a clean diaper area before putting on the new diaper.

Give your baby lots of soothing drinks, such as diluted chamomile tea, to reduce the acidity of the urine.

Aromatherapy

Add a few drops of tea tree to the rinse cycle of your machine when using cloth diapers to disinfect. Cloth diapers are much kinder to your baby's delicate skin.

A few drops of lavender or rose oil in a peach kernel carrier oil can be gently rubbed into the diaper area. Use this blend to protect against diaper rash as well.

A drop of oregano or thyme oil, in a light carrier oil, can be used to discourage thrush. (*See page 156.*)

Homeopathy

Calendula ointment can be applied to the diaper area.

Internally, you can try giving Rhus tox. for an itchy, blistered rash. (*See page 194.*)

Sulfur may be appropriate if the skin is dry and scaled. Merc. sol. can help to reduce the acidity of the urine.

Cantharis, when the urine is scalding and the skin is raw. Rhus tox., when the rash appears as mounds or pimples.

Flower Essences

Rescue Remedy cream may be gently massaged into the affected area to reduce inflammation and ease pain or itching. A few drops of Rescue Remedy on pulse points will calm a distressed baby. (*See page 229.*)

WORMS

An infestation of worms in the digestive system is quite common, particularly in young children, who usually contract them at school. Worms can sometimes be seen around the anus, or in the feces, and they inflame the area of the bowel or rectum where they attach themselves. Several types of worms can exist as parasites in humans, ranging in size from microscopic to many meters in length. Most infestations are uncommon in the U.K. and the U.S., apart from threadworms. Threadworms, which are tiny, white threadlike worms which infest the rectum, are not dangerous, although they do tend to disturb sleep. They cause itching around the anus, and sometimes mild, colicky abdominal pain. Worms may be acquired by eating undercooked, infected meat, by contact with soil or water contaminated by worm larvae, or by accidental ingestion of worm eggs from soil contaminated by infected feces.

> **CAUTION**
> Whatever treatment you give, repeat after two weeks to expel the worms that were embryos at the first treatment.

TREATMENT

Traditional Home and Folk Remedies

Raw garlic, which is toxic to worms and parasites, can be eaten, or a small piece, wrapped in some gauze, can be inserted into the anus. (*See page 70.*)

Give 5 lemon pips, ground and mixed with honey, daily for 5 days. (*See pages 74 and 87.*)

Herbalism

Cayenne pepper and senna can be combined; the former stuns the worms and the latter encourages them to be expelled. Mix in a little live yogurt, to avoid irritating the digestive tract. (*See page 103.*)

Wormwood tea will stun worms.

Aromatherapy

Rub a little black pepper oil, very diluted in grapeseed oil, into the abdominal area. (*See page 153.*)

Homeopathy

China may alter the balance of the body so that the child expels threadworms naturally. (*See page 175.*)

Teucrium, for an itchy bottom and nose, which are worse in the evening and accompanied by restless sleep patterns.

Santoninum, when all else fails.

Flower Essences

Rescue Remedy for distress caused by discomfort.

Crab Apple, if your child feels unclean or polluted.

Vitamins and Minerals

Acidophilus tablets should be taken for several weeks to improve the health of the bowel. (*See page 256.*)

WHOOPING COUGH (PERTUSSIS)

Whooping cough is an acute, highly infectious, and quite serious illness which occurs mostly in children under the age of five. The incubation period of whooping cough is seven to ten days, and the condition can last for about six weeks—sometimes longer. Pertussis, as it is known, usually begins with a normal cold, which develops into a cough. The infection is bacterial and irritates the airways, causing them to become swollen and lined with thick, infected mucus. The coughing becomes severe, with long bouts that have a characteristic "whoop" sound to them. Vomiting often accompanies the coughing. Whooping cough is more dangerous in infants, who can suffer anxiety from being unable to breathe normally. Infected children should be kept away from others.

Whooping cough is caused by a bacteria, Bordetella pertussis.

Because of mass vaccination of children, whooping cough is now relatively rare, affecting only a small proportion of the population.

After an incubation period of about a week, symptoms at first resemble those of the common cold; after 7–10 days, coughing increases and takes on the distinctive attributes of whooping cough.

The younger the patient, the greater the risk of serious illness; most deaths from whooping cough occur in the first six months of life.

> **CAUTION**
> There is a risk of secondary infection, in particular pneumonia and bronchitis. All cases of whooping cough should be seen by a physician. If the cough is accompanied by vomiting, make sure there is adequate intake of fluid to prevent dehydration. Call your physician if your child becomes blue around the lips.

TREATMENT

Traditional Home and Folk Remedies

Honey and licorice can be mixed with a little hot water to make a drink to relieve the cough.

A garlic poultice, placed on the chest and back area, is recommended to help expel the phlegm. Do not leave the poultice on for too long, because it can cause blistering.

Herbalism

A combination of coltsfoot and elecampane can prevent the infection by strengthening the body and clearing phlegm.

Sundew is very successful in treating a number of bacterial infections, and also works to relax the muscles of the breathing tubes. It should be made into an infusion and taken by the teaspoonful, as necessary.

Hyssop and lobelia should be used to help allay the spasmodic cough.

Coltsfoot can be used to loosen the cough and help to expel the mucus.

The bark of the wild cherry has a profound effect on the cough reflex.

Red clover will help to reduce any spasm of the bronchi.

A few drops of tincture of thyme should be taken to loosen and expel the mucus. Thyme also works as an antiseptic. (*See page 122.*)

Massage comfrey ointment into the chest and back to relax the lungs. (*See page 119.*)

Lemon balm tea will soothe anxiety.

Elecampane is commonly used for children's coughs, and can be purchased in easy-to-use syrup form.

Offer a little black root if there is vomiting.

After the bath, massage a little comfrey ointment into the chest and back to relax and expand the lungs.

Aromatherapy
Mix a few drops of lavender and chamomile oils in a light carrier oil, and massage into the chest and back area to calm, and to relax tensed muscles.

Tea tree, lavender, chamomile, and eucalyptus can be used in a vaporizer to help open up the lungs and reduce spasm. (*See pages 133–157.*)

A few drops of oil of thyme, in the bath, will soothe and reduce the severity of the cough. (*See page 156.*)

Homeopathy
Pertussin may be given in one dose toward the end of the disease to prevent an "echo" effect.

Aconite can be taken during an attack or at the beginning of the illness. (*See page 163.*)

Ant. tart., when there is a rattling cough with gasping. Sanguinaria, for a harsh, dry cough.

Arnica, when there is bleeding, or the child is distressed before the coughing starts. (*See page 167.*)

Drosera is useful when the cough is made worse by lying down and there are pains below the ribs. (*See page 178.*)

Bryonia, when there is a dry, painful cough and vomiting.

Flower Essences
Rescue Remedy is excellent for calming a child who has difficulty drawing breath, and who is frightened by the condition. A few drops on pulse points, or sipped in a glass of cool water, will help. (*See page 229.*)

Cherry Plum will help if there is any serious spasmodic coughing. (*See page 221.*)

Mimulus and olive are good during the later stages of the condition. (*See page 220.*)

GERMAN MEASLES (RUBELLA)

Rubella, or German measles, is a viral infection that begins with symptoms of a cold and loss of appetite, occasionally accompanied swelling of the lymph nodes. The rash will appear about a day later and consists of tiny pink spots that may be so concentrated that the overall area appears red and inflamed. There may be a mild fever. German measles is very infectious, with an incubation period of two or three weeks. The illness itself only lasts three to five days.

CAUTION

The symptoms in small children may be mild, but if a pregnant woman comes into contact with the condition there is a serious risk of miscarriage or birth defects. Sufferers are infectious from one week before the rash appears to three weeks afterward.

TREATMENT
Chinese Herbalism
Rubella is believed to be caused by external Wind and Heat. Use mulberry, honeysuckle, and chrysanthemum.

Traditional Home and Folk Remedies
Pound some anise seeds, allow them to steep in boiling water for about 30 minutes, and then offer the drink by the teaspoonful to relieve symptoms.

Honey and lemon in a little hot water can be drunk to reduce discomfort of the cold-like symptoms.

Cool baths will relieve itchiness and reduce a fever.

Herbalism
Borage stimulates the kidneys and can help with a fever.

Yarrow tea, cooled and drunk several times daily, will relieve symptoms. (*See page 97.*)

An infusion of elderflower, combined with peppermint, will cool a fever and calm your child.

Aromatherapy
A few drops of lavender oil on the bedsheets, or on a handkerchief near the bed, will help ease symptoms and calm the child. (*See page 147.*)

If there is a build-up of phlegm, use a few drops of tea tree or eucalyptus essential oil in a vaporizer to assist easier breathing. (*See pages 148 and 145.*)

Homeopathy
Pulsatilla, when there is thick, yellow discharge and hot, red eyes. (*See page 193.*)

Belladonna, for fever, a bright red rash, and a hot face.

Phytolacca, for painful ears and swollen glands which are improved by taking cool drinks.

Aconite, for a high fever without much mucus.

Merc. sol., where there is yellow discharge and a fever.

Flower Essences
Rescue Remedy will ease distress and calm the child.

Vitamins and Minerals
Eat a good amount of raw fruit and vegetables to cleanse the system.

Increase the intake of foods containing vitamin C and zinc to aid the action of the immune system.

Vitamin E oil can be applied to the spots to prevent scarring. Take vitamin E supplements for the same reason.

Acidophilus should be taken after any illness to encourage the production of healthy bacteria in the gut.

German measles is highly contagious but mild.

Many people may have had German measles without knowing it, because a skin rash is not always present.

Natural infection apparently produces lifelong immunity.

Pregnant women who become infected with rubella have a high risk of giving birth to a baby with serious birth defects, including blindness, cardiovascular disorders, deafness, or mental retardation.

MEASLES

Measles is a highly infectious disease caused by a virus which is normally inhaled. The incubation period is about 14 days, and just before the rash appears spots can be seen in the mouth. It begins like a cold, with runny nose or cough, then a fever, and occasionally conjunctivitis occurs. Fever tends to become high as the rash comes out. The rash is characterized by flat, brown-red spots, which usually begin behind the ears and on the face. The lymph nodes will become swollen and there will be little or no appetite; vomiting and diarrhea may occur in some cases. Measles spots are not itchy, but your child will feel profoundly unwell. Complications of measles are common, and they include pneumonia, middle ear infections, and bronchitis. Encephalitis may also occur.

Measles usually affects children, but the disease can occur at any age in susceptible people.

The early symptoms—fever, malaise, sore muscles, headache, eye irritation, and sensitivity to light—occur about 11 days after infection.

Nasal discharge, sneezing, and coughing develop rapidly.

Measles reduces normal resistance, making a patient susceptible to more serious secondary bacterial infections.

In rare cases, the virus causes a form of encephalitis.

Measles was once common throughout the world, but in 1963 the measles vaccine was introduced, which greatly reduced the incidence.

The 1980s saw a marked increase in measles cases in the U.S., which may have been due to the failure to vaccinate many infants at the age of 15 months.

About 5 percent of vaccinated adults are not adequately protected by a single dose of vaccine.

Infection confers lifelong immunity.

> **CAUTION**
> If fever recurs several days after the spots have begun to heal, see your physician.

TREATMENT
Chinese Herbalism
The source of the illness is believed to be excess Heat in the Blood and Stomach. Peppermint, safflower, and honeysuckle may be used to treat measles. (*See pages 44 and 52.*)

Traditional Home and Folk Remedies
Garlic will encourage the spots to "come out," which means that the body is expelling toxins. (*See page 70.*)

Ginger can be used as a compress directly on the spots.

Hot honey and lemon drinks are soothing and will encourage healing. (*See pages 87 and 74.*)

Herbalism
Garlic and echinacea can be taken to improve the action of the immune system. (*See pages 98 and 105.*)

Elderflower is also useful. (*See page 116.*)

Add chamomile or marigold to the bath water to calm your child and soothe the symptoms.

A compress of ginger may be used to help encourage the toxins to be released from the body. (*See page 126.*)

Aromatherapy
A few drops of Roman chamomile in the bath will ease symptoms and help encourage sleep. (*See page 137.*)

Lavender oil can be dropped on the bedclothes or on a handkerchief by the bed to calm. It can also be applied neat to spots to encourage healing. (*See page 147.*)

When there is a build-up of phlegm and other symptoms of a cold, a gentle chest massage with a few drops of tea tree oil in a light carrier oil base will help. (*See page 148.*)

Use essential oil of eucalyptus, tea tree, or chamomile in a vaporizer. (*See pages 133–157.*)

Homeopathy
Aconite and Belladonna can be taken for a high fever.

Pulsatilla, when there is diarrhea, yellow discharge, and a cough. (*See page 193.*)

Bryonia, when there is a hard, painful cough and a high temperature, accompanied by thirst. (*See page 170.*)

Stramonium, when there is a high fever, a red face, and convulsions.

Morbillinum can be taken for three days if your child has been in contact with a sufferer. This will help reduce the severity of the symptoms.

Flower Essences
Rescue Remedy eases distress and discomfort.

Cherry Plum, Hornbeam, and Chicory are suggested for all childhood illnesses.

Vitamins and Minerals
Eat plenty of raw fruit and vegetables every day to cleanse the system.

Increase the intake of foods containing vitamin C and zinc to aid the action of the immune system.

Vitamin E oil can be applied to the spots to prevent scarring. Take vitamin E supplements for the same reason.

Acidophilus should be taken after any illness to encourage production of the healthy bacteria in the gut.

CHICKEN POX

Chicken pox is an extremely contagious viral infection, which features a headache, fever, and general malaise, with spots starting usually on the trunk and spreading to most parts of the body, including the mouth, anus, vagina, and ears. They appear as pimples, which soon fill with fluid to become little blisters. Eventually the spots dry up and form a scab, which may cause scars. These spots are very itchy and it is important that the child does not scratch, for scarring and bacterial infection can result. The incubation period is 10 to 14 days, and sufferers are contagious from just before the spots appear.

Chicken pox is usually contracted before the age of nine.

The chicken pox virus, varicella zoster, usually lies dormant in the body. When immune activity is low, it can resurface as shingles.

The rash develops into itching blisters that break in a few days and are covered by scabs, which leave no scars unless they become infected by bacteria from scratching.

Chicken pox can be life-threatening to children with depressed immune systems.

A mother with chicken pox may transmit the virus to her baby during the last days of her pregnancy.

In 1995 a vaccine called Varivax was approved for use in children over the age of one. The vaccine is 70–90 percent effective in preventing chicken pox over the short term.

> **CAUTION**
> When fever lasts for more than a couple of days, or there is an obvious chest infection accompanying the rash, see your physician. Very rarely, chicken pox pneumonia can occur as a secondary infection.

TREATMENT

Chinese Herbalism

The illness is believed to be caused by Wind and Heat invasion. Safflower, cimicifuga, and honeysuckle may be used in the treatment. (*See pages 44 and 52.*)

Traditional Home and Folk Remedies

Add baking soda to the bath to ease itching.

Herbalism

A witch hazel compress can be applied directly to the spots, or a little added to the bath, to ease discomfort.

Tincture of comfrey or elderflower can be applied directly to the spots to encourage healing and to relieve the itching. (*See pages 116 and 119.*)

Add burdock infusion to your child's bath. (*See page 100.*)

Crushed peppermint leaves, applied to the spots, relieve symptoms. (*See page 111.*)

Aromatherapy

A few drops of Roman chamomile can be used in the bath to soothe. (*See page 137.*)

Essential oil of lavender can be dabbed directly on spots to ease the itching and encourage healing. Lavender also has an antibacterial action, which will help prevent a secondary infection. (*See page 147.*)

Homeopathy

Variolinum can be taken once before your child acquires the illness, during an epidemic of chicken pox, and symptoms should be less severe.

Rhus tox. can be taken for a few days after contact with an infected child, and then again as soon as the first spots appear. (*See page 194.*)

Aconite, in the early stages of the illness. (*See page 163.*)

Belladonna, for fever. (*See page 168.*)

Flower Essences

If the child is unreasonably demanding of attention, Chicory may be helpful. (*See page 213.*)

Impatiens can ease fractious behavior. (*See page 218.*)

Crab Apple may be diluted and applied directly to the spots to encourage healing. (*See page 219.*)

Olive will be useful for the convalescence period.

MUMPS

Mumps is a viral infection which usually affects children, causing fever and swelling of the main salivary glands, the parotids. This swelling furnishes the sufferer with the characteristic "chipmunk" appearance. The condition rarely occurs in children under two or three years of age, and takes about two or three weeks to incubate. It is infectious from a day before the glands begin to swell until about a week after they have gone down. The virus is spread by coughing and sneezing.

> ### CAUTION
> Complications can develop in teenage boys who contract mumps: inflammation of the testicles can lead to sterility. If the illness if followed by a severe headache, stiffness, or fever, see your physician immediately.

Symptoms

- fever
- headache
- pains around the neck
- swallowing will be painful

Because mumps is a systemic infection, other parts of the body may also be affected, including salivary glands, the testicles, the ovaries, the pancreas, and the nervous system.

Mumps is communicable, though less so than measles, and occurs with great frequency in heavily populated areas.

While the disease can occur at any age, it is children aged 5–15 who are primarily affected.

Once contracted, this ensures permanent immunity.

An infection involving the ovaries, oophoritis, occurs occasionally in women. It causes fever, and lower back pain.

A condition called aseptic meningitis sometimes occurs when the virus enters the central nervous system.

TREATMENT

Chinese Herbalism

The source of mumps is considered to be Wind and Damp Heat, and dandelion, honeysuckle, skullcap, and rhubarb may be suggested. (*See pages 52, 61, and 60.*)

Traditional Home and Folk Remedies

Chop fresh ginger and apply as a compress directly to the swollen glands to provide relief.

Cayenne powder, mixed with vinegar, can be warmed and applied to the affected area. (*See pages 74 and 87.*)

Herbalism

Catmint, marigold, or chamomile infusions can be sipped to reduce fever, or added to a bath of cool water.

Garlic, peppermint, and echinacea can be taken internally to boost immunity and encourage healing.

Red clover and cleavers can help to reduce the inflammation and swelling. Drink both as a lukewarm infusion.

A warm compress with poke root or marigold can be applied to the swelling. (*See page 102.*)

Aromatherapy

Eucalyptus and thyme can be used for steam inhalations and in the bath (use sparingly). (*See pages 145 and 156.*)

Massage the neck area with chamomile or lavender oil, diluted in a little grapeseed oil. Take care to do so gently.

Homeopathy

If your child has not had mumps, Phytolacca or Parotidium can be taken during an epidemic to reduce the severity of symptoms.

Rhus tox., when the left glands are more severely affected than the right. (*See page 194.*)

Belladonna, when there is a high fever, shooting pains, and a bright red face and throat. (*See page 168.*)

Merc. sol., when the patient sweats heavily and has a coated tongue. (*See page 189.*)

Pulsatilla may help to prevent orchitis, and is useful if fever continues. (*See page 193.*)

Flower Essences

Rescue Remedy can be used to ease distress caused by discomfort. (*See page 229.*)

Willow may be helpful if the child resents the fact that brothers and sisters are still well. (*See page 224.*)

Vitamins and Minerals

Eat a good selection of raw fruit and vegetables to cleanse the system.

Increase the intake of foods containing vitamin C and zinc to aid the action of the immune system.

Acidophilus should be taken after any illness to encourage production of the healthy bacteria in the gut.

FIRST AID

BITES AND STINGS

Insect bites and stings are common, and may cause discomfort, but unless you suffer from an allergic reaction, the best course of treatment is to soothe the pain and reduce swelling. The stinging insects inject a toxin through a stinger at the tail end of the abdomen. The reaction is usually local, but if the sting occurs in the mouth or throat, swelling can cut off the air supply and cause death by asphyxiation. Death can occur in individuals who are hypersensitive to bee venom. Animal bites should always be cleaned carefully and seen by a doctor. Dogs and other animals can transmit the infectious disease rabies through bites. Symptoms include fever and convulsions.

Ayurveda

Aloe vera can be applied to the bite or sting to soothe; it also has anti-inflammatory and antiseptic properties.

Bitter orange is anti-inflammatory and bactericidal.

Rub ghee on the affected area.

Place a slice of raw onion on the bite or sting for natural relief. (*See page 16.*)

Traditional Home and Folk Remedies

The juice of a spring onion or a cucumber can be applied to stings to soothe and reduce inflammation. (*See page 75.*)

The juice of daikon radish is useful for spider bites.

Bathe stings in a bowl of water with several teaspoons of baking soda. (*See page 86.*)

A slice of raw onion placed on an animal bite will discourage infection and draw out poison. (*See page 70.*)

Apply garlic and onion to ant bites, and cucumber juice to ease the discomfort. (*See page 70.*)

Make a compress from a pad of cotton wadding soaked in lemon juice or cider vinegar and apply to a wasp sting. (*See pages 74 and 87.*)

Granulated sugar can be used to prevent a bite wound from scarring. Apply a poultice of sugar to the wound, after it has been cleaned, and bandage it with gauze.

Herbalism
Marigold petals are useful on a bee sting.

Calendula cream will reduce swelling.

The leaves of wormwood, sage, or rue can be macerated and applied to spider, scorpion, or jellyfish stings.

Cover bites and stings with a wet, macerated plantain leaf. When it dries, replace with a wet leaf.

Witch hazel is useful on mosquito bites.

Aromatherapy
Use neat lavender oil on stings to reduce swelling and discomfort. (*See page 147.*)

1 drop of tea tree oil can be rubbed into an insect bite or sting. (*See page 148.*)

A few drops of geranium oil, applied to water, can be used to clean a bite wound and encourage it to heal.

Prevent insect bites by diluting essential oils of eucalyptus or citronella in half a mug of water, and then gently applying to exposed areas, avoiding the eyes and mouth. Use cider vinegar in the same way. (*See pages 145 and 144.*)

Homeopathy
Ledum is useful for animal bites. (*See page 186.*)

Clean stings and animal bites with pure tincture of Hypericum.

Aconite, for shock. (*See page 163.*)

Arnica, for bruising. (*See page 167.*)

Apis can be used for bee stings, after you have removed the sting with a pair of tweezers. (*See page 165.*)

Flower Essences
Rescue Remedy or Emergency Essence, diluted in a few ounces of cool water, or the cream, can be applied to the sting or bite. Take orally for shock, pain, or distress, or apply to pulse points. (*See page 229.*)

BRUISES
(*See page 335.*)

BLISTERS

A blister occurs when an area of the skin becomes raised and swollen by an accumulation of blood serum beneath it. If a blister is punctured, the flesh beneath it becomes open to infection. It is essential that it is kept clean and dry in order to heal. Blisters can be caused by a number of things, including injuries—such as burns, scalds, or chafing—insect bites, or infections. Some diseases will produce blisters, including chicken pox, herpes, and impetigo, and the disease can be transmitted by the virus inside the blisters.

Ayurveda
Aloe vera juice can be applied to the blister to help it heal.

Barberry can be used for an infected blister. (*See page 18.*)

Apply a basil oil poultice to the area. (*See page 29.*)

Cedar is a natural insect repellent. Spray around the room in an atomizer half full of water. (*See page 21.*)

Traditional Home and Folk Remedies
Boiled and mashed carrots can be applied to blisters to help to heal the area, and this is particularly good for infection.

Use roasted onions, applied as a poultice to blisters, particularly those which have become infected. (*See page 70.*)

Peach pit tea is recommended to heal blisters.

Ice will also reduce inflammation and itching or pain.

Bathe the blister with cold, salty water, which will discourage infection and help the blister to dry out. (*See page 88.*)

You can also apply surgical spirit, and then petroleum jelly to areas susceptible to blisters caused by chafing.

Cover blisters in the day to prevent damage and infection. Remove bandages at night to allow them to dry out.

Herbalism
Aloe vera can be applied to the blister to help it heal.

Marigold (calendula) can be applied to a blister to promote healing. (*See page 102.*)

Witch hazel, applied neat to a blister, will quickly relieve pain and swelling, and encourage healing. (*See page 109.*)

THE HEALING REMEDIES SOURCEBOOK

Aromatherapy

Neat lavender oil can be applied to blisters.

Benzoin, applied to areas which are susceptible to blisters, can prevent as well as heal them. (*See page 156.*)

Roman chamomile has antiseptic properties. Use a few drops in half a mug of water to cleanse punctured blisters and the area around them. (*See page 137.*)

Homeopathy

Urtica urens ointment can be applied to blisters caused by infection or burns. (*See page 201.*)

Hypericum ointment will encourage healing.

Cantharis, for itching, burning blisters.

Rhus tox., for red and itchy blisters, particularly those caused by the chickenpox virus. (*See page 194.*)

Punctured blisters can be cleansed with a few drops of tincture of calendula in clean water. (*See page 172.*)

Flower Essences

Rescue Remedy or Emergency Essence can be diluted in water and applied directly to the blister. (*See page 229.*)

CAUTION

Try not to burst a blister, which will leave the skin open to infection. The top layers of the skin are usually affected by blisters. See your physician if blisters become very painful and inflamed, or if blisters appear for no reason.

Herbalism

Sip chamomile tea to calm. (*See page 104.*)

Add a little powdered ginseng to warm water with honey and lemon to restore. (*See page 112.*)

Aromatherapy

Lavender, melissa, or peppermint can be dropped on a handkerchief and held under the nose until help arrives or the condition stabilizes. (*See pages 133–157.*)

Homeopathy

Aconite, for shock. Take every five minutes until it has subsided or help arrives. (*See page 163.*)

Ignatia, for shock from an emotional upset or trauma.

Flower Essences

Four drops of Rescue Remedy or Emergency Essence can be taken internally or applied to the temples and pulse points, to reduce the effects of shock and ease a feeling of panic.

Rock Rose is suitable if you are experiencing panic.

Try Mimulus for fear. (*See page 220.*)

CAUTION

Only mild shock should be treated with natural remedies.

TOOTHACHE

(*See page 308.*)

MILD SHOCK

Injury or severe emotional trauma can lead to a potentially dangerous condition we call shock, in which the blood fails to circulate properly. In serious cases of shock, the brain and other organs can be deprived of oxygen. Causes of shock include extreme pain, severe vomiting or diarrhea, blood infection, or violent allergy.

Chinese Herbalism

Ginger and black pepper are warming and will help to restore circulation in cases of mild shock.

CUTS AND ABRASIONS

Minor cuts and abrasions should be cleaned with a mild antiseptic or cooled, previously boiled water to ensure that they do not become infected. More serious cuts, with damage to the skin and structures below, should be seen by a physician.

Ayurveda

Aloe vera can be applied directly to cuts to encourage healing, reduce inflammation, and prevent infection.

Yarrow improves blood clotting and may be useful for deeper wounds. (*See page 15.*)

Myrrh can be used to clean the wound. (*See page 23.*)

Traditional Home and Folk Remedies

Lemon juice is an excellent styptic, and can be diluted and applied directly to a clean wound. (*See page 74.*)

A compress made of peach pit tea can be used on infected wounds.

Sugar is said to prevent scar tissue. Press a few teaspoons of granulated sugar into a clean wound and dress with gauze. Rinse the wound carefully and dress again. Repeat up to five times daily, but take care not to disturb the clotting action.

Direct pressure should be applied to the bleeding area, and maintained until the flow of blood ceases.

Herbalism

A few drops of marigold tincture in fresh, warm water can be used to clean the wound. This will help to prevent infection and encourage healing. (*See page 102.*)

Echinacea can be diluted and used directly on the wound to prevent infection. (*See page 105.*)

Comfrey ointment can be used on wounds which have become inflamed. (*See page 119.*)

Use a witch hazel compress on wounds and swellings.

Tincture of myrrh is an excellent antiseptic. Apply a few drops to bandages before dressing a wound.

Aromatherapy

Lavender oil, applied directly to the nostrils or massaged in a light carrier oil into the temples, will provide relief from any accompanying shock or pain.

A few drops of tea tree oil, in clear, warm water, can be used to clean a wound and act as an antiseptic.

Geranium oil can be dropped on to a dressing to encourage healing. (*See page 151.*)

Homeopathy

Ledum, for puncture wounds. This is particularly good if there is a risk of tetanus. (*See page 186.*)

Clean with calendula or hypericum tinctures.

Arnica should be used in the case of all injuries, to encourage healing and reduce the risk of bruising.

Flower Essences

Rescue Remedy or Emergency Essence can be applied neat to a graze to encourage healing and reduce pain, or applied to the temples and pulse points to calm. Use diluted in water on cuts, as the brandy may sting. (*See Shock, page 423.*) (*See page 229.*)

> **CAUTION**
> If you are unable to stop the bleeding, see emergency medical attention. Do not offer food or drink.

SPRAINS
(*See page 393.*)

TRAVEL SICKNESS
(*See page 341.*)

NOSEBLEEDS
(*See page 307.*)

BURNS AND SCALDS

A burn is an injury to the tissue of the body caused by heat, chemicals, electricity, or radiation. Serious burns must always be seen by a physician, as an emergency, but minor burns and scalds can be safely treated at home. Always cool a burn by letting cool water run over it until the pain has stopped. Try to avoid applying anything to the burn until it is cooled and you can see the extent of the damage. "Wet" burns should be dressed with a fabric, like gauze, which will "breathe." Change the dressing regularly.

Ayurveda

Aloe vera cools and prevents infection. (*See page 17.*) Onions may be used directly on the skin for instant relief.

St. John's wort can be used directly on the burn to cool and soothe. (*See page 28.*)

Traditional Folk and Home Remedies

Crush blueberries and extract the juice. Keep in the refrigerator or freezer to use on burns or scalds in the case of an emergency.

Honey can be applied directly to a burn to facilitate healing and to help prevent infection. (*See page 87.*)

Raw potatoes can be placed on a burn to provide instant relief. (*See page 84.*)

Immerse the area in cool (not freezing water) for at least 10 minutes. Then apply hypericum lotion (about 10 drops of mother tincture, in a cup of water).

Herbalism

Aloe can be applied directly to a burn in order to soothe and seal it from infection. It will also encourage healing. (*See page 99.*)

A few drops of echinacea in a liter of water, poured over the burn, will help to prevent infection. (*See page 105.*)

Marigold tincture, applied sparingly to a dressing, is a useful healing agent. (*See page 102.*)

Aromatherapy

Lavender oil is ideal for burns and can be applied neat (use sparingly). (*See page 147.*)

A few drops of geranium oil in a liter of cooled boiled water can be poured over a burn or scald to encourage healing. (*See page 151.*)

Homeopathy

Arnica can be taken to promote healing. (*See page 167.*)

Cantharis can help to relieve pain when taken immediately after the accident. (*See page 173.*)

Urtica can be used if the burn continues to be painful.

Hypericum is useful for burns affecting the ends of fingers or toes, when there are sharp, stabbing pains.

Aconite should be taken for shock. (*See page 163.*)

Urtica urens ointment may help to soothe a burn.

Use hypericum ointment or calendula to prevent injection and encourage the burn to heal. (*See page 184.*)

Flower Essences

Rescue Remedy or Emergency Essence will help to calm. A little bit of diluted tincture can be applied directly to a minor burn. (*See page 229.*)

SUNBURN

(*See page 284.*)

SUNSTROKE (HEATSTROKE)

Sunstroke is a type of heat exhaustion, with symptoms that include headache, vomiting, fever, dizziness, and physical collapse. Heat exhaustion or sunstroke is usually caused by the excessive loss of water from the body that is the result of intensive heat. It is a mild form of shock. Sunstroke is also due to the body's inability to regulate internal heat. Heatstroke is a disorder that occurs when body-temperature regulating mechanisms are overwhelmed by excessive heat or fail in otherwise tolerable heat. Early nonspecific symptoms are faintness, dizziness, staggering, headache, dry skin, thirst, and nausea, which may be specifically related to heatstroke. In the latter stages of the condition, sweating ceases. Heatstroke is a medical emergency. The body temperature may be 105°F (40.5°C) or higher.

Ayurveda

Add the juice of a lime or lemon to half a glass of soda water and sip in small doses.

Chinese Herbalism

Fresh ginger, cinnamon twigs, and peppermint may be useful. (*See page 44.*)

Traditional Home and Folk Remedies

Sip a little fresh cucumber juice to cool. (*See page 75.*)

Herbalism

Small sips of fresh ginger tea, made with root ginger, will help to ease the symptoms. (*See page 126.*)

Teas of rock rose flowers or wild rose flowers, with a little honey, will be helpful.

Homeopathy

Take Aconite initially, for symptoms of shock. (*See page 163.*) The following remedies will help in the aftermath:

- Gelsemium, when there is accompanying trembling.
- Nux, when symptoms are made worse by flickering lights.
- Calcarea, when symptoms are worse on looking up.
- Borax, for symptoms made worse by downward motion.

Flower Essences
Rescue Remedy or Emergency Essence should be offered as soon as possible to treat shock. (*See page 229.*)

Olive will help in the aftermath. (*See page 220.*)

FOOD POISONING

Food poisoning is usually caused by eating food or drinking water that has been contaminated with bacteria, usually the salmonella strain. Symptoms of this kind of poisoning include diarrhea, fever, vomiting, and possibly pain in the abdomen. Gastroenteritis, an inflammation of the digestive system, can also result.

Ayurveda
Fresh lemon juice will help to cleanse, and fight infection.

Strong spices like cayenne, curry, and turmeric have preventive properties against food poisoning.

Combine 1 teaspoon of black pepper, 2 cloves of garlic, 1 tablespoon of cumin seeds, and a little salt in 4 cups of water. Boil until the liquid has reduced to 2 cups, and drink three times daily to cleanse and treat diarrhea.

Chinese Herbalism
Fresh ginger root will help to ease the nausea.

Ping Wei Pian or Ren Dan may he useful.

Traditional Home and Folk Remedies
Drink warm water with lemon juice to cleanse the system.

Add plenty of honey to a cup of warm water and sip for its antibacterial and immune-enhancing properties.

Chew ginger root to help ease the nausea.

Cider vinegar, drunk with some warm water, will encourage vomiting to expel the poisons. (*See page 87.*)

Drink plenty of cool fresh water, and avoid any food for at least twenty-four hours. (*See page 88.*)

When the vomiting has ceased, ripe bananas can be eaten to help restore the bacterial balance in the gut. Live yogurt will have a similar effect. (*See page 79.*)

Herbalism
Make a tea of comfrey root and meadowsweet to treat infection and relieve symptoms. (*See pages 119 and 106.*)

Arrowroot or slippery elm tea can be sipped during the worst symptoms to soothe the digestive tract, and afterward to help restore bowel health. (*See page 123.*)

Golden seal and meadowsweet can be drunk as tisanes. Licorice tea will help to flush out the toxins. (*See page 108.*)

Fresh garlic, or garlic capsules, should be taken to reduce infection. (*See page 98.*)

Chamomile, drunk as a tea, will help to ease digestion and reduce inflammation. (*See page 104.*)

Aromatherapy
Chamomile oil, sprayed in the air or rubbed into the temples, will help to calm and ease symptoms. (*See page 137.*)

Tea tree, garlic, eucalyptus, and juniper all work to kill bacteria, and can be added to a cool bath or placed on a burner to help fight infection. (*See pages 133–157.*)

Rub a little diluted lavender oil into the abdomen to reduce any spasm and to help encourage healing. (*See page 147.*)

Bergamot will help to reduce any fever. Place on a cold compress on the head. (*See page 140.*)

Homeopathy
Aconite, for symptoms that come on swiftly, causing some distress and shock. (*See page 163.*)

Baptisia, for salmonella infections. (*See page 169.*)

Pulsatilla, when the symptoms are worse at night and the sufferer feels tearful. (*See page 193.*)

Phosphorus, when there is diarrhea with a burning sensation, vomiting, and a craving for cold drinks.

Arsenicum is excellent for many cases, particularly when there are burning pains and diarrhea. (*See page 167.*)

Nux vomica will help when the pain improves upon passing stools and there is a feeling of chilliness. (*See page 198.*)

Flower Essences
Take Rescue Remedy or Emergency Essence initially.

Olive will be useful as symptoms improve, to ease overwhelming exhaustion. (*See page 220.*)

THE HEALING REMEDIES SOURCEBOOK

INDEX

THE HEALING REMEDIES SOURCEBOOK